CHILDHOOD EPILEPSIES AND BRAIN DEVELOPMENT

CHILDHOOD EPILEPSIES AND BRAIN DEVELOPMENT

Editors
*Astrid Nehlig, Jacques Motte, Solomon L. Moshé and
Perrine Plouin*

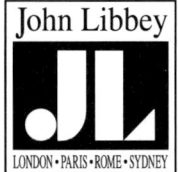

John Libbey
JL
LONDON · PARIS · ROME · SYDNEY

British Library Cataloguing in Publication Data

Childhood Epilepsies and Brain Development
  Current problems in epilepsy series: 14

  1. Epilepsy in children   2. Brain-damaged children
  I. Nehlig, A.

  618.9'2'853

ISBN: 0 86196 578 7

ISSN: 0950-4591

Published by

John Libbey & Company Ltd, 13 Smiths Yard, Summerley Street,
London SW18 4HR, England
Telephone: 081-947 2777 – Fax: 081-947 2664
 John Libbey & Company Pty Ltd,
Level 10, 15–17 Young Street, Sydney, NSW 2000, Australia
John Libbey Eurotext Ltd, 129 rue de la République, 92120 Montrouge, France
John Libbey at C.I.C. Edizioni s.r.l., via Lazzaro Spallanzani 11, 00161 Rome, Italy

© 1999 John Libbey & Company Ltd. All rights reserved.
Unauthorised duplication contravenes applicable laws.

Printed in Malaysia by Kum-Vivar Printing Sdn Bhd, 48000 Rawang, Malaysia

Contents

Preface		vii
Part I	**Brain development, changes in excitability with age and the role of neurotransmitters**	
Chapter 1	Homeobox genes in brain development *Edoardo Boncinelli, Antonio Faiella, Michela Zortea, Francesca Albani and Elena Barbaria*	3
Chapter 2	Prominent expression of glutamate decarboxylase during early hippocampal development: a review of recent findings *Carolyn R. Houser, Shannon T. Dupuy-Davies and Nianhui Zhang*	13
Chapter 3	The contribution of developmental plasticity to early-life seizures and chronic epilepsy *Martha Pierson and John Swann*	25
Chapter 4	Age-related mechanisms involved in the control of seizures *Jana Velíšková*	39
Part II	**Lesional partial epilepsies and neuronal migration disorders**	
Chapter 5	Neuronal migration disorders and epilepsies *Jean-Paul Misson, Jean-Marie Dubru, Patricia Leroy, Sandrine Pirard, T. Takahashi and Verne S. Caviness, Jr*	55
Chapter 6	Structural and functional causes of neuronal hyperexcitability in a rat model of cortical migration disorder *Heiko J. Luhmann, Nik Karpuk, Robert-Alexander Reiprich, Petra Schwarz and Christine C. Stichel*	71
Chapter 7	Prenatal treatment with methylazoxymethanol in rats: a model for cortical malformation associated with epilepsy? *N. Chevassus-au-Louis, A. Rafiki, P. Congar, I. Jorquera, Y. Ben-Ari, J.L. Gaïarsa and A. Represa*	81
Part III	**Age-specific syndromes**	
Chapter 8	Infantile spasms: a pathophysiological hypothesis *Olivier Dulac, Catherine Chiron, Olivier Robain, Perrine Plouin, Isabelle Jambaque, Jean-Marc Pinard*	93
Chapter 9	The Lennox–Gastaut syndrome: from baby to adolescent *Charlotte Dravet*	103
Chapter 10	Developmental consequences of epilepsies in infancy *Thierry Deonna*	113

Chapter 11	Cognitive and behavioural consequences of epilepsies in childhood *Marie-Noëlle Metz-Lutz and Rita Massa*	123
Chapter 12	PET studies of Landau–Kleffner syndrome and related disorders *Pierre Maquet, Edouard Hirsch, Marie-Noëlle Metz-Lutz,* *Christian Marescaux, Georges Franck*	135

Part IV   **Non-genetic experimental models of childhood epilepsies**

Chapter 13	Mechanisms of non-genetic, provoked seizures in the neonatal and infant brain *Tallie Z. Baram and Carolyn G. Hatalski*	145
Chapter 14	Excitatory amino acids and epileptogenesis during ontogenesis *Pavel Mareš*	157
Chapter 15	Acute and chronic epileptogenic effects of hypoxia in the immature brain *Frances E. Jensen*	161

Part V   **Consequences of seizures in the immature and mature brain**

Chapter 16	Hippocampal neuropathology in children with severe epilepsy *Gary W. Mathern, James K. Pretorius, Joao P. Leite, and P. David Adelson*	171
Chapter 17	$GABA_A$ receptor alterations in temporal lobe epilepsy *Douglas A. Coulter*	187
Chapter 18	Seizure-induced apoptosis and necrosis in the developing rat brain *Raman Sankar*	199
Chapter 19	Characterization of the pilocarpine model of epilepsy in developing rats *Esper A. Cavalheiro*	211
Chapter 20	Age-related metabolic and circulatory changes during seizures *Astrid Nehlig, Anne Pereira de Vasconcelos, Céline Dubé,* *Maria José da Silva Fernandes and Jacques Motte*	221
Chapter 21	Long-term effects of recurrent seizures on the developing brain *Claude G. Wasterlain, Kerry W. Thompson, Harley Kornblum, Andrey M. Mazarati,* *Yukiyoshi Shirasaka, Hiroshi Katsumori, Hantao Liu, and Raman Sankar*	237
Chapter 22	The resiliency of the immature brain to seizure induced damage *E.F. Sperber, I.M. Germano, L.K. Friedman, J. Velíšková and M.T. Romero*	255
Chapter 23	Effects of recurrent seizures in the developing brain *Gregory L. Holmes, Matthew Sarkisian, Yehezkel Ben-Ari and* *Nicolas Chevassus-Au-Louis*	263

PART VI   **Consequences of treatment on brain development**

Chapter 24	Anti-epileptic drugs and cognitive function *Catherine Billard*	279
Chapter 25	Consequences of early chronic antiepileptic treatments in animals *A. Pereira de Vasconcelos, H. Schroeder and A. Nehlig*	289

PART VII   **Concluding remarks and future plans**

Chapter 26	Concluding remarks and future plans *Solomon L. Moshé*	307
	Author Index	311

Preface

The epilepsies are quite frequent among the general population and particularly during childhood. Many childhood epilepsies are associated with abnormalities of brain development as well as with learning abilities.

During the last decade, important progress has been made towards a better understanding of epileptic seizures, including the recognition of new syndromes in children and their genetic origin, the use of new antiepileptic treatments, and epilepsy surgery. Basic science and clinical studies have clearly indicated that there are many age-specific features in (1) the seizure susceptibility of the brain to environmental stimuli; (2) the brain structures and circuits involved in seizures; (3) the clinical and EEG expression of seizures; (4) the consequences of seizures and/or epilepsy on brain development; (5) the response to and the cognitive consequences of various antiepileptic treatments. However, there is a long way to go towards the understanding of these various features. Furthermore, there is still limited knowledge as to why learning disabilities may occur in some childhood epilepsies and not in others. Are learning disabilities associated with the epilepsies the result of the seizures themselves or their underlying cause? What is the role of interictal EEG abnormalities, treatment and/or psychosocial burden of the epilepsies?

In an attempt to clarify the clinical questions and maintain the dialogue initiated during the meeting on Brain Development and Epilepsy held in Houston in 1992, we brought together clinicians and scientists in Obernai (Alsace) on 3–5 April 1997. By bringing together scientists and clinicians involved in the diagnosis, treatment and research on childhood epilepsies and in the study of specific features of brain development in relation to the pathophysiology of childhood epilepsies, we hoped that we would begin intergrating the conceptual frameworks necessary for the better understanding of the development and impact of childhood epilepsies.

This meeting was particularly succesfull because of the active participation and great interaction of the group. This volume is the logical conclusion in the symposium. The contributions to this book demonstrate the considerable advances that have been made since the 1992 meeting. This publication has been made possible by a grant from Sanofi Pharma International, which we gratefully acknowledge.

The Editors

Part I
Brain development, changes in excitability with age and the role of neurotransmitters

Chapter 1

Homeobox genes in brain development

Edoardo Boncinelli[1,2], Antonio Faiella[1], Michela Zortea[3], Francesca Albani[4] and Elena Barbaria[1]

[1]*DIBIT, Scientific Institute H San Raffaele, Via Olgettina 58, 20132 Milan, Italy;* [2]*Centre for Cellular and Molecular Pharmacology, CNR, Via Vanvitelli 32, 20129 Milan, Italy;* [3]*Department of Radiology, IRCCS Bambino Gesu' Children's Hospital, Piazza Sant'Onofrio 4, 00165 Rome, Italy;* [4]*Institute of Child Neurology and Psychiatry, IRCCS 'Stella Maris' Foundation, University of Pisa, Via dei Giacinti 2, 56018 Calambrone, Pisa, Italy*

A great diversity of neural cell types is produced from a relatively homogeneous pool of precursor cells during embryonic development. In recent years, the cellular and molecular mechanisms by which specific types of neurons are generated and organized in the CNS have been explored and a number of principles and developmental pathways have been discovered. All events of differentiation and patterning at the level of single cells or groups of cells are preceded by developmental decisions that involve entire regions of the forming nervous system. Recently, some of these events have received particular attention. Among them are the regionalization of the CNS along its anterior–posterior axis, the establishment and maintenance of a dorsal–ventral polarity of the neural tube, the process of segregation of the presumptive cerebral cortex from basal ganglia and the lamination of the cerebral cortex. Most alterations in one of these processes are likely to cause major developmental defects and generate pathology of the nervous system. The regionalization of the CNS of vertebrates along the anterior–posterior body axis appears to be of particular relevance for the specification of the identity of all regions along the body. In the neural tube of the developing vertebrate there are at least two levels of regionalization (Boncinelli, 1994): the first one subdivides the adult CNS in telencephalon, diencephalon, mesencephalon, metencephalon, myelencephalon and spinal cord. This subdivision follows the initial subdivision of the developing brain into three early vesicles, forebrain, midbrain and hindbrain. Within some of the major regions of the developing neural tube there is a second level of regionalization, which gives rise to identifiable neuroepithelial domains, sometimes called neuromeres. Subsequent differentiation of the various neuroepithelial domains within each major region of the CNS results in neural structures of distinct histologies and anatomical complexity.

Homeobox genes and neural development

A key role in the regionalization of the CNS and in the specification of the various anatomical and functional neural domains is played by regulatory genes. These genes act through the control of the expression of other genes laying hierarchically downstream from them and sometimes termed target genes. Regulatory genes generally code for transcription factors, i.e. nuclear proteins able to recognize specific DNA sequences, bind to them and modulate, through this specific binding, the level of expression of the corresponding target genes. A relatively large proportion of regulatory genes are indeed homeobox genes.

Homeobox genes are regulatory genes characterized by the presence of a specific DNA sequence termed homeobox, able to code for a protein domain of some 60 amino acid residues, termed homeodomain. It is through the action of their homeodomain that the protein products of the homeobox genes, the homeoproteins, bind to the regulatory regions of specific genes and control their expression. Among the vertebrate homeobox genes stand out those belonging to the HOX family (Krumlauf, 1994; McGinnis & Krumlauf, 1992 for reviews). Homeobox genes belonging to the *Hox* family are structurally and functionally homologous to the *Drosophila* homeotic genes. In mice and humans, they are organized in four genomic clusters of about 100 kb in length, termed HOX loci (and precisely *Hoxa, Hoxb, Hoxc* and *Hoxd* in the mouse and HOXA, HOXB, HOXC and HOXD in man), each containing several *Hox* genes arranged in a homologous sequence. Corresponding genes in the four loci belong to any one of 13 homology groups. *Hox* genes collectively control the identity of the various regions along the body axis from the branchial area through the tail. This action occurs in a collinear way, with 3' *Hox* genes expressed early in development and controlling anterior regions; and progressively more 5' genes expressed later in development and controlling progressively more posterior regions. In particular, 3' *Hox* genes of the four loci belonging to groups 1–4 primarily control the development of the branchial area and of the rhombencephalon, the embryonic region corresponding to the future hindbrain, and its orderly regionalization into 7–8 neural segments termed rhombomeres. Central *Hox* genes of groups 5–8 control the thoracic portion of the body, whereas 5' *Hox* genes of groups 9–13 control the lumbo-sacral region, including analia and genitalia. Conversely, these genes do not seem to play any significant role in the head and in brain regions anterior to the hindbrain. Actually, development of the most anterior body domain corresponding to the anterior head has remained relatively obscure also in flies (Finkelstein & Boncinelli, 1994). Nevertheless, in the last few years at least three genes have been identified that play a role in the development and regionalization of the *Drosophila* head: *empty spiracles* (*ems*), *orthodenticle* (*otd*) and *buttonhead* (*btd*). The first two are homeobox genes and four vertebrate homologues have been isolated and characterized. These four genes are *Emx1* and *Emx2* (Simeone et al., 1992a, b), related to *ems*, and *Otx1* and *Otx2* (Simeone et al., 1992a, 1993; Finkelstein & Boncinelli, 1994), related to *otd*. The four vertebrate genes are expressed in extended regions of the developing rostral brain of mouse embryos, including the presumptive cerebral cortex and olfactory bulbs.

At embryonic day 10 (E10), the developing neural tube of the mouse shows recognizable regions corresponding to the future anatomical subdivisions. The entire neural tube consists of neuroepithelial cells undergoing active proliferation and most of the specific differentiative events have not yet occurred. In E10 mouse embryos all four genes are expressed. Their expression domains (Simeone et al., 1992a) are continuous regions of the developing brain contained within each other in the sequence *Emx1* < *Emx2* < *Otx1* < *Otx2*. The *Emx1* expression domain includes the dorsal telencephalon with a posterior boundary slightly anterior to that between presumptive diencephalon and telencephalon. *Emx2* is expressed in dorsal and ventral neuroectoderm with an anterior boundary slightly anterior to that of *Emx1* and a posterior boundary within the roof of presumptive diencephalon. The *Otx1* expression domain contains the *Emx2* domain. It covers a continuous region including part of the telencephalon, the diencephalon and the mesencephalon with an anterior boundary approximately coincident with that of *Emx2*. The posterior boundary of *Otx1* domain practically coincides with that of the mesencephalon. Finally, the *Otx2* expression domain contains the *Otx1* domain, both dorsally and ventrally, and covers the entire fore- and midbrain.

In summary, the analysis of the E10 brain shows a pattern of nested expression domains of the four genes in brain regions defining an embryonic rostral, or pre-isthmic, brain, including the fore- and midbrain, as opposed to hindbrain and spinal cord. The first appearance of transcripts of the four genes is also sequential: *Otx2* is already expressed in the headfold at E7.5, followed by *Otx1* and *Emx2* in

E8–8.5 and finally by *Emx1* in E9.5 mouse embryos (Simeone *et al.*, 1992a). It seems reasonable to postulate a role of the four homeobox genes in establishing the identity of the various embryonic brain regions. In this respect, the specification of the regions of the early rostral brain seems to be a discrete process with its focal point in the dorsal telencephalon. In midgestation mouse embryos the two *Otx* genes are expressed in dorsal and basal telencephalon, in diencephalon and mesencephalon (Simeone *et al.*, 1993). Their expression domains in mesencephalon show a sharp posterior boundary, both dorsally and ventrally, approximately at the level of rhombic isthmus.

Otx1 and *Otx2* are also expressed in restricted regions of the diencephalon: epithalamus, dorsal thalamus and mammillary region of posterior hypothalamus. In these regions, the expression is almost exclusively confined to cells of the ventricular zone. Both *Otx* genes are also expressed in developing special sense organs, that is in the olfactory epithelium, as well as in the developing inner ear from early expression in the otic vesicle to epithelia in auricular ducts of sacculus and cochlea and in the developing eye, including the external sheaths of the optic nerve (Boncinelli *et al.*, 1993; Simeone *et al.*, 1993). It has to be emphasized that *Otx* and *Emx* genes are by no means the only genes expressed in the developing brain. Many other regulatory or structural genes are also expressed here, even if not exclusively here (Rubenstein & Puelles, 1994; Rubenstein *et al.*, 1994; Shimamura *et al.*, 1995 and references therein). Partly on the basis of the expression domains of all of these genes, a model has been proposed for the subdivision of the developing rostral brain in neuromeres, namely the so-called prosomeric model (Rubenstein *et al.*, 1994). It entails a subdivision of the embryonic forebrain into six neuromeres, termed prosomeres, p1 to p6, from posterior to anterior. Three of these, p1 to p3, subdivide the diencephalon and three subdivide what these authors call secondary prosencephalon, that is telencephalon and hypothalamic regions.

All four genes are expressed between E9.5 and E10.5 in the presumptive cerebral cortex. Starting from E10.75, *Otx2* expression progressively disappears from this region. This process is relatively quick and initiates in the central areas of both hemispheres. *Otx2* expression persists in the forming choroid plexus, an extremely specific *Otx2* localization (Boncinelli *et al.*, 1993), and in the septum and some regions of the ganglionic eminence.

Emx1, *Emx2* and *Otx1* are expressed in the presumptive cerebral cortex in an extended developmental period corresponding to major events in cortical neurogenesis (Simeone *et al.*, 1992b). *Emx1* expression domain comprises cortical regions including primordia of neopallium, hippocampal and parahippocampal archipallium. *Emx1* expression seems characteristic of cortical regions, mainly but not exclusively hexalaminar in nature. In the same period, the *Emx2* expression domain comprises presumptive cortical regions including the neopallium, hippocampal and parahippocampal archipallium and selected paleopallial localizations, but no basal internal grisea (Simeone *et al.*, 1992b). *Otx1* expression domain in forebrain (Simeone *et al.*, 1993; Frantz *et al.*, 1994; Gulisano *et al.*, 1996) includes dorsal telencephalon but also extends to basal regions.

It is interesting to consider the temporal pattern of expression of *Otx1* and the *Emx* genes in the various zones of the forming cerebral cortex (Frantz *et al.*, 1994; Gulisano *et al.*, 1996). Here, at least three major zones can be defined: the germinal neuroepithelium or ventricular zone, where cortical neurons proliferate, a transitional field, and finally the forming cortical plate from which the cortical gray matter will subsequently develop (Bayer & Altman, 1991). At the beginning and up to E12.5 the germinal neuroepithelium is practically the sole component of the prosencephalic wall. Then a transitional field appears. This includes the subventricular zone and the intermediate zone, to which differentiating cortical cells translocate before migrating to outer regions. As development proceeds, the thickness of the cortical plate progressively increases. Both the transitional field and the cortical plate develop at the expense of the neuroepithelium according to specific spatial and temporal gradients within the forming cortex. Two major neurogenetic and morphogenetic gradients can be observed: one progressing in an anterior to posterior direction and a second progressing in a ventrolateral to dorsomedial direction. The various cortical layers are then formed in an inside-out pattern (Bayer & Altman, 1991). Cell tracing experiments have shown that neurons destined to occupy the depth of the cortex are generated first and that the subsequently generated waves of neurons bypass the earlier ones by active migration and settle above them.

In mouse embryos of all stages *Emx2* expression coincides with cells of the germinal neuroepithelium (Gulisano *et al.*, 1996). In E12.5 embryos, *Emx2* hybridization signal is uniformly distributed across the cortex without major differences, but starting from E13.5 it appears to be confined to the germinal neuroepithelium of the ventricular zone, excluding both the transitional field and the cortical plate. From day 14.5 on, *Emx2* cortical expression progressively declines in anterior and ventrolateral regions and by the end of gestation is solely confined to specific cell layers in hippocampus. It is conceivable that *Emx2* plays a role in the control of proliferation of cortical neuroblasts, and thus, the regulation of their subsequent migration process, since it is known that these cells reach their final destination in the mature cortex according to their birthdate.

Otx1 is expressed in the ventricular zone and specifically in deeper layers of telencephalic cortex since their birth. In the adult cortex *Otx1* is expressed in a subpopulation of neurons in layer 5 and overall in layer 6 (Frantz *et al.*, 1994; Gulisano *et al.*, 1996). Conversely, *Emx1* is expressed in most cortical neurons, whether proliferating, migrating, differentiating, or fully differentiated and organized in a mature cerebral cortex (Gulisano *et al.*, 1996). On the other hand, no *Emx1* expression is detectable in ventral forebrain regions and in particular in the developing basal ganglia. These observations suggest that *Emx1* may be involved in the definition of a specific cellular identity in the cerebral cortex.

It is interesting to note that *Emx2* is expressed in the ventricular zone of midgestation mouse embryos according to an anterior–posterior gradient of intensity, higher in posterior cortical regions than in anterior ones. This expression gradient of *Emx2* is suggestive of a contribution of *Emx2* to cortical polarization in the framework of an arealization process taking place in the ventricular zone (O'Leary *et al.*, 1994). As a regulatory gene encoding a transcription factor, *Emx2* is an ideal candidate for generating and/or maintaining a position-dependent signal within the cortex. *Emx1* is in turn highly expressed in at least a subset of subplate neurons. The subplate (Allendoerfer & Shatz, 1994) is a layer of early generated neurons lying just beneath the cortical plate. Subplate neurons seem to participate in early functional circuitry: they receive synaptic inputs from waiting thalamic afferents and make axonal projections onto the cortical plate. Some experiments suggest that the subplate shows basic features of cortical organization later projected onto the layers of the adult cerebral cortex. *Emx1* gene products might play a role in some of these crucial events.

Preliminary data are available about the phenotypes exhibited by mice bearing null mutations in these four genes. Transgenic mice lacking *Otx2* gene products are lethal at early embryonic stages (Acampora *et al.*, 1995; Matsuo *et al.*, 1995; Ang *et al.*, 1996). Therefore, they do not provide useful information about the role of this gene in late brain development. Conversely, transgenic mice lacking the gene products of *Otx1*, *Emx1* and *Emx2* are born and their brain can be analysed. All of them show major disturbances in the architecture of various brain regions, including the cerebral cortex. Particularly noticeable is the altered patterning of the hippocampus and the total absence of dentate gyrus in *Emx2* null mice (Pellegrini *et al.*, 1996). A detailed anatomical and functional analysis of these mutants is underway. Plenty of useful information about the role of these genes may hopefully derive from this study even if it can be anticipated that these studies will require quite a long time, mainly due to the complexity of the cortical functional architecture.

Homeobox genes and pathology

In the meantime, mutations in the human *Emx2* gene, more correctly designated EMX2, have been reported (Brunelli *et al.*, 1996; Faiella *et al.* 1997; Granata *et al.*, 1997) in sporadic cases of schizencephaly, a human congenital defect of the cerebral cortex. The schizencephalies are congenital brain malformations characterized by clefts of the cerebral mantle, extending from the pial surface to the lateral ventricles and lined by heterotopic polymicrogyric gray matter (Yakovlev & Wadsworth, 1946a, b). The schizencephaly patients are clinically characterized by motor and mental deficits of varying degree, according to the severity and extent of the brain malformation, and they are frequently affected by epilepsy (Table 1). The malformation may be unilateral or bilateral, the latter being usually symmetric in location, but not in size (Guerrini *et al.*, 1996). Based on the space separating the walls of the fissure, an open-lip form and a closed-lip form can be distinguished. The external opening is covered with cortex showing stellate convolutions with unlayered polymicrogyria (Ferrer, 1984), covering the lips of the fissure and proceeding down to the ventricular wall. The cortex is covered with a membrane resulting from the fusion between the pia and the ventricular ependyma (pial–ependymal seam). The cleft can be detected in any encephalic site, but it is far more frequent in the perisylvian area (Barkovich & Kjos, 1992). In 80 per cent of cases the septum pellucidum is also absent (Chamberlain *et al.*, 1990). Septo-optic dysplasia (agenesis of the septum pellucidum and optic nerve hypoplasia) is observed in about one/three of cases (Barkovich & Norman, 1988; Hosley *et al.*, 1992). The description of a few familial cases of schizencephaly raised the possibility that genetics factors could play a relevant role in the pathogenesis of this brain malformation. The hypothesis that the schizencephalies are due to a malformative origin occurring during early ontogenesis is countered by Barkovich and collaborators who believe schizencephaly and polymicrogyria are the result of the same ischaemic cortical damage in the early postmigrational period. The Barkovich hypothesis is supported by the frequent association of areas of polymicrogyria contralaterally and symmetrically located to unilateral schizencephalies. Conversely, the finding of EMX2 mutations in two siblings, and not in their neurologically normal parents, provides further evidence that, at least in some cases, schizencephalies are determined by deleterious mutations of this homeobox gene (Granata *et al.*, 1997). The genetic hypothesis does not rule out the possibility of alternative pathogenetic mechanisms. A genetic analysis of a larger series of schizencephaly patients (Faiella *et al.*, 1997) demonstrated that only some schizencephaly patients carried EMX2 mutations. Therefore, some cases of schizencephaly may not be related to loss of function of the EMX2 gene, but may be acquired encephaloclastic lesions resulting, like porencephalies, from focal infarction in the territory of a major cerebral artery (Sarnat, 1992).

Table 1. Summary of cases analysed

Patient	Schizencephaly	Association	Nature/position of the mutation	Mechanism
BA	Severe, bilateral	Agenesis cc, sp	ins A at +107 of the hb	Nonsense
DZ	Severe, bilateral	Agenesis cc, sp	A→G (syn) at +15 of the hb (arg→arg)	Unknown
GM	Severe, bilateral	Agenesis cc, sp	ΔGT at +89–90 of *i2*	Unknown
ME	Severe, bilateral	Agenesis cc, sp	G→T at −4 at 3' end *i1/e2*	Splice site
MI	Severe, bilateral	Agenesis cc, sp	G→T at +1 of *e2* (gly→val)	Splice site, missense
MM	Severe, bilateral	Hypoplasia cc	G→T at +1 of *e2* (gly→val)	Splice site, missense
PN	Severe, bilateral	Hydr, dysgenesis cc	G→A at −1 of *i1/e2*	Splice site
Fa	Severe, bilateral	Polymicrogyria		
BV	Mild, unilateral	Partial epilepsy	C→A (syn) at +7 of the hb (arg→arg)	Unknown
DCS	Mild, unilateral	Partial epilepsy	C→A (syn) at +7 of the hb (arg→arg)	Unknown
PC	Mild, unilateral	Partial epilepsy	C→A (syn) at +7 of the hb (arg→arg)	Unknown
VF	Mild, unilateral	Partial epilepsy, mMR	C→A (syn) at +7 of the hb (arg→arg)	Unknown
MB	Mild, unilateral	Partial epilepsy	ΔGT at +58 of *i2*	Unknown
PB	Mild, unilateral	Partial epilepsy	C→A at +73 of *i2*	Unknown
Rb	Mild, unilateral	Partial epilepsy	–	
Mc	Mild, unilateral	Partial epilepsy	–	
Od	Mild, unilateral	Partial epilepsy	–	
CG	Mild, unilateral	Partial epilepsy	–	

Ins, insertion; hb, homeobox; syn, synonymous; cc, corpus callosum; sp, septum pellucidum; *il–i2*, intron 1–2; *el–e2*, exon 1–2; fl, frontal lobe; mMR, mild mental retardation; hydr, hrdrocephalus; Δ, deletion.

Patients with bilateral clefts usually have microcephaly, and severe developmental delay with spastic quadriparesis (Barkovich & Kjos, 1992; Granata et al., 1996). Openlip clefts result in more severe impairment, with seizures being present in most patients, usually beginning before 3 years of age. Unilateral clefts are accompanied by a much less severe clinical phenotype. Small, unilateral closedlip clefts may be discovered on MRI performed after the onset of seizures in otherwise normal individuals (Barkovich & Kjos, 1992). Epilepsy is estimated to occur in equal proportion in patients with unilateral or bilateral cleft (about 80 per cent) (Granata et al., 1996). However, early seizure onset and seizure intractability are much more frequent when the malformation is bilateral (81 per cent vs. 63 per cent and 50 per cent vs. 27 per cent, respectively). Epilepsy is always partial, and there are no distinctive electroclinical patterns. The presence of *Emx2* mutations in cases of schizencephaly lends support to the hypothesis that *Emx2* gene products are required for the correct formation of the human cerebral cortex.

Classification and molecular analysis of the various *Emx2* mutations implicated in schizencephaly are likely to provide useful information for both clinical practice and understanding of the pathogenesis of these types of diseases (Table 1). Preliminary data (Capra et al., 1997; Faiella et al., 1997; Granata et al., 1997) point in the direction of a correlation between the nature of the molecular defect, the severity of the phenotype and the presence of particular clinical features. In fact, severe molecular defects, like frameshift mutations or mutations affecting the splicing pattern are invariably associated with severe, openlip, bilateral schizencephaly, whereas subtle or leaky mutations are associated with mild, closedlip, seemingly unilateral schizencephaly (Table 1). In view of the difficulties of the differential diagnosis of schizencephaly versus similar cortical dysplasias, it is extremely important to devise a molecular differential diagnosis to distiguish schizencephaly from other similar cortical dysplasias and to further discriminate between different clinical forms of schizencephaly. Finally, it is conceivable to produce transgenic mice carrying specific mutations in their *Emx2* gene in order to investigate their cortical phenotype.

Emx and *Otx* genes represent powerful tools for the study of the developing brain, and in particular of the developing cerebral cortex. Their expression patterns during mammalian embryogenesis allow us to closely follow major events in cortical neurogenesis and differentiation. It is also conceivable that mutational events, either germ line or somatic, in these genes or in some of their targets underlie a number of brain defects and in particular cortical dysplasias (Guerrini et al., 1996). Therefore, it seems useful to investigate the possible implication of mutations of these genes in pathological entities such as, for example, in various forms of gray matter heterotopia, agyria–pachygyria, polymicrogyrias, hemimegalencephaly and focal cortical dysplasia. These defects are characterized by abnormal cortical architecture with either normal or dysplastic neurons in aberrant positions implying in turn abnormal connectivity.

Epileptic seizures are present in schizencephaly, as well as in most defects of cortical development (Guerrini et al., 1996). It is still unknown whether seizure activity in the schizencephalic brain originates directly from intrinsic epileptogenic properties of cortical neurons bordering the cleft, from possible abnormalities in signalling systems (Eksioglu et al., 1996) or abnormal connectivity and circuitry (Ferrer et al., 1992). Seizure activity has been demonstrated to arise directly from abnormal neuronal aggregates in both gray matter heterotopia (Morrell et al., 1992; Munari et al., 1996) and focal cortical dysplasia. In the latter case, it has been related to intrinsic neuronal properties (Mattia et al., 1995). However, unlike other non-dysplastic epileptogenic lesions in which epileptic activity originates from normal neurons bordering the abnormal tissue, in gray matter heterotopia and focal cortical dysplasia the seizure-generating neurons are those within the abnormal area. Therefore, the genetic abnormalities which may cause such malformations (Dobyns et al., 1996; Eksioglu et al., 1996; Robain, 1996) have a direct involvement in epileptogenesis as well. Whether these considerations also apply to schizencephaly is still unknown. Further insight into the epileptogenic properties of neurons forming the schizencephalic cleft may arise from electrocorticography or depth electrode studies in patients who are candidates for epilepsy surgery. Functional MRI or direct electrophysiologic studies of tissue slices obtained from surgical specimens may provide additional information. Identification of epilepsy genes has profound implications for therapy as well as pathophysiology, but it has proven a difficult task mainly due to extreme genetic and phenotypic heterogeneity. For this reason it will be of interest to examine the structure and expression of specific developmental genes such as the *Otx* and *Emx* genes in these pathological entities causing human epilepsy. Results of this analysis are likely to be of primary relevance for our understanding of the genetic component of some multifactorial congenital defects of the brain.

Acknowledgement: We are indebted to G. Battaglia, A. Cama, T. Granata and R. Guerrini for a number of helpful comments and suggestions. This work was supported by grants from EC BIOTECH and BIOMED Programmes, the Telethon-Italia Programme and the Italian Association for Cancer Research (AIRC).

References

Acampora, D., Mazan, S., Lallemand, Y., Avantaggiato, V., Maury, M., Simeone, A. & Brulet, P. (1995): Forebrain and midbrain regions are deleted in *Otx2-/-* mutants due to a defective anterior neuroectoderm specification during gastrulation. *Development* **121**, 3279–3290.

Allendoerfer, K.L. & Shatz, C.J. (1994): The subplate, a transient neocortical structure: its role in the development of connection between thalamus and cortex. *Annu. Rev. Neurosci.* **17**, 185–218.

Ang, S.-L., Jin, O., Rhinn, M., Daigle, N., Stevenson, L. & Rossant, J. (1996): A targeted mouse *Otx2* mutation leads to severe defects in gastrulation and formation of axial mesoderm and to deletion of rostral brain. *Development* **122**, 243–252.

Bally-Cuif, L. & Boncinelli, E. (1997): Transcription factors and head formation in vertebrates. *Bioessays* **19**, 127–135.

Bally-Cuif, L. & Wassef, M. (1995): Determination events in the nervous system of the vertebrate embryo. *Curr. Opin. Genet. Dev.* **5**, 450–458.

Barkovich, A.J. & Kjos, B.O. (1992): Schizencephaly: correlation of clinical findings with MR characteristics. *AJNR.* **13**, 85–94

Barkovich, A.J. & Norman, D. (1988): MR of schizencephaly. *AJNR.* **9**, 297–302.

Barkovich, A.J., Gressens, P. & Evrard, P. (1992): Formation, maturation and disorders of brain neocortex. *AJNR*, 13, 423–446.

Bayer, S.A. & Altman, J. (1991): *Neocortical development.* New York: Raven Press.

Boncinelli, E. (1994): Early CNS development: *Distal-less* related genes and forebrain development. *Curr. Opin. Neurobiol.* **4**, 29–36.

Boncinelli, E. (1997): Homeobox genes and disease. *Curr. Opin. Genet. Dev.* **7**, 331–337.

Boncinelli, E. & Mallamaci, A. (1995): Homeobox genes in vertebrate gastrulation. *Curr. Opin. Genet. Dev.* **5**, 619–627.

Boncinelli, E., Gulisano, M. & Broccoli, V. (1993): Emx and Otx genes in the developing mouse brain. *J. Neurobiol.* **24**, 1356–1366.

Brunelli, S., Faiella, A., Capra, V., Nigro, V., Simeone, A., Cama, A. & Boncinelli, E. (1996): Germline mutations in the homeobox gene EMX2 in patients with severe schizencephaly. *Nat. Genet.* **12**, 94–96.

Capra, V., De Marco, P., Moroni, A., Faiella, A., Brunelli, S., Tortori-Donati, P., Andreussi, I, Boncinelli, E. & Cama, A. (1997): Schizencephaly: surgical features and new molecular genetic results. *Eur. J. Ped. Surg.* **6** (Suppl.), 27–29.

Chamberlain, M.C., Press, G.A. & Bejar, R.F. (1990): Neonatal schizencephaly: comparison of brain imaging. *Pediatr. Neurol.* **6**, 382–387.

Dobyns, W.B., Andermann, E., Andermann, F., Czapansky-Beilman, D., Dubeau, F., Dulac, O., Guerrini, R., Hirsch, B., Ledbetter, D.H., Lee, N.S., Motte, J., Pinard, J.-M., Radtke, R.A., Ross, M.E., Tampieri, D., Walsh, C.A. & Truwit, C.L. (1996): X-linked malformations of neuronal migration. *Neurology* **47**, 331–339.

Eksioglu, Y.Z., Scheffer, I.E., Cardenas, P., Knoll, J., DiMario, F., Ramsby, G., Berg, M., Kamuro, K., Berkovic, S.F., Duyk, G.M., Parisi, J., Huttenlocher, P.R. & Walsh, C.A. (1996): Periventricular heterotopia: an X-linked dominant epilepsy locus causing aberrant cerebral cortical development. *Neuron* **16**, 77–78.

Faiella, A., Brunelli, S., Granata, T., D'Incerti, L., Cardini, R., Lenti, C., Battaglia, G. & Boncinelli, E. (1997): A number of schizencephaly patients including two brothers are heterozygous for germline mutations in the homeobox gene EMX2. *Eur. J. Hum. Genet.* **5**, 186–190.

Ferrer, I. (1984): A Golgi analysis of unlayered polymicrogyria. *Acta Neuropathol.* **65**, 69–76.

Ferrer, I., Pineda, M., Tallada, M., Olivier, B., Russi, A., Oller, L., Noboa, R., Zujar, M.J. & Alcantara, S. (1992): Abnormal local circuit neurons in epilepsia partialis continua associated with focal cortical dysplasia. *Acta Neuropathol.* **83**, 647–652.

Finkelstein, R. & Boncinelli, E. (1994): From fly head to mammalian forebrain: the story of *otd* and *Otx*. *Trends Genet.* **10**, 310–315.

Frantz, G.D., Weimann, J.M., Levine, M.E. & McConnell, S.K. (1994): *Otx1* and *Otx2* define layers and regions in developing cerebral cortex and cerebellum. *J. Neurosci.* **14**, 5725–5740.

Granata, T., Battaglia, G., D'Incerti, L., Franceschetti, S., Spreafico, R., Savoiardo, M. & Avanzini, G. (1996): Schizencephaly: clinical findings. In: *Dysplasias of cerebral cortex and epilepsy*, Guerrini, R., Andermann, F., Canapicchi, R., Roger, J., Zifkin, B. & Pfanner, P. (eds), pp. 407–415. Philadelphia: Lippincott-Raven.

Granata, T., Farina, L., Faiella, A., Cardini, R., D'Incerti, L., Boncinelli, E. & Battaglia, G. (1997): Familial schizencephaly associated with EMX2 mutation. *Neurology* **48**, 1403–1406

Guerrini, R., Andermann, F., Canapicchi, R., Roger, J., Zifkin, B. & Pfanner, P. (eds) (1996): *Dysplasias of cerebral cortex and epilepsy*. Philadelphia: Lippincott-Raven.

Gulisano, M., Broccoli, V., Pardini, C. & Boncinelli, E. (1996): *Emx1* and *Emx2* show different patterns of expression during proliferation and differentiation of the developing cerebral cortex. *Eur. J. Neurosci.* **8**, 1037–1050.

Guthrie, S. (1995): The status of the neural segment. *Trends Neurosci.* **18**, 74–79.

Harding, B.N. (1992): Malformations of the nervous system. In: *Greenfield's neuropathology*, Adams, J.H. & Duchen, L.W. (eds), pp. 521–638. London: Edward Arnold.

Hosley, M.A., Abroms, I.F. & Ragland, R.L. (1992): Schizencephaly: case report of familial incidence. *Pediatr. Neurol.* **8**, 148–150.

Krumlauf, R. (1994): *Hox* genes in vertebrate development. *Cell* **78**, 191–201.

Matsuo, I., Kuratani, S., Kimura, C., Takeda, N. & Aizawa, S. (1995): Mouse *Otx2* functions in the formation and patterning of rostral head. *Genes Dev.* **9**, 2646–2658.

Mattia, D., Olivier, A. & Avoli, M. (1995): Seizure-like discharges recorded in the human dysplastic neocortex maintained *in vitro*. *Neurology* **45**, 1391–1395.

McGinnis, W. & Krumlauf, R. (1992): Homeobox genes and axial patterning. *Cell* **68**, 283–302.

Morrell, F., Whisler, W. & Hoeppner, T. (1992): Electrophysiology of heterotopic gray matter in the 'double cortex' syndrome. *Epilepsia* **33**, (Suppl. 3), 76.

Munari, C., Francione, S., Kahane, P., Tassi, L., Hoffmann, D., Garrel, S. & Pasquier, B. (1996): Usefulness of stereo EEG investigations in partial epilepsy associated with cortical dysplastic lesions and gray matter heterotopia. In: *Dysplasias of cerebral cortex and epilepsy* Guerrini, R., Andermann, F., Canapicchi, R., Roger, J., Zifkin, B. & Pfanner, P. (eds), pp. 383–394. Philadelphia: Lippincott-Raven.

O'Leary, D.D.M., Schlaggar, B.L. & Tuttle, R. (1994): Specification of neocortical areas and thalamocortical connections. *Annu. Rev. Neurosci.* **17**, 419–439.

Pellegrini, M., Mansouri, A., Simeone, A., Boncinelli, E. & Gruss, P. (1996): Dentate gyrus formation requires *Emx2*. *Development* **122**, 3893–3898.

Robain, O. (1996): Introduction to the pathology of cerebral cortical dysplasia. In: *Dysplasias of cerebral cortex and epilepsy*, Guerrini, R., Andermann, F., Canapicchi, R., Roger, J., Zifkin, B.G. & Pfanner, P. (eds), pp. 1–9. Philadelphia: Lippincott-Raven.

Rubenstein, J.L.R., Martinez, S., Shimamura, K. & Puelles, L. (1994): The embryonic vertebrate forebrain: The prosomeric model. *Science* **266**, 578–580.

Sarnat, H.B. (1992): *Cerebral dysgenesis: embryology and clinical expression*. New York: Oxford Univ. Press.

Shimamura, K., Hartigan, D.J., Martinez, S., Puelles, L. & Rubenstein, J.L.R. (1995): Longitudinal organization of the anterior neural plate and neural tube. *Development* **121**, 3923–3933.

Simeone, A., Acampora, D., Gulisano, M., Stornaiuolo, A. & Boncinelli, E. (1992a): Nested expression domains of four homeobox genes in developing rostral brain. *Nature* **358**, 687–690.

Simeone, A., Gulisano, M., Acampora, D., Stornaiuolo, A., Rambaldi, M. & Boncinelli, E. (1992b): Two vertebrate homeobox genes related to the *Drosophila empty spiracles* gene are expressed in the embryonic cerebral cortex. *EMBO J.* **11,** 2541–2550.

Simeone, A., Acampora, D., Mallamaci, A., Stornaiuolo, A., D'Apice, M.R., Nigro, V. & Boncinelli, E. (1993): A vertebrate gene related to *orthodenticle* contains a homeodomain of the *bicoid* class and demarcates anterior neuroectoderm in the gastrulating mouse embryo. *EMBO J.* **12,** 2735–2747.

Yakovlev, P. & Wadsworth, R.C. (1946a): Schizencephalies: a study of the congenital clefts in the cerebral mantle, I. Clefts with fused lips. *J. Neuropathol. Exp. Neurol.* **5,** 116–130.

Yakovlev, P.L. & Wadsworth, R.C. (1946b): Schizencephalies: a study of congenital clefts in the cerebral mantle, II. Clefts with hydrocephalus and lips separated. *J. Neuropathol. Exp. Neurol.* **5,** 169–206.

Chapter 2

Prominent expression of glutamate decarboxylase during early hippocampal development: a review of recent findings

Carolyn R. Houser[1], Shannon T. Dupuy-Davies[2] and Nianhui Zhang[3]

[1,2,3]*Department of Neurobiology and* [1]*Brain Research Institute, University of California at Los Angeles, and* [1]*Comprehensive Epilepsy Center, Neurology Service, Department of Veterans Affairs Medical Center, West Los Angeles, Los Angeles, CA 90095, USA*

Summary

Numerous investigations have suggested that GABA may have critical influences during CNS development. The present studies were designed to identify the morphological substrates for GABAergic influences in the developing hippocampal formation. Two forms of glutamate decarboxylase, GAD65 and GAD67, were used as markers for GABA neurons in immunohistochemical studies, and several new views of GABA neuron development have emerged. First, GAD-labelled neurons in the hippocampal formation were detected during the embryonic period, and this was substantially earlier than previously demonstrated. Second, the patterns of GAD localization changed rapidly during the early phases of hippocampal development and progressed from predominant labelling of neuronal cell bodies to pronounced labelling of fibres and terminal-like structures during late embryonic and early postnatal ages. Electron microscopy demonstrated that, as early as PN1, GAD immunoreactivity was concentrated in vesicle-filled regions of axon-like processes. Finally, the labelled cell bodies and processes were first detected in dendritic regions of the hippocampus and dentate gyrus, and this distribution differs considerably from that of the adult in which GAD-labelled terminals are highly concentrated in the principal cell body layers. These findings provide morphological support for important and changing roles for GABA neurons during the early development of the hippocampal formation.

Introduction

Considerable evidence from physiological and biochemical studies suggests that GABA may have important roles in the development of many brain regions prior to the establishment of its role as a major neurotransmitter with inhibitory actions in most regions of the adult central nervous system (CNS). The variety of proposed effects of GABA during development include promotion of neuronal differentiation and neurite outgrowth (Hansen *et al.*, 1984; Spoerri, 1988; Michler, 1990; Barbin *et al.*, 1993); stimulation of synaptogenesis (Spoerri & Wolff, 1981; Gordon-Weeks, 1984); induction of $GABA_A$ receptors (Meier *et al.*, 1984); stimulation of chemotaxis (Behar *et al.*, 1996); regulation of some neuronal phenotypes (Marty *et al.*, 1996); and inhibition of DNA synthesis (LoTurco *et al.*, 1995). While most of these effects have been demonstrated in neuronal cultures, unique physiological actions of GABA have also been observed in slice preparations of the developing hippocampus as well as other brain regions. Specifically, GABA has strong depolarizing actions in the hippocampus during early postnatal life (Mueller *et al.*, 1984; Janigro & Schwartzkroin, 1988; Ben-Ari *et al.*, 1989; Cherubini *et al.*, 1991; Zhang *et al.*, 1991), and similar depolarizing effects of GABA have been observed in *in vitro* slice preparations of the developing cerebral cortex as well as cultured cerebellar and hypothalamic neurons (Connor *et al.*, 1987; Obrietan & van den Pol, 1995; Owens *et al.*, 1996). These depolarizing, excitatory actions of GABA are particularly significant because they occur at a time when the excitatory glutamate system is still poorly developed (Ben-Ari *et al.*, 1989; Hosokawa *et al.*, 1994). Thus, the GABA system may be the major source of depolarization during early development, and this depolarization and the associated increase in intracellular calcium may be the key to GABA's trophic actions (Connor *et al.*, 1987; Yuste & Katz, 1991; Obrietan & van den Pol, 1996; Huang & Redburn, 1996; Ben-Ari *et al.*, 1997). It is therefore important to identify the possible early sources of GABA *in vivo* and to determine if GABA neurons are present and appropriately positioned for the roles that have been suggested by previous *in vitro* studies.

The first goal was to determine if glutamate decarboxylase (GAD), the synthesizing enzyme for GABA, is present in neurons of the hippocampal formation during the early development of this region. Although GAD is responsible for most GABA synthesis in the adult, GAD levels have been reported to lag behind those of GABA during early brain development (Coyle & Enna, 1976), and it has been suggested that alternative routes of GABA synthesis may be used in developing neural regions (Lauder *et al.*, 1986; Eliasson *et al.*, 1997). The recent identification of two isoforms of GAD, GAD65 and GAD67 (Erlander & Tobin, 1991; Erlander *et al.*, 1991; Kaufman *et al.*, 1991), has raised further questions as to whether either or both GAD isoforms are present during early hippocampal development.

The second goal was to determine the characteristics and distribution of GAD-containing neurons in the developing hippocampal formation and to determine if such neurons are present in locations that would be compatible with their influence on the development of other hippocampal neurons. In the adult, GABA neurons and their axon terminals are most prominent in or near the principal cell body layers of the hippocampus and dentate gyrus (Barber & Saito, 1976; Ribak *et al.*, 1978; Mugnaini & Oertel, 1985). Thus, it was anticipated that these would be the sites at which GABA neurons would first be detected in the developing hippocampal formation.

We used immunohistochemical localization of both forms of GAD to determine the earliest ages at which GAD could be detected in the hippocampal formation and to determine the locations and characteristics of the labelled structures. These studies have resulted in several new and unexpected findings that are consistent with changing roles for GABA neurons during the maturation of the hippocampal formation. The present report reviews several of our previously published findings on the development of GAD-containing neurons in the hippocampal formation (Dupuy & Houser, 1995, 1996, 1997; Zhang *et al.*, 1996).

Methods

Experimental animals

Sprague Dawley rats (Harlan Sprague Dawley, Indianapolis, IN) were used in these studies. Female rats were mated overnight, and insemination was verified by vaginal smears. The day a positive smear was obtained was considered embryonic day 0 (E0). Birth usually occurred on E22 and was designated as postnatal day 0 (PN0). For the light microscopic immunohistochemical studies, E16–E21 embryos, PN1 pups, and adult animals were used. Tissue from PN1 animals was used for the electron microscopic studies.

Light and electron microscopy

Tissue preparation. Pregnant rats were deeply anaesthetized with sodium pentobarbital (60 mg/kg, i.p.) before removal of the embryos from the uterus. Young postnatal animals were anaesthetized by cooling or ether inhalation, and adults were anaesthetized with sodium pentobarbital, as above, before perfusion. For light microscopy, all animals were perfused intracardially with a freshly prepared fixative solution of 4 per cent paraformaldehyde in 0.12 M sodium phosphate buffer, pH 7.3. After removal from the skull, the brains were rinsed, cryoprotected, frozen on dry ice, and sectioned in the coronal plane on a cryostat. For electron microscopy, PN1 rat pups were perfused with a fixative solution of 2 per cent paraformaldehyde and 2.5 per cent glutaraldehyde in 0.12 M phosphate buffer, pH 7.3. After rinsing, forebrain sections were cut on a vibratome.

Immunohistochemistry. Two isoforms of GAD were localized with immunohistochemical methods. These isoforms have different molecular weights, 65 kD and 67 kD, and are thus referred to as GAD65 and GAD67 respectively (Erlander & Tobin, 1991). A monoclonal antibody, GAD–6 (Chang & Gottlieb, 1988), was used to localize GAD65, and a polyclonal antiserum, K2 (Kaufman et al., 1991), was used to localize GAD67. The characteristics and specificity of the antibodies have been described previously (Chang & Gottlieb, 1988; Kaufman et al., 1991; Esclapez et al., 1994).

For light and electron microscopy, free-floating sections were processed with unlabelled primary antibodies, K2 and GAD–6, and standard avidin–biotin immunolabelling methods (Vectastain Elite ABC, Vector Laboratories, Burlingame, CA). These methods have been described in detail previously (Esclapez et al., 1994; Dupuy & Houser, 1996). The additional steps that were used in preparing the tissue for electron microscopy were identical to those described in Dupuy and Houser (1996).

Results

Three major findings have emerged from our immunohistochemical studies of GAD localization in the developing hippocampal formation. First, both forms of GAD are present quite early in hippo-

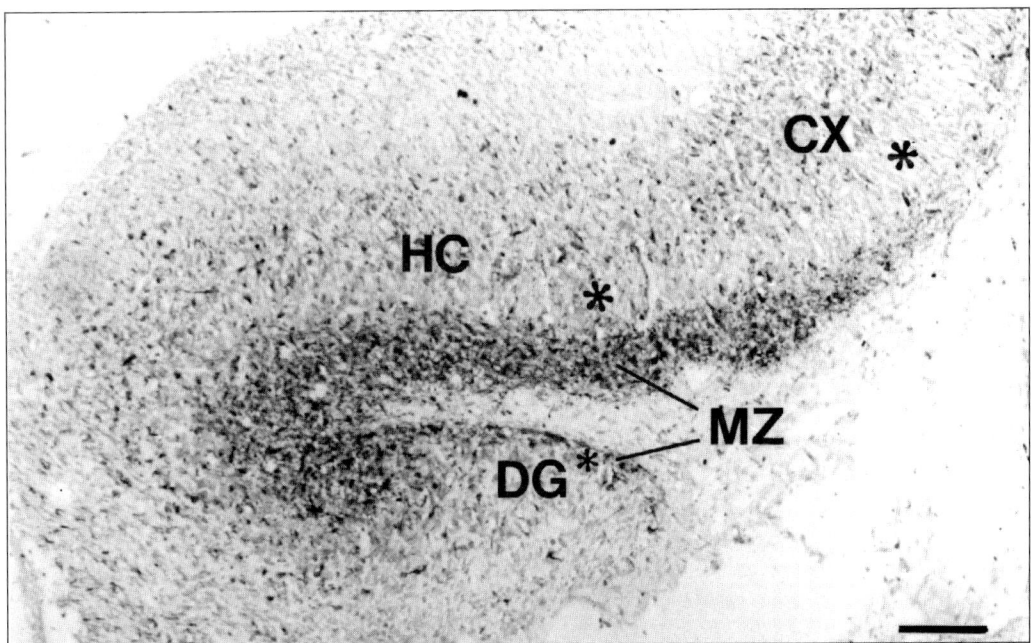

Fig. 1. GAD67-labelled neurons in a coronal section of the rat hippocampal formation at E20. Labelled neurons are highly concentrated in the marginal zone (MZ) which represents the future apical dendritic regions of the hippocampus (HC) and dentate gyrus (DG), and this layer merges with the marginal zone of the neocortex (CX). At this age, GAD-labelled neurons are sparse within the adjacent principal cell body layers and cortical plate (asterisks), but some labelled neurons are scattered throughout the prospective basilar dendritic regions of the hippocampus (future stratum oriens). Scale bar, 100 μm.

campal development, and the initial times of detection, at late embryonic ages, parallel those at which GABA is first observed in this region. Second, the distribution of GAD shifts from a predominant localization in cell bodies to localization in putative axons and terminals during the late embryonic to early postnatal period. Third, the early GAD-labelled cell bodies and terminals are concentrated in locations that are quite different from those of the adult.

Early appearance of GAD

GAD-labelled neurons in the rat hippocampal formation were detected substantially earlier than we had anticipated. Both GAD67- and GAD65-containing neurons were observed as early as E17 in the hippocampus and E19 in the dentate gyrus. The cell bodies of the early-appearing population of GAD-containing neurons were particularly prominent at E20. At this age, GAD-labelled cell bodies extended in a continuous band from the marginal zone of the neocortex through the marginal zone of the hippocampus (future strata radiatum and lacunosum moleculare) and, finally, into the marginal zone of the dentate gyrus (future molecular layer) (Fig. 1). A distinct but less prominent group of GAD-labelled cell bodies was present in the region that will become the stratum oriens in the hippocampal formation.

Transition from cell body to terminal labelling

GAD was initially prominent in the *cell bodies* of neurons within the marginal zones of the hippocampal formation (Fig. 2). However, over a short period of two to three days, there were changes in the labelling patterns for both GAD65 and GAD67 in these regions. At E21 to PN1, GAD labelling shifted from a predominance of cell body labelling to labelling of numerous fibres with varicosities in the same region (Fig. 3). This meshwork of GAD-labelled processes was pronounced throughout much

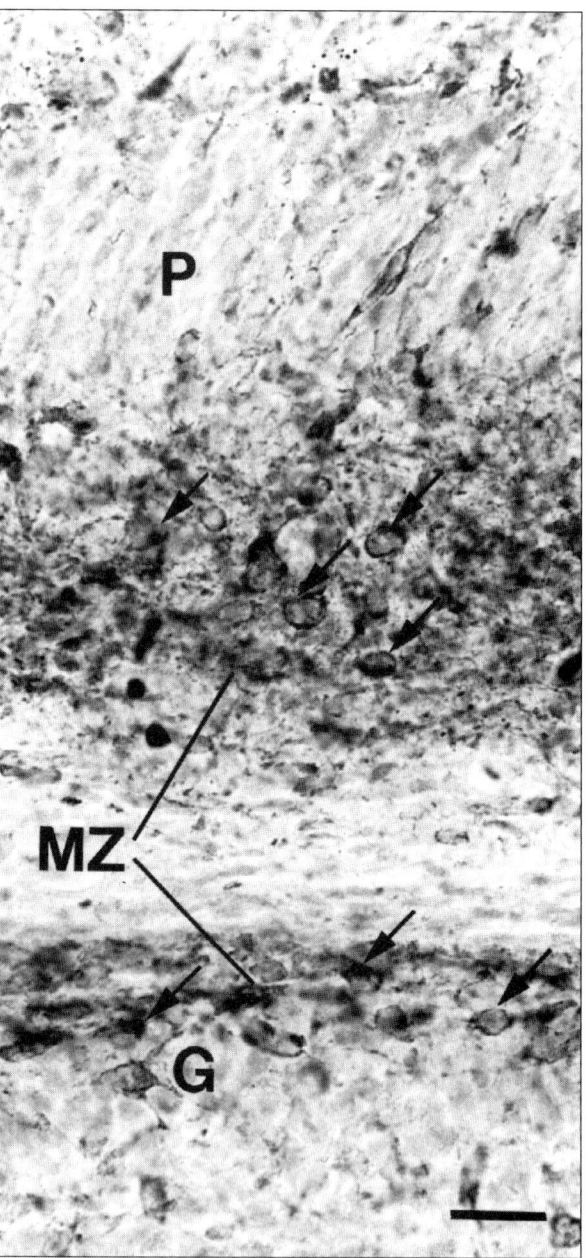

Fig. 2. Higher magnification of GAD67-labelled neurons in the hippocampal formation at E20. GAD-containing cell bodies (examples at arrows) are highly concentrated in the marginal zones (MZ) of the hippocampus and dentate gyrus at E20. The numerous labelled cell bodies in these future dendritic regions contrast with the relatively small number of labelled neurons in the adjacent pyramidal (P) and granule (G) cell layers. This figure is modified from Fig. 3 of Dupuy and Houser (1996). Scale bar, 25 µm.

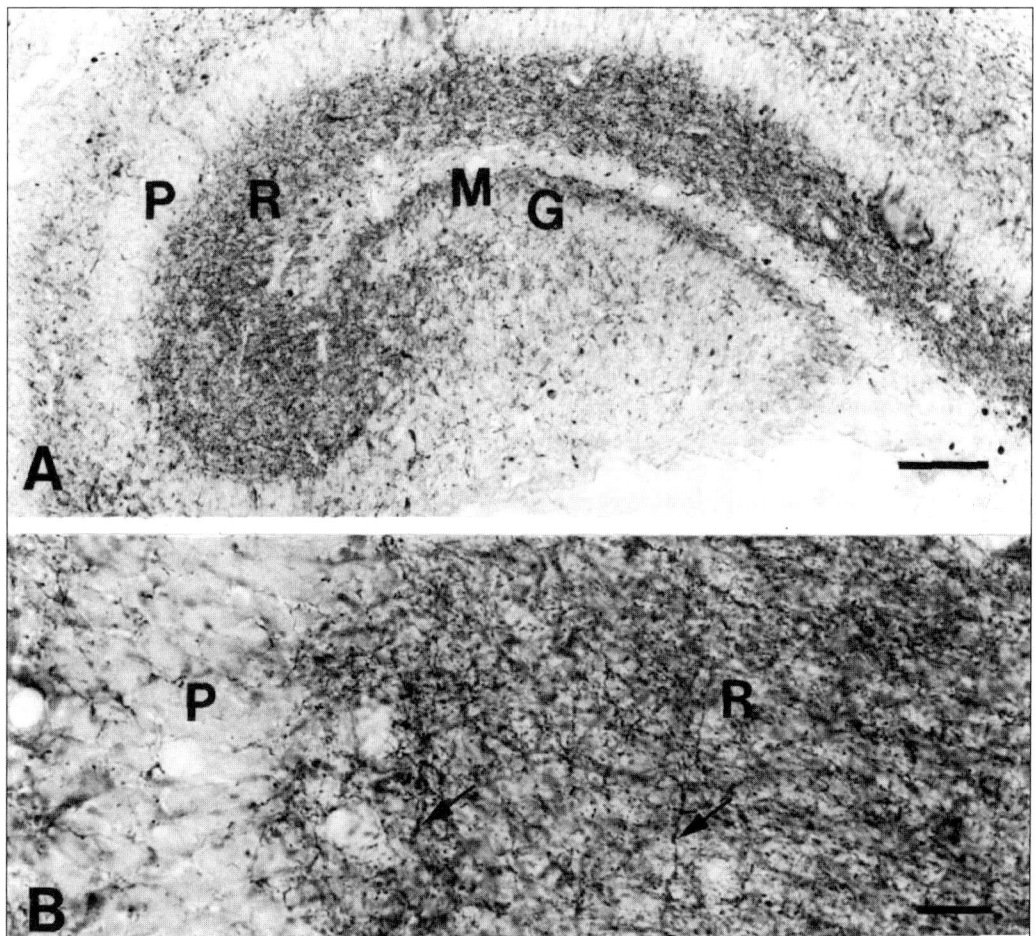

Fig. 3. GAD65-labelled processes in the developing dendritic regions of the hippocampal formation at PN1. A. Labelled processes are highly concentrated in the stratum radiatum (R) of the hippocampus and in the molecular layer (M) of the dentate gyrus. The pyramidal cell (P) and granule cell (G) layers contain very few labelled structures. B. At high magnification, a meshwork of GAD-labelled fibres, many of which display periodic varicosities (examples at arrows) are evident in stratum radiatum (R) of CA3. The abundance of axon-like structures in the developing apical dendritic layer contrasts with the paucity of labelled structures in the pyramidal cell layer (P). Scale bars, A, 100 μm; B, 25 μm.

of the developing dendritic regions of the dentate gyrus and hippocampus (Fig. 3) and was continuous with a similar rich plexus of GAD-labelled fibres in the developing molecular layer of the cerebral cortex. The fine fibres with periodic varicosities appeared to be axons *en passant* (Fig. 3).

Electron microscopic findings support the axonal identity of the GAD-labelled processes. As early as PN1, GAD immunoreactivity was concentrated in vesicle-filled regions of small diameter axon-like structures (Figs. 4A, B). In some instances, the GAD-containing terminal-like structures were found adjacent to immature dendritic processes that displayed a flocculent cytoplasm and lacked the microtubule arrays that characterize more mature dendrites (Fig. 4B). However, GAD-labelled terminal-like structures were also located near more mature dendrites with well-developed microtubules (Fig. 4A). At PN1, some of the GAD-labelled terminals already displayed morphological synapses. However, in many instances, the GAD-labelled terminals contained numerous synaptic-like

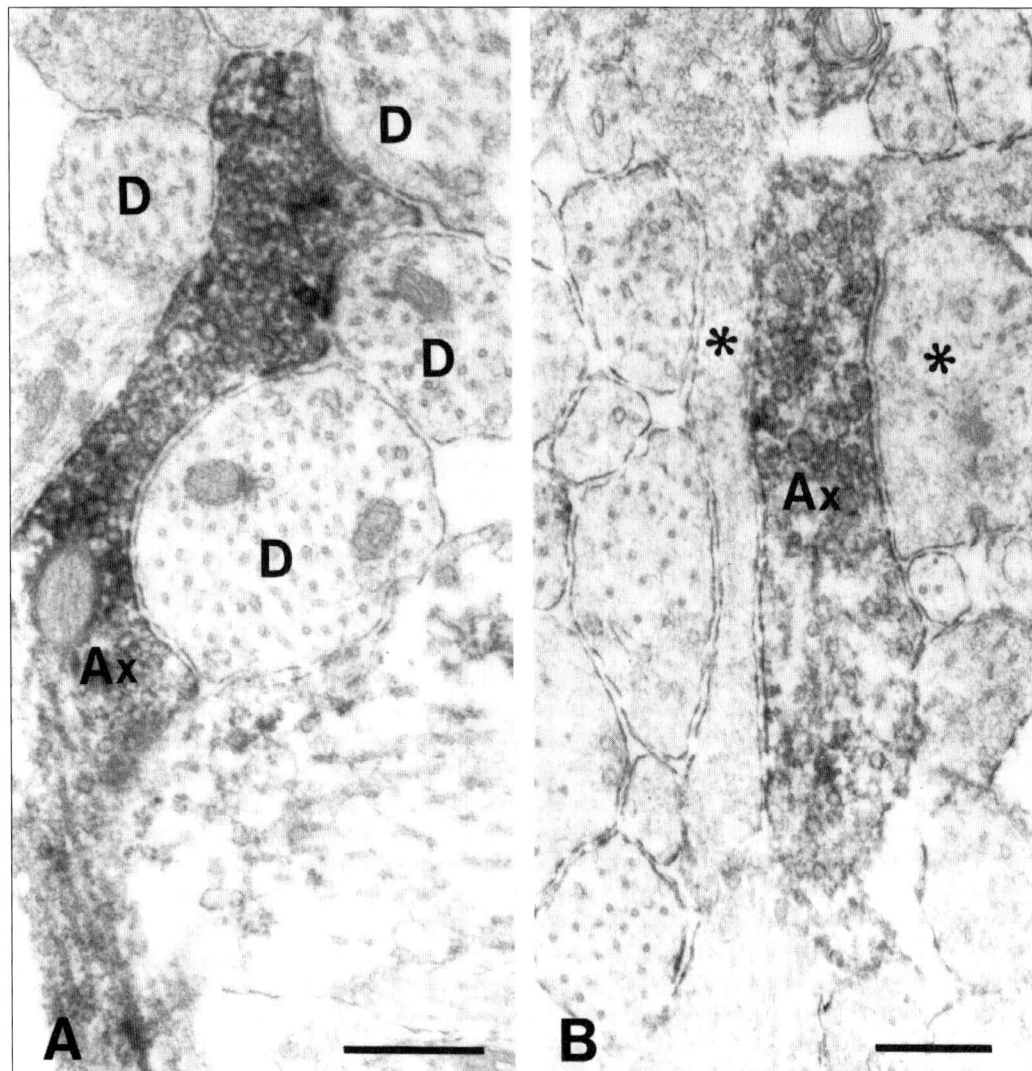

Fig. 4. Ultrastructural characteristics of GAD65-labelled fibres in the hippocampus at PN1. A. A GAD65-labelled axonal process (Ax) courses between several dendritic profiles (D) in the CA3 field. Numerous vesicles are present within the process, and GAD immunoreactivity is highly concentrated at these sites. B. In another GAD-labelled process (Ax) from CA1, vesicles are highly concentrated near developing processes (*) that lack the typical arrays of mature organelles. Scale bars, 0.4 µm for both panels.

vesicles but were not apposed to distinct postsynaptic densities that are characteristic of mature synapses (Figs. 4A, B).

Different GAD localization patterns in developing and adult tissue

At late prenatal and early postnatal ages, the distribution of GAD-labelled structures was distinctly different from that of the mature hippocampal formation (Fig. 5). In the adult, GAD-labelled terminals are highly concentrated around the cell bodies of the majority of pyramidal cells in the hippocampus (Fig. 5B) and granule cells of the dentate gyrus. This creates distinct laminae with the most intense

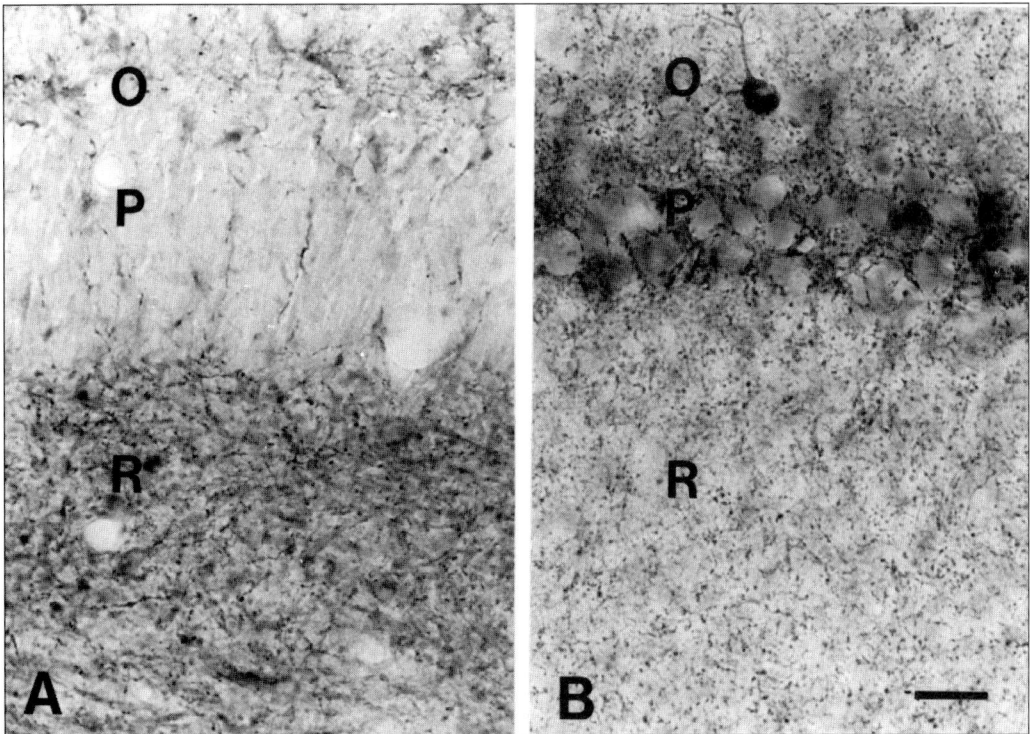

Fig. 5. Comparison of GAD65-labelled structures in the CA1 field of the hippocampus in PN1 (A) and adult (B) rats. A. At PN1, labelled axon-like processes with varicosities are abundant in stratum radiatum (R) but are virtually absent from the pyramidal cell layer (P) which is relatively wide at this early stage of development. B. In contrast, in the adult, labelled axons and terminals are highly concentrated in the pyramidal cell layer (P) and are comparatively less numerous in stratum radiatum (R). Labelled terminals and some cell bodies are also evident in stratum oriens (O). Scale bars, 25 μm for both panels.

GAD-immunoreactivity in the cell body layers, even though numerous small-diameter fibres and terminals are also distributed throughout all dendritic regions. In contrast to the above pattern, GAD-labelled processes in the embryonic and early postnatal hippocampal formation were most highly concentrated in the future apical dendritic layers (Fig. 5A), i.e. strata radiatum and lacunosum moleculare of the hippocampus and stratum moleculare of the dentate gyrus. Surprisingly, at these ages, the cell body layers contained relatively few GAD-containing cell bodies or processes (Fig. 5A). Thus, the regions with high and low densities of GAD-labelled structures in the early developing hippocampal formation were reversed from those in the adult (compare Figs. 5A, B).

Discussion

A central finding of our recent studies is that GAD-containing neurons are present quite early in hippocampal development in the rat and can be detected at prenatal ages in both the hippocampus and dentate gyrus (Dupuy & Houser, 1995). GABA-containing cell bodies have been described at similar ages and in similar locations in the rat (Lauder *et al.*, 1986; Rozenberg *et al.*, 1989). The presence of both forms of GAD in groups of neurons that appear comparable to the GABA neurons suggests that GAD is likely to be responsible for the synthesis of GABA during the early development of the hippocampal formation. Thus, it does not appear necessary to hypothesize an alternate pathway for GABA synthesis as has been suggested in several neural regions (Lauder *et al.*, 1986; Swann *et al.*,

1989; Eliasson *et al.*, 1997). This is significant because some earlier biochemical and immunohistochemical studies have suggested that the appearance of GAD might lag behind that of GABA in the development of the hippocampus as well as other brain regions (Swann *et al.*, 1989; Coyle & Enna, 1976). In previous immunohistochemical studies of the hippocampal formation, GAD was first detected at PN2–PN5 (Seress & Ribak, 1988; Seress *et al.*, 1989; Nitsch *et al.*, 1990), whereas GABA was detected during the late prenatal period (Lauder *et al.*, 1986; Rozenberg *et al.*, 1989). However, due to the availability of increasingly sensitive reagents and methods for GAD localization, it is now clear that both GAD forms appear early in CNS development and are likely to be responsible for GABA synthesis from the earliest ages that GABA is detected (Dupuy & Houser, 1995, 1996).

The early expression of GAD by neurons in the hippocampus and dentate gyrus may be related to previous findings that GAD-labelled neurons in the adult are born comparatively early in the hippocampal formation (Amaral & Kurz, 1985; Lübbers *et al.*, 1985; Soriano *et al.*, 1986). Birthdating studies of the dentate gyrus have demonstrated that the peak birthdate of GAD-containing neurons, identified in the adult, is E14 in the rat (Amaral & Kurz, 1985), and this is considerably earlier than the birthdates of the granule cells that are born predominantly during postnatal life (Altman & Das, 1965; Schlessinger *et al.*, 1975). Both the early birthdates of GABA neurons and the early expression of GAD are consistent with a precocious development of interneurons in the hippocampus as compared with the principal neurons.

Since we could not be certain that the early GAD-labelled neurons were the same as those with early birthdates in the adult, we conducted birthdating studies of the early GAD-containing population (Dupuy & Houser, 1995, 1996). The animals were injected with BrdU, a thymidine analogue that labels dividing neurons during the S-phase, at E10 to E16, and the birthdates of the GAD-labelled cells in the dentate gyrus were determined at E20. These studies demonstrated that the early-appearing GAD-containing neurons were born over a relatively wide range of ages but had their peak birthdates at E14 and E15. These early birthdates are similar to the birthdates of GAD-containing neurons in the dentate gyrus in the adult rat (Amaral & Kurz, 1985), and, therefore, it is likely that the two populations are the same. Both their early birthdates and early appearance are consistent with a role for GAD-containing neurons in the early development of the hippocampal formation.

In addition to their early appearance, two features of the GAD localization patterns were particularly interesting and unexpected. The first was the change in the GAD-containing structures from a predominance of labelled cell bodies at the earliest times of detection to a predominance of labelled axons and terminal-like structures a few days later, at early postnatal ages. Our interpretation of these findings is that the presumptive axons and terminal-like structures are derived from the initially observed cell bodies and that the changes in the patterns of immunoreactivity represent a shift in the concentration of GAD from the cell bodies to the terminals as the neurons develop. The similarities in the distribution of the two types of structures support this suggestion. The presence of GAD in axon-like processes is consistent with previous reports of extensive axonal arborizations of some interneurons in dendritic regions of the hippocampus at early postnatal ages (Ben-Ari *et al.*, 1994). However, an extrinsic source of some of the labelled fibres remains a possibility, and the septum could be one such source (Linke & Frotscher, 1993).

It now appears that the early expression of GAD and GABA in developing axon-like processes may be a common feature of GABA neuron development in several brain regions. Van den Pol (1997) has recently demonstrated high levels of GABA immunoreactivity in presumptive axons and their growth cones at embryonic ages in the hypothalamus, and previous ultrastructural studies demonstrated GAD immunoreactivity in developing axons and growth cones in the cerebellum (McLaughlin *et al.*, 1975). GABA-labelled fibres were also described by Lauder *et al.* (1986) in several brain regions in an early study of prenatal development of the GABA system.

The punctate localization of GAD in the hippocampal formation suggests that GABA could be synthesized and released at focal sites during early development in contrast to being released more diffusely from neuronal cell bodies and dendritic processes. This is supported by the ultrastructural findings of high concentrations of GAD immunoreactivity in vesicle-rich regions of axonal processes. Furthermore, the electron microscopic findings are consistent with release from nonsynaptic as well as synaptic sites. Importantly, some GAD-labelled terminals are located in close apposition to dendritic growth cones and developing dendritic processes, and these findings provide *in vivo* support for previous suggestions of trophic roles for GABA in the differentiation and maturation of neuronal processes (Spoerri, 1988; Barbin *et al*., 1993).

A second feature of the early GAD localization patterns that was quite striking was the high concentration of labelled fibres and terminals in the developing *dendritic* regions of the hippocampus and dentate gyrus and the paucity of GAD-labelled terminals in the principal cell body layers. Physiological studies have demonstrated that the earliest GABA actions in the hippocampal formation are depolarizing rather than hyperpolarizing (Mueller *et al*., 1984; Ben-Ari *et al*., 1989; Cherubini *et al*., 1991), and our findings would suggest that these actions are exerted through axonal processes primarily in dendritic regions of the developing hippocampal formation. This contrasts with the hyperpolarizing, inhibitory effects of GABA that predominate at axosomatic sites in the adult hippocampus. Interestingly, despite the early appearance of GAD-containing fibres and terminals in the developing dendritic regions, the completely mature pattern of high concentrations of labelled axon terminals around neuronal cell bodies and the characteristic laminar patterns of GAD-labelled terminals in the molecular layer of the dentate gyrus and strata radiatum and lacunosum moleculare of the hippocampus are not evident until relatively late in hippocampal development, between PN20 and PN30 (C.R. Houser and S.T. Dupuy, unpublished findings). Such observations are consistent with the relatively late maturation of several aspects of inhibitory GABAergic function in the hippocampal formation (Swann *et al*., 1989; Michelson & Lothman, 1989; Hollrigel & Soltesz, 1997).

The precise roles of GABA in early hippocampal development have not been determined *in vivo*, but the presently observed distributions of GAD-containing neurons suggest that they are in ideal locations to influence dendritic outgrowth and maturation of the principal cells. This idea can be related to previous studies of the effects of GABA in several *in vitro* experiments. One of the earliest demonstrations of GABAergic effects during development was the stimulation of neurite outgrowth in neuroblastoma cells (Spoerri & Wolff, 1981), and these effects were later replicated in cerebral cortical and retinal neurons in culture (Spoerri, 1988). Subsequent studies of cultured hippocampal neurons showed that the presence of a $GABA_A$ receptor antagonist led to a substantial decrease in neurite length and branching, thus supporting the suggestion that GABA, acting through $GABA_A$ receptors, promotes the outgrowth of neuronal processes (Barbin *et al*., 1993). The presently observed concentration of GAD-containing processes in the future dendritic regions of the hippocampus could serve as a GABA-rich field toward which the growing apical dendrites might be directed. Electron microscopic demonstrations of vesicle-filled terminals that display GAD immunoreactivity near immature dendrites are consistent with this suggestion. Electrophysiological studies have demonstrated that embryonic hippocampal neurons are extremely sensitive to GABA (Fiszman *et al*., 1990), and thus even small amounts of GABA could have effects on nearby neuronal processes. If, as anticipated, GABA release at the terminal-like sites were to produce depolarization of the adjacent processes, this could lead to increases in intracellular calcium which, in turn, could have trophic effects such as stimulation of dendritic outgrowth.

Other developmental effects of the early GABA neurons in the hippocampal formation are also possible. GABA release by these neurons could stimulate synaptogenesis, as has been demonstrated in cultured neurons and the retina (Spoerri, 1988; Messersmith & Redburn, 1993; Wolff *et al*., 1993). Another possibility is that the early GABA neurons could serve as temporary targets for hippocampal afferents prior to development of their ultimate postsynaptic targets such as the dendrites of the developing principal cell. Similar functions have been proposed for calretinin and GABA neurons in the developing mouse hippocampus (Soriano *et al*., 1994). Finally the initial, close proximity of the early population of GABA neurons to the developing principal cell layers suggests that the GABA neurons could help establish the proper alignment of the pyramidal cells and granule cells in their respective cell body layers and thus have architectural influences, similar to those that have been described in the retina (Messersmith & Redburn, 1993).

Just as the precise functional roles of the early-appearing GABA neurons have not been determined, neither has their subsequent fate. These neurons could undergo cell death, become the mature population of GABA neurons in the molecular layers, change their transmitter phenotype or migrate to new positions in the developing hippocampal formation.

In summary, the early-appearing populations of GAD-containing neurons are likely to be the major source of GABA during early periods of hippocampal development, and, as such, may be critical for the normal development of the hippocampal formation. A loss or deficit of these neurons could lead to alterations in the normal organization of the hippocampal formation and, potentially, to altered excitability and increased seizure susceptibility within the region. These possibilities are worth exploring in the search for early developmental causes of seizure disorders that affect the hippocampus and cerebral cortex.

Acknowledgements: We thank Donald Chang, Bruce Havens and Eric Walker for excellent immunohistochemical and photographic assistance. This research was supported by a grant from the National Institutes of Health, National Institute of Neurological Disorders and Stroke, NS33360.

References

Altman, J. & Das, G.D. (1965): Autoradiographic and histological evidence of postnatal hippocampal neurogenesis in rats. *J. Comp. Neurol.* **124**, 319–336.

Amaral, D.G. & Kurz, J. (1985): The time of origin of cells demonstrating glutamic acid decarboxylase-like immunoreactivity in the hippocampal formation of the rat. *Neurosci. Lett.* **59**, 33–39.

Barber, R. & Saito, K. (1976): Light microscopic visualization of GAD and GABA-T in immunocytochemical preparations of rodent CNS. In: *GABA in Nervous System Function*, Roberts, E., Chase, T.N. & Tower, D.B. (eds), pp. 113–132. New York: Raven Press.

Barbin, G., Pollard, H., Gaïarsa, J.L. & Ben-Ari, Y. (1993): Involvement of GABA$_A$ receptors in the outgrowth of cultured hippocampal neurons. *Neurosci. Lett.* **152**, 150–154.

Behar, T.N., Li, Y.-X., Tran, H.T., Ma, W., Dunlap, V., Scott, C. & Barker, J.L. (1996): GABA stimulates chemotaxis and chemokinesis of embryonic cortical neurons via calcium-dependent mechanisms. *J. Neurosci.* **16**, 1808–1818.

Ben-Ari, Y., Cherubini, C., Corradetti, R. & Gaiarsa, J.-L. (1989): Giant synaptic potentials in immature rat CA3 hippocampal neurones. *J. Physiol.* **416**, 303–325.

Ben-Ari, Y., Tseeb, V., Raggozzino, D., Khazipov, R. & Gaiarsa, J.-L. (1994): γ-Aminobutyric acid (GABA): a fast excitatory transmitter which may regulate the development of hippocampal neurons in early postnatal life. *Prog. Brain Res.* **102**, 261–273.

Ben-Ari, Y., Khazipov, R., Leinekugel, X., Caillard, O. & Gaiarsa, J.-L. (1997): GABA$_A$, NMDA and AMPA receptors: a developmentally regulated 'ménage à trois'. *Trends Neurosci.* **20**, 523–529.

Chang, Y.-C. & Gottlieb, D.I. (1988): Characterization of the proteins purified with monoclonal antibodies to glutamic acid decarboxylase. *J. Neurosci.* **8**, 2123–2130.

Cherubini, E., Gaiarsa, J.L. & Ben-Ari, Y. (1991): GABA: an excitatory transmitter in early postnatal life. *Trends Neurosci.* **14**, 515–519.

Connor, J.A., Tseng, H.-Y. & Hockberger, P.E. (1987): Depolarization- and transmitter-induced changes in intracellular Ca^{2+} of rat cerebellar granule cells in explant cultures. *J. Neurosci.* **7**, 1384–1400.

Coyle, J.T. & Enna, S.J. (1976): Neurochemical aspects of the ontogenesis of GABAnergic neurons in the rat brain. *Brain Res.* **111**, 119–133.

Dupuy, S.T. & Houser, C.R. (1995): Early appearance and generation of a prominent population of GAD67-containing neurons in the developing rat hippocampal formation. *Soc. Neurosci. Abstr.* **21**, 307.

Dupuy, S.T. & Houser, C.R. (1996): Prominent expression of two forms of glutamate decarboxylase in the embryonic and early postnatal rat hippocampal formation. *J. Neurosci.* **16**, 6919–6932.

Dupuy, S.T. & Houser, C.R. (1997): Developmental changes in GAD67 mRNA-containing neurons of the rat dentate gyrus: an *in situ* hybridization and birthdating study. *J. Comp. Neurol.* **389**, 402–418.

Eliasson, M.J.L., McCaffery, P., Baughman, R.W. & Dräger, U.C. (1997): A ventrodorsal GABA gradient in the embryonic retina prior to expression of glutamate decarboxylase. *Neuroscience* **79**, 863–869.

Erlander, M.G. & Tobin, A.J. (1991): The structural and functional heterogeneity of glutamic acid decarboxylase: a review. *Neurochem. Res.* **16**, 215–226.

Erlander, M.G., Tillakaratne, N.J.K., Feldblum, S., Patel, N. & Tobin, A.J. (1991): Two genes encode distinct glutamate decarboxylases. *Neuron* **7**, 91–100.

Esclapez, M., Tillakaratne, N.J.K., Kaufman, D.L., Tobin, A.J. & Houser, C.R. (1994): Comparative localization of two forms of glutamic acid decarboxylase and their mRNAs in rat brain supports the concept of functional differences between the forms. *J. Neurosci.* **14**, 1834–1855.

Fiszman, M.L., Novotny, E.A., Lange, G.D. & Barker, J.L. (1990): Embryonic and early postnatal hippocampal cells respond to nanomolar concentrations of muscimol. *Dev. Brain Res.* **53**, 186–193.

Gordon-Weeks, P.R. (1984): Uptake and release of [^{3}H]GABA by growth cones isolated from neonatal rat brain. *Neurosci. Lett.* **52**, 205–210.

Hansen, G.H., Meier, E. & Shousboe, A. (1984): GABA influences the ultrastructure composition of cerebellar granule cells during development in culture. *Int. J. Dev. Neurosci.* **2**, 247–257.

Hollrigel, G.S. & Soltesz, I. (1997): Slow kinetics of miniature IPSCs during early postnatal development in granule cells of the dentate gyrus. *J. Neurosci.* **17**, 5119–5128.

Hosokawa, Y., Sciancalepore, M., Stratta, F., Martina, M. & Cherubini, E. (1994): Developmental changes in spontaneous GABA$_A$-mediated synaptic events in rat hippocampal CA3 neurons. *Eur. J. Neurosci.* **6**, 805–813.

Huang, B. & Redburn, D. (1996): GABA-mediated increases in [Ca^{2+}]$_i$ in retinal neurons of postnatal rabbits. *Vis. Neurosci.* **13**, 441–447.

Janigro, D. & Schwartzkroin, P.A. (1988): Effects of GABA and baclofen on pyramidal cells in the developing rabbit hippocampus: an '*in vitro*' study. *Dev. Brain Res.* **41**, 171–184.

Kaufman, D.L., Houser, C.R. & Tobin, A.J. (1991): Two forms of the gamma-aminobutyric acid synthetic enzyme glutamate decarboxylase have distinct intraneuronal distributions and cofactor interactions. *J. Neurochem.* **56**, 720–723.

Lauder, J.M., Han, V.K.M., Henderson, P., Verdoorn, T. & Towle, A.C. (1986): Prenatal ontogeny of the GABAergic system in the rat brain: an immunocytochemical study. *Neuroscience* **19**, 465–493.

Linke, R. & Frotscher, M. (1993): Development of the rat septohippocampal projection: tracing with DiI and electron microscopy of identified growth cones. *J. Comp. Neurol.* **332**, 69–88.

LoTurco, J.J., Owens, D.F., Heath, M.J.S., Davis, M.B.E. & Kriegstein, A.R. (1995): GABA and glutamate depolarize cortical progenitor cells and inhibit DNA synthesis. *Neuron* **15**, 1287–1298.

Lübbers, K., Wolff, J.R. & Frotscher, M. (1985): Neurogenesis of GABAergic neurons in the rat dentate gyrus: a combined autoradiographic and immunocytochemical study. *Neurosci. Lett.* **62**, 317–322.

Marty, S., Berninger, B., Carroll, P. & Thoenen, H. (1996): GABAergic stimulation regulates the phenotype of hippocampal interneurons through the regulation of brain-derived neurotrophic factor. *Neuron* **16**, 565–570.

McLaughlin, B.J., Wood, J.G., Saito, K., Roberts, E. & Wu, J.-Y. (1975): The fine structural localization of glutamate decarboxylase in developing axonal processes and presynaptic terminals of rodent cerebellum. *Brain Res.* **85**, 355–371.

Meier, E., Drejer, J. & Schousboe, A. (1984): GABA induces functionally active low-affinity GABA receptors on cultured cerebellar granule cells. *J. Neurochem.* **43**, 1737–1744.

Messersmith, E.K. & Redburn, D.A. (1993): The role of GABA during development of the outer retina in the rabbit. *Neurochem. Res.* **18**, 463–470.

Michelson, H.B. & Lothman, E.W. (1989): An in vivo electrophysiological study of the ontogeny of excitatory and inhibitory processes in the rat hippocampus. *Dev. Brain Res.* **47**, 113–122.

Michler, A. (1990): Involvement of GABA receptors in the regulation of neurite growth in cultured embryonic chick tectum. *Int. J. Dev. Neurosci.* **8**, 463–472.

Mueller, A.L., Taube, J.S. & Schwartzkroin, P.A. (1984): Development of hyperpolarizing inhibitory postsynaptic potentials and hyperpolarizing response to γ-aminobutyric acid in rabbit hippocampus studied *in vitro*. *J. Neurosci.* **4**, 860–867.

Mugnaini, E. & Oertel, W.H. (1985): An atlas of the distribution of GABAergic neurons and terminals in the rat CNS as revealed by GAD immunohistochemistry. In: *Handbook of Chemical Neuroanatomy, Vol.4: GABA and Neuropeptides in the CNS, Part I*, Björklund, A. & Hökfelt, T. (eds), pp. 436–608. Amsterdam: Elsevier.

Nitsch, R., Bergmann, I., Küppers, K., Mueller, G. & Frotscher, M. (1990): Late appearance of parvalbumin immunoreactivity in the development of GABAergic neurons in the rat hippocampus. *Neurosci. Lett.* **118**, 147–150.

Obrietan, K. & van den Pol, A.N. (1995): GABA neurotransmission in the hypothalamus: developmental reversal from Ca^{2+} elevating to depressing. *J. Neurosci.* **15**, 5065–5077.

Obrietan, K. & van den Pol, A.N. (1996): Growth cone calcium elevation by GABA. *J. Comp. Neurol.* **372**, 167–175.

Owens, D.F., Boyce, L.H., Davis, M.B.E. & Kriegstein, R. (1996): Excitatory GABA responses in embryonic and neonatal cortical slices demonstrated by gramicidin perforated-patch recordings and calcium imaging. *J. Neurosci.* **16**, 6414–6423.

Ribak, C.E., Vaughn, J.E. & Saito, K. (1978): Immunocytochemical localization of glutamic acid decarboxylase in neuronal somata following colchicine inhibition of axonal transport. *Brain Res.* **140**, 315–332.

Rozenberg, F., Robain, O., Jardin, L. & Ben-Ari, Y. (1989): Distribution of GABAergic neurons in late fetal and early postnatal rat hippocampus. *Dev. Brain Res.* **50**, 177–187.

Schlessinger, A.R., Cowan, W.M. & Gottlieb, D.I. (1975): An autoradiographic study of the time of origin and the pattern of granule cell migration in the dentate gyrus of the rat. *J. Comp. Neurol.* **159**, 149–175.

Seress, L., Frotscher, M. & Ribak, C.E. (1989): Local circuit neurons in both the dentate gyrus and Ammon's horn establish synaptic connections with principal neurons in five day old rats: a morphological basis for inhibition in early development. *Exp. Brain Res.* **78**, 1–9.

Seress, L. & Ribak, C.E. (1988): The development of GABAergic neurons in the rat hippocampal formation. An immunocytochemical study. *Dev. Brain Res.* **44**, 197–209.

Soriano, E., Cobas, A. & Fairén, A. (1986): Asynchronism in the neurogenesis of GABAergic and non-GABAergic neurons in the mouse hippocampus. *Dev. Brain Res.* **30**, 88–92.

Soriano, E., Del Río, J.A., Martínez, A. & Supèr, H. (1994): Organization of the embryonic and early postnatal murine hippocampus. I. Immunocytochemical characterization of neuronal populations in the subplate and marginal zone. *J. Comp. Neurol.* **342**, 571–595.

Spoerri, P.E. (1988): Neurotrophic effects of GABA in cultures of embryonic chick brain and retina. *Synapse* **2**, 11–22.

Spoerri, P.E. & Wolff, J.R. (1981): Effect of GABA-administration on murine neuroblastoma cells in culture. I. Increased membrane dynamics and formation of specialized contacts. *Cell Tissue Res.* **218**, 567–579.

Swann, J.W., Brady, R.J. & Martin, D.L. (1989): Postnatal development of GABA-mediated synaptic inhibition in rat hippocampus. *Neuroscience* **28**, 551–561.

van den Pol, A.N. (1997): GABA immunoreactivity in hypothalamic neurons and growth cones in early development *in vitro* before synapse formation. *J. Comp. Neurol.* **383**, 178–188.

Wolff, J.R., Joó, F. & Kása, P. (1993): Modulation by GABA of neuroplasticity in the central and peripheral nervous system. *Neurochem. Res.* **18**, 453–461.

Yuste, R. & Katz, L.C. (1991): Control of postsynaptic Ca^{2+} influx in developing neocortex by excitatory and inhibitory neurotransmitters. *Neuron* **6**, 333–344.

Zhang, L., Spigelman, I. & Carlen, P.L. (1991): Development of GABA-mediated, chloride-dependent inhibition in CA1 pyramidal neurons of immature rat hippocampal slices. *J. Physiol.* **444**, 25–49.

Zhang, N., Dupuy, S.T. & Houser, C.R. (1996): Ultrastructure of GAD-immunoreactive processes in the early postnatal rat hippocampal formation. *Soc. Neurosci. Abstr.* **22**, 1972.

Chapter 3

The contribution of developmental plasticity to early-life seizures and chronic epilepsy

Martha Pierson and John Swann

The Cain Foundation Laboratories, Department of Paediatrics; and Division of Neuroscience, Baylor College of Medicine, Houston, Texas 77030, USA

Not only is there a critical developmental period of enhanced vulnerability to seizures in humans, but there is also such a window in experimental animals. For example, under conditions of GABAergic disinhibition, brain slices, taken from rats and studied *in vitro*, exhibit maximum epileptogenicity between postnatal days (PNDs) 9 and 19. By contrast, prolonged epileptiform discharges do not occur at all in tissues from rats of earlier or later ages. Figure 1 demonstrates this difference in recordings of CA3 neurons in brain slices which were disinhibited by picrotoxin (Swann & Brady, 1984). Extracellular field recordings were obtained from small microdissected segments of the hippocampal CA3 subfield. Segments, which were called mini slices, measured approximately 600 μm along stratum pyramidale. Mini slices were taken from rats on postnatal day 5, 10 and in adulthood (day 43). During the first postnatal week (panel A), epileptiform activity was not observed. However, starting on day 9 large prolonged electrographic seizures were routinely observed (panel B). In adulthood, brief interictal discharges were recorded that were approximately 100 ms in duration. Not only is this phenomenon observed in CA3 region of hippocampus, but an age-dependent propensity for epileptiform activity is also observed in brain slice studies of the CA1 region (Schwartzkroin, 1984; Hamon & Heinemann, 1988) and of neocortex (Hablitz, 1987). Correspondingly, behavioural studies of rat also demonstrate a profound developmental peak in seizure susceptibility. A partial list of these *in vivo* studies includes the following observations. Rat pups have a lower threshold to seizures induced by chemical convulsants (e.g. kainic acid (Albala *et al.*, 1984; Tremblay *et al.*, 1984), pilocarpine (Cavalheiro *et al.*, 1987), or picrotoxin (Woodbury, 1977)). Moreover, pups are more susceptible to neocortical focal epileptogenesis (Mares, 1973), to amygdala kindling (Moshé, 1981), to hippocampal kindling (Haas *et al.*, 1990; Michelson & Lothman, 1991), to hippocampal electrical stimulations (Velisek & Mares, 1991), to tetanus toxin-induced epileptogenesis (Anderson *et al.*, 1997), and to induction and expression of audiogenic seizure susceptibility (Pierson & Swann, 1991) than are adults.

Numerous studies have sought to understand the basis of the exceptional proneness of developing brain to seizures. This is an important question, not only because it may help to identify those transient elements which contribute to developmental seizures, but because it may delineate characteristics which may be abnormally preserved into adulthood in instances of chronic epilepsy. In this charac-

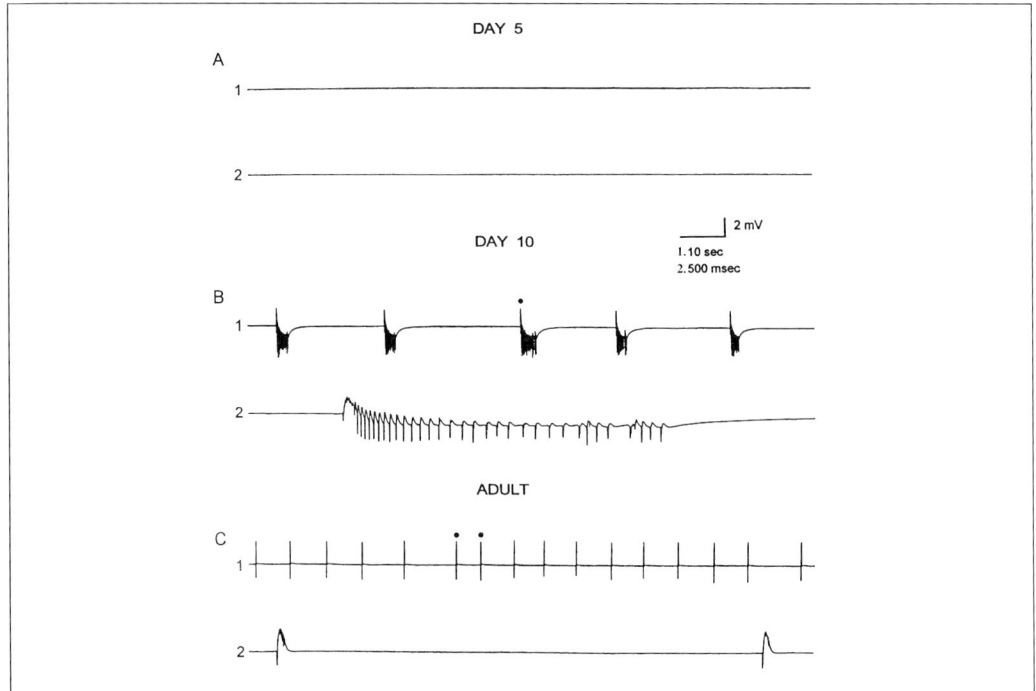

Fig. 1. Age-dependent alterations in epileptiform discharges induced in area CA3 by bath application of picrotoxin (20 μM). In panel A, extracellular field recordings were made from a slice taken on postnatal day 5. Synchronized discharges of the CA3 population were not observed. Panel B: by postnatal day 10, prolonged network-based discharges are readily recorded. Panel C: in adult tissues (PND 43), only brief synchronized discharges are observed. The event marked by dots in traces 1 are shown in traces 2 at a faster time base.

terization of physiology and anatomy of developing brain, two issues have received focussed attention. It has been asked whether there exists inadequate inhibition or excessive excitation during the critical period of vulnerability. Findings regarding these opposing possibilities are reviewed in the following.

Ontogeny of inhibitory synapses

Gamma aminobutyric acid (GABA) is the main inhibitory neurotransmitter in brain and studies have considered whether there exist age-dependent differences, either in GABAergic neurons or in postsynaptic responses. In rat hippocampus, GABAergic interneurons are 'born' relatively early, around embryonic day 12 (E12) (Amaral & Kurz, 1985; Soriano et al., 1989). Although at birth, the activity of glutamic acid decarboxylase (GAD), the synthetic enzyme for GABA, and the corresponding GABA levels are only a fraction of those measured in adult, these biochemical markers of inhibition become substantial after birth (Coyle & Enna, 1976; Swann et al., 1989). Furthermore, the number of synapses with immunoreactivity to antibodies to either GABA or GAD is also less at birth (Kunkel et al., 1966; Seress & Ribak, 1988). In addition, Dupuy & Houser (1996) reported the existence of a transient population of GABAergic neurons in hippocampus of embryos and neonatal rats (e.g. on E17 or PND 0) (see also Rozenberg et al., 1989). Neurons in this population are located in stratum oriens as well as in stratum radiatum. It was demonstrated that axo-dendritic rather than axo-somatic contacts are prevalent. It is probable that some of these GABA interneurons die prior to or in the first week after birth due to a developmental programmed cell death (apoptosis). It is noteworthy that transient cell populations (such as the Cajal–Retzius neurons in the outer marginal zone of neocortex and hippocampus), present only during the first week of rat postnatal life (Del Rio et al., 1995; Jiang & Swann, 1997), have been proposed previously to play a role in guiding brain maturation (Marin-Padilla, 1990; Allendoerfer & Shatz, 1994). Nonetheless, it remains to be explored whether the transient population of GABAergic cells in E17 rats plays a similar role.

Not only are there differences in inhibitory interneurons, but there are differences in postsynaptic responses to GABA in embryonic and neonatal hippocampus and neocortex when compared with those of adult tissue. The GABAa receptor is a heteropentamer which forms a chloride (Cl^-) channel. In mature brain, ligand binding causes Cl^- to rush into the postsynaptic cell (Zhang et al., 1990, 1991; Luhmann & Prince, 1991). However a surprising finding has been that in embryonic and neonatal hippocampus and neocortex, an outward Cl^- transporter appears to remain incompetent until the second postnatal week (Luhmann & Prince, 1991; LoTurco et al., 1995). Because Cl^- concentrations are higher inside cells, immature responses to GABA are actually depolarizing (excitatory) rather than hyperpolarizing until rats become approximately 6–8 days old. Not only does this mean there is a major lack of inhibition, but it confers GABA with the ability to induce low threshold voltage-activated calcium (Ca^{2+}) conductances. In fact, Fura–2 -based Ca^{2+} imaging has shown that both GABA and GABA-mediated synaptic potentials can increase Ca^{2+} intracellularly (Yuste & Katz, 1991; LoTurco et al., 1995; Owens et al., 1996). Taken together, these findings have led to speculation that early in life, GABA may act as a neurotrophic factor (via intracellular signaling). In that capacity, GABA could potentially regulate such diverse processes as neuronal proliferation, migration and differentiation.

So, are any of the above age-dependent differences in inhibition responsible for the pronounced seizure susceptibility that occurs between the ages of day 9 and day 19 in rat? Most likely the answer is negative. All of the above differences occur too early, generally during the embryonic and neonatal periods. And, whereas GABA postsynaptic potentials are depolarizing during the start of the neonatal period, both the Cl^- equilibrium potential and the GABA reversal potential have achieved adult characteristics by the start of the stage of heightened epileptogenicity. Even indirect evidence such as that presented in Fig. 1 suggests GABAergic inhibition is competent to regulate neuronal excitability and to prevent early life seizures. That is, the epileptiform discharges, demonstrated in both panels B and C, occurred only after bath application of the GABAa receptor antagonist, picrotoxin. In short, while epileptiform discharges may be dramatically more severe in brain slices taken during the vulnerable period (panel b), the need for a chemical blockade of constitutive GABAergic inhibition suggests such inhibition is nominally adequate for the prevention of seizure activity in both 10-day-old and adult tissues. Thus, a different hypothesis – one not related to the late onset of synaptic inhibition – must be sought in order to account for the pronounced generation of seizures in developing hippocampus and neocortex.

Ontogeny of excitatory connections within local circuits of hippocampus

The fact that similar sorts of age-dependency occur in intact animals as well as in microdissected pieces of tissue (see Fig. 1, above) indicates several things. First, it suggests that the basis of enhanced vulnerability may reasonably be sought within the local circuit elements and the neuronal connectivity contained within the 300 to 500 μm thick sections of brain that are studied in vitro. Second, data suggest there may be transiently hyperexcitable circuit elements which support the inordinate seizure-like activity during the vulnerable period. And, third, because in vitro brain slice studies of developing brain involve the use of tissues from behaviourally normal (non-epileptic) rats, it may be inferred that phases of excessive epileptogenicity are actually a feature of normal development. The primary issue in studies of immature brain is, therefore, the identification of those transient excitatory characteristics of local circuit anatomy and physiology that are most likely to underlie the propensity for seizures early in life. Thus it is worthwhile to review developmental excitatory characteristics of those tissues which have the capacity to sustain seizure activity. So far, such tissue has been found exclusively to be cortical in nature and to include hippocampus, neocortex, or cortex of the inferior colliculus (in midbrain). Pharmacological studies have revealed that the excitatory synapses which underlie behavioural seizures or epileptiform events (*in vitro*) are glutamatergic in nature. Excitatory amino acid antagonists suppress both the interictal spikes and prolonged electrographic seizures in adult hippocampus, neocortex, and inferior colliculus. In addition, these same agents block the ictal events that are characteristic of both EEGs and *in vitro* recordings made during the period of developmentally enhanced epileptogenesis. (Jones *et al.*, 1984; Brady & Swann, 1986, 1988; Pierson (*et al.*, 1989). Thus, if one wishes to hypothesize that excitation is in some manner excessive in the developing brain, it is toward the glutamatergic excitatory synapses that one's attention turns.

Neuronal networks of both adult neocortex and hippocampus possess recurrent excitatory synapses that have been implicated in seizure generation. Within cortical networks, pyramidal cells not only activate each other, but under ordinary conditions, they also activate inhibitory interneurons which produce powerful feedforward (or recurrent) inhibitory postsynaptic potentials. It is this disynaptic GABAergic inhibition which prevents epileptic discharges under ordinary circumstances. However, this synaptic inhibition also makes it impossible to study the full extent of excitatory interactions among the principal neurons. In order to study the extent of recurrent excitation, it is necessary to block GABA receptors on pyramidal cells using antagonists (Connors, 1984; Miles & Wong, 1987). In one such study, dual intracellular recordings provided a detailed demonstration of such connections in the CA3 subfield of hippocampus (Miles & Wong, 1986). In their report, they showed that action potentials in one pyramidal cell do not usually produce responses in other pyramidal cells. However, when GABAa receptors were suppressed, polysynaptic excitatory postsynaptic potentials (EPSPs) were often produced in other cells. Because each cell now excites many others, there soon occurs a cascade of synaptic excitations until the whole CA3 network becomes involved in a synchronous discharge (Miles & Wong, 1983). Thus, it is the mutuality of excitation, made possible by recurrent excitatory connections, which enables cortical tissues to sustain epileptiform discharges.

Similar neurophysiological studies of local excitatory interactions in developing hippocampus (i.e. in *in vitro* brain slice studies) have suggested differences in the basic physiological properties of recurrent excitation may contribute to the prominent epileptogenicity observed during the early postnatal period in rat. When studied during the second neonatal week, dual intracellular recordings have revealed that a majority (85 per cent) of impaled CA3 pyramidal cells are able to initiate synchronous discharges in the entire CA3 population (Smith *et al.*, 1995). By contrast, in similar studies made of adult tissue, only 28 per cent of cells were found to have this ability (Miles & Wong, 1983). Second, a larger percentage of impaled immature pyramidal cell pairs were found to demonstrate monosynaptic recurrent EPSPs compared to adult pairs (8 per cent vs. 2 per cent). And, third, there are fewer instances of transmission failures between recorded pairs of polysynaptically coupled cells in the immature brain. These observations underscore the importance in the study of developmental epilepsy of achieving an understanding of the anatomy and formation of recurrent excitatory networks during early life.

Three identifiable stages of neuronal development determine patterns of connectivity. First, neurons, under growth cone guidance, extend axons to make synaptic contacts. In this process, initial arbors are unusually exuberant and have projection fields much broader than are characteristic in adult brain. In a second developmental step, many of these provisional synapses undergo a selective regression – a 'pruning' process which leads more closely to the adult pattern of innervation. That is, maturation is not simply an age-dependent increase in the complexity of connectivity. Quite the opposite, pathways are often overexpressed perinatally. A third stage of development involves localized elaborations of axons and synapses (for reviews, see Goodman & Shatz, 1993; O'Leary & Koester, 1993). It has been examined, as shown in Fig. 2, whether these three stages characterize the maturation of axon arbors in hippocampal area CA3. Gomez-DiCesare *et al.* (1997) examined recurrent collateral connectivity by analysis of computer reconstructions of axons from single pyramidal cells filled by intracellular injections of biocytin in 500 μm thick *in vitro* brain slices of rat. Such reconstructions were made of tissues of rats before, during and after the period of enhanced seizure susceptibility (e.g.

Chapter 3 Developmental plasticity in early-life seizures and chronic epilepsy

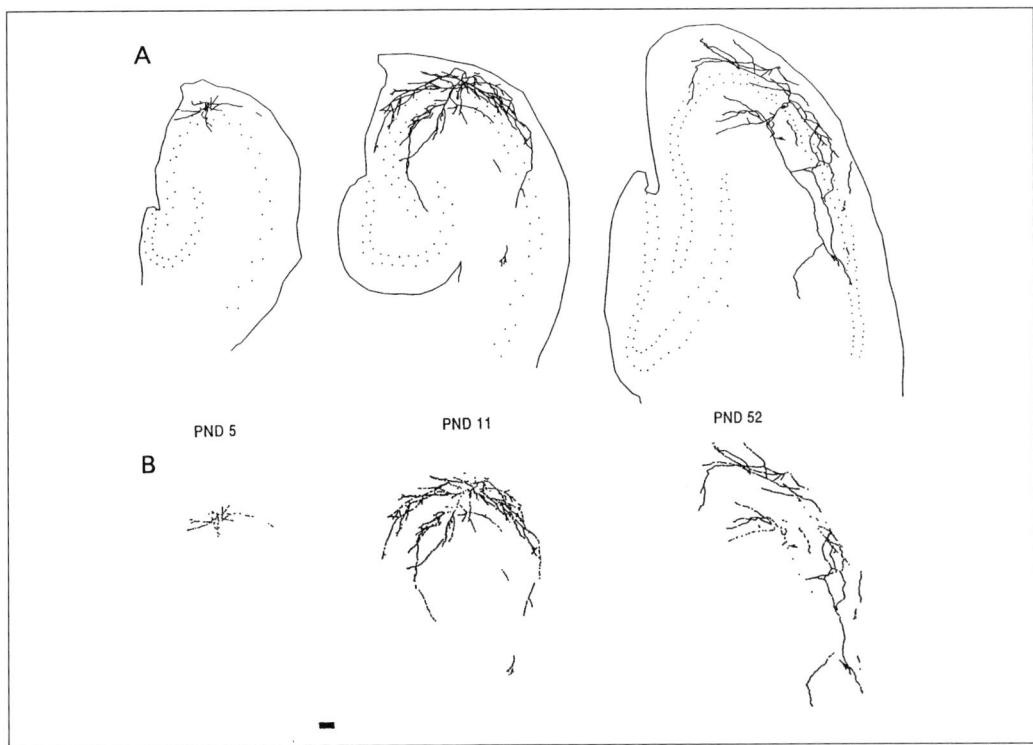

Fig. 2. Comparison of axon arbors arising from three CA3 pyramidal cells that were filled with biocytin at three different postnatal ages (days 5, 11, or 52). Panel A: computer reconstruction of axon arbors; the soma are also represented. The natural surfaces of the slices are indicated by solid lines while the pyramidal and granule cell body layers are denoted by dotted lines. Panel B: the location of varicosities seen along the axon arbors in panel A.. Each varicosity is represented by a dot and each is the likely location of a synaptic contact. Scale = 100 μm.

PND 5 vs. PND 11 vs. PND 52). The results suggest that prior to the critical epileptogenic period, CA3 neurons have few axon collaterals. For example, axons from single cells branch an average of only 9 times. However, by the critical period, there occurs a great increase in the complexity of such arbors. By PND 11 there are approximately 5 to 6 times more branch points. With further maturation (to adulthood), axons appeared to undergo a major simplification; arbors demonstrate only half the number of branch points observed in hippocampi of rats during the second week. However, while it was true that the period of greatest vulnerability to seizures is indeed the period when axons are most branched, it could not be said that this was a period when total axon length or total number of axonal varicosities is greatest [note: varicosities are axonal fibre swellings which have been shown at the ultrastructural level to be sites of synaptic contact (Deitch *et al.*, 1991)]. When the parameters of branching, axon length and synaptic number were measured and corrected for volume increase of hippocampal tissue as a function of age, it was found that the dramatic decrease in axonal branching between postnatal week 2 and adulthood is not accompanied by a complementary decrease in total axon length or total number of varicosities. It is believed that as the hippocampus expands in volume, neurons not only grow, they move away from each other. Under such circumstances, axons must lengthen in order to remain in contact with a given complement of cells. Thus, long simple arbors replace the short branched arbors of immature hippocampus. To maintain the same number of varicosities while branches of axons are being eliminated (along with their early synaptic contacts) would require a relatively late elaboration of new varicosities, presumably on the now lengthening surviving axons. It is clear that one cannot ascribe early life seizure susceptibility to an excess of recurrent excitatory contacts. And while it cannot be ruled out whether an increased density of synapses during the critical period is an important issue, it may be judicious to turn to age-dependent differences in the biophysical properties of early-formed synapses and/or their relative location on dendritic arbors in order to account for the prodigious seizure generation in developing hippocampus. Indeed, numerous studies have shown that EPSPs in immature neocortex and hippocampus are strikingly different from their mature counterparts (Schwartzkroin, 1982; Kriegstein et al., 1987; Burgard & Hablitz, 1993). Not only can such events be unusually large, they are notable for their long durations.

Comparisons of seizure-related events in immature and mature brain is not the only issue of interest in the basic science of developmental epilepsy. Other studies attempt to understand specific brain alterations that follow certain early life events – especially those which result in chronic epilepsy in non-genetic animal models. In such studies, the experimenter provides subjects with an abnormal experience during a critical developmental period. When the animal matures, it exhibits seizure susceptibility or recurrent seizures. Thereupon, the experimenter compares behavioural responses, neurophysiological events and anatomical features in treated and untreated (or sham-treated) litter mates. The goal is to understand the pathogenesis of epilepsy. One common expectation is that epileptic adults will exhibit responses and features of neuronal circuitry which are present in early life. There is a reason for this hypothesis.

As is apparent in Fig. 2, between PNDs 10 and 19, the rat is in a period of dramatic synaptic reorganization. Initially, each pyramidal cell axon begins with a certain complement of synaptic contacts. However, by adulthood the axon not only has fewer branches but it demonstrates a modified array of synaptic swellings. How does this occur? To answer this, we recall what were perhaps the most elegant studies of developmental synaptic plasticity – those involving the formation of ocular dominance columns in brain. Initially eye-specific regions do not exist in layer IV of cat striate cortex. However, with maturation, projection regions become dedicated to one or the other eye. In their first experiments, Hubel and Wiesel found that transiently blinding kittens at birth (before eye-opening) caused cortex to fail to develop an afferent innervation pattern that organizes cortex into eye-specific regions (columns) (Hubel & Wiesel, 1970). Furthermore, if they sutured only one eye shut, the resulting innervation pattern was such that all regions developed a responsiveness primarily to the eye which was initially open (Wiesel & Hubel, 1965). Others later discovered this process was not only 'use'-dependent, but was dependent on use of glutamatergic synapses of the NMDA type. When aminophosphonovalerate (APV), a selective NMDA receptor antagonist, was locally applied (by minipump) to the cortex, ocular dominance columns also failed to form – even when kittens had never been visually deprived (Kleinschmidt et al., 1987). With subsequent experiments, it was discovered that synapse consolidation also required time-correlated activation like that which is most likely to occur in afferents arising from a single eye (Stryker & Strickland, 1984). The above scheme, involving correlated use- and NMDA receptor-dependent synaptic remodelling, has now been shown to apply to the development of projection fields in other sensory systems as well. In each instance, prevention of the selective withdrawal of some of the initial (provisional) synapses leaves target tissues non-specifically innervated – a pattern that is characteristic of immature, but not mature brain.

So what does this have to do with the origins of epilepsy? In fact, it has been specifically demonstrated that prevention of normal afferent remodelling does result in at least one epileptic disorder. Audiogenic seizure (AGS) susceptibility is a reflex epilepsy afflicting murine species and in which seizures are initiated in cortical regions of inferior colliculus (IC), an auditory nucleus in midbrain. In susceptible rodents, exposure to loud, high-frequency sounds triggers tonic/clonic seizures. There are genetic models of this epilepsy, but it can also be experimentally induced by the transient deafening of rats or mice during a critical period of early postnatal development (Pierson & Swann, 1991). At the same time, the auditory deprivation, on or about PND 14, results in a failure of a developmental organization of IC into frequency-specific domains (Snyder-Keller & Pierson, 1992; Pierson & Snyder-Keller,

Chapter 3 Developmental plasticity in early-life seizures and chronic epilepsy

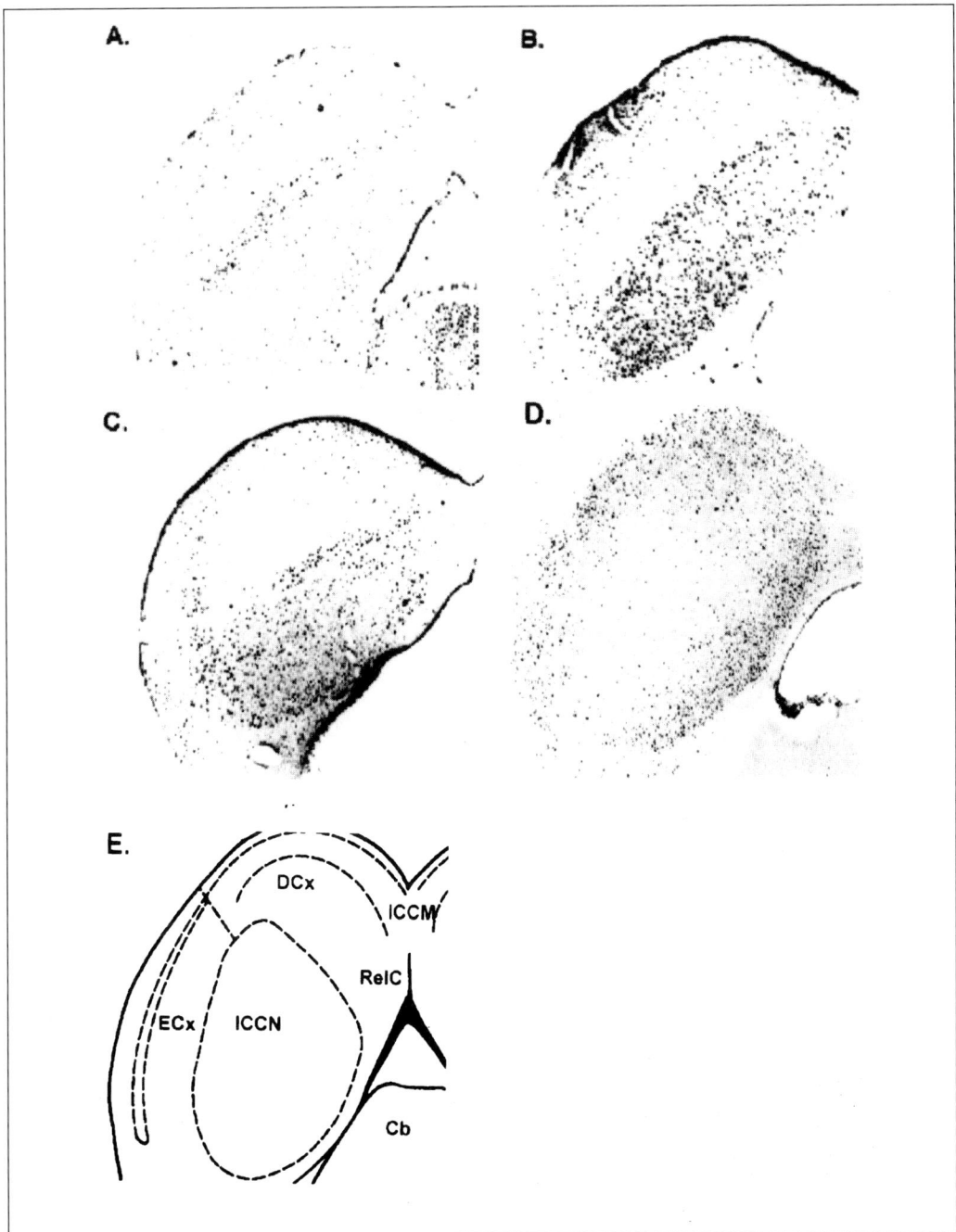

Fig. 3. Comparison of 15 kHz pure tone Fos-immunoreactive responses in inferior colliculus (IC) of: (A) normal adult, (B) AGS susceptible adult, and (C) normal 14-day rat. Panel D shows a cortical Fos-immunoreactive pattern after an audiogenic seizure stimulated by a 10-s exposure to a manually controlled fire-alarm bell. Also shown (E), is a diagram of midbrain anatomy: ICCN = central nucleus of IC; DCx = dorsal cortex of IC; ECx = external cortex of IC; PAG = periaquaductal grey; ICCM + commissure of IC; ReIC + recess of IC; Cb = cerebellum.

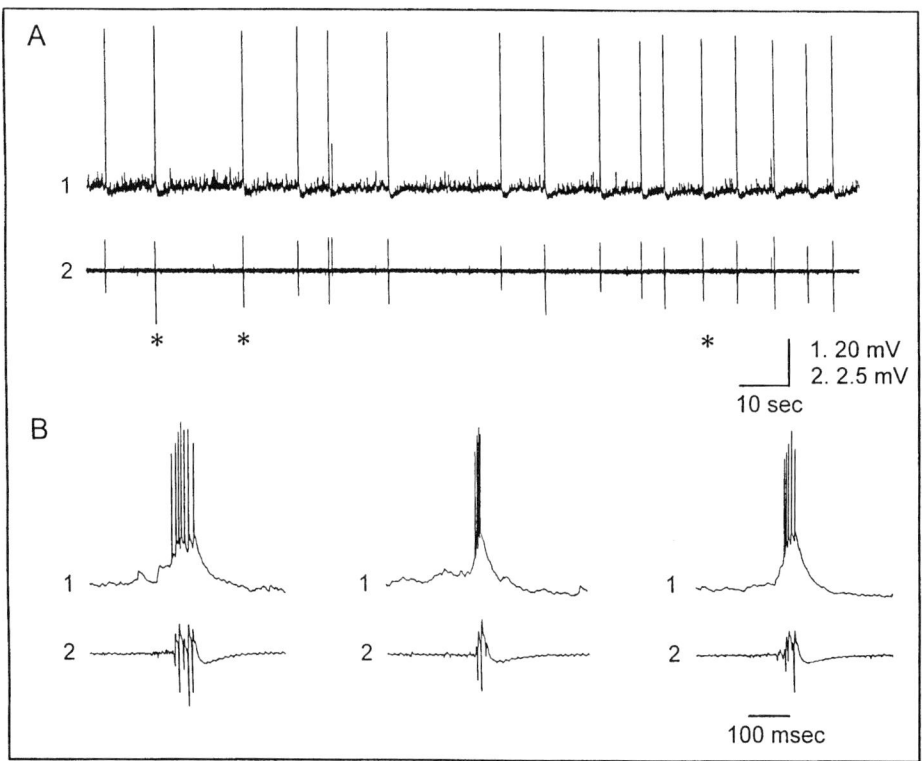

Fig. 4. Interictal discharges recorded in an adult rat hippocampal slice after tetanus toxin injection in infancy. Simultaneous intracellular (1) and extracellular field (2) recordings illustrate spontaneous discharges that occurred in normal artificial cerebrospinal fluid. Selected events (*) in slow-time base recordings in A are expanded in time in B. This slice was taken on postnatal day 55 from hippocampus contralateral to tetanus toxin injection. Recordings were made in area CA_{3C}. Resting potential and input resistance: -58 mV and 32 MΩ.

1994). The effect is specifically correlated with susceptibility. If only one ear is transiently deafened, only the contralateral IC exhibits disorganization during adulthood and, correspondingly, it is only this IC which participates in adult seizures (Pierson et al., 1996). Notably, the pattern of disorganization observed in susceptible ICs is indistinguishable from that present normally in immature rats on PND 14 – the age when sound deprivation is capable of engendering susceptibility. These findings are demonstrated in Fig. 3. Panel A demonstrates the normal band-like response field in IC of an adult rat which was stimulated by a continuous, 85 dB SPL, 15 kHz pure tone for 2 h prior to perfusion. All such responses involve both the central nucleus and the dorsal cortex (DCx) of IC. Panel B shows such response patterns are excessively broad in rats made susceptible to AGSs on PND14. Nonetheless, as shown in panel C, this unsegregated response pattern is normal in PND 14 rats, suggesting a failure of developmental synaptic remodelling. Seizures induce transcription of the c-fos gene in exclusively cortical regions, as shown in panel D. A comparison of puretone-stimulated (A and C), and seizure-stimulated Fos immuno-reactivity (D) indicate that DCx is the area excited in common by these two events. This, in itself, suggests that sound-triggered seizures are initiated in DCx.

For one to use induction of AGS susceptibility as a prototype for what goes on in the pathogenesis of temporal lobe epilepsy, certain differences between epilepsies involving the IC and the hippocampus must be appreciated. In IC the triggering of a seizure is probably due to the giant population EPSP that results from high-frequency stimulation. By contrast, in hippocampus, the feature of immature brain which appears to engender hyperexcitability is the pattern of recurrent innervation among pyramidal cells. Thus, consider the following. How would one go about experimentally promoting an error of development which affected not the long range afferents such as exist in the auditory pathway, but the local innervation that exists between pyramidal cells via recurrent collaterals? Are there developmental experiences which would cause recurrent innervation patterns to persist with their hyperexcitable juvenile features? (After all, one cannot exactly provide the hippocampus with sensory deprivation as was done easily in the instance of the IC, nor would one expect local circuit effects from such a treatment.)

It will be recalled that in studies of visual development, time-correlated use of synapses was found to promote the preservation of, or conversely, to prevent the selective elimination of synapses. If both eyes of kittens were simultaneously and strongly stimulated (using a strobe light), highly correlated activity arose bilaterally and among most visual afferents. The result was just as if both eyes had been sight-deprived; there was a failure of formation of ocular dominance columns. This is notable because if one cannot provide the hippocampus with a transient signal deprivation, it can nonetheless be provided with experiences which involve inordinately time-correlated excitations. That is, seizures themselves involve synchronous activity within a population of neurons, and induced seizures can be imposed transiently during a critical developmental period. The question, then, for epilepsy studies might be: would the correlated activity inherent in juvenile hippocampal seizures result in chronic epilepsy? If so, the anatomical and physiological correlates in the adult epileptic brain could then be assessed in order to understand pathogenesis.

Recently, a model of recurrent postnatal hippocampal seizures was developed using rats (Lee *et al.*, 1995; Smith *et al.*, 1998). Tetanus toxin acts to inactivate synaptobrevin, a docking protein that permits the fusing of GABA-filled synaptic vesicles with presynaptic membranes. It is by this prevention of GABA release that tetanus toxin is thought to produce seizures. When tetanus toxin is stereotaxically injected into the CA3 region of dorsal hippocampus, recurrent, short lasting (approximately 2 min) seizures begin in 2 days and continue for 1 week at a rate of about 1 seizure/h. Typically rat pups so-injected on PND 10 experience multiple seizures which occur between PNDs 12 and 19, the most vulnerable period for epileptogenesis in rat hippocampus. Subsequently, when the rats mature, a time long after the tetanus toxin has been metabolized, it has been found that they exhibit spontaneous seizures. Thus, it is concluded that early life seizures can result in chronic epilepsy.

Tissues from such adults, both the injected and the contralateral hippocampi, have been examined in *in vitro* brain slice preparations along with tissues from sham-injected litter mates. Figure 4 shows that in normal artificial cerebrospinal fluid, brain slices from those adult rats which were neonatally tetanus toxin injected, exhibit spontaneous epileptiform discharges that are typically in the form of interictal discharges. In panel A, a slow time base recording shows the frequency of these epileptiform events. Trace 1 is an intracellular recording from a CA_3 pyramidal cell while trace 2 is an extracellular field recording obtained nearby in the pyramidal cell body layer. Events marked by an asterisk are shown below at a faster time base. Recordings in trace 1 show that individual neurons undergo an intense 'depolarization shift' that is coincident with the synchronous discharging of the CA_3 population observed in Trace 2. Results from detailed mapping of the extracellular field potential suggest these epileptiform discharges arise in the $CA3_C$ subfield.

An even more remarkable finding has been that when slices of epileptic rats were bathed in picrotoxin, a $GABA_A$ receptor antagonist, they sustained prolonged electrographic seizures as shown in Fig. 5. As noted previously (see Fig. 1), brain slices from normal adults typically exhibit only interictal bursts when exposed to $GABA_A$ receptor antagonist. Control traces in Fig. 5 are an illustration of this type of discharge recorded in a slice from a sham-injected control rat. However, in experimental adult rats that had recurrent seizures in infancy, blockade of the $GABA_A$ receptor leads to prolonged electrographic seizures which can be seen in the upper traces of Fig. 5A and 5B. Panel C compares the maximum duration of epileptiform discharges recorded in 12 slices taken from control rats and 23

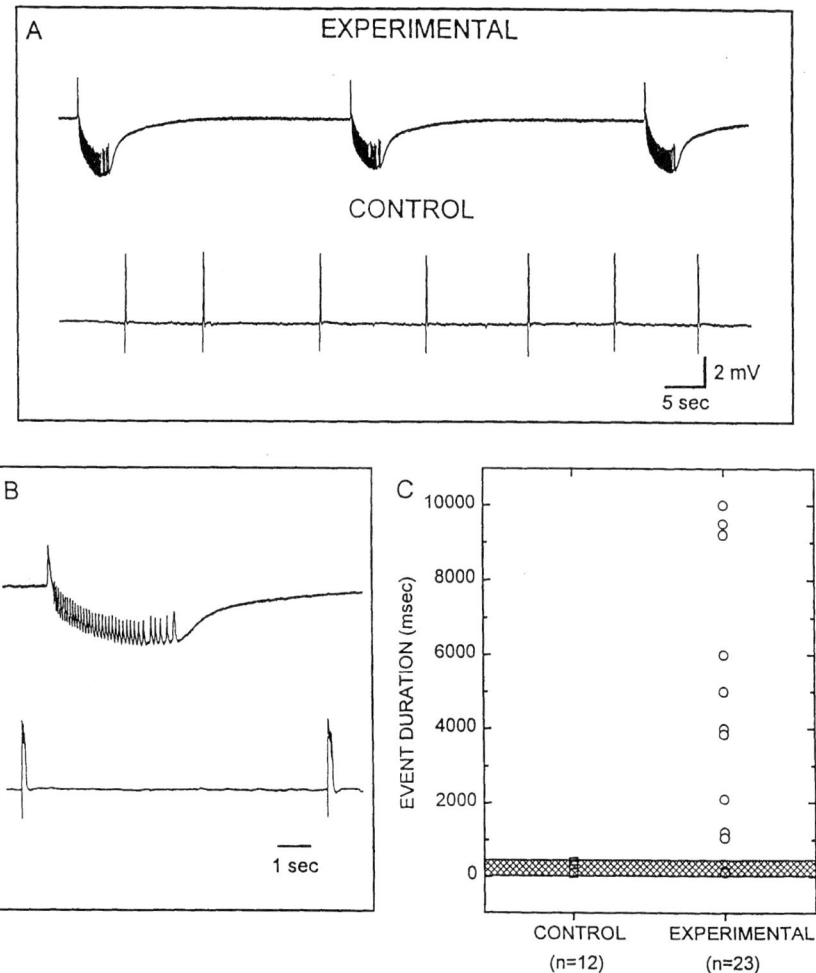

Fig. 5. *Comparison of epileptiform discharging produced by picrotoxin in slices from experimental and control rats. (A) Slow-time base extracellular field recordings during bath application of picrotoxin (20 µM). (B) Representative events at a faster time base. Although slices from control rat (day 64) produced brief burst discharges, slices from experimental rat (day 46) underwent prolonged afterdischarges. In scatter diagram (C), duration of longest epileptiform discharges recorded in 12 and 23 slices taken from six control and eight experimental rats, respectively, is plotted. Hatched area shows range of durations recorded in slices from control rats.*

slices from experimental rats. Discharges were considerably more prolonged in the epileptic rats than in slices from their controls.

Because brain slices of neonatally tetanus toxin injected adult rats appear to be as hyperexcitable as juvenile tissues, studies of anatomical alterations in the hippocampi of these epileptic adults will be of great interest as they become available. It seems plausible that ongoing seizure activity during development may alter the normal remodelling of recurrent excitatory collaterals. A hyperinnervation network involving CA3 hippocampal pyramidal cells may underlie seizures in this chronic model of early onset epilepsy.

Summary and discussion

It is appreciated, both behaviourally and physiologically at the local circuit level, that in rodents (as in humans) there is a narrow developmental window of extreme vulnerability to epileptic events. This pivotal observation has fueled the study of developmental epilepsy in non-genetic models. Two main approaches have been taken. The first has been phenomenological in nature. Studies have addressed and compared the hyperexcitable properties, behavioural seizures, and neuroanatomical features of brains of young *vs* old rodents. The second, newer wave of studies has concerned the development of chronic epilepsy in animals without genetic predisposition. In such studies young rodents are: (1) experimentally induced to become susceptible, (2) are allowed to grow up, (3) confirmed as adults to exhibit behavioural or electroencephalographic evidence of epilepsy, and then (4) neurophysiologically and neuroanatomically compared to untreated or sham-treated litter mates in order to determine pathogenic alterations. In a sense, the first type of study asks 'which brain differences are likely to account for the seizure propensity of all young animals?'. The second studies ask 'what kind of brain differences correspond to pathogenesis in epilepsies with experimental and developmental origins?'. Address of each of these sets of questions has begun with specific hypotheses as discussed below.

It has been asked whether GABAergic inhibition is inadequate during the juvenile period of pronounced seizure susceptibility. And indeed, it has been found that hyperpolarizing responses to GABA are not present until about 1 week after birth in rat due to an immature Cl^- transport in hippocampal neurons. It has also been found that there are unique, transient populations of GABAergic neurons in developing hippocampus. Nonetheless, by day 10, when the vulnerable period begins, GABA responses are both vigorous and hyperpolarizing and the transient GAD-immunoreactive population of neurons has vanished. Thus, at present there is no reason to believe that the seizure proneness of ordinary PND 10 to PND 19 rats depends on any sort of relative immaturity of inhibitory systems. It has also been asked whether an excess of excitatory connectivity or a difference in excitatory responses might underlie the pronounced juvenile epileptogenicity. In experiments aimed at these possibilities, it has been found that the morphological remodelling of pyramidal cell axons in hippocampus, whereby nearly 50 per cent of branches of axonal arbors are lost, corresponding to the decrease in seizure susceptibility that is seen by puberty. Conversely, it is during the period of exuberant developmental outgrowth of these recurrent excitatory axon collaterals that seizures become pronounced. Thus, it appears that hyperexcitability of excitatory connectivity may well be the basis of the window of enhanced epileptogenicity during postnatal development in rat.

It has been tested whether the pathogenesis of epilepsy involves, in some manner, the preservation of an immature, inherently epileptogenic form of connectivity in brain. Not only is developmental remodelling of axonal arbors a common feature in most areas of the central nervous system, but results from an audiogenic seizure model of early onset epilepsy suggest that prevention of such remodelling (due to transient sensory deprivation) may leave the animal in a permanently immature state characterized by an overinnervation of target nuclei. Importantly, what arises at the same time is a chronic susceptibility to sound-triggered seizures. When it was recently examined whether site-specific interruption of use-dependent remodelling similarly induced epileptic pathogenesis in hippocampus, it was found that the outcome was similar. Repeated seizures, induced by a single tetanus toxin injection into the CA3 region of hippocampus of PND 10 rat, induce chronic temporal lobe epilepsy. Further studies are needed in order to demonstrate whether the overly synchronized activity inherent in early-life seizures prevents the normal developmental remodelling of neuronal connectivity in postnatal hippocampus. It may well be that some temporal lobe epilepsies are due to hyperinnervated networks that leave hippocampi chronically hyperexcitable.

Acknowledgements: Work in our laboratories was supported by grants from NINDS NS18309, NS11535 (J. Swann) and NS34504 (M. Pierson).

References

Albala, B.J., Moshé, S.L. & Okada, R. (1984): Kainic acid induced seizures: A developmental study. *Dev. Brain Res.* **13**, 139–148.

Allendoerfer, K.L. & Shatz, C.J. (1994): The subplate transient neocortical structure: Its role in the development of connections between thalamus and cortex. *Annu. Rev. Neurosci.* **17**, 185–218.

Amaral, D.G. & Kurz, J. (1985): The time of origin of cells demonstrating glutamic acid decarboxylase-like immunoreactivity in the hippocampal formation of the rat. *Neurosci. Lett.* **59**, 33–39.

Anderson, A.E., Hrachovy, R.A. & Swann, J.W. (1997): Increased susceptibility to tetanus toxin-induced seizures in immature rats. *Epilepsy Res.* **26**, 433–442.

Brady, R.J. & Swann, J.W. (1986): Ketamine selectively suppresses synchronized afterdischarges in immature hippocampus. *Neurosci. Lett.* **69**, 143–149.

Brady, R.J. & Swann, J.W. (1988): Suppression of ictal-like activity by kynurenic acid does not correlate with its efficacy as an NMDA receptor antagonist. *Epilepsy Res.* **2**, 232–238.

Burgard, E.C. & Hablitz, J.J. (1993): Developmental changes in NMDA and non-NMDA receptor-mediated synaptic potentials in rat neocortex. *J. Neurophysiol.* **69**, 230–240.

Cavalheiro, E.A., Silva, D.F., Turski, W.A., Calderazzo-Filho, L.S., Bortolotto, Z.A. & Turski, L. (1987): The susceptibility of rats to pilocarpine-induced seizures is age-dependent. *Dev. Brain Res.* **37**, 43–58.

Connors, B.W. (1984): Initiation of synchronized neuronal bursting in neocortex. *Nature* **310**, 685–687.

Coyle, J.T. & Enna, S.J. (1976): Neurochemical aspects of the ontogenesis of GABAnergic neurons in the rat brain. *Brain Res.* **111**, 119–133.

Deitch, J.S., Smith, K.L., Swann, J.W. & Turner, J.N. (1991): Ultrastructural investigation of neurons identified and localized using the confocal scanning laser microscope. *J. Electron Microsc. Techn.* **18**, 82–90.

Del Rio, J.A., Martinez, A., Fonseca, M., Auladell, C. & Soriano, E. (1995): Glutamate-like immunoreactivity and fate of Cajal–Retzius cells in the murine cortex as identified with calretinin antibody. *Cerebral Cortex* **1**, 13–21.

Dupuy, S.T. & Houser, C.R. (1996): Prominent expression of two forms of glutamate decarboxylase in the embryonic and early postnatal rat hippocampal formation. *J. Neurosci.* **16**, 6919–6932.

Gomez-DiCesare, C.M., Smith, K.L., Rice, F. & Swann, J. (1997): Axonal remodeling during postnatal maturation of CA_3 hippocampal pyramidal neurons. *J. Comp. Neurol.* **384**, 165–180.

Goodman, C.S. & Shatz, C.J. (1993): Developmental mechanisms that generate precise patterns of neuronal activity. *Cell* **10**, 77–98.

Haas, K.Z., Sperber, E.F. & Moshé, S.L. (1990): Kindling in developing animals: expression of severe seizures and enhanced development of bilateral foci. *Dev. Brain Res.* **56**, 275–280.

Hablitz, J.J. (1987): Spontaneous ictal-like discharges and sustained depolarization shifts in the developing rat neocortex. *Neurophysiology* **58**, 1052–1065.

Hamon, B. & Heinemann, U. (1988): Developmental changes in neuronal sensitivity to excitatory amino acids in area CA1 of the rat hippocampus. *Brain Res.* **466**, 286–290.

Hubel, D.H. & Wiesel, T.N. (1970): The period of susceptibility to the physiological effects of unilateral eye closure in kittens. *J. Physiol.* **206**, 419–436.

Jiang, M. & Swann, J. (1997): Expression of calretinin in diverse neuronal populations during development of rat hippocampus. *Neuroscience* **81**, 1137–1154.

Jones, A.W., Croucher, M.J., Meldrum, B.S. & Watkins, J.C. (1984): Suppression of audiogenic seizures in DBA/2 mice by two new dipeptide NMDA receptor antagonists. *Neurosci. Lett.* **45**, 157–161.

Kleinschmidt, A., Bear, M.F. & Singer, W. (1987): Blockade of 'NMDA' receptors disrupts experience-dependent plasticity of kitten striate cortex. *Science* **238**, 355–358.

Kriegstein, A.R., Suppes, T. & Prince, D.A. (1987): Cellular and synaptic physiology and epileptogenesis of developing rat neocortical neurons *in vitro*. *Dev. Brain Res.* **34**, 161–171.

Kunkel, D.D., Hendrickson, A.E., Wu, J. & Schwartzkroin, A. (1966): Glutamic acid decarboxylase (GAD) immunocytochemistry of developing rabbit hippocampus. *J. Neurosci.* **6**, 541–552.

Lee, C.L., Hrachovy, R.A., Smith, K.L., Frost Jr., J.D. & Swann, J.W. (1995): Tetanus toxin-induced seizures in infant rats and their effects on hippocampal excitability in adulthood. *Brain Res.* **677**, 97–109.

LoTurco, J.J., Owens, D.F., Heath, M.J.S., Davis, M.B.E. & Kriegstein, A.R. (1995): GABA and glutamate depolarize cortical progenitor cells and inhibit DNA synthesis. *Neuron* **15**, 1287–1298.

Luhmann, H.J. & Prince, D.A. (1991): Postnatal maturation of the GABAergic system in rat neocortex. *J. Neurophysiol.* **65**, 247–263.

Mares, P. (1973): Ontogenetic development of bioelectrical activity of the epileptogenic focus in rat neocortex. *Neuropadiatrie* **4**, 434–445.

Marin-Padilla, M. (1990): Three-dimensional structural organization of layer I of the human cerebral cortex: A Golgi study. *J. Comp. Neurol.* **299**, 89–105.

Michelson, H. & Lothman, E. (1991): An ontogenetic study of kindling using rapidly recurring hippocampal seizures. *Dev. Brain Res.* **61**, 79–85.

Miles, R. & Wong, R.K.S. (1983): Single neurones can initiate synchronized population discharge in the hippocampus. *Nature* **306**, 371–373.

Miles, R. & Wong, R.K.S. (1986): Excitatory synaptic interactions between CA3 neurones in the guinea-pig hippocampus. *J. Physiol. (Lond.)* **373**, 397–418.

Miles, R. & Wong, R.K.S. (1987): Inhibitory control of local excitatory circuits in the guinea-pig hippocampus. *J. Physiol. (Lond.)* **388**, 611–629.

Moshé, S.L. (1981): The effects of age on the kindling phenomenon. *Dev. Psychobiol.* **14**, 75–81.

O'Leary, D.D.M. & Koester, S.E. (1993): Development of projection neuron types, axon pathways, and patterned connections of the mammalian cortex. *Neuron* **10**, 991–1006.

Owens, D.F., Boyce, L.H., Davis, M.B.E. & Kriegstein, A.R. (1996): Excitatory GABA responses in embryonic and neonatal cortical slices demonstrated by gramicidin perforated-patch recordings and calcium imaging. *J. Neurosci.* **16**, 6414–6423.

Pierson, M. & Snyder-Keller, A. (1994): Development of frequency-selective domains in inferior colliculus of normal and neonatally noise-exposed rats. *Brain Res.* **636**, 55–67.

Pierson, M., Snyder-Keller, A. & Kwon, J. (1996): Abnormal frequency-selective domains in inferior colliculus of audiogenic seizure susceptible rats. *Epilepsy Res.* **12**, 101–109.

Pierson, M.G. & Swann, J.W. (1991): Ontogenetic features of audiogenic seizure susceptibility induced in immature rats by noise. *Epilepsia* **32**, 1–9.

Pierson, M.G., Smith, K.L. & Swann, J.W. (1989): A slow NMDA-mediated synaptic potential underlies seizures originating from midbrain. *Brain Res.* **486**, 381–386.

Rozenberg, F., Robain, O., Jardin, L. & Ben-Ari, Y. (1989): Distribution of GABAergic neurons in late fetal and early postnatal rat hippocampus. *Dev. Brain Res.* **50**, 177–187.

Schwartzkroin, P.A. (1982): Development of rabbit hippocampus: Physiology. *Dev. Brain Res.* **2**, 469–486.

Schwartzkroin, P.A. (1984): Epileptogenesis in the immature CNS. In: *Electrophysiology of epilepsy*, Schwartzkroin, P.A. and Wheal, H.V. (eds), pp. 389–412. London: Academic Press.

Seress, L. & Ribak, C.E. (1988): The development of GABAergic neurons in the rat hippocampal formation. An immunocytochemical study. *Dev. Brain Res.* **44**, 197–209.

Smith, K.L., Szarowski, D.H., Turner, J.N. & Swann, J.W. (1995): Diverse neuronal populations mediate local circuit excitation in area CA3 of developing hippocampus. *J. Neurophysiol.* **74**, 650–672.

Smith, K.L., Lee, C.L. & Swann, J.S. (1998): Local circuit abnormalities in chronically epileptic rats after intrahippocampal tetanus toxin injection in infancy. *J. Neurophysiol.* **79**, 106–116.

Snyder-Keller, A. & Pierson, M. (1992): Audiogenic seizures induce *c-fos* in model of developmental epilepsy. *Neurosci. Lett.* **135**, 108–112.

Soriano, E., Cobas, A. & Fairen, A. (1989): Neurogenesis of glutamic acid decarboxylase immunoreactive cells in the hippocampus of the mouse. I: Regio superior and regio inferior. *J. Comp. Neurol.* **281**, 586–602.

Stryker, M.P. & Strickland, S.L. (1984): Physiological segregation of ocular dominance columns depends on the pattern of afferent electrical activity. *Invest. Opthalmol. Vis. Sci.* **25** (Suppl.), 278.

Swann, J.W. & Brady, R.J. (1984): Penicillin-induced epileptogenesis in immature rat CA3 hippocampal pyramidal cells. *Dev. Brain Res.* **12**, 243–254.

Swann, J.W., Brady, R.J. & Martin, D. (1989): Postnatal development of GABA-mediated synaptic inhibition in rat hippocampus. *Neuroscience* **28**, 551–561.

Tremblay, E., Nitecka, L., Berger, M.L. & Ben-Ari, Y. (1984): Maturation of kainic acid seizure-brain damage syndrome in the rat. I. Clinical electrographic and metabolic observations. *Neuroscience* **13**, 1051–1072.

Velisek, L. & Mares, P. (1991): Increased epileptogenesis in the immature hippocampus. *Exp. Brain Res. Series* **20**, 183–185.

Wiesel, T.N. & Hubel, D.H. (1965): Comparison of the effects of unilateral and bilateral eye closure on cortical unit responses in kittens. *J. Neurophysiol.* **28**, 1029–1040.

Woodbury, L.A. (1977): Incidence and prevalence of seizure disorders including the epilepsies in the U.S.A. A review and analysis of the literature. In: *Anonymous plan for the nationwide action on epilepsy*, pp. 24–77. DEW Publication No. (NH) 78–276, Volume IV.

Yuste, R. & Katz, L.C. (1991): Control of postsynaptic Ca^{2+} influx in developing neocortex by excitatory and inhibitory neurotransmitters. *Neuron* **6**, 333–344.

Zhang, L., Spigelman, I. & Carlen, P.L. (1990): Whole-cell patch study of GABAergic inhibition in CA1 neurons of immature rat hippocampal slices. *Dev. Brain Res.* **56**, 127–130.

Zhang, L., Spigelman, I. & Carlen, P.L. (1991): Development of GABA-mediated, chloride-dependent inhibition in CA1 pyramidal neurones of immature rat hippocampal slices. *J. Physiol. (Lond.)* **444**, 25–49.

Chapter 4

Age-related mechanisms involved in the control of seizures

Jana Velíšková

Department of Neurology, Albert Einstein College of Medicine, Bronx, NY, USA

Summary

Steroid hormones play an important role in seizure susceptibility. Hormones influence maturation of the brain. During embryonic and early postnatal development, gonadal hormones can induce the differentiation of discrete brain regions. Substantia nigra pars reticulata (SNR) plays a critical role in the control of seizures and changes its features during development.

Our recent studies in adult male rats revealed that there are two distinct $GABA_A$-sensitive regions within the SNR, which mediate opposite effects on flurothyl seizures. Thus, muscimol infused into the anterior region of the SNR ($SNR_{anterior}$) mediates anticonvulsant effects while similar infusions into the posterior region of the SNR ($SNR_{posterior}$) mediate proconvulsant effects. These two regions differ morphologically and involve different efferent networks. In contrast, in PN (postnatal day) 15 rats, there is no such differentiation. At this age, muscimol infusions have only proconvulsant effects. The SNR efferent network in PN 15 rats seems to utilize similar structures as the adult $SNR_{posterior}$ network.

The development of $SNR_{anterior}$ and $SNR_{posterior}$ follows different patterns. The $SNR_{anterior}$ starts to differentiate around PN 25 and emerges with its 'anticonvulsant' features between PN 25 and 30. In male rats, there is a sudden drop in testosterone levels between PN 20 and 25 just prior to the age when the $SNR_{anterior}$ assumes its anticonvulsant features. This observation raises the possibility that the maturation of the $SNR_{anterior}$ may be under the influence of postnatal testosterone. Studies in neonatal castrated male rats indicate that testosterone depletion accelerates the development of the $SNR_{anterior}$ with its 'anticonvulsant' features following muscimol infusions. The $SNR_{posterior}$ with its 'proconvulsant' features is already functional by PN 15; its effects remain proconvulsant throughout the maturation process. Neonatal castration does not alter the development of the $SNR_{posterior}$. Thus, speculation exists that prenatal testosterone may influence the development of the $SNR_{posterior}$. Our experiments in female rats, which do not have the prenatal testosterone surge, support our hypothesis. There is only one region within the female SNR, which mediates the anticonvulsant effects of muscimol already at PN 25. The 'proconvulsant' SNR region could not be demonstrated.

Better knowledge of hormonal effects on brain development and neuronal activity may have significant influence on future therapy of age-dependent epilepsy syndromes and especially for use of hormonal treatments.

The substantia nigra (SN) was first described by Vicq d'Azyr in 1786 (Vicq d'Azyr, 1786). Initial studies concerning the function of the SN discovered its key role in the extrapyramidal control of movements (Tretiakof, 1919). As a major output station of the basal ganglia, the SN coordinates motor functions and may also be involved in seizure control (Hayashi, 1952, 1953; Iadarola & Gale, 1982).

The SN has two major parts: pars reticulata (SNR) and pars compacta (SNC). The SNR is involved in the control of seizures via its GABAergic (γ-aminobutyric acid) neurotransmission (Depaulis *et al.*, 1988, 1989, 1990b; Gale, 1985; Iadarola & Gale, 1982; Löscher & Schwark, 1985; McNamara *et al.*, 1983, 1984; Moshé & Sperber, 1990) especially through $GABA_A$ receptors. The SNC is rich in dopaminergic neurons. There are reports suggesting that SNC may be also involved in seizure control (De Sarro *et al.*, 1986, 1991; Fariello *et al.*, 1987; Turski *et al.*, 1988, 1990). However, the data about its role in propagation of seizures are discordant and will be discussed later in this chapter.

In this chapter I will describe the effects of SNR infusions of $GABA_A$ergic agents on flurothyl seizures in adult and in developing male rats as well as in neonatally castrated male rats. Finally, I will describe preliminary data on the role of the SNR in the control of seizures in female rats.

Our data suggest that microinfusions of $GABA_A$ergic drugs in the SNR have region-, age- and gender-specific effects on flurothyl-induced seizures (Moshé & Albala, 1984; Moshé *et al.*, 1994; Sperber *et al.*, 1987; Velíšková *et al.*, 1996; Xu *et al.*, 1992).

For studying the involvement of the $GABA_A$ system in the SNR in seizure control, we originally used muscimol, an agonist of the low- and high-affinity $GABA_A$ receptor sites (Bartholini *et al.*, 1985; Meldrum, 1981). In further studies, we used bicuculline, an antagonist of the low-affinity $GABA_A$ receptor site (Heyer *et al.*, 1981), ZAPA (Z)–3-[(aminoiminomethyl)thio]prop–2-enoic acid, an agonist of the low-affinity $GABA_A$ receptor site (Allan *et al.*, 1991) and THIP (4,5,6,7-tetrahydroisoxazolo[5,4-c]pyridin–3-ol) (Krogsgaard-Larsen, 1984), an agonist of the high-affinity $GABA_A$ receptor site. The drugs were infused bilaterally in the SNR. There was a special requirement that both cannulae were placed symmetrically into the anterior or posterior part of the SNR. Rats with unilateral SNR microinfusions or asymmetric placements were excluded. The drugs were infused via the implanted cannulae over a 2 min interval using Hamilton microsyringes and an infusion pump, and the volume was 0.25 μl per SNR. For site-specificity of the effects we examined rats with infusions dorsal to the SNR. In this group of animals, the drug infusions did not alter the threshold to flurothyl seizures.

The flurothyl seizure model

Flurothyl is a volatile convulsant agent established as an effective tool to measure the brain's threshold to primary generalized seizures (Fang *et al.*, 1997; Prichard *et al.*, 1969). The real mechanism of how flurothyl produces seizures is unknown. Flurothyl appears to act by primary action on the protein and lipid layers of the synaptic membrane. It can act either presynaptically and influence the release of a neurotransmitter or postsynaptically by influencing ionic fluxes (Schuck & Shulman, 1971). There is also indirect evidence that the GABAergic system, especially inhibition of GABA synthesis, may be involved in its presynaptic action (Bowdler and Green, 1982; Green *et al.*, 1987a, b). The procedure used for flurothyl eliminates the stress of the injection associated with other systemic convulsants.

Flurothyl produces two sequential types of seizures: *clonic seizures* consisting of facial and forelimb clonus (with or without tonic forelimb flexion) with preservation of the righting reflex, followed by *tonic–clonic seizures* consisting of loss of righting reflex, tonic flexion or extension of all four limbs followed by long clonus of all four limbs (Velíšek *et al.*, 1995). For seizure testing, the rats are challenged with flurothyl at a constant flow rate (20 μl/min) in an air-tight chamber (9.38 l) until tonic–clonic seizures occur. We record the latency to the onset of a first clonic and a first tonic–clonic seizure. Because flurothyl is infused at a constant rate, the latency to the onset of seizures allows us to calculate the amount of infused flurothyl necessary to elicit the seizure and thus determine the flurothyl seizure threshold for our chamber size. Eventually, it is possible to calculate threshold amounts of inhaled flurothyl for individual types of seizures (Lánský *et al.*, 1997).

The flurothyl seizure manifestations have age-specific behavioural patterns (Franck *et al.*, 1989; Sperber & Moshé, 1988). Rats on postnatal day 25 (PN) and younger, experience just one episode of a clonic seizure followed shortly after by a tonic–clonic seizure. In these age groups, the clonic seizure does not contain the initial tonic extension seen in older rats. The interval between clonic and tonic–clonic seizures increases with age. In PN 15 rats, seizures consist of one short episode of a clonic seizure, which progresses almost instantly into a tonic–clonic seizure. In PN 21 and PN 25 rats, the clonic seizure is clearly separated from the tonic–clonic seizure. The PN 30 and 35 rats have already the 'adult like' seizure pattern. The rats at this age as well as adult rats experience several episodes of clonic seizures, which usually start with tonic extension of forelimbs and are finally followed by the tonic–clonic seizure (Veliškova et al., unpublished observations).

Region-specific effects of microinfusions of GABA$_A$ergic agents in the SNR of adult male rats

In the adult male rat SNR, there are two GABA$_A$ sensitive, topographically distinct functional regions located in the anterior and posterior SNR (SNR$_{anterior}$ and SNR$_{posterior}$, respectively) (Moshé et al., 1994; Velíšková et al., 1996). These two SNR regions mediate differential effects of infused GABA$_A$ergic drugs on clonic flurothyl seizures. In contrast, the tonic–clonic seizures are not affected by the GABA$_A$ergic drug infusions. Initially, we microinfused 100 ng of muscimol (in 0.25 µl saline) or saline symmetrically into both nigral regions to determine site-specific effects on seizures. In the SNR$_{anterior}$, bilateral microinfusions of muscimol have anticonvulsant effects, while in the SNR$_{posterior}$, muscimol microinfusions have proconvulsant effects. Furthermore, to determine which of the GABA$_A$ receptor sites are involved in the control of seizures, we infused specific antagonists and agonists of the low- and high-affinity GABA$_A$ receptor sites in the two SNR regions (Table 1).

Table 1. Region- and age-specific effects of GABAergic drug infusions in the SNR

	Adult rats		Postnatal day 15 rats
	SNR$_{anterior}$	SNR$_{posterior}$	SNR$_{anterior}$ or SNR$_{posterior}$
Muscimol	Anticonvulsant	Proconvulsant	Proconvulsant
Bicuculline	Proconvulsant	No effect	Proconvulsant
ZAPA	Anticonvulsant	Proconvulsant	Biphasic effect
THIP	Anticonvulsant	Not available	Proconvulsant

Microinfusions of bicuculline, ZAPA and THIP influence the seizure threshold in a region-specific manner. In the SNR$_{anterior}$, bicuculline (an antagonist of low-affinity GABA$_A$ receptor sites) has proconvulsant effect, i.e. opposite to the effect of muscimol (an agonist of both high- and low- affinity GABA$_A$ receptor sites) (Velíšková et al., 1996). The effects of ZAPA (an agonist of low-affinity GABA$_A$ receptor sites) and THIP (an agonist of high-affinity GABA$_A$ receptor sites) are in the opposite direction from the bicuculline effects, as ZAPA and THIP have anticonvulsant effects (Velíšková et al., 1996). We thus propose that, in adult male rats, GABAmimetic stimulation of the SNR$_{anterior}$ induces anticonvulsant effects in the flurothyl seizure model by activating both high- and low-affinity GABA$_A$ receptors (Velíšková et al., 1996).

However in the SNR$_{posterior}$, the effects of ZAPA and bicuculline on seizures are not in the opposite direction. Bicuculline does not alter the seizure threshold while ZAPA is proconvulsant (Velíšková et al., 1996). The effect of ZAPA in this region may be direct via its weak action on high-affinity GABA$_A$ receptors or by competing with endogenous GABA for transport (Allan et al., 1991), thus enhancing GABA concentration in the synaptic cleft. Thus, the incongruent effects of ZAPA and bicuculline infusions suggest that there may be a differential distribution of low-affinity GABA$_A$ receptors along the SNR. Low-affinity GABA$_A$ receptors may be absent or not functional in the SNR$_{posterior}$. Therefore, the influence of the SNR$_{posterior}$ on flurothyl seizures may be via its high-affinity GABA$_A$ receptors (Velíšková et al., 1996). However, infusions of GABA$_A$ receptor agonists in the SNR$_{posterior}$ produce proconvulsant effect, suggesting that the high-affinity GABA$_A$ receptors may be heterogeneous in the two SNR regions (GABA$_A$ receptor heterogeneity).

In mammals, central $GABA_A$ receptors are a heterogeneous family of related proteins comprising several subunits (α1–6, β1–4, γ1–3, δE, and probably ρ1–2) (Lüddens et al., 1995). Studies using patch-clamp techniques show different functional properties of $GABA_A$ receptors depending on the subunit composition (Saxena & MacDonald, 1996; Sigel et al., 1990; Verdoorn et al., 1990; Wafford et al., 1992). It is therefore likely that neuronal responsiveness to GABAergic input is influenced by differential expression of various subunit genes (Levitan et al., 1988a, b). In situ hybridization and immunohistochemistry studies have revealed that the different subunits have a characteristic topographic distribution in the brain (Araki & Tohyama, 1992; Dunn et al., 1994; Wisden et al., 1989, 1992). Using in situ histochemistry, we have demonstrated that in adult male rats, the two SNR functional regions differ in the distribution of the $GABA_A$ receptor α1 subunit mRNA (Moshé et al., 1994), which is the most abundant $GABA_A$ receptor subunit in the adult SNR (Wisden et al., 1992). Optical density measurements of film autoradiograms revealed the highest optical density in the $SNR_{posterior}$ (Moshé et al., 1994). However, these data should be interpreted with caution. The higher optical density on film autoradiograms may not represent the real number of mRNA per cell but rather the amount of cells in that particular region. Anatomical studies suggest that the $SNR_{anterior}$ contains fewer cells than the $SNR_{posterior}$. For example, at the cellular level we found that in the $SNR_{anterior}$, there are spare large clusters of labelled cells with high expression of hybridization grains. In the $SNR_{posterior}$, there is a high density of labelled cells, which have, however, moderate expression of the α1 hybridization grains (Velíšková et al., 1998).

The different effects of $GABA_A$ergic agonists in the two SNR regions may also be the result of divergent SNR output pathways involved in these effects. The GABAergic manipulation can affect all four major outputs of the SN: striatum, thalamus, tectal and tegmental areas.

Although the nigrostriatal pathway is dopaminergic, the GABAergic projection neurons of the SNR are mediators of the disinhibition of the nigrostriatal dopaminergic neurons (Grace & Bunney, 1979; Tepper et al., 1995). The GABAergic axon terminals are in direct synaptic contact with cell bodies and dendrites of dopaminergic neurons in the SNC (Tepper et al., 1995; van den Pol et al., 1985). There are several studies using microinfusions in the SNC suggesting that the nigrostriatal pathway may be involved in the control of seizures (De Sarro et al., 1986, 1991; Fariello et al., 1987; Turski et al., 1988, 1990). But the question remains of whether the effects of the infused agents are specific for the SNC. For example, the volume of infused drugs in the cited papers was too large to avoid diffusion to the SNR or to nearby structures. Several authors deny the involvement of the SNC in seizure protection, based on the studies using microinfusions of dopaminergic antagonists or neurotoxic lesions which failed to affect seizure susceptibility (Albala et al., 1986; Depaulis et al., 1990b; Gale, 1985; Garant & Gale, 1987; Iadarola & Gale, 1982; N'Gouemo et al., 1990).

Similar incongruent results have been found by investigating the involvement of the nigrothalamic pathway in seizure control. The nigrothalamic projection is GABAergic with nerve terminals ending mainly in the ventromedial thalamic nucleus (VTM) (MacLeod et al., 1980). There is also evidence of direct projection from the SNR to the reticular nucleus of the thalamus (Paré et al., 1990), which exerts a dynamic regulatory influence over other thalamic nuclei (Crick, 1984). There are studies showing the involvement of the thalamic nuclei in seizures (Garant et al., 1993; Miller, 1992). However, lesions of the VTM or interruption of the nigrothalamic pathway does not modify the anticonvulsant effects of SNR GABAergic drug infusions (Depaulis et al., 1990a; Garant and Gale, 1987; Garant et al., 1993; Moshé et al., 1985).

The integrity of the nigral projection to the superior colliculus may be essential for mediating the SNR effects on seizures following infusions of GABAergic agonists (Depaulis et al., 1990b; Garant & Gale, 1987). Pharmacological manipulation of the superior colliculus modulates seizure susceptibility in several seizure models (Depaulis et al., 1990a; Gale et al., 1993; Redgrave et al., 1992; Shehab et al., 1993).

Few data have been collected concerning the involvement of the nigrotegmental pathway. GABAergic manipulations in the pedunculopontine nucleus affects pentylenetetrazol-induced seizures (Okada et

Chapter 4 Age-related mechanisms involved in the control of seizures

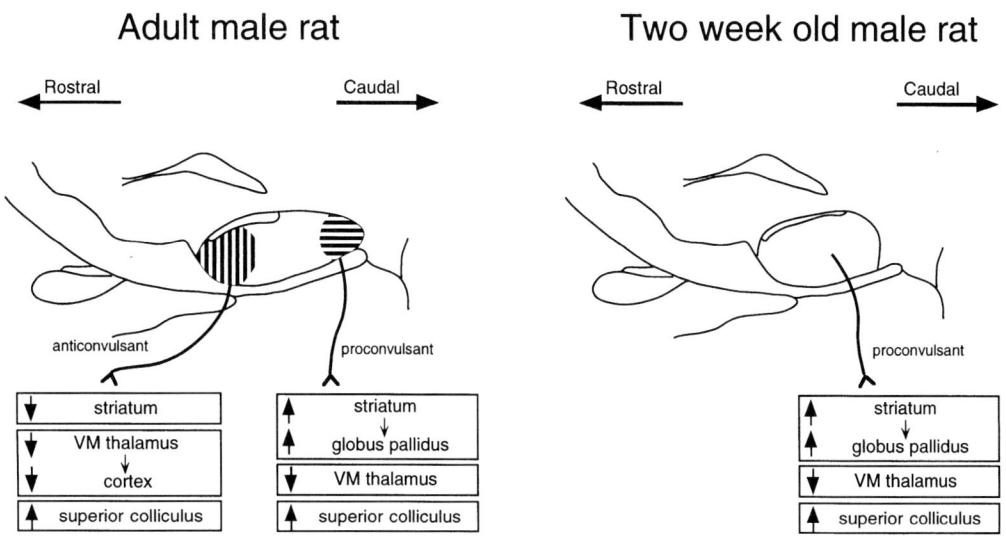

Fig. 1. Age-related differences in SNR region-specific effects and in the networks involved in seizures in male rats.

al., 1989). On the other hand, Miller et al. (1991) demonstrated the role of the laterodorsal tegmental nucleus in seizure control but not of the pedunculopontine nucleus.

To test the functional network differences in adult male rats, we used [^{14}C]2-deoxyglucose autoradiography to determine which output projections are metabolically altered by unilateral muscimol infusions in the $SNR_{anterior}$ or $SNR_{posterior}$. The metabolic changes are region-specific (Fig. 1). In the $SNR_{anterior}$, muscimol infusions decreased glucose utilization in the striatum, sensorimotor cortex and ventromedial thalamus, and increased glucose utilization in superior colliculus (Moshé et al., 1994). In contrast, in the $SNR_{posterior}$ muscimol infusions increased glucose utilization in the dorsal striatum, globus pallidus and superior colliculus, and decreased glucose utilization in thalamus (Moshé et al., 1994). These data support the findings of the topographic and functional segregation of the SNR in adult male rats.

Our results are also supported by anatomical and electrophysiological studies. In the adult rat SNR, Poirier et al. (1983) describe three populations of neurons. While the small-globular type is uniformly distributed in the SNR, the two larger types (reticulata and intermediary) have region-specific distribution. In the $SNR_{anterior}$, the majority of neurons are represented by the reticulata type while in the $SNR_{posterior}$, the intermediary type is most abundant (Poirier et al., 1983). This cytoarchitectonic heterogeneity of the adult SNR may be a substrate for the distinct physiological properties of the two SNR regions. In the electrophysiological study, Niemi et al. (1994) demonstrated that GABA application in the $SNR_{anterior}$ produced mostly disinhibition of neuronal activity in the superior colliculus, one of the major projection sites of the SNR. On the other hand, GABA application in the $SNR_{posterior}$ produced inhibition of collicular activity (Niemi et al., 1994). Hajós & Greenfield (1993) also showed distinct physiological properties of the neurons in the $SNR_{anterior}$ and in the $SNR_{posterior}$.

Age-specific effects of microinfusions of GABA$_A$ergic agents in the SNR of developing male rats

As described earlier, the behavioural manifestations of flurothyl seizures are different in immature rats compared to adult animals. Accordingly, the properties of the SNR appear to change as a function of age (Moshé et al., 1986; Sperber & Moshé, 1988). In the PN 15 SNR, we found the following disparities from adult SNR:

The organization of the SNR into two functional regions, which was described for adult male rats, is absent in PN 15 male rats (Moshé et al., 1994; Velíšková et al., 1996). In PN 15 rats, there is only one functional region within the SNR with respect to the effects of microinfusions of $GABA_A$ergic drug on seizures (Table 1).

Pharmacological manipulations in the SNR in PN 15 rats affected both clonic and tonic–clonic seizures. This may be explained by the underdevelopment of inhibitory mechanisms and therefore rapid propagation of seizures to the brainstem structures responsible for the tonic–clonic seizures (Browning, 1985) as well as the immaturity of the SN circuitry in rat pups (Garant et al., 1992).

Another interesting finding is that in PN 15 rats, activation of high-affinity $GABA_A$ receptors (using muscimol or THIP) mediates only proconvulsant effects (Moshé & Albala, 1984; Xu et al., 1992). The anticonvulsant effect of high-affinity $GABA_A$ receptor agonists could not be demonstrated, even after the administration of several different doses of these agonists (Garant et al., 1995). In addition, in PN 15 rats, blockade of low-affinity $GABA_A$ receptors by bicuculline has proconvulsant effects (Sperber et al., 1987; Velíšková et al., 1996), while in adult rats, bicuculline does not alter the seizure threshold (Velíšková et al., 1996). To determine whether the activation of low-affinity $GABA_A$ receptors in PN 15 rats might mediate anticonvulsant effects, we tested the effect of ZAPA. We found that in PN 15 rats, ZAPA has biphasic effects. An intermediate dose of ZAPA (2 µg per site) has anticonvulsant effects against seizures, while a larger dose (8 µg per site) is proconvulsant (Velíšková et al., 1996). The anticonvulsant action of ZAPA may be mediated by $GABA_A$ low-affinity receptors either by ZAPA's direct action or indirectly due to blockade of $GABA_A$ uptake. The latter may result in an increased amount of endogenous GABA in the synaptic cleft which enhances GABA action at the abundant low-affinity $GABA_A$ receptor. Indeed, previous studies indicate that these receptors are present in the PN 15 old SNR at slightly higher densities (130 per cent) than in the adult substantia nigra (Wurpel et al., 1988). The proconvulsant effect of the higher dose may be due to the action of ZAPA on high-affinity receptors as described earlier for the adult $SNR_{posterior}$. These results suggest that the immature, undifferentiated SNR has some similarities with the $SNR_{posterior}$ in terms of the presence of the 'proconvulsant' high-affinity $GABA_A$ receptor subtype. However, in the immature substantia nigra, the $GABA_A$ low-affinity receptors are also present and functional (Velíšková et al., 1996; Wurpel et al., 1988).

In situ hybridization and immunohistochemistry studies have revealed that the expression of different subunits for $GABA_A$ receptors is developmentally regulated (Dunn et al., 1994; Fritschy et al., 1994; Laurie et al., 1992; MacLennan et al., 1991; Wisden & Seeburg, 1992). Therefore, we also looked at the distribution of $\alpha 1$ subunit for $GABA_A$ receptors in PN 15 rats. The film autoradiograms revealed uniform distribution of the $\alpha 1$ subunit signal in the SNR. At the cellular level, we found that the silver grains of $\alpha 1$ subunit are clustered over the labelled cells and uniformly distributed throughout the SNR. There is a moderate amount of the hybridization grains in these clusters. The distribution and the density of these clusters resembles the pattern described in the $SNR_{posterior}$ in adult male rats (Velíšková et al., 1996).

In $[14_C]$-deoxyglucose studies, muscimol infusions in the SNR also produced specific regional metabolic changes compared to controls (Fig. 1). Irrespective of the site of muscimol infusion, glucose utilization is increased in the ipsilateral dorsal striatum and not changed in the sensorimotor cortex. Glucose utilization is also increased in the globus pallidus and superior colliculus. In contrast, muscimol infusion decreases glucose utilization in the ipsilateral ventromedial thalamus (Moshé et al., 1994). The data suggest that at PN 15, there is only one output network, which may resemble the one observed in the $SNR_{posterior}$ in adult rats.

Based on these data, we hypothesized that, in the flurothyl model, the full 'anticonvulsant' properties of the $SNR_{anterior}$ emerge with development as the density of high-affinity receptors, which may have different subunit composition, rises to its mature levels. For this purpose, we determined the developmental profile of the SNR with respect to the effects of muscimol infusions on flurothyl-induced seizures. In PN 15 and PN 21 rats, muscimol infusions have uniform proconvulsant effects compared to saline-infused controls, irrespective of the site of infusion. At PN 25, the SNR starts to differentiate; infusions of muscimol in the $SNR_{anterior}$ have no effects on flurothyl seizures, while infusions in the $SNR_{posterior}$ have proconvulsant effects. In PN 30 and older rats, there is a clear difference between muscimol infusions into the $SNR_{anterior}$ and the $SNR_{posterior}$. Muscimol infusions into the $SNR_{anterior}$ have anticonvulsant effects and muscimol infusions into the $SNR_{posterior}$ retain the proconvulsant effects.

Gender-specific effects of microinfusions of $GABA_A$ergic agents in the SNR in rats

The maturation of the 'anticonvulsant' SNR region strikingly coincides with the sexual maturation (Ojeda & Urbanski, 1994). In male rats, there is a sudden drop in plasma testosterone levels (PN 20–25) (Döhler & Wuttke, 1975; Lee *et al.*, 1975; Piacsek & Goodspeed, 1978) just prior to the age when the $SNR_{anterior}$ assumes its 'anticonvulsant' characteristics. Thus, we speculate that the functional maturation of the SNR regions may be under the influence of testosterone. Testosterone, as other gonadal steroids, plays a significant role in the formation of neuronal circuits as well as in modulation of neuronal development (Arnold & Gorski, 1984; Breedlove, 1984; Goy & McEwen, 1980; Toran-Allerand, 1984). To test the hypothesis that testosterone may play a role in formation of the 'anticonvulsant' $SNR_{anterior}$, male rats were castrated on the day of birth. The rats were exposed to flurothyl at ages PN 15 and PN 25 following bilateral infusions of muscimol in the $SNR_{anterior}$ or $SNR_{posterior}$ (Table 2). In the $SNR_{anterior}$ in PN 15 neonatally castrated male rats, muscimol infusions have no effects on seizures; in PN 25, muscimol infusions have anticonvulsant effects compared to saline-infused neonatally castrated controls. Thus, in neonatally castrated male rats the emergence of the 'anticonvulsant' $SNR_{anterior}$ shifts to an earlier time point than that observed in intact or sham-operated male rats. Our data suggest that the depletion of postnatal testosterone may accelerate the appearance of the 'anticonvulsant' $SNR_{anterior}$.

Table 2. Gender-specific effects of muscimol infusions in the SNR

	Postnatal day 15		Postnatal day 25	
	$SNR_{anterior}$	$SNR_{posterior}$	$SNR_{anterior}$	$SNR_{posterior}$
Intact males	Proconvulsant	Proconvulsant	No effect	Proconvulsant
Gonadectomized males	No effect	Proconvulsant	Anticonvulsant	Proconvulsant
Females	No effect	No effect	Anticonvulsant	Anticonvulsant

In the $SNR_{posterior}$ in PN 15 and PN 25 rats, muscimol infusions have proconvulsant effects compared to saline-infused neonatally castrated controls. These data suggest that the postnatal testosterone surge does not influence the emergence of the $SNR_{posterior}$. On the other hand, the prenatal testosterone surge may be responsible for the formation of the $SNR_{posterior}$.

During embryonic and postnatal development, steroid hormones can induce the differentiation of discrete brain regions. They also influence the differentiation of specific neuronal and glial components directly involved in synaptogenesis and myelinogenesis (Timiras & Hill, 1980). Depending on the steroid hormones involved, there are many sex differences in the nervous system, including the size of nucleus and nucleolus in neurons, size of synaptic vesicles and terminals, synaptic organization, dendritic branching pattern, gross nuclear volume and neurotransmitter distribution (Breedlove, 1992;

Dyer et al., 1976; Kelly, 1991; MacLusky & Naftolin, 1981; Sakuma & Pfaff, 1981; Toran-Allerand, 1978). These gonadal hormone-dependent sexual dimorphisms occur in many areas in the CNS. These include not only areas well recognized for involvement in sexual behaviour such as preoptic area, hypothalamus and lumbar spinal cord, but also structures involved in the initiation or control of seizures like the amygdala, hippocampus and substantia nigra (Kawata, 1995; Toran-Allerand, 1978).

Steroid hormones can influence the brain at the non-genomic or the genomic level. The non-genomic effect involves the action of hormones on the pre- or post-synaptic membrane, such as changing the permeability of neurotransmitters and the functioning of neurotransmitter receptors. The genomic effect of the steroid hormone leads to alteration of protein synthesis, which may participate in pre- or postsynaptic events (McEwen, 1991a,b). In the CNS, genomic effects are mediated through interaction with the intracellular receptors. The influence of gonadal steroid hormones on the nervous system can be divided in two categories: *organizational effects,* which develop during embryonic or neonatal life (the 'critical period' for sexual differentiation), and are permanent, or *activational effects*, which can occur at any time during life and are mostly reversible (McEwen et al., 1990).

In mammals, the sex chromosome assembly determines the development of ovaries in the presence of X chromosomes, while the role of the Y chromosome is the determination of gonad differentiation into testes. The testes can secrete testosterone during the 'critical period', while ovaries stay inactive at this time. The phenotype of the individual depends on the exposure to testosterone during the critical period irrespective of the genotype. Testosterone can act on a variety of tissues, including the brain, and can even turn a genotypic female into a phenotypic male (McEwen et al., 1990). On the other hand, neonatal castration can turn a genotypic male into a phenotypic female (Breedlove & Arnold, 1983; Breedlove et al., 1982).

The results with neonatally castrated male rats prompted us to test the hypothesis, whether the shift in development of the SNR in neonatally castrated male rats (in terms of its GABAergic effects on seizures) can be reproduced in female rats. We infused muscimol in PN 15 and PN 25 rats and determined its effects on flurothyl seizures (Table 2). At PN 15, muscimol infusions in the $SNR_{anterior}$ had no effect on flurothyl seizures compared to saline-infused females. At PN 25, muscimol infusions had anticonvulsant effects irrespective of the infusion site. The data suggest that maturation of the 'anticonvulsant' SNR network in females is accelerated and perhaps similar to that of castrated males. However, in female rats at PN 25, there is no difference between the muscimol effects whether infused in the $SNR_{anterior}$ or $SNR_{posterior}$. Infusions in either SNR region produce anticonvulsant effects. The data may suggest that in female rats there is no functional separation of the SNR into $SNR_{anterior}$ and $SNR_{posterior}$ region as it is in male rats. The data in neonatally castrated male rats (the presence of the 'proconvulsant' $SNR_{posterior}$) and in females (the absence of the 'proconvulsant' $SNR_{posterior}$) support the hypothesis that the prenatal testosterone surge is important for forming the 'proconvulsant' $SNR_{posterior}$ region in male rats.

Preliminary data regarding the distribution of $\alpha 1$ subunit for GABAA receptors in female rats show that at the cellular level in the $SNR_{anterior}$, there are spare clusters of high-density hybridization grains over some cells, similar as in the $SNR_{anterior}$ of male rats. In the female $SNR_{posterior}$, there are also clusters of high-density hybridization grains alternating with the clusters of moderate density. This is different from the male $SNR_{posterior}$, where only the moderate-density clusters of silver grains are present.

Conclusions

In the SNR of male rats over PN 25, there are two regions mediating opposite effects of $GABA_A$ergic agents. These regions differ in sensitivity to the low- and high-affinity $GABA_A$ receptor sites, in the distribution of the $\alpha 1$ subunit for $GABA_A$ receptors and use divergent output networks. These two regions begin to emerge around PN 25. The natural prepubertal decrease in testosterone level may be the signal for the emergence for the 'anticonvulsant' SNR region, which is located in the $SNR_{anterior}$.

Our studies in neonatally castrated male rats suggest that early *postnatal* depletion of testosterone may accelerate the development of the 'anticonvulsant' SNR region. However, the emergence of the 'proconvulsant' SNR region is independent of early *postnatal* testosterone and probably the *prenatal* testosterone surge is responsible for the development of the 'proconvulsant' SNR region. Lack of *prenatal* testosterone leads to the female type of the SNR with only one $GABA_A$ sensitive region.

Our data may have a significant influence on prospective therapy of age-dependent epileptic syndromes and especially for use of hormonal treatment. Better knowledge of the influence of the endocrine system on brain development and neuronal activity may bring new insights in the therapy of age-dependent seizure disorders.

Acknowledgements: This work was supported by grants NS–36238 and NS–20253 from NINDS and Epilepsy Foundation of America Research Grant. I would like to thank Dr. Solomon L. Moshé for helpful comments regarding the chapter.

References

Albala, B.J., Moshé, S.L., Cubells, J.F., Sharpless, N.S. & Makman, M.H. (1986): Unilateral perisubstantia nigra catecholaminergic lesion and amygdala kindling. *Brain Res.* **370**, 388–392.

Allan, R.D., Dickenson, H.W., Duke, R.K. & Johnston, G.A.R. (1991): ZAPA, a substrate for the neuronal high affinity GABA uptake system in rat brain slices. *Neurochem. Int.* **18**, 63–67.

Araki, T. & Tohyama, M. (1992): Region-specific expression of $GABA_A$ receptor $\alpha 3$ and $\alpha 4$ subunits mRNAs in the rat brain. *Mol. Brain Res.* **12**, 293–314.

Arnold, A.P. & Gorski, R.A. (1984): Gonadal steroid induction of structural sex differences in the central nervous system. *Ann. Rev. Neurosci.* **7**, 413–442.

Bartholini, G., Scatton, B., Zivkovic, K.G., Depoortere, H., Langer, S.Z. & Morselli, P.L. (1985): GABA receptor agonists as a new therapeutic class. In: *Epilepsy and GABA receptor agonists*, Bartholini, G., Bossi, L., Lloyd, K.G. & Morselli, P.L. (eds), pp. 1–30. New York: Raven Press.

Bowdler, J.M. & Green, A.R. (1982): Regional rat brain benzodiazepine receptor number and gamma-aminobutyric acid concentration following a convulsion. *Brit. J. Pharmacol.* **76**, 291–298.

Breedlove, S.M. (1984): Steroid influences on the development and function of a neuromuscular system. *Progr. Brain Res.* **61**, 147–170.

Breedlove, S.M. (1992): Sexual dimorphism in the vertebrate nervous system. *J. Neurosci.* **12**, 4133–4142.

Breedlove, S.M. & Arnold, A.P. (1983): Hormonal control of a developing neuromuscular system I. Complete demasculinization of the male rat spinal nucleus of the bulbocavernosus using the anti-androgen flutamide. *J. Neurosci.* **3**, 417–423.

Breedlove, S.M., Jacobson, C.D., Gorski, R.A. & Arnold, A.P. (1982): Masculinization of the female rat spinal cord following a single injection of testosterone propionate but not estradiol benzoate. *Brain Res.* **237**, 173–181.

Browning, R.A. (1985): Role of the brain-stem reticular formation in tonic–clonic seizures: lesion and pharmacological studies. *Fed. Proc.* **44**, 2425–2431.

Cavalheiro, E.A. & Turski, L. (1986): Intrastriatal N-methyl-D-aspartate prevents amygdala kindled seizures in rats. *Brain Res.* **377**, 173–176.

Chevalier, G., Vacher, S., Deniau, J.M. & Desban, M. (1985): Disinhibition as a basic process in the expression of striatal functions. I. The striato-nigral influence on tecto-spinal/tecto-diencephalic neurons. *Brain Res.* **334**, 215–226.

Crick, F. (1984): The function of the thalamic reticular complex: the searchlight hypothesis. *Proc. Natl. Acad. Sci.* **81**, 4586–4590.

De Sarro, G., De Sarro, A. & Meldrum, B.S. (1991): Anticonvulsant action of 2-chloroadenosine injected focally into the inferior colliculus and substantia nigra. *Eur. J. Pharmacol.* **194**, 145–152.

De Sarro, G., Patel, S. & Meldrum, B.S. (1986): Anticonvulsant action of a kainate antagonist γ-D-glutamyl aminomethylsulphonic acid injected focally into the substantia nigra and antopeduncular nucleus. *Eur. J. Pharmacol.* **132**, 229–236.

Depaulis, A., Vergnes, M., Marescaux, C., Lannes, B. & Warter, J.M. (1988): Evidence that activation of GABA receptors in the substantia nigra suppressses spontaneous spike and wave discharges in the rat. *Brain Res.* **448**, 20–29.

Depaulis, A., Snead, O.C.I., Marescaux, C. & Vergnes, M. (1989): Suppressive effects of intranigral injection of muscimol in three models of generalized non-convulsive epilepsy induced by chemical agents. *Brain Res.* **498,** 64–72.

Depaulis, A., Liu, Z., Vergnes, M., Marescaux, C., Micheletti, G. & Warter, J.M. (1990a): Suppression of spontaneous generalized non-convulsive seizures in the rat by microinjection of GABA antagonists into the superior colliculus. *Epilepsy Res.* **5,** 192–198.

Depaulis, A., Vergnes, M., Liu, Z., Kempf, E. & Marescaux, C. (1990b): Involvement of the nigral output pathways in the inhibitory control of the substantia nigra over generalized non-convulsive seizures in the rat. *Neuroscience* **39,** 339–349.

Döhler, K.D. & Wuttke, W. (1975): Changes with age in levels of serum gonadotropins, prolactin, and gonadal steroids in prepubertal male and female rats. *Endocrinology* **97,** 898–907.

Dunn, S.J., Bateson, A.N. & Martin, I.L. (1994): Molecular neurobiology of the $GABA_A$ receptor. *Int. Rev. Neurobiol.* **36,** 51–98.

Dyer, R.G., MacLeod, N.K. & Ellendorff, F. (1976): Electrophysiological evidence for sexual dimorphism and synaptic convergence in the preoptic and anterior. *Proc. R. Soc. Lond.* **193,** 4 21–440.

Fang, Z., Laster, M.J., Gong, D., Ionescu, P., Koblin, D.D., Sonner, J., Eger, E.I. 2nd & Halsey, M.J. (1997): Convulsant activity of nonanesthetic gas combinations. *Anesthesia & Analgesia* **84,** 634–460.

Fariello, R.G., DeMattei, M., Catorina, M., Ferraro, T.N. & Golden, G.T (1987): MPTP and convulsive responses in rodents. *Brain Res.* **426,** 373–376.

Franck, J.E., Ginter, K.L. & Schwartzkroin, P.A. (1989): Developing genetically epilepsy-prone rats have an abnormal seizure response to flurothyl. *Epilepsia* **30,** 1–6.

Fritschy, J.-M., Paysan, J., Enna, A. & Möhler, H. (1994): Switch in the expression of rat $GABA_A$-receptor subtypes during postnatal development: An immunohistochemical study. *J. Neurosci.* **14,** 5302–5324.

Gale, K. (1985): Mechanisms of seizure control mediated by gamma-aminobutyric acid: a role of the substantia nigra. *Fed. Proc. Fed. Am. Soc. Exp. Biol.* **44,** 2414–2424.

Gale, K., Pazos, A., Maggio, R., Japikse, K. & Pritchard, P. (1993): Blockade of GABA receptors in superior colliculus protects against focally evoked limbic motor seizures. *Brain Res.* **603,** 279–283.

Garant, D.S. & Gale, K. (1987): Substantia nigra-mediated anticonvulsant actions: Role of nigral output pathways. *Exp. Neurol.* **97,** 143–159.

Garant, D.S., Velíšek, L., Sperber, E. & Moshé, S.L. (1992): Why do infants have seizures? *Int. Pediatrics* **7,** 199–212.

Garant, D.S., Xu, S.G., Sperber, E.F. & Moshé, S.L. (1993): The influence of thalamic GABA transmission on the susceptibility of adult rats to flurothyl induced seizures. *Epilepsy Res.* **15,** 185–192.

Garant, D.S., Xu, S.G., Sperber, E.F. & Moshé, S.L. (1995): Age-related differences in the effects of $GABA_A$ agonists microinjected into rat substantia nigra: Pro- and anticonvulsant actions. *Epilepsia* **36,** 960–965.

Goy, R.W. & McEwen, B.S. (1980): *Sexual differentiation of the brain.* Cambridge: MIT Press, 223.

Grace, A.A. & Bunney, B.S. (1979): Paradoxical GABA excitation of nigral dopaminergic cell: indirect mediation through reticulata inhibitory neurons. *Eur. J. Pharmacol.* **59,** 211–218.

Green, A.R., Metz, A., Minchin, M.C. & Vincent, N.D. (1987a): Inhibition of the rate of GABA synthesis in regions of rat brain following a convulsion. *Brit. J. Pharmacol.* **92,** 5–11.

Green, A.R., Minchin, M.C. & Vincent, N.D. (1987b): Inhibition of GABA release from slices prepared from several brain regions of rats at various times following a convulsion. *Brit. J. Pharmacol.* **92,** 13–18.

Hajós, M. & Greenfield, S.A. (1993): Topographic heterogeneity of substantia nigra neurons: diversity in intrinsic membrane properties and synaptic inputs. *Neuroscience* **55,** 919–934.

Hayashi, T. (1952): A physiological study of epileptic seizures following cortical stimulation in animals and its aplication to human clinics. *Jap. J. Pharmacol.* **3,** 46–64.

Hayashi, T. (1953): The efferent pathway of epileptic seizures for the face following cortical stimulation differs from that for limbs. *Jap. J. Pharmacol.* **4,** 306–321.

Heyer, E.J., Nowak, L.M. & MacDonald, R.L. (1981): Bicuculline: A convulsant with synaptic and nonsynaptic actions. *Neurology* **31,** 1381–1390.

Iadarola, M.J. & Gale, K. (1982): Substantia nigra: site of anticonvulsant activity mediated by γ-aminobutyric acid. *Science* **218,** 1237–1240.

Jung, M.J., Lippert, B., Metcalf, B.W., Böhlen, P. & Schechter, J.P. (1977): γ-vinyl GABA (4-aminohex-5-enoic acid), a new selective irreversible inhibitor of GABA-T: effects on brain GABA metabolism in mice. *J. Neurochem.* **29**, 797–802.

Kawata, M. (1995): Roles of steroid hormones and their receptors in structural organization in the nervous system. *Neurosci. Res.* **24**, 1–46.

Kelly, D.D. (1991): Sexual Differentiation of the Nervous System. In: *Principles of neural science*, Kandel, E.R., Schwartz, J.H. & Jessell, T.M. (eds), pp. 959–973. New York: Elsevier.

Krogsgaard-Larsen, P. (1984): THIP, a specific and clinically active GABA agonist. *Neuropharmacology* **23**, 837–838.

Lánský, P., Velíšková, J. & Velíšek, L. (1997): An indirect method for absorption rate estimation: Flurothyl-induced seizures. *Bull. Math. Biol.* **59**, 569–579.

Laurie, D.J., Wisden, W. & Seeburg, P.H. (1992): The distribution of thirteen GABAA receptor subunit mRNAs in the rat brain. III. Embryonic and postnatal development. *J. Neurosci.* **12**, 4151–4172.

Lee, V.W.K., de Kretser, D.M., Hudson, B. & Wang, C. (1975): Variations in serum FSH, LH and testosterone levels in male rats from birth to sexual maturity. *J. Reprod. Fert.* **42**, 121–126.

Levitan, E.S., Blair, L.A.C., Dionne, V.E. & Barnard, E.A. (1988a): Biophysical and pharmacological properties of cloned GABAA receptor subunits expressed in xenopus oocytes. *Neuron* **1**, 773–781.

Levitan, E.S., Schofield, P.R., Burt, D.R., Rhee, L.M., Wisden, W., Kohler, M., Fujita, N., Rogriguez, H., Stephenson, F.A., Darlison, M.G., Barnard, E.A. & Seeburg, P.H. (1988b): Structural and functional basis for $GABA_A$ receptor heterogeneity. *Nature* **335**, 76–79.

Löscher, W. & Schwark, W.S. (1985): Evidence for impaired GABA-ergic activity in the substantia nigra in amygdaloid kindled rats. *Brain Res.* **339**, 146–150.

Lüddens, H., Korpi, E.R. & Seeburg, P.H. (1995): $GABA_A$/benzodiazepine receptor heterogeneity: neurophysiological implications. *Neuropharmacology* **34**, 245–254.

MacLennan, A.J., Brecha, N., Khrestchatisky, M., Sternini, C., Tillakaratne, N.J.K., Chiang, M.Y., Anderson, K., Lai, M. & Tobin, A.J. (1991): Independent cellular and ontogenetic expression of mRNAs encoding three polypeptides of the rat $GABA_A$ receptor. *Neuroscience* **43**, 369–380.

MacLeod, N.K., James, T.A., Kilpatrick, I.C. & Starr, M.S. (1980): Evidence for a GABAergic nigrothalamic pathway in the rat. II. Electrophysiological studies. *Brain Res.* **40**, 55–61.

MacLusky, N.J. & Naftolin, F. (1981): Sexual differentiation of the central nervous system. *Science* **211**, 1294–1303.

McEwen, B.S. (1991a): Non-genomic and genomic effects of steroids on neural activity. *Trends Pharmacol. Sci.* **12**, 141–144.

McEwen, B.S. (1991b): Steorids affect neuronal activity by acting on the membrane and the genom. *Trends Pharmacol. Sci.* **12**, 141–147.

McEwen, B.S., Coirini, H. & Schumacher, M. (1990): Steroid effects on neuronal activity: when is the genome involved? In: *Steroids and neuronal activity CIBA Foundation Symposium*, pp. 3–21. Chichester: Wiley.

McNamara, J.O., Rigsbee, L.C. & Galloway, M.T. (1983): Evidence that the substantia nigra is crucial to the network of kindled seizures. *Eur. J. Pharmacol.* **86**, 485–486.

McNamara, J.O., Galloway, M.T., Rigsbee, L.C. & Shin, C. (1984): Evidence implicating substantia nigra in regulation of kindled seizure threshold. *J. Neurosci.* **4**, 2410–2417.

Meldrum, B.S. (1981): GABA-agonists as antiepileptic agents. In: *GABA and benzodiazepine receptor*, Costa, E. (ed.), pp. 207–217. New York: Raven Press.

Miller, J.W. (1992): The role of mesencephalic and thalamic arousal systems in experimental seizures. *Prog. Neurobiol.* **39**, 155–178.

Miller, J.W., Bardgett, M.E. & Gray, B.C. (1991): The role of the laterodorsal tegmental nucleus of the rat in experimental seizures. *Neuroscience* **43**, 41–49.

Moshé, S.L. & Albala, B.J. (1984): Nigral muscimol infusions facilitate the development of seizures in immature rats. *Dev. Brain Res.* **13**, 305–308.

Moshé, S.L. & Sperber, E.F. (1990): Substantia nigra-mediated control of generalized seizures. In: *Generalized epilepsy:cellular, molecular and pharmacological approaches*, Gloor, G., Kostopoulos, R., Naquet, M. & Avoli, P. (eds), pp. 355–367. Boston: Birkhauser Inc.

Moshé, S.L., Brown, L.L., Kubová, H., Velíšková, J., Zukin, R.S. & Sperber, E.F. (1994): Maturation and segregation of brain networks that modify seizures. *Brain Res.* **665**, 141–146.

Moshé, S.L., Ackermann, R.F., Albala, B.J. & Okada, R. (1986): The role of substantia nigra in seizures of developing animals. In: *Kindling 3*, Wada, J.A. (ed.), pp. 91–106. New York: Raven Press.

Moshé, S.L., Okada, R. & Albala, B.J. (1985): Ventromedial thalamic lesions and seizure susceptibility. *Brain Res.* **337**, 368–372.

N'Gouemo, P., Lerner-Natoli, M., Rondouin, G., Sandillon, F., Privat, A. & Baldy-Moulinier, M. (1990): Catecholaminergic systems and amygdala kindling development. Effects of bilateral lesions of substantia nigra dopaminergic or locus coeruleus noradrenergic neurons. *Epilepsy Res.* **5**, 92–102.

Niemi, U.J., Redgrave, P. & Westby, G.W.M. (1994): Regional variation in the effects of nigral GABA on collicular neuronal activity: implications for the role of the nigrotectal pathway. *Eur. J. Neurosci.* Suppl. **7**, 213.

Ojeda, S.R. & Urbanski, H.F. (1994): Puberty in the rat. In: *The physiology of reproduction*, Knobil, E. (ed.), pp. 363–411. New York: Raven Press.

Okada, R., Nagishi, N. & Nagaya, H. (1989): The role of the nigrotegmental GABAergic pathway in the propagation of pentylenetetrazol induced seizures. *Brain Res.* **480**, 383–387.

Paré, D., Hazrati, L.-N., Parent, A. & Steriade, M. (1990): Substantia nigra pars reticulata projects to the reticular thalamic nucleus of the cat: a morphological and electrophysiological study. *Brain Res.* **535**, 139–146.

Piacsek, B.E. & Goodspeed, M.P. (1978): Maturation of the pituitary-gonadal system in the male rat. *J. Reprod. Fert.* **52**, 29–35.

Poirier, L., Giguere, M. & Marchand, R. (1983): Comparative morphology of the substantia nigra and ventral tegmental area in the monkey, cat and rat. *Brain Res. Bull.* **11**, 371–397.

Prichard, J.W., Gallagher, B.B. & Glaser, G.H. (1969): Experimental seizure threshold testing with flurothyl. *J. Pharm. Exp. Ther.* **166**, 170–178.

Redgrave, P., Marrow, L. & Dean, P. (1992): Anticonvulsant role of nigrotectal projection in the maximal electroshock model of epilepsy – II. Pathways from substantia nigra pars lateralis and adjacent peripeduncular area to the dorsal midbrain. *Neuroscience* **46**, 391–406.

Sakuma, Y. & Pfaff, D.W. (1981): Electrophysiologic determination of projections from ventromedial hypothalamus to midbrain central gray: difference between female and male rats. *Brain Res.* **225**, 184–188.

Saxena, N.C. & MacDonald, R.L. (1996): Properties of putative cerebellar gamma-aminobutyric acid A receptor isoforms. *Mol. Pharmacol.* **49**, 567–79.

Schuck, S.L. & Shulman, A. (1971): A study of the central action of flurothyl and methoxyflurane. *Aust. J. Exp. Biol. Med. Sci.* **49**, 501–512.

Shehab, S., Simkins, M., Dean, P. & Redgrave, P. (1993): The dorsal midbrain anticonvulsant zone – I. Effects of locally administered excitatory amino acids or bicuculline on maximal electroshock seizures. *Neuroscience* **65**, 671–679.

Sigel, E., Baur, R., Trube, G., Möhler, H. & Malherbe, P. (1990): The effect of subunit composition of rat brain $GABA_A$ receptors on chanel function. *Neuron* **5**, 703–711.

Sperber, E.F. & Moshé, S.L. (1988): Age-related differences in seizure susceptibility to flurothyl. *Dev. Brain Res.* **39**, 295–297.

Sperber, E.F., Wong, B.Y., Wurpel, J.N. & Moshé, S.L. (1987): Nigral infusions of muscimol or bicuculline facilitate seizures in developing rats. *Brain Res.* **465**, 243–250.

Tepper, J.M., Martin, L.P. & Anderson, D.R. (1995): $GABA_A$ receptor-mediated inhibition of rat substantia nigra dopaminergic neurons by pars reticulata projection neurons. *J. Neurosci.* **15**, 3092–3103.

Timiras, P.S. & Hill, H.F. (1980): Antiepileptic drugs – hormones and epilepsy. In: *Antiepileptic drugs: mechanisms of action*, Glaser, G.H., Penry, J.K. & Woodbury, D.M. (eds), pp. 655–666. New York: Raven Press.

Toran-Allerand, C.D. (1978): Gonadal hormones and brain development: cellular aspects of sexual differentiation. *Amer. Zool.* **18**, 553–565.

Toran-Allerand, C.D. (1984): On the genesis of sexual differentiation of the central nervous system: morphologic consequences of steroid exposure, role of alpha-fetoprotein. *Progr. Brain Res.* **61**, 63–98.

Tretiakof, C., Thèse, No. 293, Paris, 1919.

Turski, L., Meldrum, B.S., Cavalheiro, E.A., Calderazzo-Filho, L.S., Bortolotto, Z.A., Ikonomidou-Turski, C. & Turski, W.A. (1987): Paradoxical anticonvulsant activity of the excitatory amino acid N-methyl-D-aspartate in the rat caudate-putamen. *Proc. Natl. Acad. Sci.* **84,** 1689–1693.

Turski, L., Cavalheiro, E.A., Bortolotto, Z.A., Ikonomidou Turski, I., Kleinrok, Z. & Turski, W.A. (1988): Dopamine-sensitive anticonvulsant site in the rat striatum. *J. Neurosci.* **8,** 4027–4037.

Turski, W.A., Cavalheiro, E.A., Ikonomidou, C., Bortolotto, Z.A., Klockgether, T. & Turski, L. (1990): Dopamine control of seizure propagation: intranigral dopamine D1 agonist SKF–38393 enhances susceptibility to seizures. *Synapse* **5,** 113–119.

van den Pol, A.N., Smith, A.D. & Powell, J.F. (1985): GABA axons in synaptic contact with dopamine neurons in the substantia nigra: double immunocytochemistry with biotin-peroxidase and protein A-colloidal gold. *Brain Res.* **348,** 146–154.

Velíšek, L., Velíšková, J., Ptachewich, Y., Ortíz, J., Shinnar, S. & Moshé, S.L. (1995): Age-dependent effects of GABA agents on flurothyl seizures. *Epilepsia* **36,** 636–643.

Velíšková, J., Velíšek, L., Nunes, M. & Moshé, S. (1996): Developmental regulation of regional functionality of substantia nigra $GABA_A$ receptors involved in seizures. *Eur. J. Pharmacol.* **309,** 167–173.

Velíšková, J., Kubová, H., Friedman, L.F., Wu, R., Sperber, E.F., Zukin, R.Z. and Moshé, S.L. (1998): The expression of $GABA_A$ receptor subunits in the substantia migra is developmentally regulated and region specific. *Ital. J. Neurol. Sci.* **19,** 201–206.

Verdoorn, T.A., Draguhn, A., Ymer, S., Seeburg, P.H. & Sakmann, B. (1990): Functional properties of recombinant rat $GABA_A$ receptors depend upon subunit composition. *Neuron* **4,** 919–928.

Vicq d'Azyr, F. (1786): In: *Traité d'anatomie et de physiologie,* pp. 72–81, 96. Paris.

Wafford, K., Whiting, P. & Kemp, J. (1992): Differences in affinity and efficacy of benzodiazepine receptor ligands at recombinant γ-aminobutyric acid A receptor subtypes. *Mol. Pharmacol.* **43,** 240–244.

Wisden, W. & Seeburg, P. (1992): $GABA_A$ receptor channels: from subunits to functional entities. *Current Opinion in Neurobiology* **2,** 263–269.

Wisden, W., Laurie, D.J., Monyer, H. & Seeburg, P.H. (1992): The distribution of 13 $GABA_A$ receptor subunit mRNAs in the rat brain. I. Telencephalon, diencephalon, mesencephalon. *J. Neurosci.* **12,** 1040–1062.

Wisden, W., Morris, B.J., Darlison, M.G., Hunt, S.P. & Barnard, E.A. (1989): Localization of $GABA_A$ receptor α-subunit mRNAs in relation to receptor subtypes. *Mol. Brain Res.* **5,** 305–10.

Wurpel, J.N.D., Tempel, A., Sperber, E.F. & Moshé, S.L. (1988): Age-related changes of muscimol binding in the substantia nigra. *Dev. Brain Res.* **43,** 305–308.

Xu, S.G., Garant, D.S., Sperber, E.F. & Moshé, S.L. (1992): The proconvulsant effect of nigral infusion of THIP on flurothyl-induced seizures in rat pups. *Dev. Brain Res.* **68,** 275–277.

Part II
Lesional partial epilepsies and neuronal migration disorders

Chapter 5

Neuronal migration disorders and epilepsies

Jean-Paul Misson[1], Jean-Marie Dubru[2], Patricia Leroy[2], Sandrine Pirard[3], T. Takahashi[4] and Verne S. Caviness, Jr[5]

[1]*Professor of Paediatric Neurology;* [2]*Paediatric Neurology;* [3]*Research Fellow, Paediatric Neurology, University of Liège, Belgium;* [4]*Professor of Paediatric Neurology, Department of Paediatrics, Keio University School of Medecine, Tokyo, Japan; and* [6]*Professor of Paediatric Neurology, Massachusetts General Hospital, Harvard Medical School, Boston, USA*

The cerebral neocortex is the dominant structure of the cerebral hemisphere. It is essential to all domains of cognition, behaviour and conscious experience, and plays a critical role in skilled motor activity and perception of sensory stimuli. Abnormalities of the developing neocortex are characteristically associated with mental, sensorimotor retardation and epilepsy. In some instances developmental disorders of the neocortex associated with mental retardation or epilepsy reflect abnormalities in the earliest events of histogenesis and are expressed as abnormalities in the neocortical architectonic patterns. Disturbances have been documented to affect each of the major steps of the early neocortical histogenetic sequence: neuronal production, migration and final distribution within the cortex. At each of these steps, the development of neuronal and glial cells is closely interdependent, and early developmental disorders of the neocortex may be expected to affect both neuronal and glial cell lineages. In particular, disruptions of neuronal migration are prominent among the early histogenetic events which critically affect the behaviour and integrity of both the neuronal and glial population. In this chapter we will review the principles which regulate the process of neuronal migration and which are responsible from the earliest stages of development for appropriate distribution of neurons in the cortex. The role and function of glial cells will be discussed with respect both to architectonic abnormalities and mechanisms of epileptogenesis.

Principles of neuroglial proliferation and neuronal migration

During development the ventricular zone where neuronal production occurs and the cortical anlagen where young neurons come to be positioned become progressively separated (Takahashi *et al.*, 1995a, 1996). Architectonic evolution of the cerebral wall results in stratification and intracortical laminar organization. At its earliest stage of development the cerebral wall is bilaminate, comprised of the ventricular zone (VZ), including the pseudostratified proliferative ventricular epithelium (PVE), and the plexiform marginal zone (Takahashi *et al.*, 1995a, 1996b). As neuronal proliferation and migration of postmitotic neurons proceed, the cortical strata (marginal zone, cortical plate and subplate) emerge in the outer plexiform marginal zone, and these are separated from the VZ by the intermediate zone (IZ) with the more densely cellular and fibrous subventricular zone (SVZ) at the interface of VZ and

IZ. Eventually subcortical axonal systems, including the projection, associational and commissural systems, expand within the intermediate zone (Marin-Padilla, 1978). The external sagittal stratum, a dense fascicle of projection fibres, marks the inferior limit of the developing cortex at its interface with the intermediate zone (Crandall & Caviness, 1984). Proliferative activity during the early and principal phase of cell generation is limited to the PVE and a secondary proliferative population (SPP) distributed more diffusely from the outer VZ through the full width of SVZ and IZ (Takahashi *et al.*, 1995b). The PVE is principally, if not exclusively, the source of neocortical neurons but also seeds cells to the SPP. The SPP gives rise to the glial populations of the neocortex and subjacent cerebral wall (Levinson & Goldman, 1993).

Neurons arising from the neuroepithelium of the VZ are distributed within the cortex of all mammalian species thus far investigated in an inside-out sequence with respect to their sequence of origin (Angevine & Sidman, 1961; Caviness, 1982; Rakic, 1974; Sidman & Rakic, 1973). Thus, the first to be formed are destined for the deepest layers, VI and V, while successively later formed neurons come to populate in turn layers IV, III and II. Particularly the later formed neurons must migrate great distances relative to their size to attain their neocortical positions. The hypothesis of Rakic (Rakic, 1972), supported by electron microscopic study of migrating cells in monkey, that neurons are guided in their migrations by following the ascending process of a special class of glial cells, the radial glial cells, has been abundantly confirmed by subsequent investigations based upon a variety of techniques (Misson *et al.*, 1991e; Pinto-Lord *et al.*, 1982; Rakic *et al.*, 1974).

In our own investigations, for example, we have tracked β-galactosidase marked migrating neurons in their ascent along RC–2 marked radial glial fibres (Misson *et al.*, 1991b). β-Galactosidase positive migrating neurons are readily identified because of their elongate or fusiform somatic shape preceded by the gradually tapering leading process (Fig 1,C–D). In some instances a finer trailing process may also be identified. This general configuration and disposition with respect to the radial glial fibre are characteristic at every level of their journey through the intermediate zone and the cortical plate, although the cell may increase in size (Rakic *et al.*, 1974) and in primates some cells may give rise to an axon even before migration is completed (Schwartz *et al.*, 1991). The young neuron detaches from the radial glial guide upon reaching the interface of cortical plate and plexiform layer (Pinto-Lord *et al.*, 1982).

The radial glial cells may be the earliest cell form to differentiate within the vertebrate central nervous system. The differentiated radial form is fully elaborated and fitted with differentiation antigens RC–1 and RC–2 at least as early as neurulation, corresponding to embryonic day 8–9 in mouse (Edwards *et al.*, 1990; Misson *et al.*, 1988b). The earliest of these cells to be identified are part of the original proliferative population of the neuroepithelium in the VZ, and the somata of these cells undergo interkinetic nuclear migration within the neuroepithelium in the VZ (Misson *et al.*, 1988a). During the histogenetic phase of active neuronal migration, large numbers of these cells exit the cell cycle and their somata are displaced into the SVZ or overlying levels of the IZ (Schmechel & Rakic, 1979a,b). There they remain in G_0 phase until after the completion of migration. Subsequently they are transformed into astrocytes of the cerebral wall (Misson *et al.*, 1991a; Takahashi *et al.*, 1991).

Whether the radial glial cell is in active proliferative or G_0 mode, the configuration of the individual ascending process is the same, ascending through the IZ and cortical strata where it arborizes terminally in the molecular layer to terminate at the pial surface in endfeet varicosities (Misson *et al.*, 1988b, 1991a; Rakic, 1972). Laterally directed branches which contact blood vessel arise from the ascending fibre. At a secondary level of organization, radial glial fibres are organized in fascicles which span the entire thickness of the cerebral wall and the features of these fascicles are variable in their ascent through the strata of the cerebral wall and with respect to stage of development (Gadisseux & Evrard, 1985; Gadisseux *et al.*, 1987, 1989a, b, 1990). As development proceeds and the cortex expands, the fascicles break up into single fibres (defasciculation) which span the cortex. The defasciculation appears to be initiated at the level of the ESS and to extend progressively through the successive layers of the cortex, beginning first in the subplate (future layers VI and V) and eventually involving the fibres in their span across layers III/II. By the end of the migratory epoch only single fibres are observed in the superficial layers of the cortex, and it is characteristic to observe a drop in the fibre density throughout the cortical span (Fig. 2).

In addition to these modifications in the fascicular architecture of the radial glial fibre system, there are also developmental stage-dependent alterations in the pattern of fibre alignment reflecting patterns of tissue expansion in the growing cerebrum (Edwards *et al.*, 1990; Misson *et al.*, 1991a) (Fig.1 A–B). At the earliest stages of cerebral development the fascicles are uniformly radially aligned throughout the full neocortical anlagen. However, with time there is differential expansion of the cortical strata with respect to the VZ, with regard to both the medial to lateral and the anterior posterior axes of the hemisphere. With respect to the medial to lateral axis, radial fibres with progressively lateral insertion in the VZ will have a progressively medial to lateral curving ascent across the cerebral wall, and similar patterns of curving ascent also develop along the rostral to caudal axis of the hemisphere. This divergence from true radial alignment is particularly obvious in the lateral portion of the cerebral wall where the fibres follow a trajectory which is almost tangential to the cerebral surface in their course across the intermediate zone. As they reach the EES they undergo reorientation and realign in a radial fashion in their final ascent towards the pia. β-Galactosidase marked migrating cells have been observed to follow faithfully these dramatically curving pathways of the more laterally positioned radial glial fibres (Fig.1 D) (Misson *et al.*, 1991b).

Multiple lines of evidence suggest that the neocortical architectonic map is already instantiated within the proliferative epithelium that gives rise to neocortical neurons (Rakic, 1988). Thus, from the outset of neuronogenesis, the patterns of expression of genes involved in spatial encoding already recognize the major forebrain boundaries (Bulfone *et al.*, 1993, 1995; Puelles & Rubenstein, 1993; Shimamura *et al.*, 1995). At a finer grained level, patterns of proliferation in adjacent regions of the epithelium which give rise to areas 17 and 18 in monkey are different in ways that anticipate the different neuronal complement to characterize these adjacent neocortical areas (Dehay *et al.*, 1993). Finally, current evidence suggests that the neocortical map is already instantiated with respect to the earliest postmigratory neurons and that this occurs independently of the instantiation of the thalamic map with which it early becomes registered through reciprocal connections (Erzurumlu & Jhaveri, 1992; Molnar & Blakemore, 1995; O'Leary *et al.*, 1994). It is a critical element of this general hypothesis that the epithelial protomap is translated upon the neocortex by orderly radial migration of neurons assured by the radial organization of the glial system (Rakic, 1988). Although some lateral mixing of migrating neurons clearly does occur (Fishell *et al.*, 1993; O'Rourke *et al.*, 1995; Tan & Breen, 1993; Tan *et al.*, 1995; Walsh, 1996; Walsh & Kepko, 1993), for most the neighbourhood relationships of proliferating progenitors corresponds to that of postmigratory progeny, and this is particularly rigorous for the early formed population of neurons with respect to which the map appears to be instantiated (Kornack & Rakic, 1995; Mione *et al.*, 1994).

Neuronal production within the VZ is developmentally regulated and this regulation is essential to correct neuronal migration and neocortical histogenesis (Caviness *et al.*, 1994, 1995a, b; Takahashi *et al.*, 1996, 1997; Waechter & Jaensch, 1972). The proliferative epithelium is a pseudostratified epithelium with the consequence that the location of cell nuclei is systematically related to the phase of the cell cycle (Sauer, 1936; Sauer & Walker, 1959; Takahashi *et al.*, 1992, 1993). Thus, S phase occurs with nuclei in the outer half of the epithelium while mitoses occur at the ventricular margin. The gap phases, G1 and G2, occur as the nuclei ascend and descend between these two extreme levels of the epithelium. Studies of neocortical cell cycle kinetics in mouse, based upon cumulative S phase labelling with Brdu, have provided the basis for a comprehensive quantitative model of neuronal production (Caviness *et al.*, 1995b; Takahashi *et al.*, 1996). In this species, the period of neuronogenesis is 6 days and is divisible into 11 integer cell cycles. The duration of the cell cycle (T_C) essentially doubles over this interval, increasing from approximately 10 to nearly 20 h in the course of the 11 cycles. The increase in T_C is due essentially to increase in the duration of the G1 phase (T_{G1}); the other phases of the cycle have no systematic change in the course of the neuronogenetic interval.

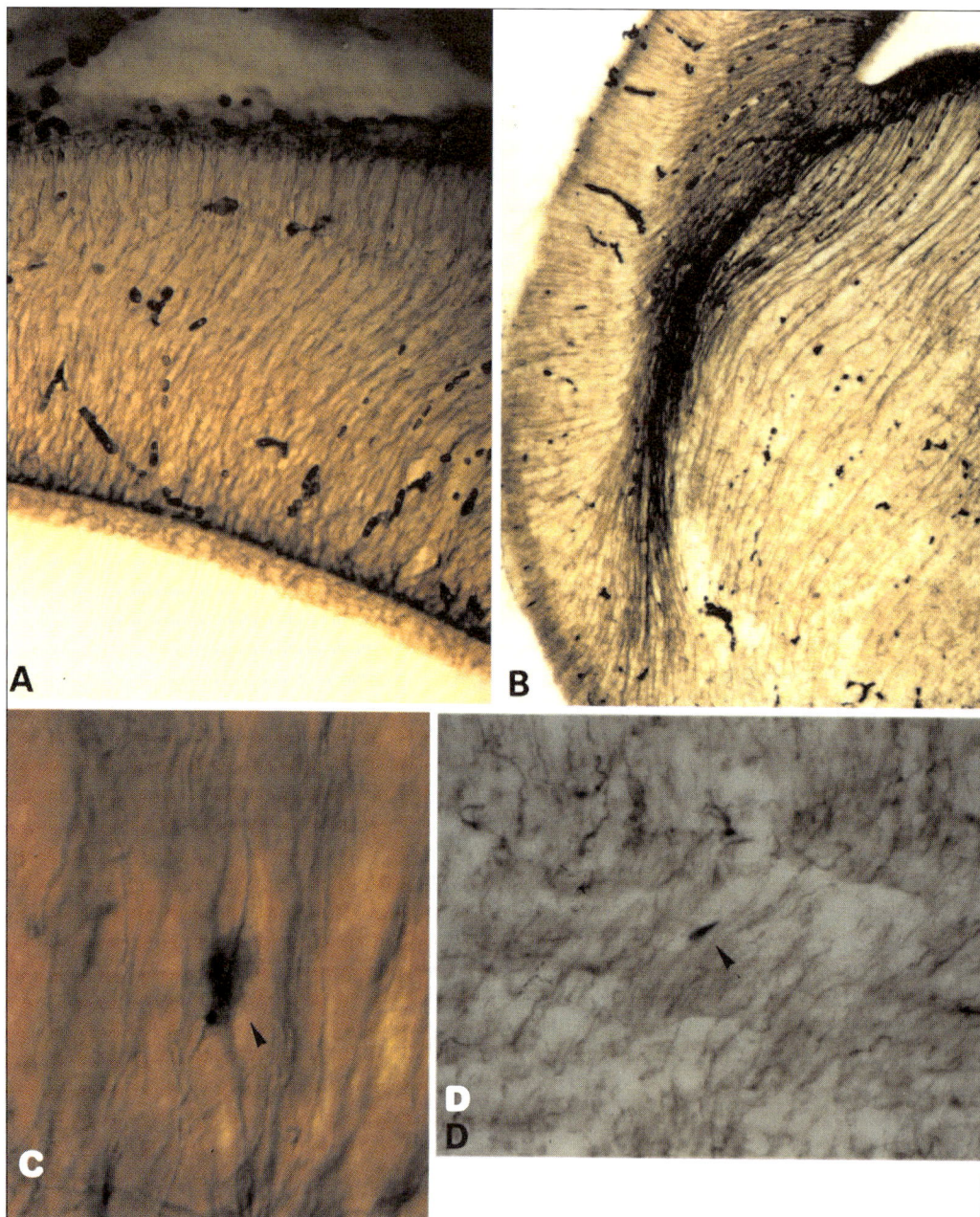

Fig. 1. Identification of radial glia and migrating neurons in mouse cerebral wall. (A) At E 14, radial glia immunostained with RC2 appear organized in perpendicular fascicles spanning all the width of the cerebral wall. (B) At E17 the cerebral wall has expanded from medial to laterally. Radial glial fibres are deflected from their radial trajectory in their span through the intermediate zone. In the most lateral portion of the wall they are coursing tangentially to the pial surface but are radially reoriented throughout the cortical strata. (C–D) β-galactosidase marked migrating neurons (arrowhead) not only appear closely apposed to RC2 immunolabelled radial glia (C) but are oriented in parallel to the pathway determined by the radial glial system (D).

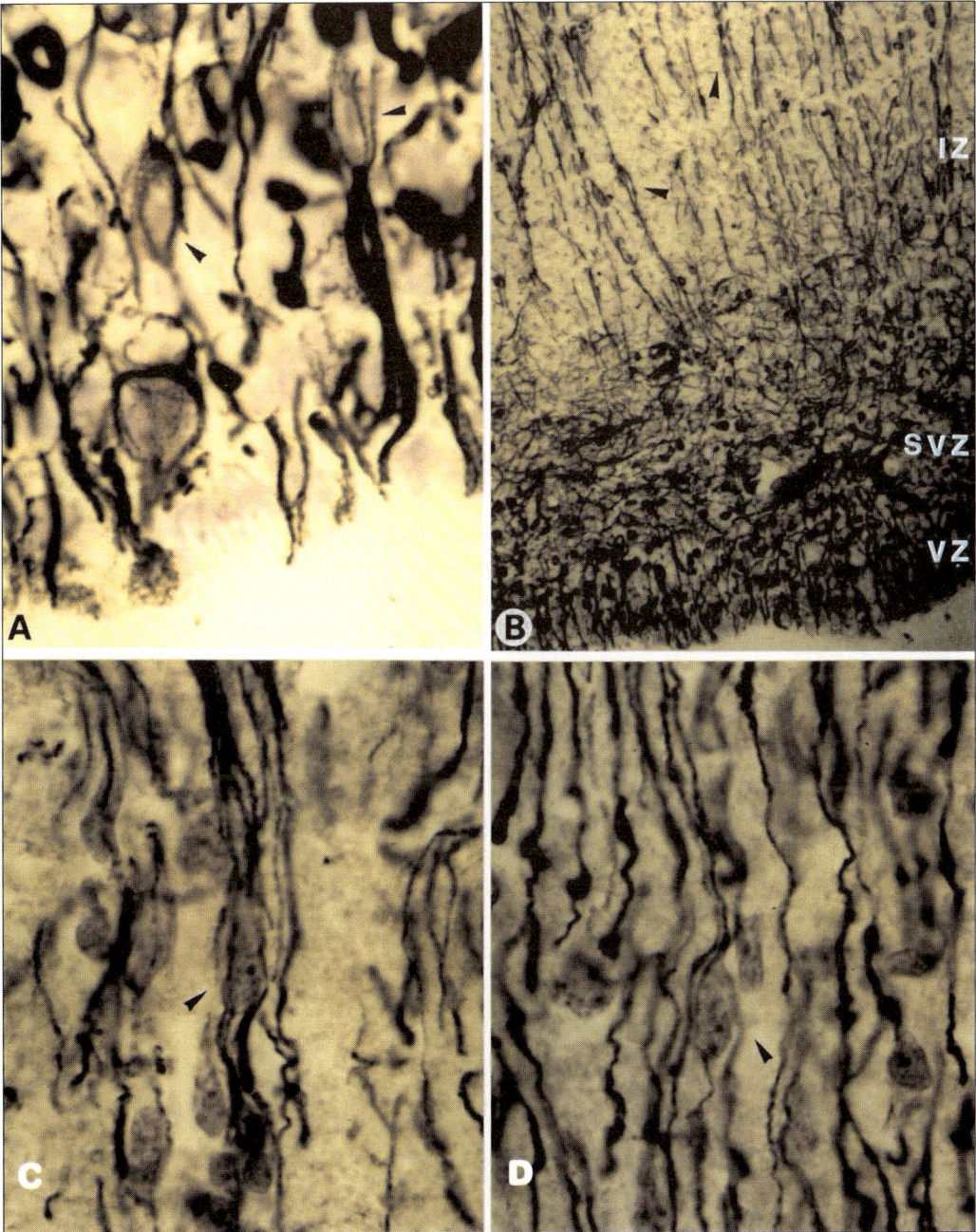

Fig. 2. Organization of the radial glial system in the human cerebral wall at 20 weeks. (A) In the ventricular zone: bipolar radial glial cells (arrowhead) identified with RC1 form a dense neuroepithelium. Descending processes form the ventricular margin. (B) In the intermediate zone, ascending processes appear grouped in parallel fascicular arrays (arrowheads) oriented towards the pia. (C) At higher magnification migrating neurons (arrowhead) appear incorporated within the glial fascicles. (D) Defasciculation occurs above the ESS. Glial fascicles break down into individual fibres. Migrating neurons (arrowhead) remain closely apposed to fibres in their final span through the cortical plate.

The fraction of postmitotic cells which exits the proliferative process increases progressively from 0.0 to 1.0 in the course of the neuronogenetic interval, with values less than 0.5 until the interval is nearly 75 per cent completed in the course of integer cycle 8. The fraction that returns to the proliferative process, P, complementary to Q decreases from 1.0 to 0.0 over the neuronogenetic interval. It is an implication of this pattern of progression of P and Q that through the initial 7–8 cycles until Q = P = 0.5, the size of the epithelium increases and the rate of neuronal exit is relatively low. It is these cycles which give rise to the infragranular layers of the cortex, layers VI and V. Subsequently, over the final three cycles with the formation of the neurons of layers IV–II, the size of the epithelium decreases and there is massive acceleration in the rate of neuronal exit. In mouse the epithelium expands approximately 50 fold before it reaches its maximum size in the course of cell cycle 8 (Takahashi *et al.*, 1996). The total multiplicative force of a single founder cell over the course of the total 11 cycles in mouse is approximately 150 fold. It may be confidently predicted that the multiplicative force of a unit of founder cells in the human brain where the neuronogenetic interval is a matter of months must be orders of magnitude greater than that in mouse (Caviness *et al.*, 1995b).

Mitosis, migration and transformation of radial glia

Neuronal migration which is associated with transformation of radial glial cells is critical to normal neocortical histogenesis. As described, the bipolar radial glia are the prevalent glial cell form during the early phase of neocortical histogenesis when neuronal migration and the assembly of the neocortical laminae are underway. At the end of the migratory epoch the radial glia are rapidly transformed into astrocytes which are prevalent through adult life. Intermediary forms in the process of transformation are monopolar forms which elaborate astrocytic processes (Misson *et al.*, 1991a; Takahashi *et al.*, 1991). The classic astrocyte then becomes the most prominent form through the remainder of development and into adult life. The present section will address this sequence of transformations and will consider their significance to histogenetic events.

Dramatic adaptations and changes in the radial glial system are reflected in the overall pattern of distribution of the radial fibres. These changes occur sequentially as development proceeds. In the interval E11 to E13 in mouse, which we will refer to as Stage I of neocortical histogenesis, there is divergence of neuronal and glial lineage. During this stage, the system of glial fascicles spanning the entire cerebral wall is already well established. Stage 2, extending from E13 to E17, corresponds to the migratory epoch. In this interval bipolar radial glial fibres become organized into fascicles. Progressively through Stage 2, there is increasing lateral deflection and divergence in the span of fibre fascicles in their ascent through the intermediate zone. The population of radial glial cells increases dramatically in number in this stage. Growth cone-tipped radial glial fibres, elaborated from postmitotic somata which are located in the VZ and probably also in the SVZ, are abundant at all levels of the intermediate zone, but there is a sharp drop in the density of the fibres in transition from IZ to the cortical strata. Stage 3 extends from E17 to the end of neuronal migration during the first two days of postnatal life in mouse. This terminal phase of migration corresponds to the period when neurons of the supragranular layers enter the cortex. This period is marked by a massive ingrowth of fibres from subcortical levels, such that the fibre density at both cortical and subcortical levels is essentially uniform. Stage 4 extends from the end of migration to the first postnatal week and is characterized by the disappearance of radial glial forms from the cerebral wall as these cells are transformed first into monopolar and finally into the classic multipolar mature astrocytic cell. The multipolar astrocytic forms contribute to the establishment of the non-radial glial network, first in the infragranular layers than in the supragranular layers.

Disorders of neuronal migration associated with epilepsy

Neuropathological studies have revealed disturbances of neuronal migration in many syndromes associated with mental and behavioural delay and epilepsy (Caviness *et al.*, 1995a). The defining neuropathological lesion is neuronal heterotopia, i.e. a clustering of neurons in abnormal position along the migratory route. Generally heterotopias are subcortical but some may extend into the cortex

(Caviness *et al.*, 1989). Heterotopia is distinguished from ectopia in which neurons have migrated beyond their appropriate cortical positions to enter the molecular layer or to form extracerebral collections within the leptomeninges (Caviness *et al.*, 1978). For some no disorder of the nervous system is suspected prior to the appearance of seizures. For others, epilepsy with seizures, varying widely in character and attack pattern, is only one feature of a gravely disabling disorder of all cerebral functions. In all instances epilepsy is a major factor in management and prognosis for adaptive existence.

In this section we will present developmental malformations associated with disordered neuronal migration. The objective will be to describe the malformations and their clinical as well as neurological presentations. We will also consider hypotheses as to mechanisms leading to these malformations. Finally, we will review the characteristics of the epilepsy associated with each of the disorders.

Periventricular heterotopia (Fig. 3-A)

Periventricular heterotopia has only recently been recognized to be associated with a specific syndrome which includes epilepsy (Raymond *et al.*, 1994; Smith, *et al.*, 1988). Although periventricular nodules have in the past been suspected on the basis of CT scans, it was the advent of MR imaging with its high sensitivity for discrimination of gray and white matter structures which has allowed confident delineation and characterization of the periventricular heterotopia in the living patient. The heterotopia may be distributed as either a discontinuous series of nodules or as a continuous band at the ventricular margin. Usually the heterotopias project into the ventricles giving rise to irregularities of the ventricular surface. They are most prevalent in the occipital horns of the lateral ventricles but may also be encountered in the temporal and frontal horns as well. There is a slightly higher proportion of bilateral cases. Typically the thickness of the neocortex appears to be normal and there are no gyral abnormalities.

Microscopically, band and nodular heterotopias appear to be formed of normally differentiated cortical neurons including both pyramidal and non-pyramidal cell forms. Several hypothesis might be proposed to explain the failure of this limited set of cells to migrate away from their site of origin in the VZ in a condition in which the majority of neurons do migrate normally. For example, it might be that the heteropic cells represent a set of late forming neurons which are defective in their cytoskeletal mechanisms of migration or neurons defective in the adhesion molecules necessary for normal neuronal to radial glial apposition and migration. The recent demonstration by Eksioglu *et al.* (1996) that periventricular heterotopia is linked to gene abnormalities in the Xq28 locus favours a mechanism of the second variety in that the Xq28 locus includes a gene responsible for synthesis of L1CAM, a molecule which is implicated in neuronal migration.

With respect to its clinical characteristics there is a female predominance supporting an X-linked dominant mode of inheritance (Dobyns *et al.*, 1996; Eksioglu *et al.*, 1996; Huttenlocher *et al.*, 1994). This would imply that the hemizygous state of the defective allele is an early embryonic lethal to affected males. Seizure characteristics are variable though partial or partial complex seizures are predominant. There is no specific EEG pattern but bursts of 3–4 Hz spike and wave activity mimicking the EEG patterns of generalized epilepsy can be observed. Usually epilepsy is delayed in appearance until the second decade of life though a few cases are described in which seizures have appeared before the age of 10. Most patients have normal early development milestones and achievements, but it is our personal experience that the disorder may be associated with learning difficulties and attention deficit disorder. Slight cognitive impairment is present in cases where migration abnormalities are diffuse.

Aicardi syndrome

The Aicardi syndrome (1965) is encountered only in females, and, like periventricular nodular heterotopia, may be an X-linked dominant disorder which is an embryonic lethal in males. Subependymal periventricular and subcortical heteropia are also characteristic of the Aicardi syndrome which

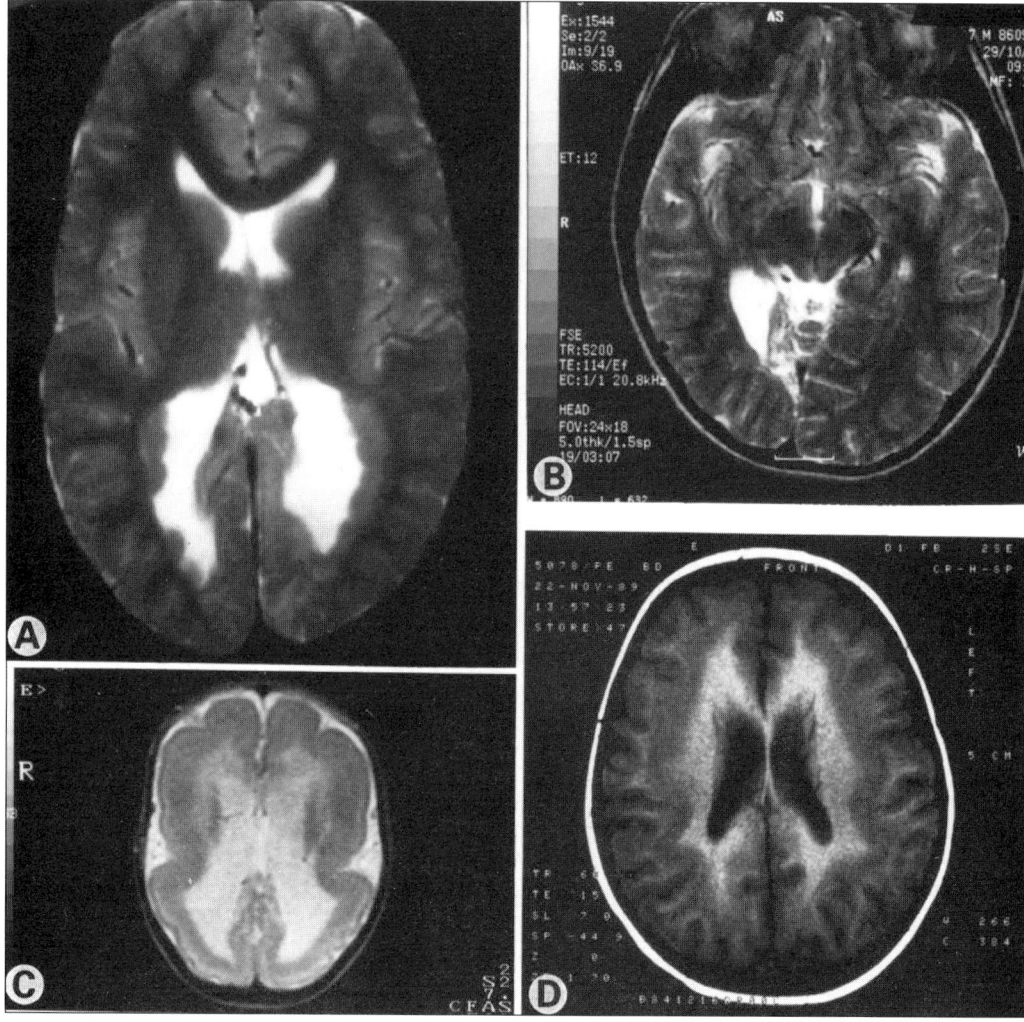

Fig. 3. Neuronal migration disorders: (A) Periventricular heterotopia: axial T1 MRI showing confluent subependymal heterotopic nodules. (B) Focal cortical dysplasia: axial T2-weighted MRI showing an increased signal in the inner face of the occipital lobe. (C) Lissencephaly–pachygyria: Surface of the brain appear smooth especially in the occipital lobes. Few broad gyri are seen in the frontal lobes. The sylvian gyri exhibit very characteristic vertical orientation. (D) Double cortex: T2-weighted images show normal cortex underlined by a continuous band of heterotopic neurons.

also includes pachygyria and polymicrogyria, agenesis of corpus callosum and retinal lacunae. The anomalies of gyrification are interpreted as resulting from abnormal neuronal migration. There is no obvious proliferation of glial cells within the cortical malformation. Affected patients are profoundly delayed in acquisition of developmental milestones. Typically the early occurrence of infantile spasms and hypsarrythmia leads to the diagnosis (Donnenfeld *et al.*, 1989).

Tuberous sclerosis

Tuberous sclerosis has a complex phenotype, variable in expression, which includes cutaneous lesions and ocular and visceral anomalies. Although the disorder is typically associated with developmental delay, cognition and behaviour may be normal and the disorder may not be suspected until revealed by the advent of seizures. In the more severely affected, seizures may be grave and intractable and may be the most disabling of the phenotypic features of tuberous sclerosis. Not uncommonly infantile spasms occur early in life and are followed by complex partial seizures as the child grows older.

Neuropathological features include, in addition to the characteristic cortical tubers, cortical dysplasia with subcortical heterotopia, subependymal heterotopic nodules and subependymal giant cell astrocytoma. In all of these lesions the density of astroglial cells is high and probably reflects glial transformation or a glial proliferation process resulting in some way from the autosomal dominant mutant gene. It is probable that early glial transformation plays a role in the disruption of neuronal migration that gives rise to heterotopia (Caviness & Takahashi, 1990).

Focal cortical dysplasia (Fig. 3-B)

The focal cortical dysplasias include a heterogeneous set of focal cortical abnormalities which are typically associated with severe epileptic disorders. Certain of these associated with giant multinucleated neuronal and glial forms with heterotopic neurons distributed both within and below the cortex are also associated with the polymorphic histological phenotype of tuberous sclerosis. The cytological features of these cells, in particular the astrocytes, suggests a disturbance of the astroglial transformation process. In other focal cortical dysplasias there is a more limited disruption of neuronal position within the cortex with malregistration of cortical laminae (Caviness *et al.*, 1995). Locally the cortex may be abnormally firm and pachygyric in appearance.

Because of focal increase in cortical width and cellularity and the typically associated signal abnormality, this malformation can be revealed by an increase in signal on MRI (Marchal *et al.*, 1989; Raymond *et al.*, 1995; Sellier *et al.*, 1987). There is no preferential regional cerebral distribution of these abnormalities. They have been encountered in frontal areas as well as in perisylvian and mesiotemporal/hippocampal and occipital cortical regions. Although this class of malformation is not common, it is important clinically because of the often associated severe and even intractable epilepsy which typically has its onset early in life. These patients have partial seizures and focal EEG abnormalities although no specific EEG pattern has been described. Some of these lesions associated with intractable epilepsy are amenable to therapeutic surgical resection.

Lissencephalic syndromes

Lissencephaly is the generic name given to a broad spectrum of malformations in which the gyrification of the cerebral surface is reduced. The degree is variable (Fig. 3-C), ranging from the presence of a few broad gyri (pachygyria) to a condition of complete absence of gyri (agyria). Modern classification recognizes two broad groups of lissencephalic disorders: the classical type I lissencephaly (agyria–pachygyria of Bielschowski and the double cortex syndrome) and type II (cobblestone lissencephaly) (Dobyns & Truwit 1995).

Type I lissencephaly. The architectonic features of type I lissencephaly are highly characteristic. The outer cerebral wall has four strata with a thick zone of heterotopic neurons (stratum 1) lying most deeply and separated from the true cortex (strata 3 and 4: marginal layer and neuronal layer) by a cell sparse zone (stratum 2). The heterotopic neurons of stratum 1 are arrested within the corona radiata, lying above the external sagittal stratum of the cerebral wall. The heterotopic population includes pyramidal and non-pyramidal cells, many of which are aligned radially with normally appearing ascending orientation (Caviness & Williams, 1979). The type I lissencephalic malformation has been associated with a heterogeneous set of genetic abnormalities, suggesting that a variety of genetic mechanisms contribute to the essential cellular events of neuronal migration.

Miller–Dieker syndrome. The prototypic genetic disorder associated with type I lissencephaly is the Miller–Dieker syndrome which has characteristic facial dysmorphic features including retrognathism, long philtrum, prominent nostrils and narrow forehead. The infant may be considered as normal or slightly hypotonic at birth, but inevitably there is severe psychomotor delay and mental retardation.

Epilepsy is virtually invariant in this syndrome and may be the first recognized manifestation. Seizures may start in the first days of life, but usually begin only after a few months. This disorder should be considered in the differential diagnosis of West Syndrome in that more than 50 per cent of infants with the Miller–Dieker malformation manifest infantile spasms. Myoclonic jerks may precede the appearance of frank spasms. At later ages seizures will be of the partial type in most patients but generalized tonic–clonic seizures are also common (Alvarez et al., 1986; Dobyns et al., 1991; Miller, 1963).

The EEG is gravely deranged and no underlying basic rhythm may be recognizable. The presence of fast activity is highly characteristic (Gastaut et al., 1987). This may be distributed as short bursts or may be continuous. This pattern usually coexists with slow irregular high voltage activity in the delta frequency range, with intermixed episodes of slow spike–wave complexes. A hypsarrythmic pattern may evolve.

A chromosomal abnormality within the 17p13.3 region is typically associated with the Miller–Dieker syndrome (Vantuinen et al., 1988). In isolated type I lissencephaly, that is, where the typical cerebral malformation is not associated with the other dysmorphic features associated with the Miller–Dieker syndrome, chromosome 17 appears 'macroscopically' normal. However, Ledbetter et al. (1992) have recently described submicroscopic deletions within the 17p13.3 region in association with non-Miller–Dieker lissencephaly I. It now appears that there is a mutated single allele located in this region, now designated the Lis-I gene, which encodes the B-subunit (45kD) of the heterotrimeric protein G, also known as platelet-activating factor (PAF) (Hattori et al., 1994; Renier et al., 1993). Recently Mizuguchi et al. (1995) have demonstrated the loss of immunoreactivity for the 45kD Lis-I protein in the brain of Miller–Dieker patients. The finding suggests that this protein is in some way essential to the cellular events of migration disrupted in the entire group of lissencephaly malformations. Multiple genetic loci in addition to the Lis-I gene may be expected to support these same cellular mechanisms. Thus, it has also recently become apparent that the lissencephalic I malformation and also the milder anomaly referred to as band heterotopia or the double cortex syndrome may also be transmitted through an X-linked mode rather than by the allele on 17p.

Subcortical band heterotopia (Fig. 3-D). Subcortical band heterotopia or the 'double-cortex syndrome' appears to represent a relatively mild extreme of the general class of migration disorder typified by the more severe classic lissencephaly type I and Miller–Dieker malformation. Though characterized architectonically as early as the late 18th and early 19th century (Mattel, 1893), it has in modern times been amenable to diagnosis in life by MRI (Barkovich et al., 1989; Livingston & Aicardi, 1990). In the 'double-cortex syndrome' as in classic lissencephaly there is a zone of heterotopic neurons positioned in the corona radiata, above the external sagittal stratum. In 'double-cortex syndrome' this zone is relatively much more narrow than the heterotopic zone in classic lissencephaly type I. Further, the true cortex is little if at all reduced in width and the pattern of gyral folding is somewhat broadened whereas in lissencephaly the true cortex is relatively narrow and there may be no gyral folding. MR imaging may suggest that the heterotopic band is separated from the cortex by a zone of apparently normal corona radiata, although such an intervening zone of white matter is not always observed.

As with periventricular nodular heterotopia most cases are female. Psychomotor development is typically delayed, and there may be severe retardation. From early school age these patients have learning difficulties and additional behavioural problems. Epilepsy makes its appearance in early childhood and may be mild or it may be intractable and gravely disabling. Patients with mild as well as severe epilepsy have been described. According to some authors increasing size of the heterotopic band and decreasing width of the true cerebral cortex are correlated with increasing gravity of mental retardation and severity of epilepsy (Barkovich et al., 1992, 1994). Several types of seizures and epilepsy have been reported. These conditions include both West and Lennox–Gastaut syndromes (Ricci et al., 1992) and also partial and generalized seizures. No specific EEG pattern has been described. Partial and generalized seizures are thought to be characteristic of cases in which there is discontinuity within the band of heterotopia so that precision in characterization of the malformation in MR images may aid in prognostic predictions.

The relatively small size of the subcortical heterotopia suggests that the disorder of migration affects a limited population of neurons undergoing migrations relatively late in the migratory epoch. The occurrence of this disorder in females, as in the case of Aicardi syndrome and subependymal nodular heterotopia, suggests that it is linked to the X chromosome, and it may be a dominant lethal with the result that affected males are eliminated early after conception (des Portes *et al.*, 1997; Pinard *et al.*, 1994).

Cobblestone type II lissencephaly and Walker–Warburg syndrome: The architecture of the cerebral wall is more severely disrupted in type II than in type I lissencephaly. The gravest of this set of disorders is the Walker–Warburg malformation which also includes the much milder though still grave cerebro–oculo–muscular or Fukuyama syndrome or HARD+/–E Fukuyama syndrome (Dobyns *et al.*, 1985, 1989; Valane *et al.*, 1994; Williams *et al.*, 1984). In the Walker–Warburg malformation the surface is faintly cobbled or frankly smooth without normal gyrification. There is a densely adherent meningoglial cicatrix which tightly encases the entire brain and penetrates as septa deeply into the brain substance. The ventricles are massively dilated. In the cerebrum septa of meningoglial tissue penetrate deeply through the cortical and subcortical plane partitioning the neuronal populations. A rudimentary true cortex of postmigratory neurons is appropriately positioned near the cerebral surface. Larger numbers of heterotopic neurons are spread through a subcortical zone, which like that in lissencephaly I appears to lie above the rudimentary external sagittal stratum within the corona radiata. In the Fukuyama disorder, there are also adhesions at the surface and disruptions of cortical laminar architecture, but these are much less severe and there is no subcortical heterotopic field. The origin of these malformations, certainly the Walker–Warburg malformation, must be early in gestation, perhaps even as early as the end of the first trimester when vigorous neuronal migration is underway.

The characteristic architectural abnormality of the Walker–Warburg malformation has been recognized in a fetus of 16 weeks personally examined by us. In this specimen no radial glial fibre system could be seen but instead there was an extensive network of astroglial fibres. Because multiple members of a sibship have been affected with the Walker–Warburg malformation the disorder may be transmitted by autosomal inheritance. This mechanism of transmission has been already established for the Fukuyama disorder.

Both the Walker–Warburg and Fukuyama malformations are associated with congenital muscular dystrophy (Rodgers, 1994; Sasaki *et al.*, 1989). Because of its extreme gravity the Walker–Warburg disorder is typically associated with still birth or death soon after birth. There is, therefore, essentially no clinical neurology of this condition. The Fukuyama condition, by contrast, is compatible with a longer survival which may extend through the third decade of life in exceptional cases. Whereas a severe and unusually generalized muscular dystrophy is the hallmark of this condition, it is important to emphasize that it is also associated with psychomotor retardation and infrequently also with seizures. The seizures are of different types and no typical EEG pattern has been described.

Zellweger syndrome

The Zellweger syndrome is associated with a characteristically anomalous gyral pattern as well subcortical and intracortical heterotopia (Evrard *et al.*, 1978; Volpe & Adams, 1972). The gyral abnormalities are restricted to the central and perisylvian regions and are bilaterally symmetrical. In the perisylvian region the pattern is microgyric and associated with a well developed cortical lamination pattern and a relatively small degree of heterotopia. By contrast, higher on the convexity in the central region the pattern becomes pachygyric, and this gyral pattern is associated with a more substantial reduction in cortical width and a larger degree of heterotopia. The distribution of the heterotopic neurons differs dramatically from patterns observed in the lissencephalic syndromes. Thus, in the Zellweger malformation heterotopic neurons are scattered through a uniform field which extends from the corona radiata subcortically into the cortex itself where the fundamental laminar patterns are reasonably well preserved. Heterotopic neurons are distributed both diffusely and as columnar aggregates through the subcortical and intracortical heterotopic region. The presence of multipolar astrocytes among the heterotopic neurons in affected fetal specimens of around 20 weeks gestation suggests that the disorder in some way provokes a premature transformation of radial glial cells into multipolar astrocytes, a transformation which might underlie the disruption of the migratory process for many of the neurons. Intact radial glial fibres are to some extent preserved, however, and may be observed coursing around neuronal aggregates (Caviness *et al.*, 1989).

Zellweger malformation is a manifestation of a defect of the peroxisomal functions, β-oxidation of very long chain fatty acids and synthesis of plasmalogen. It is probable that both of these metabolic operations, essential both to cellular energetics and membrane synthesis, are necessary to the integrity and normal operation of the neuronal and glial interactions critical to the migratory process.

The clinical phenotype of Zellweger syndrome includes high forehead, large anterior fontanelle, low nasal bridge, micrognathia and hepatomegaly. Neurological examination is dominated by severe hypotonia and poor reactivity. Stippled calcification of the patella visualized in radiographs is pathognomonic. There is also severe psychomotor retardation and generally an active seizure disorder becomes established early in infancy.

Epileptogenesis and disorders of neuronal migration

The strongest generalization that comes from this survey is that disorders of neuronal migration are characteristically associated with epilepsy. Typically seizures appear early in life and the associated seizure disorders are varied in their seizure patterns, their attack patterns and their tractability. No single feature of the epilepsy patterns appears to correlate with the specific features of the migration disorder. The migration disorders themselves are protean in nature. Although many and perhaps most reflect disordered gene action, the fundamental cellular and molecular biological mechanisms that have failed are certainly protean. An incomplete roster of the plausible attack points, the entire spectrum considered, should include disorders of cellular membranous or cytoskeletal structure, of ionic channel function, of cellular energetics, of cell–cell adhesion and of cell positional signalling.

The common feature of the entire group of malformations is that neocortical cells are malpositioned, that is, the cellular interrelationships of the final neuronal community are aberrant. This suggests that the fundamental contribution to the epileptic state, arising indirectly as a consequence of disordered migration, is perversion of cellular interrelationships. By implication, the epileptic state associated with these malformations very probably arises from the aspect of disordered cellular interactions where cellular interactions are broadly considered. Thus, a host of perverted cellular interactions might be expected to derive from the heterotopic state and to contribute to the onset and propagation of epilepsy. Among these would be those interactions which assure the normal formation of proximate and remote connections, including axonal guidance and the formation of a pattern of synaptogenesis where excitatory and inhibitory systems are appropriately balanced. Other cellular interactions that might be aberrant as a consequence of neuronal malposition might be those neuronal–glial interactions essential to normal membrane stability. Finally to be considered are those interactions with the progression of programmed cell death. A neuronal degenerative process, such as that underlying the epilepsies of the lysosomal disease, on the other hand is a less likely contributor to the epileptic state in this spectrum of disorders associated with disordered neuronal migration. With the possible exception of the Aicardi syndrome, the spectrum considered here appears to be associated with populations of neurons which are stable throughout the life span of the patient. In summary, we view the epileptic state in these disorders of migration as probably only incidental to the specific gene-determined cellular and molecular mechanisms which lead to failure of migration and heterotopia. Rather it is likely, we feel, that the epileptic state reflects the consequences of aberrancy of cellular interactions incidental to the abnormal community relationships of neurons stranded in alien territory in the course of their aborted ascent to the cortex.

Acknowledgements: The authors wish to thank Professor G. Moonen and P. Leprince for their comments, Maguy Beduin and Ginny Tosney for editing the manuscript. This work was supported by the Fonds National de la Recherche Scientifique in Belgium and a NIH Grant NS 12005.

References

Aicardi, J., Chevrie, J.-J. & Lerique-Koechlin, A. (1965): A new syndrome: Spasms in flexion, callosal agenesis, ocular abnormalities. *Electrencephal. Clin. Neurophysiol.* **19**, 609–610.

Alvarez, L.A., Yamamoto, T., Wong, B., Resnick, T.J., Liena, J.F. & Moshé, S.L. (1986): Miller–Dieker Syndrome: A disorder affecting specific pathways of neuronal migration. *Neurology* **36**, 489–493.

Angevine, J. B. & Sidman, R.L. (1961): Autoradiographic study of cell migration during histogenesis of the cerebral cortex in the mouse. *Nature* **192**, 766–768.

Barkovich, A.J. & Kjos, B.O. (1992): Gray matter heterotopis: MR characteristcs and correlation with developmental and neurologic manifestations. *Radiology* **182**, 493–499.

Barkovich, A.J., Jackson, D.E. & Boyer, R.S. (1989): Band heterotopia: a newly recognized neuronal migration anomaly. *Radiology* **171**, 455–458.

Barkovich, A.J., Gressens, P. & Evrard, Ph. (1992): Formation, maturation and disorders of brain neocortex. *AJNR* **13**, 423–446.

Barkovich, A.J., Guerrini, R., Battaglia, G., Kalifa, G., N'Guyen, T., Parmeggiani, A., Santucci, M., Givanardi-Rossi, P., Garanata,T. & D'Incerti, L. (1994): Band heterotopia: correlation of outcome with magnetic resonance immaging parameters. *Ann. Neurol.* **36**, 609–617.

Bulfone, A., Puelles, L., Porteus, M., Frohman, M., Martin, G. & Rubenstein, J. (1993): Spatially restricted expression of Dlx–1, Dlx–2 (Tes–1), Gbx–2, and Wnt–3 in the embryonic day 12.5 mouse forebrain defines potential transverse and longitudinal segmental boundaries. *J. Neurosci.* **13**, 3155–3172.

Bulfone, A., Smiga, S., Shimamura, K., Peterson, A., Puelles, L. & Rubenstein, J. (1995): T-brain–1: a homolog of brachyury whose expression defines molecularly distinct domains within the cerebral cortex. *Neuron* **15**, 63–78.

Caviness, V.S., Jr. (1982): Neocortical histogenesis in normal and reeler mice: a developmental study based upon [3H]thymidine autoradiography. *Dev. Brain Res.* **4**, 293–302.

Caviness, V.S., Jr., Misson, J.-P. & Gadisseux, J.-F. (1989): Abnormal neuronal patterns and disorders of neocortical development. In: *From Reading to Neurons*, Galaburda, A. M. (ed.), pp. 405–439. Cambridge, MA: MIT Press.

Caviness, V.S., Jr. & Takahashi, T. (1990): Cerebral lesions of tuberous sclerosis in relation to normal histogenesis. *Ann. NY Acad. Sci.* 187–194.

Caviness, V., Jr., & Williams, R. S. (1979): Cellular pathology of developing human cortex. *Research Publications Association for Research in Nervous & Mental Disease* **57**, 69–98.

Caviness, V.S., Jr., Evrard, P. & Lyon, G. (1978): Radial neuronal assemblies, ectopia and necrosis of developing cortex: a case analysis. *Acta Neuropathol. (Berl.)* **41**, 67–72.

Caviness, V.S., Jr., Takahashi, T., Nowakowski, R.S. & Tsai, L.-H. (1994): Regulated and nonregulated parameters of neocortical cytogenesis. In: *Structural and functional organization of the neocortex*, Albowitz, B., Albus, K., Kuhnt, U., Nothdurft, H.-C. & Wahle, P. (eds), pp. 8–22. Berlin: Springer Verlag.

Caviness, V.S. Jr., Hatten, M.E., McConnell, S.K. & Takahashi, T. (1995a): Epilepsy of childhood: perspectives from neurobiology. In: *Brain development and epilepsy*,Schwartzkroin, P.A., Moshé, S. L., Noebels, J. L. & Swann, J. W. (eds), pp. 94–121. Oxford: Oxford University Press.

Caviness, V.S.J., Takahashi, T. & Nowakowski, R.S. (1995b): Numbers, time and neocortical neuronogeneis: A general developmental and evolutionary model. *Trends Neurosci.* **18**, 379–383.

Crandall, J.E. & Caviness, V.S. (1984): Axon strata of the cerebral wall in embryonic mice. *Dev. Brain Res.* **14**, 185–195.

Dehay, C., Giroud, P., Berland, M., Smart, I. & Kennedy, H. (1993): Modulation of the cell cycle contributes to the parcellation of the primate visual cortex. *Nature* **366**, 464–466.

des Portes, V., Pinard, J.M., Smadja, D., Motte, J. *et al.* (1997): Dominant X linked subcortical laminar heterotopia and lissencephaly syndrome: evidence for the occurence of mutation in males and mapping of potential locus in Xq22. *J. Med. Genet.* **34**, 177–183.

Dobyns, W.B. and Truwit, C.L. (1995): Lissencephaly and other malformations of cortical development. *Neuropediatrics* **26**, 132–147.

Dobyns, W.B., Kirkpatrick, J.B., Hittner, H.M., Roberts, R.M. & Kretzer, F.L. (1985): Syndromes with lissencephaly II: Walker-Warburg and cerebro-oculo-muscular syndromes and a new syndrome with type II lissencephaly. *Am. J. Med. Genet.* **22**, 157–195.

Dobyns, W.B., Pagon, R.A., Armstrong, D., Curry, C.J.R., Greenberg, F., Grix, A. *et al.* (1989): Diagnostic criteria for Walker–Warburg Syndrome. *Am. J. Med. Genet.* **32**, 195–210.

Dobyns, W.B., Curry, C.J., Hoyme, H.E., Turlington, L. & Ledbetter, D.H. (1991): Clinical and molecular diagnosis of Miller–Dieker syndrome. *Am. J. Hum. Genet.* **48**, 584–594.

Dobyns, W.B. *et al.* (1996): X-linked malformations of neuronal migration. *Neurology* **47**, 331–339.

Donnenfeld, A.E., Packer, R.J., Zachai, E.H., Chee, C.M., Sellinger, B. & Emmanuel, B.S. (1989): Clinical, cytogenetic and pedigree findings in 18 cases of Aicardi syndrome. *Am. J. Med. Genet.* **32**, 461–467.

Edwards, M.A., Yamamoto, M. & Caviness, V.S. (1990): Organization of radial glial and related cells in the developing murine CNS. *Neuroscience* **36**, 121–144.

Eksioglu, Y.Z., Scheffer, I.E. *et al.* (1996): Periventricular heterotopia: An X-linked dominant epilepsy locus causing aberrant cerebral cortical development. *Neuron* **16**, 77–87

Erzurumlu, R.S. & Jhaveri, S. (1992): Emergence of connectivity in the embryonic rat parietal cortex. *Cereb. Cortex* **2**, 336–352.

Evrard, P., Caviness, V.S., Jr., Prats-Vinas, J. & Lyons, G. (1978): The mechanism of arrest of neuronal migration in the Zellweger malformation; an hypothesis based upon cytoarchitechtonic analysis. *Acta Neuropath.* **41**, 109–117.

Fishell, G., Mason, C.A. & Hatten, M.E. (1993): Dispersion of neural progenitors within the germinal zones of the forebrain. *Nature* **362**, 636–638.

Gadisseux, J.F. & Evrard, P. (1985): Glial neuronal relationship in the developing central nervous system: a histochemical electron microscope study of radial glial cell particulate glycogen in normal and reeler mice and the human fetus. *Dev. Neurosci.* **7**, 12–32.

Gadisseux, J.F., Evrard, P., Misson, J.P. & Caviness, V.S. (1987): Fascicular organization of radial glial fibers in developing murine neocortex: an immunocytochemical study combined with 3H-thymidine autoradiography. *Soc. Neurosci. Abst.* **13**, 1117.

Gadisseux, J.F., Evrard, P., Misson, J.P. & Caviness, V.S. J. (1989a): Dynamic changes in the density of radial glial fibers of the developing murine cerebral wall: a quantitative immunohistological analysis. *J. Comp. Neurol.* **322**, 246–254.

Gadisseux, J.-F., Evrard, P., Misson, J.-P. & Caviness, V.S. (1989b): Dynamic structure of the radial glial fiber system of the developing murine cerebral wall. An immunocytochemical analysis. *Dev. Brain Res.* **50**, 56–67.

Gadisseux, J.F., Kadhim, H.J., van den Bosch, P., Caviness, V.S.J. & Evrard, P. (1990): Neuron migration within the radial glial fiber system of the developing murine cerebrum: an electron microscopic autoradiographic analysis. *Dev. Brain Res.* **52**, 39–56.

Gastaut, H., Pinsard, N., Raybaud, C., Aicardi, J. & Zifkin, B. (1987): Lissencephaly (agyria-pachygyria): Clinical findings and serial EEG studies. *Dev. Med. Child Neurol.* **29**, 167–180.

Hattori, M., Adachi, H., Tsujimoto, M., Arai, H. & Inoue, K. (1994): Miller–Dieker lissencephaly gene encodes a subunit of brain platelet-activating factor. *Nature* **370**, 216–218.

Huttenlocker, P.R., Taravath, S. & Mojtahedi, S. (1994): Periventricular heterotopia and epilepsy. *Neurology* **44**, 51–55.

Kornack, D.R. & Rakic, P. (1995): Radial and horizontal deployment of clonally related cells in the primate neocortex: relationship to distinct mitotic lineages. *Neuron* **15**, 311–321.

Ledbetter, S.A., Kuwano, A., Dobynsm W,B. & Ledbetter, D.H. (1992): Microdeletions of chromosome 17p13 as a cuase of isolated lissencephaly. *Am. J. Hum. Genet.* **50**, 182–189.

Levinson, S.W. & Goldman, J.E. (1993): Both oligodendrocytes and astrocytes develop from progenitors in the subventricular zone of the postnatal rat forebrain. *Neuron* **10**, 201–212.

Livingston, J.H. & Aicardi, J. (1990): Unusual MRI appearance of diffuse subcortical heterotopia or 'double cortex' in two children. *J. Neurol. Neurosurg. Psychiatry* **53**, 617–620

Marchal, G., Andermann, F., Tampieri, D., Robitaille, Y., Melanson, D., Sinclair, B., Olivier, A., Silver, K. & Langevin, P. (1989): Generalized cortical dysplasia manifested by diffusely thick cerebral cortex. *Arch. Neurol.* **46**, 430–434.

Marin-Padilla, M. (1978): Dual origin of the mammalian neocortex and evolution of the cortical plate. *Anat. Embryol.* **159**, 161–206.

Mattel, M. (1893): Ein Fall von Heterotopie der grauen Substanz in den beiden Hemispheren des Grosshirns. *Arch. Psychiatr. Nevenkr.* **25**, 124–136.

Miller, J.Q. (1963): Lissencephaly in two siblings. *Neurol.* **13**, 841–856.

Mione, M.C., Danevic, C., Boardman, P., Harris, B. & Parnavelas, J.G. (1994): Lineage analysis reveals neurotransmitter (GABA or glutamate) but not calcium-binding protein homogeneity in clonally related cortical neurons. *J. Neurosci.* **14**, 107–123.

Misson, J.-P., Edwards, M.A., Yamamoto, M. and Caviness, V.C., Jr. (1988): Mitotic cycling of radial glial cells of the fetal murine cerebral wall: A combined autographic and immunohistochemical study. *Dev. Brain Res.* **38**, 183–190.

Misson, J-P., Edwards, M.A., Yamamoto, M. & Caviness, V.S., Jr. (1998b): Identification of radial glial cells within the developing murine central nervous system. Studies based upon a new immunohistochemical marker. *Dev. Brain Res.* **44**, 95–108.

Misson, J.-P., Takahashi, T. & Caviness, V.S., Jr. (1991a): Ontogeny of radial and other astroglial cells in murine cerebral cortex. *Glia* **4**, 138–148.

Misson, J.-P., Austin, C.P., Takahashi, T., Cepko, C.L. & Caviness, V.S. (1991b): The alignment of migrating neural cells in relation to the murine neopallial radial glial fiber system. *Cerebral Cortex* **1**, 221–229.

Mizuguchi, M., Takashima, S., Kakita, A., Yamada, M. & Ikeda, K. (1995): Lissencephaly gene product: localizationin the central nervous system and loss of immunoreactivity in Miller–Dieker syndrome. *Am. J. Pathol.* **147**, 1142–1151.

Molnar, Z. & Blakemore, C. (1995): How do thalamic axons find their way to the cortex? *Trends Neurosci.* **18**, 389–397.

O'Leary, D.D.M., Schlaggar, B.L. & Tuttle, R. (1994): Specification of neocortical areas and thalamocortical connections. In: *Annual Rev. Neurosci.*, Cowan, W.M., Shooter, E.M., Stevens, C.F. &. Thompson, R.F. (eds), pp. 419–439. Palo Alto, CA: Annual Reviews, Inc.

O'Rourke, N.A., Sullivan, D.P., Kaznowski, C., Jacobs, A.A. & McConnell, S.K. (1995): Tangential migration of neurons in the developing cerebral cortex. *Development* **121**, 2165–2176.

Pinard, J.M., Motte, J., Chiron, C., Brian, R., Andermann, E. & Dulac, O. (1994): Subcortical laminar heterotopia and lissencephaly in two families: a single X linked dominant gene. *J. Neurol. Neurosurg. Psychiatry* **57**, 914–920.

Pinto-Lord, M.C., Evrard, P. & Caviness, V.S. (1982): Obstructed neuronal migration along radial glial fibers in the neocortex of the reeler mouse: a Golgi-EM analysis. *Dev. Brain Res.* **4**, 379–393.

Puelles, L & Rubenstein, J. (1993): Expression patterns of homeobox and other putative regulatory genes in the embryonic mouse forebrain suggest a neuromeric organization. *Trends Neurosci.* **16**, 472–479.

Rakic, P. (1972): Mode of cell migration to the superficial layers of fetal monkey neocortex. *J. Comp. Neurol.* **145**, 61–84.

Rakic, P. (1974): Neurons in rhesus monkey visual cortex: systematic relation between time of origin and eventual disposition. *Science* **183**, 425–427.

Rakic, P. (1988): Specification of cerebral cortical areas. *Science* **241**, 170–176.

Rakic, P., Stensaas, L.J., Sayer, E.P. & Sidman, R.L. (1974): Computer aided 3-dimensional reconstruction and quantitative analysis of cells from serial electron microscopic montage of foetal monkey brain. *Nature* **250**, 31–34.

Raymond, A.A., Fish, D.R., Stevens, J.M., Sisodiya, S.M., Alsajari, N. & Shorvon, S.D. (1994): Subependymal eheterotopia: A distinct neuronal migration disorder associated with epilepsy. *J. Neurol. Neurosurg. Psychiatry* **57**, 1195–1202.

Raymond, A.A., Fish, D.R., Sisodiya, S.M., Alsanjari, N., Stevens, J.M. & Shorvon, S.D. (1995): Anormalities of gyration, heterotopias, focal cortical dysplasia, microdysgenesis, dysembryoplastic neuroepithelial tumour and dysgenesis of the archicortex in epilepsy. *Brain* **118**, 629–660.

Reiner, O., Carrozo, R., Shen, Y., Wehnert, M., Faustinella, F., Dobyns, W.B., Caskey, C.T. & Ledbetter, D.H. (1993): Isolation of a Miller–Dieker lissencephaly gene containing G Protein B-Subunit-like repeats. *Nature* **364**, 717–721.

Ricci, S., Cusmai, R., Fariello, G., Fusco, L. & Vigevano, F. (1992): Double cortex: a neuronal migration anomaly as possible cause of Lennox–Gastaut syndrome. *Arch. Neurol.* **49**, 61–64.

Rodgers, B.L., Vanner, L.V., Pai, G.S. & Sens, M.A. (1994): Walker-Warbury syndrome: Report of three affected sibs. *Am. J. Med. Genet.* **49**, 198–201.

Sasaki, M., Yoshioka, K., Yanagisawa, T., Nemoto, A., Takasago, Y. & Nagano, T. (1989): Lissencephaly with congenital muscular dystrophy and ocular abnormalities: Ceebro–oculo–muscular syndrome. *Child's Nerv. Syst.* **5**, 35–37.

Sauer, F.C. (1936): The interkinetic migration of embryonic epithelial nuclei. *J. Morphol.* **60**, 1–11.

Sauer, M.E. & Walker, B.E. (1959): Radioautographic study of interkinetic nuclear migration in the neural tube. *Proc. Soc. Ext. Biol. (NY)* **101**, 557–560.

Schmechel, D.E. & Rakic, P. (1979a): A Golgi study of radial glial cells in developing monkey telencephalon: morphogenesis and transformation into astrocytes. *Anat. Embryol.* **156**, 115–152.

Schmechel, D.E. & Rakic, R. (1979b): Arrested proliferation of radial glial cells during midgestation in rhesus monkey. *Nature* **277**, 303–305.

Schwartz, M.L., Rakic, P. & Goldman-Rakic, P. S. (1991): Early phenotype expression of cortical neruons: evidence that a subclass of migrating neurons have callosal axons. *Proc. Nat. Acad. Sci. (USA)* **88**, 1354–1358.

Sellier, N., Kalifa, G., Lalande, G., Demange, P., Ponsot, G., Dulac, O. & Robain, O. (1987): Focal cortical dysplasia. A rare cause of epilepsy. *Ann. Radiol.* **30**, 439–445.

Shimamura, K., Hartigan, D., Martinez, S., Puelles, L. & Rubenstein, J. (1995): Longitudinal organization of the anterior neural plate and neural tube. *Development* **121**, 3923–3933.

Sidman, R. L. & Rakic, P. (1973): Neuronal migration, with special reference to developing human brain: a review. *Brain Res.* **62**, 1–35.

Smith, A.S., Weinstein, M.A., Quencer, R.M. *et al.* (1988): Association of heterotopic gray matter with seizures. *MR Imaging Radiology* **168**, 195–198.

Takahashi, T., Misson, J.-P. & Caviness, V. S. (1991): Glial process elongation and branching in the developing murine neocortex: a qualitative and quantitative immunohistochemical analysis. *J. Comp. Neurol.* **302**, 15–28.

Takahashi, T., Nowakowski, R.S. & Caviness, V.S., Jr. (1992): BUdR as an S-phase marker for quantitative studies of cytokinetic behaviour in the murine cerebral ventricular zone. *J. Neurocytol.* **21**, 185–197.

Takahashi, T., Nowakowski, R.S. & Caviness, V.S., Jr. (1993): Cell cycle parameters and patterns of nuclear movement in the neocortical proliferative zone of the fetal mouse. *J. Neurosci.* **13**, 820–833.

Takahashi, T., Nowakowski, R.S. & Caviness, V.S.J. (1995a): The cell cycle of the pseudostratified ventricular epithelium of the murine cerebral wall. *J. Neurosci.* **15**, 6046–6057.

Takahashi, T., Nowakowski, R.S. & Caviness, V.S.J. (1995b): Early ontogeny of the secondary proliferative population of the embryonic murine cerebral wall. *J. Neurosci.* **15**, 6058–6068.

Takahashi, T., Nowakowski, R.S. & Caviness, V.S.J. (1996b): The leaving or Q fraction of the murine cerebral proliferative epithelium: a general computational model of neocortical neuronogenesis. *J. Neurosci.* **16**, 6183–6196.

Takahashi, T., Nowakowski, R. & Caviness, V. (1997): The mathematics of neocortical neuronogenesis. *Dev. Neurosci.* **19**, 17–22.

Tan, S.-S. & Breen, S. (1993): Radial mosaicism and tangential cell dispersion both contribute to mouse neocortical development. *Nature* **362**, 638–640.

Tan, S.-S., Faulkner-Jones, B., Breen, S.J., Walsh, M., Bertram, J.F. & Reese, B.E. (1995): Cell dispersion patterns in different cortical regions studied with an X-inactivated transgenic marker. *Development* **121**, 1029–1039.

Valane, L., Pihko, H., Katevuo, K., Karttunen, P., Somer, H. & Santavuori, P. (1994): MRI of the brian inmuscle-eye-brain disease. *Neuroradiol.* **36**, 473–476

Vantuinen, P., Dobyns, W.B., Rich, D.C., Summers, K.M., Robinson, T.J., Nakamura, Y. & Ledbetter, D.H. (1988): Lolecular detection of microscopic and submicroscopic demetions associated with Miller–Dieker syndrome. *Am. J. Hum. Genet.* **43**, 587–596.

Volpe, J.J. & Adams, R.D. (1972): Cerebro-hepato renal syndrome of Zellweger. An inherited disorder of neuronal migration. *Acta Neuropath.* **20**, 175–198.

Waechter, R.V. & Jaensch, B. (1972): Generation times of the matrix cells during embryonic brain development: an autoradiographic study in rats. *Brain Res.* **46**, 235–250.

Walsh, C.A. (1996): Neural development: identical twins separated at birth? *Curr. Biol.* **6**, 26–28.

Walsh, C. & Cepko, C.L. (1993): Clonal dispersion in proliferative layers of developing cerebral cortex. *Nature* **362**, 632–635.

Williams, R.S., Swisher, C.N., Jennings, M., Ambler, M. & Caviness, V.S.J. (1984): Cerebro-ocular dysgenesis (Walker–Warburg syndrome): neuropathologic and etiologic analysis. *Neurology* **34**, 1531–1541.

Chapter 6

Structural and functional causes of neuronal hyperexcitability in a rat model of cortical migration disorder

Heiko J. Luhmann[1], Nik Karpuk[1], Robert-Alexander Reiprich[1], Petra Schwarz[1] and Christine C. Stichel[2]

[1]*Institute of Neurophysiology, and* [2]*Department of Neurology, University of Düsseldorf, PO Box 101007, D–40001 Düsseldorf, Germany*

Summary

Neocortical structural abnormalities due to developmental disturbances are often the cause of therapy-resistant seizure activity. Since clinical studies are technically limited in the analysis of the cellular mechanisms underlying this hyperexcitability, animal models of cortical dysplasia are useful tools to study structural and functional modifications associated with neuronal migration disorders. A focal freeze lesion to the cerebral cortex of the newborn rat produces a cortical malformation, which resembles in its anatomy human polymicrogyria. As in humans, the rat dysplastic cortex is characterized by an atypical lamination and irregular neurons. Intracellular *in vitro* recordings in neocortical slices from freeze-lesioned rats reveal an unusual spontaneous activity and upon orthodromic synaptic stimulation epileptiform responses. This recurrent epileptiform activity is predominantly mediated by activation of N-methyl-D-aspartate receptors. In contrast to previous observations in human dysplastic cortex, our immunocytochemical studies in the rat model did not reveal a significant loss in the number of parvalbumin-labelled neurons. Other factors, like changes in the density of postsynaptic receptors, may contribute to the enhanced excitability of the dysplastic cortex.

The recent advances in neuroimaging permit the recognition of structural malformations, which were previously unrecognized or only detected by neuropathologists after neurosurgical interventions or after the patient's death (Palmini *et al.,* 1991a; Lee *et al.,* 1994). Developmental malformations can be observed in a large number of central nervous structures, like the cerebellum, hippocampus and cerebral cortex (for review see Barth, 1987; Barkovich *et al.,* 1992). Recent imaging data indicate that these malformations are much more common than was previously estimated and that they are involved in different mental disorders and diseases, like learning disabilities, autism and especially epilepsy (for review see Aicardi, 1994; Ciaranello & Ciaranello, 1995). Developmental malformations are most prominent in pharmaco-resistant epilepsy, which represents 20–30 per cent of all epileptic syndromes. Approximately 20 per cent of the adult patients with therapy-resistant epilepsy who underwent neurosurgery showed obvious structural abnormalities in cortical structures referred to as neuronal migration disorders (NMD). In children, the relative proportion was even higher (Kuzniecky *et al.,* 1993), indicating that pharmaco-resistant epilepsy due to NMD represents a major problem during early ontogenesis. Although the improvement in neuroimaging techniques emphasized the abundance of these structural disorders in the developing brain, hardly anything is known about the cellular mechanisms underlying the hyperexcitability of tissue showing NMD. In this chapter we address the question, which structural and functional factors may contribute to long-term hyperexcitability in cerebral cortex showing NMD? To answer this question, we use an animal model initially described by Dvorak and Feit in 1977 (Dvorak & Feit, 1977; Dvorak *et al.,* 1978).

Methods

Induction of focal cortical malformation

The techniques used to induce focal NMD in rat cerebral cortex were similar to those described in our previous report (Luhmann & Raabe, 1996). We used a modification of the model described by Dvorak & Feit (1977). Newborn Wistar rats were anaesthetized by hypothermia, the skin above the frontoparietal cortex was cut and a small liquid nitrogen-cooled copper cylinder was brought into contact with the exposed calvarium for 2–10 s. The wound was closed with histoacryl tissue glue. Sham-operated animals were operated in the same way with the exception that the copper cylinder was not cooled. Animals survived for 1–4 months before they were used for anatomical, immunocytochemical or *in vitro* electrophysiological studies.

Slice preparation and recording techniques

The methods used for preparing and maintaining neocortical slices *in vitro* were similar to those described previously (Luhmann & Heinemann, 1992). Coronal 400 µm thick slices of the frontoparietal cortex were cut in cold oxygenated artificial cerebrospinal fluid (aCSF) with a Dosaka vibratome. The bathing solution (aCSF) contained (in mM): 124 NaCl, 3 KCl, 1.25 NaH_2PO_4, 1.8 $MgSO_4$, 1.6 $CaCl_2$, 26 $NaHCO_3$, 10 glucose, pH 7.4 when saturated with 95 per cent O_2–5 per cent CO_2. Intracellular recordings were obtained from cells located in the upper layers with sharp microelectrodes filled with 2 M potassium acetate (60 to 120 MΩ). In dysplastic cortex, intracellular recordings were performed at 200–800 µm lateral and medial to the malformation. Cells were examined in their excitatory and inhibitory synaptic input. A bipolar tungsten stimulating electrode (3–5 MΩ, FHC, Brunswick, USA) was positioned below the recording site at the border with the white matter. Voltage pulses of 200 µs duration and 5–20 V in amplitude were delivered to the stimulating electrode at a frequency of ≤ 0.1 Hz. The stimulus intensity was gradually increased and adjusted to a value which elicited an excitatory postsynaptic potential (EPSP) of 5–15 mV in peak amplitude. To elicit an inhibitory postsynaptic potential (IPSP), stimulus intensity was increased to twice the threshold value for orthodromically evoking an action potential at resting membrane potential. This protocol is appropriate to reveal a biphasic IPSP, consisting of the $GABA_A$ receptor-mediated fast (f-) IPSP and the $GABA_B$-mediated late (l-) IPSP (Luhmann & Prince, 1991). The participation of N-methyl-D-aspartate (NMDA) and (±)-α-amino–3-hydroxy–5-methylisoxazole–4-propionic acid (AMPA) receptors in stimulus-evoked synaptic responses was studied by applying the selective antagonist DL–2-amino–5-phosphonovaleric acid (APV, Sigma, Basel, Switzerland) and 6-nitro–7-sulphamoyl-benzo(f)quinoxaline–2,3-dione (NBQX, Novo Nordisk), respectively. APV (300 µM) and NBQX (100 µM) were dissolved in aCSF and applied locally on the slice surface close to the recording site via a broken micropipette with a tip diameter of 5–10 µm.

Anatomy and immunocytochemistry

For anatomical studies, sham-operated and NMD animals were perfusion-fixed with 4 per cent paraformaldehyde and the cortical regions showing the malformations were cut along the coronal plane on a cryotome at 40–50 μm. These sections were Nissl-stained and analysed by the use of a light microscope.

For immunocytochemistry, animals were perfused transcardially with a saline flush followed by ice-cold 4 per cent paraformaldehyde. Brains were removed and post-fixed for 2–4 h. After cryoprotection with 30 per cent sucrose at 4 °C overnight, 40–50 μm coronal sections were cut on a cryotome and washed with 0.01 per cent phosphate-buffered saline (PBS). Endogenous peroxidase was blocked with 0.5 per cent H_2O_2 in PBS for 30 min. Sections were preincubated at room temperature for 30–60 min in 10 per cent normal horse serum (Vector Labs, Camon, Wiesbaden, Germany) with 0.3 per cent Triton X–100 in PBS and then washed with 0.01 M PBS (pH 7.4). Sections were incubated overnight at 4 °C in anti-parvalbumin (mouse, clone PA–235, Sigma) at a dilution of 1:1000 in PBS with 0.3 per cent Triton X–100 and 10 per cent normal horse serum. After washing in PBS, sections were incubated for 1 h at room temperature in a biotinylated anti-mouse antibody (Vector Labs) at a dilution of 1:100 and then in an avidin-biotin complex (1:100, PK–4000 kit, Vector Labs). The reaction product was visualized with 0.02 per cent 3,3´-diaminobenzidine (Sigma) as the chromogen.

Extracellular biocytin staining and histological procedures

Neurons were labelled extracellularly by injecting small biocytin (Sigma) crystals with a needle into the slice at various locations (white matter or different cortical layers). Slices were kept in the recording chamber for at least 6 h to optimize the quality of the staining. After that period, slices were immersion-fixed in 4 per cent paraformaldehyde in 0.1 M phosphate buffer, pH 7.4, for > 24 h. After washing and cryoprotection, slices were resectioned at 40–50 μm on a freezing vibratome, processed overnight with ABC peroxidase reagent (PK–4000 kit, Vector Labs) and air-dried before mounting them on gelatine-coated slides. For a detailed description of the histological protocol see Schröder & Luhmann (1997).

Results and discussion

Malformations and atypical cellular morphology

Local freeze lesions to the cerebral cortex of newborn rats caused focal malformations in the cortical architecture which resembled in their pathology some forms of neuronal migration disorders (NMD) described in humans (for review see Barth, 1987; Kuzniecky, 1994). Neuropathological studies on neocortical tissue removed surgically for the treatment of pharmaco-resistant epilepsy (Taylor et al., 1971; Cordero et al., 1994) as well as post mortem examinations (Virchow, 1867; Matell, 1893; McBride & Kemper, 1982; Meencke & Janz, 1984; Meencke & Gerhard, 1985) indicate that 'malformations of cortical development' (Kuzniecky & Barkovich, 1996) may have a focal or more diffuse appearance. The cortical malformation obtained with the present animal model resembles in many aspects the pathological pattern described in human polymicrogyria. However, we succeeded in producing other forms of cortical abnormalities, like clefts in the cerebral cortex from the pia to the white matter (schizencephaly) and local ectopic cell aggregates (focal heterotopia), by modifying our freezing protocol. Polymicrogyria refers to irregular cortical gyration with small abnomal gyri and loss of the normal six-layered structure (one, two, three or four laminae). Figure 1 illustrates a focal malformation in adult rat cerebral cortex showing the appearance of a three-layered cortex. As in humans, the upper lamina shows the normal low density of neurons, followed by a cell-rich middle layer and a cell-sparse third lamina (see for comparison Figs. 5 and 6 in Kuzniecky & Barkovich, 1996). Toxoplasmosis, maternal hypoxia, chromosomal modifications (Hattori et al., 1994), metabolic disorders, lesions and other conditions have been associated with polymicrogyria, suggesting that this cortical malformation may be caused by a large number of different processes.

Morphological studies on individual neurons obtained from human dysplastic cortex have shown that NMD are often associated with an atypical organization and position of neuronal and glial cells. Giant bipolar or pyramidal so-called *balloon cells* are present in large numbers in the white and grey matter

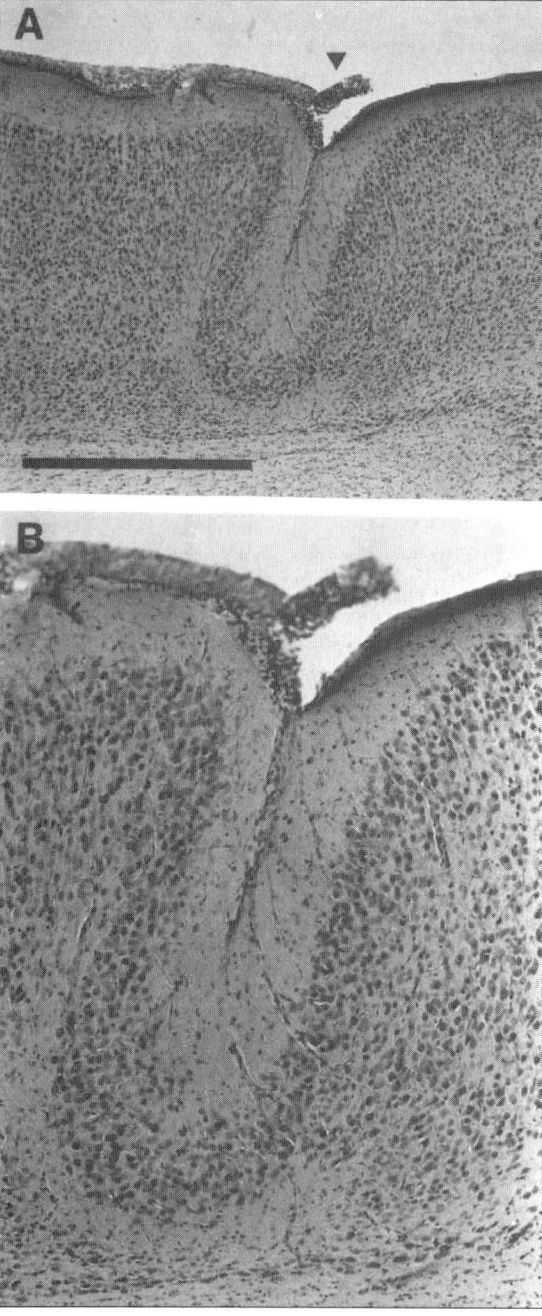

Fig. 1. Nissl-stained coronal section of focal cortical malfomation in adult rat somatosensory cortex following neonatal freeze lesioning. Note abnormal infolding and loss of normal six-layered structure (▼). This experimentally induced malformation resembles in its structural appearance human polymicrogyria. Scale bar in A refers to 800 μm in A and 400 μm in B.

(Taylor et al., 1971; Palmini et al., 1991b). These cells have soma diameters of up to 80 μm, reveal abnormal dendritic arborizations and are reactive to neuronal and glial markers. Confocal laser scanning and subsequent three-dimensional reconstructions of single Lucifer yellow-stained neurons in surgically resected specimens from epileptic patients have shown that pyramidal-like neurons in dysplastic cortex often show an atypical orientation and two or three thick apical dendrites ('*dinosaur cells*') (Belichenko et al., 1994). These large bizarre cells are immunoreactive for antibodies against microtubule-associated protein 2 (MAP2) (Yamanouchi et al., 1996). Since MAP2 plays an important role in the generation of neuronal processes during early development (Ferreira et al., 1990), the increased expression of MAP2 in adult dysplastic cortex may reflect a sustained plasticity of these large neurons. Pyramidal-like cells with atypical orientation and thick dendrites can be also observed in our rat model of focal cortical dysplasia (see ⇑ in Fig. 2B). These cells can be detected in the grey and white matter, where they transverse with their dendritic processes over large territories through the white matter (not shown).

Pathophysiology of the dysplastic cortex

In humans, NMD in cortical structures are often associated with severe hyperexcitability, like pharmaco-resistant epilepsy (Palmini et al., 1991c). Surgical removal of the focal abnormalities frequently results in a significant improvement and a marked reduction in seizure frequency, when 50 per cent or more of the structural lesion can be removed (Palmini et al., 1991b). These data indicate that the structural abnormalities observed in dysplastic cortex, like the atypical *balloon* and *dinosaur cells*, may represent the cellular basis for the pronounced hyperexcitability and pharmaco-resistance. In order to understand the cellular physiology and network interactions of the dysplastic cortex, we performed intracellular recordings in neocortical slices obtained from sham-operated and freeze-lesioned rats. In agreement with our previous extracellular observations (Luhmann & Raabe, 1996), single cells in dysplastic cortex were characterized by their unusual spontaneous activity (Fig. 3). Depolarizing spontaneous postsynaptic potentials (PSPs) could be recorded at membrane potentials between –100 and –50 mV (Fig. 3B). These events increased in amplitude and duration at membrane potentials positive to –60 mV (compare PSP recorded at –95 mV [⇑] with PSP at –59 mV [↓]), indicating a voltage-dependence in the activation of the postsynaptic receptor–ionophore complex. The pharmacology of the postsynaptic responses was studied in stimulus-evoked PSPs. Orthodromic synaptic stimulation of supragranular neurons recorded in neocortical slices from sham-operated rats elicited at resting membrane potentials the characteristic monophasic EPSP, which did not last longer than 50–80 ms (Fig. 4A1). Application of APV did not influence the amplitude or time course of this response (Fig. 4A2), indicating that NMDA receptors were not activated at resting membrane potentials in normal cortex. Addition of NBQX to the bathing solution completely

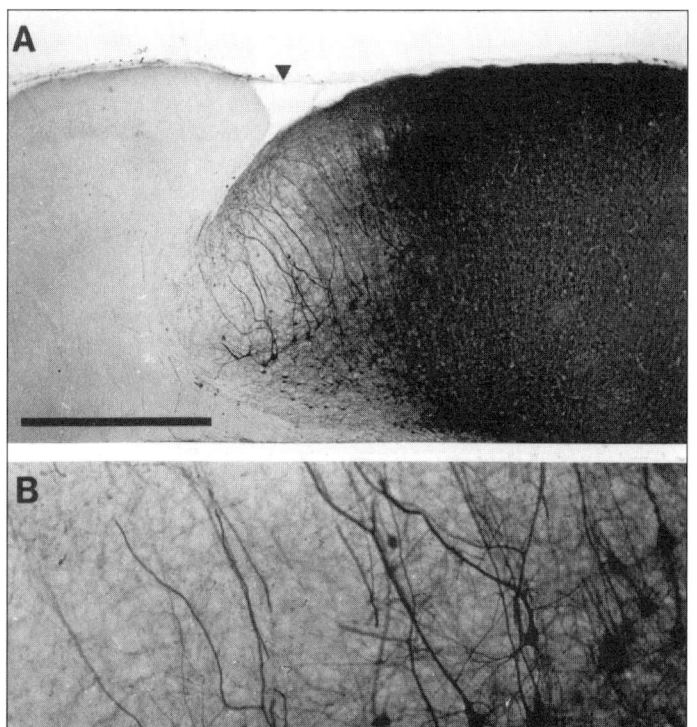

Fig. 2. Abnormal morphology of neurons in rat dysplastic cortex. Cells were labelled in a neocortical slice preparation by a large extracellular biocytin injection lateral to the focal malformation (▼). Panel B shows at a higher magnification the biocytin-labelled cells from A. Note horizontally oriented pyramidal-type neuron (⇑), which lies in close vicinity to other pyramidal neurons with relatively normal morphology. Scale bar in A corresponds to 800 μm in A and 200 μm in B.

blocked the stimulus-evoked response, suggesting that the EPSP was exclusively mediated by AMPA receptors (Fig. 4A3). Very similar synaptic stimulus protocols elicited in neurons recorded in dysplastic cortex led to a different response. In normal ACSF and at resting membrane potentials negative to –80 mV, low intensity stimuli evoked polyphasic responses lasting more than 300 ms (Fig. 4B1). These delayed and large depolarizing potentials often activated one or several action potentials (see arrow in Fig. 4B1). Application of APV blocked most of the delayed and long-lasting response, however, the initial EPSP was still polyphasic and longer in duration as compared to the controls (Fig. 4B2). Addition of NBQX to the APV-containing bathing solution blocked all postsynaptic responses, suggesting that stimulus-evoked EPSPs recorded in dysplastic cortex are mediated by AMPA and NMDA receptors (Fig. 4B3). These results are in very good agreement with previous observations by Jacobs et al. (1996), using the same freeze lesion model in rat cerebral cortex. Whether a similar pathophysiological and APV-sensitive pattern also exists in human dysplastic cortex remains to be

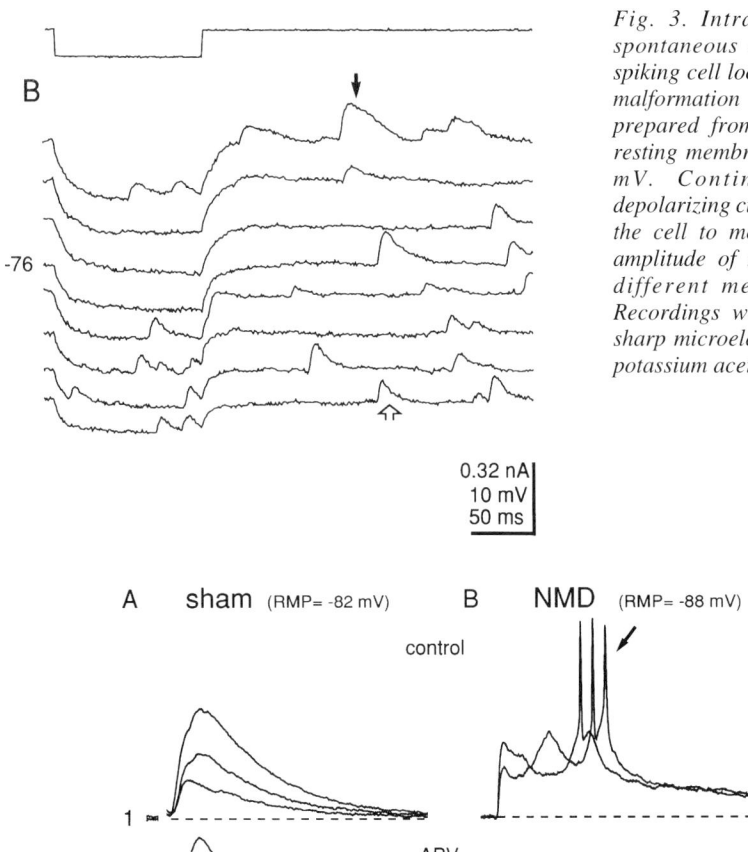

Fig. 3. Intracellularly recorded spontaneous activity in a regular spiking cell located close to the focal malformation in a neocortical slice prepared from an adult rat. Cell's resting membrane potential was –76 mV. Continuous hyper- and depolarizing current was injected into the cell to monitor changes in the amplitude of spontaneous events at different membrane potentials. Recordings were performed with a sharp microelectrode filled with 2 M potassium acetate.

Fig. 4. Stimulus-evoked excitatory postsynaptic potentials (EPSPs) recorded in a neocortical slice obtained from an adult sham-operated rat (A) and an age-matched animal with focal neuronal migration disorders (NMD) (B). Resting membrane potential (RMP) was –82 and –88 mV, respectively. Orthodromic synaptic stimulation of the afferents at three different stimulus intensities elicits in the slice from the sham-operated rat under control conditions a monophasic EPSP which lasts approximately 70 ms (A1). In the animal with NMD, a comparable stimulation evokes a multiphasic EPSP which persists for more than 200 ms and triggers delayed action potentials (B1). Application of the NMDA receptor antagonist APV does not profoundly influence the EPSP recorded in the cell from the sham-operated rat (A2), but blocks the delayed epileptiform responses in the NMD cortex (B2). Addition of the AMPA antagonist NBQX to the APV-containing bathing solution blocks all stimulus-evoked responses.

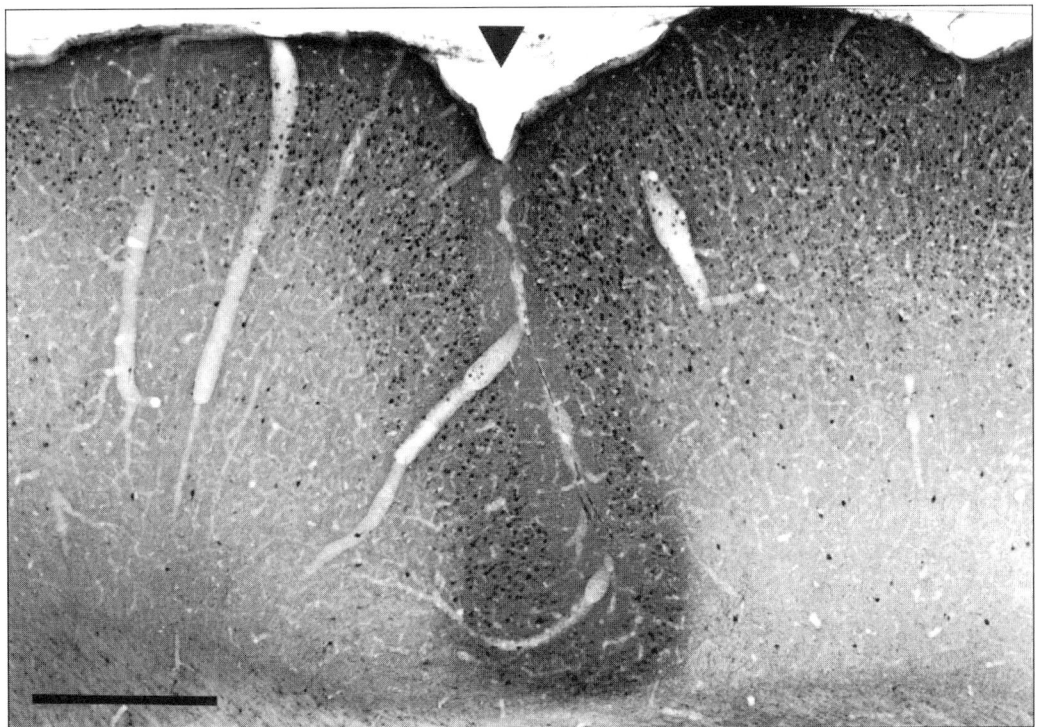

Fig. 5. Distribution of parvalbumin (PV)-stained neurons in a coronal section through the parietal cortex of a rat with focal cortical malformation (▼). High densities of PV-labelled cells can be detected in the microgyrus due to local infolding and in layers II/III of the surrounding cortex with normal layering. Scale bar refers to 500 μm.

analysed. Mattia *et al.* (1995) performed extra- and intracellular *in vitro* recordings from human dysplastic temporal neocortical slices and observed in 4-aminopyridine containing aCSF spontaneous epileptiform discharges, which were absent in slices obtained from patients suffering from temporal lobe epilepsy with Ammon's horn sclerosis and normal neocortex. These observations suggest that the human dysplastic cerebral cortex shows severe pathophysiolgical activity under *in vitro* conditions.

Role of the GABAergic system

An NMDA receptor-mediated hyperexcitability can be easily observed in slices prepared from normal rodent cerebral cortex when the efficacy of the intracortical inhibitory system is slightly reduced by application of minor concentrations of γ-aminobutyric acid (GABA) antagonists. A 10–20 per cent blockade of the $GABA_A$ receptor by low concentrations of bicuculline methiodide causes propagating epileptiform activity in rat neocortical slices (Chagnac-Amitai & Connors, 1989). In immature cortex and partially disinhibited adult cortex, these responses can be blocked by NMDA antagonists, suggesting that the activation of NMDA receptors is controlled by the GABAergic system (Luhmann & Prince, 1990). Therefore a structural and/or functional impairment of GABAergic inhibition may be involved in the generation of epileptiform NMDA receptor-mediated activity in dysplastic cortex. Abnormalities in the morphology and a loss of parvalbumin- and calbindin D–28k-immunoreactive neurons have been described in human neocortical dysplasia associated with focal drug-resistant epilepsy (Ferrer *et al.*, 1992, 1994), suggesting that a loss of at least these two subpopulations of inhibitory interneurons may contribute to a local disinhibition. A marked reduction in the number of parvalbumin-labelled neurons in dysplastic cortex has been also described in the rat freeze lesion model (Jacobs et al., 1996), indicating that similar structural modifications occur in experimentally induced NMD. In contrast to these results, our own immunocytochemical studies did not reveal a loss of parvalbumin-positive neurons in dysplastic cortex (Fig. 5). Counts of parvalbumin-labelled neurons up to 3 mm lateral and medial from the focal malformation did not reveal a statistically significant difference when compared to the controls. Our results suggest that at least this subpopulation of inhibitory local circuit neurons shows a relatively normal distribution and that other GABAergic cell types may contribute to a loss of inhibitory function in dysplastic cortex.

In summary, the clinical and experimental observations obtained from human dysplastic cortex and animal models of NMD suggest that the pronounced hyperexcitability results from a number of structural and functional modifications. (1) Large neurons with an atypical dendritic branching pattern are located throughout the cortex and in the underlying white matter. These neurons may form local excitatory networks which may act as trigger zones for pathophysiological activity. (2) Glutamate receptors may be altered in their functional properties, thereby causing enhanced excitability. The prominent activation of NMDA receptors at hyperpolarized membrane potentials (negative to −80 mV) may suggest molecular changes in the receptor subunit composition (Monyer et al., 1994). (3) The inhibitory control function of the GABAergic system may be impaired in dysplastic cortex. This disinhibition may result from functional and/or molecular changes in $GABA_A$ and $GABA_B$ receptors or loss of inhibitory interneurons.

Acknowledgements: This work was supported by DFG grant SFB 194/B4 to H.J.L.

References

Aicardi, J. (1994): The place of neuronal migration abnormalities in child neurology. *Can. J. Neurol. Sci.* **21**, 185–193.

Barkovich, A. J., Gressens, P. & Evrard, P. (1992): Formation, maturation, and disorders of brain neocortex. *Am. J. Neuroradiol.* **13**, 423–446.

Barth, P. G. (1987): Disorders of neuronal migration. *Can. J. Neurol. Sci.* **14**, 1–16.

Belichenko, P., Sourander, P. & Dahlström, A. (1994): Morphological aberrations in therapy-resistant partial epilepsy (TRPE): Confocal laser scanning and 3D reconstructions of Lucifer Yellow injected atypical pyramidal neurons in epileptic human cortex. *Mol. Neurobiol.* **9**, 245–252.

Chagnac-Amitai, Y. & Connors, B. W. (1989): Horizontal spread of synchronized activity in neocortex and its control by GABA-mediated inhibition. *J. Neurophysiol.* **61**, 747–758.

Ciaranello, A. L. & Ciaranello, R. D. (1995): The neurobiology of infantile autism. *Annu. Rev. Neurosci.* **18**, 101–128.

Cordero, M. L., Ortiz, J. G., Santiago, G., Negrón, A. & Moreira, J. A. (1994): Altered GABAergic and glutamatergic transmission in audiogenic seizure-susceptible mice. *Mol. Neurobiol.* **9**, 253–258.

Dvorak, K. & Feit, J. (1977): Migration of neuroblasts through partial necrosis of the cerebral cortex in newborn rats – contribution to the problems of morphological development and developmental period of cerebral microgyria. *Acta Neuropathol. (Berl.)* **38**, 203–212.

Dvorak, K., Feit, J. & Jurankova, Z. (1978): Experimentally induced focal microgyria and status verrucosus deformis in rats – pathogenesis and interrelation. Histological and autoradiographical study. *Acta Neuropathol. (Berl.)* **44**, 121–129.

Ferreira, A., Busciglio, J., Landa, C. & Caceres, A. (1990): Ganglioside-enhanced neurite growth: evidence for a selective induction of high-molecular-weight MAP-2. *J. Neurosci.* **10**, 293–302.

Ferrer, I., Pineda, M., Tallada, M., Oliver, B., Russi, A., Oller, L., Noboa, R., Zujar, M. J. & Alcantara, S. (1992): Abnormal local-circuit neurons in epilepsia partialis continua associated with focal cortical dysplasia. *Acta Neuropathol. (Berl.)* **83**, 647–652.

Ferrer, I., Oliver, B., Russi, A., Casas, R. & Rivera, R. (1994): Parvalbumin and calbindin-D28k immunocytochemistry in human neocortical epileptic foci. *J. Neurol. Sci.* **123**, 18–25.

Hattori, M., Adachi, H., Tsujimoto, M., Arai, H. & Inoue, K. (1994): Miller–Dieker lissencephaly gene encodes a subunit of brain platelet-activating factor. *Nature* **370**, 216–218.

Jacobs, K. M., Gutnick, M. J. & Prince, D. A. (1996): Hyperexcitability in a model of cortical maldevelopment. *Cereb. Cortex* **6**, 514–523.

Kuzniecky, R. I. (1994): Magnetic resonance imaging in developmental disorders of the cerebral cortex. *Epilepsia* **35**, S44-S56.

Kuzniecky, R. I. & Barkovich, A. J. (1996): Pathogenesis and pathology of focal malformations of cortical development and epilepsy. *J. Clin. Neurophysiol.* **13**, 468–480.

Kuzniecky, R., Murro, A., King, D., Morawetz, R., Smith, J., Powers, R., Yaghmai, F., Faught, E., Gallagher, B. & Snead, O. C. (1993): Magnetic resonance imaging in childhood intractable partial epilepsies: pathologic correlations. *Neurol.* **43**, 681–687.

Lee, N., Radtke, R. A., Gray, L., Burger, P. C., Montine, T. J., DeLong, G. R., Lewis, D. V., Oakes, W. J., Friedma, A. H. & Hoffaman, J. M. (1994): Neuronal migrations disorders: positron emission tomography correlations. *Ann. Neurol.* **35**, 290–297.

Luhmann, H. J. & Heinemann, U. (1992): Hypoxia-induced functional alterations in adult rat neocortex. *J. Neurophysiol.* **67**, 798–811.

Luhmann, H. J. & Prince, D. A. (1990): Control of NMDA receptor-mediated activity by GABAergic mechanisms in mature and developing rat neocortex. *Dev. Brain Res.* **54**, 287–290.

Luhmann, H. J. & Prince, D. A. (1991): Postnatal maturation of the GABAergic system in rat neocortex. *J. Neurophysiol.* **65**, 247–263.

Luhmann, H. J. & Raabe, K. (1996): Characterization of neuronal migration disorders in neocortical structures. I. Expression of epileptiform activity in an animal model. *Epilepsy Res.* **26**, 67–74.

Matell, M. (1893): Ein Fall von Heterotopie der grauen Substanz in den beiden Hemisphären des Grosshirns. *Arch. Psychiatr. Nervenkr.* **25**, 124–136.

Mattia, D., Olivier, A. & Avoli, M. (1995): Seizure-like discharges recorded in human dysplastic neocortex maintained in vitro. *Neurol.* **45**, 1391–1395.

McBride, M. C. & Kemper, T. L. (1982): Pathogenesis of four-layered mycrogyric cortex in man. *Acta Neuropathol. (Berl.)* **57**, 93–98.

Meencke, H. J. & Gerhard, C. (1985): Morphological aspects of aetiology and the course of infantile spasms (West syndrome). *Neuropediatrics* **16**, 59–66.

Meencke, H. J. & Janz, D. (1984): Neuropathological findings in primary generalized epilepsy: a study of eight cases. *Epilepsia* **25**, 8–21.

Monyer, H., Burnashev, N., Laurie, D. J., Sakmann, B. & Seeburg, P. H. (1994): Developmental and regional expression in the rat brain and functional properties of four NMDA receptors. *Neuron* **12**, 529–540.

Palmini, A., Andermann, F., Aicardi, J., Dulac, O., Chaves, F., Ponsot, G., Pinard, J. M., Goutières, F., Livingston, J., Tampieri, D., Andermann, E. & Robitaille, Y. (1991a): Diffuse cortical dysplasia, or the 'double cortex' syndrome: the clinical and epileptic spectrum in 10 patients. *Neurol.* **41**, 1656–1662.

Palmini, A., Andermann, F., Olivier, A., Tampieri, D. & Robitaille, Y. (1991b): Focal neuronal migration disorders and intractable partial epilepsy: results of surgical treatment. *Ann. Neurol.* **30**, 750–757.

Palmini, A., Andermann, F., Olivier, A., Tampieri, D., Robitaille, Y., Andermann, E. & Wright, G. (1991c): Focal neuronal migration disorders and intractable partial epilepsy: a study of 30 patients. *Ann. Neurol.* **30**, 741–749.

Schröder, R. & Luhmann, H. J. (1997): Morphology, electrophysiology and pathophysiology of supragranular neurons in rat primary somatosensory cortex. *Eur. J. Neurosci.* **9**, 163–176.

Taylor, D. C., Falconer, M. A., Bruton, C. J. & Corsellis, J. A. N. (1971): Focal dysplasia of the cerebral cortex in epilepsy. *J. Neurol. Neurosur. Psychiat.* **34**, 369–387.

Virchow, R. (1867): Heterotopie der grauen Hirnsubstanz. *Arch. Path. Anat. Physiol.* **38**, 138–142.

Yamanouchi, H., Zhang, W. X., Jay, V. & Becker, L. E. (1996): Enhanced expression of microtubule associated protein 2 in large neurons of cortical dysplasia. *Ann. Neurol.* **39**, 57–61.

Chapter 7

Prenatal treatment with methylazoxymethanol in rats: a model for cortical malformation associated with epilepsy?

N. Chevassus-au-Louis, A. Rafiki, P. Congar, I. Jorquera, Y. Ben-Ari, J.L. Gaïarsa and A. Represa

INSERM U29, Université Paris 5, 123 Bd Port-Royal, 75 014 Paris, France

Summary

Pharmaco-resistant childhood epilepsies are frequently associated with cortical malformations. Here, we review arguments supporting the idea that prenatal treatment with methylazoxymethanol (MAM) in rats provides a valuable model for the study of these disorders. These arguments include: (i) morphological studies indicating that MAM rats have microcephaly, disorganization of cortical lamination and presence of cortical heterotopiae; (ii) behavioural studies showing that MAM rats have learning disabilities and a lower seizure threshold, but no spontaneous seizures; (iii) electrophysiological data suggesting that the cortex of MAM rats is hyperexcitable, although no epileptogenic focus was identified. We conclude that MAM rats are appropriate model to study the propagation, but not the initiation, of paroxysmal activity in malformed brains.

In humans, cortical malformations are one of the most severe causes of childhood epilepsy (Taylor *et al.*, 1971; Mischel *et al.*, 1995; see also Chapter 8 in the present volume). These epilepsies are often drug-resistant and their treatment require surgical ablation of the dysplasic regions. However the outcome of these interventions is not fully successful, and surgery cannot be performed in case of very diffuse malformation. Therefore, new drugs efficient on children with epileptogenic cortical malformations are to be developed, which require an appropriate animal model to test them. Here, we review data showing that prenatal treatment with methylazoxymethanol (MAM) in rats provides such a model of cortical malformation associated with epilepsy.

Methylazoxymethanol disrupts neurogenesis

Methylazoxymethanol is a natural compound isolated from nuts and leaves of tropical cycads, which is highly carcinogen due to its ability to alkylate nucleic acids. As a consequence, MAM is specifically toxic to cells in the course of DNA replication, and is therefore an antimitotic agent. For presently unknown reasons, this antimitotic effect seems to be observed only with neuroblasts and not with other cell types such as myoblasts (Cattaneo *et al.*, 1995). These properties have allowed its use as a tool for experimentally targeted cellular ablation by injecting MAM at the peak of neurogenesis of

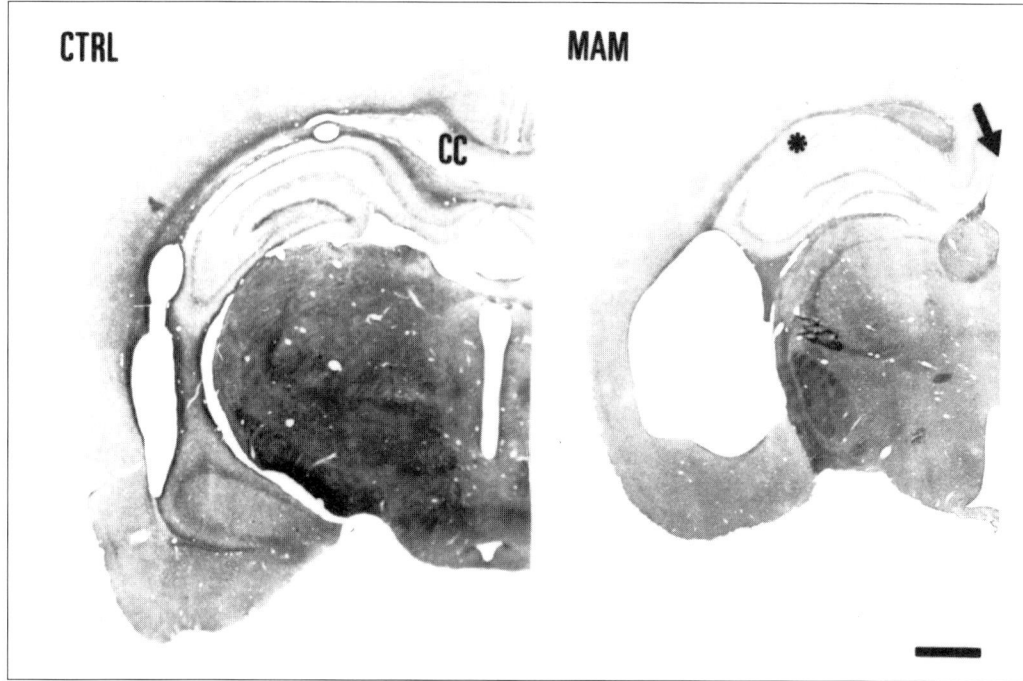

Fig. 1. Luxol staining of coronal sections of adult control and MAM rats. Note the microcephaly, the partial corpus callosum (CC) agenesis (arrow), the ventricle enlargement and the presence of periventricular and hippocampal heterotopiae (star). Scale bar: 800 µ.

the population to be ablated (Cattabeni & Di Luca, 1997). When injected intraperitoneally at embryonic day 14 to the pregnant female, MAM is able to pass the placental barrier within 2 h, and remains available for 24 h (Matsumoto et al., 1972). The main action of MAM is to kill dividing cells in the proliferative neuroepithelium that gives rise at this date to telencephalic structures such as striatum and neocortex.

Cerebral alterations in MAM animals[*]

Histopathological features

When examined 48 h after MAM injection, the brains of foetuses show a marked cell death in the proliferative neuroepithelium (Johnston & Coyle, 1979a), which confirms the antimitotic effect of MAM. This is further confirmed by the fact that dying cells are those that incorporated thymidine just before the MAM injection (Yurkewicz et al., 1984). By contrast, postmitotic cells, such as neuroblats of the cortical plate and radial glia, are spared (Zhang et al., 1995). This is an important difference with another popular model of diffuse cortical malformation obtained by prenatal X-ray irradiation at E14. In this model, the pattern of malformation is roughly similar to that of MAM rats, but embryologic studies have shown that young postmitotic neurons were also affected by the treatment (Hicks et al., 1959; Ferrer et al., 1984). At E18, the necrotic regions in the neuroepithelium have been cleaned by microglia (Ashwell, 1992), and the proliferative neuroepithelium has regenerated (Zhang et al., 1995). Therefore, the production of cells of cerebral structures formed after this date, such as the cerebellum, is not primarily affected by the MAM injection (Chen et al., 1986).

---

[*] In the rest of this Chapter, MAM rats refer to rats with prenatal injection of 25 mg/kg MAM at E14 or E15 with first gestation day as E0.

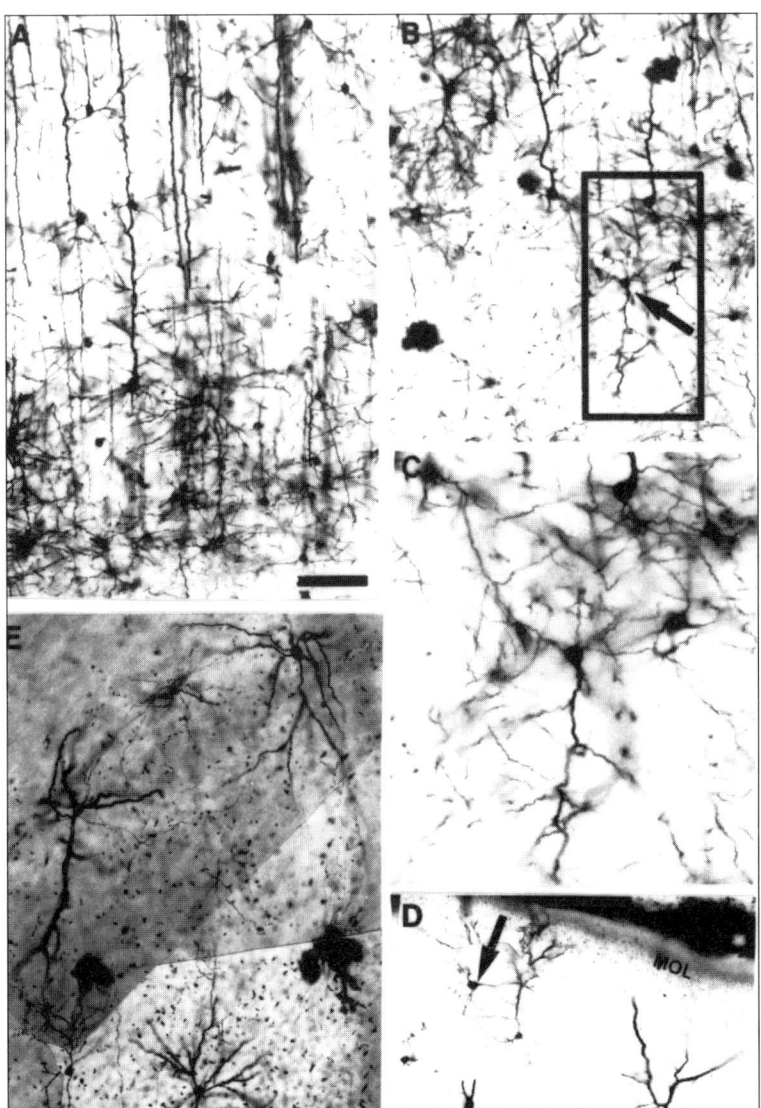

Fig. 2. Golgi staining in the neocortex of an adult control rat (A), in the neocortex of a MAM animal (B and D) and in a periventricular heterotopiae of a MAM rat (E). Note the presence of abnormally oriented (arrow in D) or even inversely oriented neuron (arrow in B, shown at a higher magnification in (C) in the neocortex of MAM rats. Periventricular heterotopiae contain pyramidal spiny neurons with abnormal shape and non-pyramidal neurons.
Scale bar: 100 μ. MOL: molecular layer.

In adult MAM animals, a clear reproducible pattern of diffuse cortical malformation is observed (Johnston & Coyle, 1979; Dambska et al., 1982). It includes (Fig. 1) microcephaly, cortical thinning with alterations of the laminar organization and abnormal dendritic orientations, ventricle enlargement, partial agenesis of the corpus callosum and presence of numerous heterotopic masses (Collier & Ashwell, 1993). Neocortical alteration is not uniform: frontal regions that have been formed earlier in neurogenesis have been spared by MAM injection and are organized almost normally (Ferrer et al., 1982). Cortical heterotopiae are found beneath the corpus callosum and in the hippocampal CA1 region. It should be noted that giant abnormal neurons characteristic of cortical dysplasia (Taylor et al., 1971) have never been described in MAM rats, which indicates that MAM brains are malformed but not dysplasic (Robain, 1996).

There is secondary damage to structures connected with the malformed neocortex (Ashwell, 1987). For example, a marked size reduction of the thalamic dorsal lateral geniculate nucleus, which was spared by initial MAM injection, was demonstrated as a consequence of the alteration of its main projection target, the visual cortex (Ashwell, 1987).

Astrocytes appear normal (Eriksdotter-Nilsson et al., 1986). Vascular abnormalities including modifications of sinovenous junctions (Bardosi et al., 1985) and high variability in the density of radial vessels (Bardosi et al., 1987) were noted. This pattern of malformation can be analysed as a consequence of a neurogenesis disorder further associated with neuronal migration disorders (heterotopiae) and neuronal differenciation disorders (abnormal neuronal shape, see Fig. 2).This pattern is very close to what is observed in several human syndromes interpreted as early neurogenesis troubles such as Aicardi syndromes or holoprosencephaly (Billette de Villemeur et al., 1992; Robain, 1996).

How does cortical connectivity establish in such an altered neocortex? Tract tracing studies have shown that the main cortical afferent projections were conserved and tended to reorganize in a smaller volume. For instance, callosal connections conserved a bilaminar organization in layers 5 and 6 instead of two/three and five/six (Yurkewicz et al., 1984). However, fine connectivity tuning such as that of thalamic afferents in the barrel neocortex was lost as a consequence of cellular disorganization in the target area, the granular somatosensory neocortex (Jones et al., 1982; Robertson et al., 1990). Another example of finely abnormal projections concerns the retinofugal projection which connects to its normal target, the thalamic dorsal lateral geniculate nucleus, but also to the adjacent dorso-parietal nucleus (Ashwell, 1986). A normal pattern of efferent projections was also conserved. For example, large pyramidal cells of layer 5 normally projected to the spinal cord, even when heterotopically situated in periventricular cortical heterotopiae (Jensen & Killackey, 1984; Yurkewicz et al., 1984). This indicates that despite marked laminar desorganization, the pattern of connections is essentially conserved in the malformed neocortex.

Neurochemical disorders

Cortical malformation in MAM animals is associated with several neurochemical disorders. Biochemical studies have long shown that MAM cortex contains an excessive amount of catecholamine and serotonin per weight unit of brain tissue, but a normal amount per whole brain (Johnston et al., 1981; Jonsson & Hallman, 1982; Matsutani et al., 1980). This was interpreted as a consequence of the fact that spared catecholaminergic and serotoninergic nuclei (locus coeruleus and raphe), which were formed before MAM injection, send the same number of fibres to the reduced cortex. Anatomical studies have confirmed this hyperdensity of catecholaminergic fibres in the cortex of MAM animals (Johnston et al., 1979; Zoli et al., 1990). The functional consequences of this abnormality are poorly understood, and actually depend on the extent of catecholaminergic receptors down-regulation (Beaulieu & Coyle, 1982; Watanabe et al., 1990, 1992). This feature is of great clinical relevance because hyperinnervation by serotoninergic and noradrenalinergic fibres was also found in human dysplasic cortex resected from patients with temporal lobe epilepsy (Trottier et al., 1994; Trottier et al., 1996).

An other important neurochemical disorder in MAM brains involves the presynaptic mechanisms of glutamate release. In normal brain, glutamate release is controled at the presynaptic level by the GAP 43/B50 protein, which can be regulated by phosphorylation by the membrane protein Phosphokinase C (PKC). In MAM cortex, a permanently altered translocation of PKC (Caputi et al., 1996) increasing the membrane bound fraction of the enzyme was noted, in addition to a permanent low level of phosphorylation of GAP 43/B50 (Di Luca et al., 1991, 1995). These biochemical alterations lead to a permanent upregulation of synaptic glutamate release (Di Luca et al., 1997) in both control and evoked conditions. The physiological consequences of these abnormalities, which are not associated with glutamate receptors down-regulation (Tamaru et al., 1992; Rafiki et al., 1998), are under investigation, and may support hyperexcitability and lack of plasticity in malformed brains (Cattabeni et al., 1994).

Behavioural disorders and epileptic syndromes in MAM animals

For two decades, prenatal treatment with MAM has been used as a model for the study of mental retardation associated with cortical malformations (Haddad et al., 1969). Indeed, juvenile as well as adult MAM animals exhibit learning impairments and cognitive disorders (Rabe & Haddad, 1972; Vorhees et al., 1984). This is reminiscent of the dramatic mental retardation found in patients with diffuse cortical malformation. By contrast, some other neonatal disorders in MAM rats such as hyperkinesy have a favourable evolution and are no longer observed in adults (Balduini et al., 1986).

The use of MAM animals as an experimental model for epilepsy was initially rejected because spontaneous behavioural seizures have never been reported at any age in these animals. However, several recent investigations on threshold for seizure induction in MAM animals have challenged this view. The main results are summarized on Table 1. Together, they show that the seizure threshold of MAM animals is decreased at a certain age for all convulsants tested to date. This decreased seizure threshold mimics the situation prevailing in humans where the presence of a cortical malformation is revealed after a first seizure caused by a usually non-convulsant stimulus, such as hyperventilation, fever or stress.

Table 1. A summary of litterature on seizure threshold in P15 and adult MAM rats. Together, they suggest that MAM animals have a lower threshold but that the maturation of this increased sensitivity depends on the type of convulsant that is used

Convulsant	Kainic acid	Pentylenetetrazole	Biccuculine	Hyperthermia	Flurothyl
P15	Increased De Feo et al.(1995)	Decreased Chevassus-au-Louis (unpublished data)	Increased De Feo et al.(1995)	Increased Germano et al. (1996b)	Not tested
Adults	Unchanged De Feo et al., 1995 Chevassus-au-Louis et al. (1998)	Increased Chevassus-au-Louis et al. (1998)	Unchanged De Feo et al.(1995)	Not tested	Increased Baraban & Schwartzkroin (1996)

It is important to emphasize that the maturation of MAM rats' seizure threshold varies with the convulsant agents. For example, the sensitivity to kainic acid (KA), a glutamate agonist, is increased at P15 (De Feo et al., 1995; Germano et al., 1996a) but normal in adults (De Feo et al., 1995; Chevassus-au-Louis et al., 1998a), whereas the sensitivity to pentylenetetrazole (PTZ), a $GABA_A$ antagonist, is decreased at P15 (unpublished data) but increased in adults (Chevassus-au-Louis et al., 1998a). This situation can be related to the high variability in the age of occurrence of the first seizure in children with cortical malformation.

However, these results suffer a major criticism: this increased seizure threshold may only reflect an increased cerebral concentration of injected drug in the microcephalic MAM brain (same amount of drug in a smaller brain leading to increased concentration). Electroencephalographic studies coupled with a study of seizure threshold for non-chemical convulsants such as kindling are required to determine if there is indeed hyperexcitability in the MAM brain (Roper et al., 1995, 1997).

Pathophysiological mechanisms of epilepsy in MAM animals

There are two distinct ways to approach the issue of the pathophysiological mechanisms of epileptogenesis in malformed cortex. It is possible either to investigate the cellular endogenous properties of neurons in the malformed regions or to study the properties of abnormal networks. Reports with both these approaches have appeared in the last two years.

The cellular approach: are there intrinsic bursting cells in the cortex of MAM animals?

This approach relies on the demonstration that cortical neurons from surgically resected human neocortex (Palmini et al., 1995) display spontaneous burst discharges in the presence of 4-amino pyridine, suggesting an alteration of endogenous cellular properties supporting epileptogenic discharges. However, the unability to perform fine pharmacological investigations in this technically difficult preparation as well as the absence of appropriate control tissue have raised the interest for animal models.

Indeed, similar abnormal bursting properties have been found in MAM animals in some pyramidal neurons of the CA1 region (Baraban & Schwartzkroin, 1995), and in the abnormal pyramidal neurons of neocortical periventricular heterotopiae (Franceschetti *et al.*, 1996) in the presence of a high K^+ concentration. These data suggest that these regions could constitute epileptic foci. However, a major condition for the formation of an epileptogenic focus would be the ability of these neurons to fire synchronously, which has never been demonstrated to date.

The network approach: is the MAM rat hippocampus intrinsequely epileptogenic?

Given the key role played by hippocampus in epilepsy, our group has focused its interests on the role played by hippocampal heterotopiae in epileptogenic disorders. We have shown that these regions are formed by supragranular neocortical neurons that settle in the CA1 field of the hippocampus after an abnormal migration. Anatomical studies show that these heterotopic neurons conserve a neocortical phenotype and do not express hippocampal markers (Chevassus-au-Louis *et al.*, 1998a). They also retain an afferent functional projection from the corpus callosum, as if they were normally situated. Furthermore, they are integrated in the hippocampal network, and receive functional connections from the perforant pathway and the Schaffer's collaterals. We conclude that neocortical heterotopiae situated in the hippocampus are integrated in both the neocortical and the hippocampal circuitry (Chevassus-au-Louis *et al.*, 1998b), which offers them a key role for facilitating the spreading of hippocampal discharges to the neocortex and therefore the generalization of seizures.

Functional consequences of this dual integration have been investigated by monitoring cerebral activation by fos immunohistochemistry in vivo after seizure induction in adult MAM animals (Chevassus-au-Louis *et al.*, 1998a). When clonic seizures were caused by PTZ injection, fos expression was noted in the thalamus, in the whole neocortex and in CA1 heterotopiae, but not in the rest of the hippocampus. This confirms the integration of CA1 heterotopiae in the neocortical circuitry. By contrast, after limbic seizures induced by KA, fos expression was noted in the hippocampus and in the neocortex, but was five-fold more important in CA1 heterotopiae as compared to the adjacent neocortex. This indicates that cortical heterotopiae are metabolically hyperactive during seizures, and this is in agreement with the assumption that cortical heterotopiae contribute to the generalization of seizures. Further electroencephalographic studies are necessary to confirm this point. Three days after the KA-induced status epilepticus, cell death was observed in the CA1 region and was very prominent in CA1 cortical heterotopiae, which confirms that they are integrated in the hippocampal network.

Concluding remarks

Prenatal treatment with MAM provides rats with neuropathological alterations reminiscent of severe human neurogenesis disorders. These animals suffer cognitive disorders and have a lower seizure threshold. These MAM animals offer a convenient, reproducible and inexpensive model for the study of the physiological consequences of cortical malformation, including epilepsy. Since these animals have a lower seizure threshold, they may offer interesting clues on the mechanisms of propagation of paroxysmal activity in the malformed neocortex. However, little is known about the regions where paroxysmal activity is initiated, which may be related to the absence of spontaneous seizures in MAM rats.

References

Ashwell, K.W.S. (1986): An abnormal retinal projection to the lateral posterior nucleus in micrencephalic rats. *Neurosci. Lett.* **72**, 7–13.

Ashwell, K.W.S. (1987): Direct and indirect effects on the lateral geniculate nucleus neurons of prenatal exposure to methylazoxymethanol acetate. *Dev. Brain Res.* **35**, 199–214.

Ashwell, K.W.S. (1992): The effects of prenatal exposure to methylazoxymethanol acetate on microglia. *Neuropathol. Appl. Neurobiol.* **18**, 610–618.

Balduini, W., Cimino, M., Lombardelli, G., Abbrachio, M.P., Peruzzi, G., Cecchini, T., Gazzanelli, G.C. & Cattabeni, F. (1986): Microencephalic rats as a model for cognitive disorders. *Clin. Neuropharmacol.* **9**, S8-S18.

Baraban, S.C. & Schwartzkroin, P.A. (1995): Electrophysiology of CA1 pyramidal neurons in an animal model of neuronal migration disorders: prenatal methylazoxymethanol treatment. *Epilepsy Res.* **22**, 145–156.

Baraban, S.C. & Schwartzkroin, P.A. (1996): Flurothyl seizure susceptibility in rats following prenatal methylazoxymethanol treatment. *Epilepsy Res.* **23**, 189–194.

Bardosi, A., Ambach, G. & Fiede, R.L. (1985): The angiogenesis of microencephalic rat brains caused by methylazoxymethanol acetate. I: Superficial venous system. A quantitative analysis. *Acta Neuropathol. (Berl.)* **66**, 253–263.

Bardosi, A., Ambach, G. & Hann, P. (1987): The angiogenesis of the micencephalic rat brains caused by methylazoxymethanol acetate. III. Internal angioarchitecture of cortex. *Acta Neuropathol. (Berl.)* **75**, 85–91.

Beaulieu, M. & Coyle, J.T. (1982): Fetally-induced noradrenergic hyperinnervation of cerebral cortex results in persistent down-regulation of beta-receptors. *Dev. Brain Res.* **4**, 491–494.

Billette de Villemeur, T., Chiron, C. & Robain, O. (1992): Unlayered polymicrogyria and agenesis of the corpus callosum: a relevant association. *Acta Neuropathol. (Berl.)* **83**, 265–270.

Caputi, A., Rurale, S., Pastorino, L., Cimino, M., Cattabeni, F.N. & Di Luca, M. (1996): Differential translocation of protein kinase C isozymes in rats characterized by a chronic lack of LTP induction and cognitive impairment. *FEBS Lett.* **393**, 121–123.

Cattabeni, F. & Di Luca, M. (1997): Developmental models of brain dysfunctions induced by targeted cellular ablations with methylazoxymethanol. *Physiol. Rev.* **77**, 199–215.

Cattabeni, F., Cinquanta, M. & Di Luca, M. (1994): Protein kinase C-dependent phosphorylation in prenatally induced microencephaly. *Neurotoxicol.* **15**, 161–170.

Cattaneo, E., Reinach, B., Caputi, A., Cattabeni, F. & Di Luca, M. (1995): Selective *in vitro* blockade of neuroepithelial cells proliferation by methylazoxymethanol acetate, a molecule capable of inducing long lasting functional impairements. *J. Neurosci. Res.* **41**, 640–647.

Chen, S. & Hullman, D.E. (1986): Selective ablation of neurons by methylazoxymethanol during pre- and postnatal brain development. *Exp. Neurol.* **94**, 103–119.

Chevassus-au-Louis, N., Rafiki, I., Jorquera, I., Ben-Ari, Y. & Represa, A. (1998): Neocortex in the hippocampus: an anatomical and functional study of CA1 heterotopiae after prenatal treatment with methylazoxymethanol in rats. *J. Comp. Neurol.* **394**, 520–536.

Chevassus-au-Louis, N., Congar, P., Ben-Ari, Y., Represa, A. & Gaïarsa, J.-L. (1998): Neuronal migration disorders: neocortical heterotopic neurons in CA1 provide a bridge between the hippocampus and the neocortex. *Proc. Nate. Acod. Sci USA* **95**, 10263–10268.

Collier, P.A. & Ashwell, K.W. (1993): Distribution of neuronal heterotopiae following prenatal exposure to methylazoxymethanol. *Neurotoxicol. Teratol.* **15**, 439–444.

Dambska, M., Haddad, R., Kozlowski, P.B., Lee, M.H. & Shek, J. (1982): Telencephalic cytoarchitectonics in the brains of rats with graded degrees of micrencephaly. *Acta Neuropathol. (Berl.)* **58**, 203–209.

De Feo, M.R., Mecarelli, O. & Ricci, G.F. (1995): Seizure susceptibility in immature rats with micrencephaly induced by prenatal exposure to methylazoxymethanol acetate. *Pharmacol. Res.* **31**, 109–114.

Di Luca, M., Cimino, M., De Graan, P.N.E., Oestraeicher, A.B., Gispen, W.H. & Cattabeni, F. (1991): Microencephaly reduces the phosphorylation of the PKC substrate B–50/GAP 43 in rat cortex and hippocampus. *Brain Res.* **538**, 95–101.

Di Luca, M., Caputi, A., Cinquanta, M., Cimino, M., Marini, P., Princivalle, A., De Graan, P.N.E., Gispen, W.H. & Cattabeni, F. (1995): Changes in protein kinase C and its presynaptic substrate B–50/GAP 43 after intrauterine exposure to methylazoxymethanol, a treatment inducing cortical and hippocampal damage and cognitive deficits in rats. *Eur. J. Neurosci.* **7**, 899–906.

Di Luca, M., Caputti, A., Cattabeni, F., De Graan, P.N.E., Gispen, W.H., Raiteri, M., Fassio, A., Schmid, G. & Bonanno, G. (1997): Increased presynaptic protein kinase C activity and glutamate release in rats with prenataly induced hippocampal lesion. *Eur. J. Neurosci.* **9**, 472–479.

Eriksdotter-Nilsson, M., Jonsson, G., Dahl, D. & Björklund, H. (1986): Astroglial development in microencephalic rat brain after fetal methylazoxymethanol treatment. *Int. J. Dev. Neurosci.* **4**, 353–362.

Ferrer, I., Fabregues, I. & Palacios, G. (1982): An autoradiographic study of methylazoxymethanol acetate-induced cortical malformation. *Acta Neuropathol. (Berl.)* **57**, 313–315.

Ferrer, I., Xumetra, A. & Santamaria, J. (1984): Cerebral malformation induced by prenatal X-irradiation: an autoradiographic and Golgi study. *J. Anat.* **138**, 81–93.

Franceschetti, S., Sancini, G., Battaglia, G., Spreafico, R., Di Luca, M. & Avanzini, G. (1996): Aberrant firing pattern of neocortical neurons from methylazoxymethanol (MAM)-treated rats in utero. *Epilepsia* **37** (Suppl. 5), 72.

Germano, I.M., Sperber, E.F. & Moshé, S.L. (1996a). Molecular and experimental aspects of neuronal migration disorders. In: *Malformations of cerebral cortex and epilepsy*, Guerrini, R. (ed.), pp. 27–34. Philadelphia: Lippincott-Raven.

Germano, I.M., Zhang, Y.F., Sperber, E.F. & Moshé, S.L. (1996b). Neuronal migration disorders increase susceptibility to hyperthermia induced seizures in developing rats. *Epilepsia* **37**, 902–910.

Haddad, R.K., Rabe, A., Laquer, G.L., Spatz, M. & Valsamis, M.P. (1969): Intellectual deficit associated with transplacentally induced microcephaly in the rat. *Science* **163**, 88–90.

Hicks, S.P., D'Amato, C.J. & Lowe, M.J. (1959): The development of the mammalian nervous system: I. Malformation of the brain, especially the cerebral cortex, induced in rats by radiation. II. Some mechanisms of the malformations of the cortex. *J. Comp. Neurol.* **113**, 435–469.

Jensen, K.F. & Killackey, H.P. (1984): Subcortical projections from ectopic cortical neurons. *Proc. Natl. Acad. Sci. USA* **81**, 964–968.

Johnston, M.V., Carman, A.B. & Coyle, J.T. (1981): Effects of fetal treatment with methylazoxymethanol acetate at various gestational dates on the neurochemistry of the adult neocortex of the rat. *J. Neurochem* **36**, 124–128.

Johnston, M.V. & Coyle, J.T. (1979): Histological and neurochemical effects of fetal treatment with metylazoxymethanol on rat neocortex in adulthood. *Brain Res.* **170**, 135–155.

Johnston, M.V., Grzanna, R. & Coyle, J.T. (1979): Methylazoxymethanol treatment to fetal rats results in abnormally dense innervation of neocortex. *Science* **203**, 369–371.

Jones, E.G., Valentino, K.L. & Fleshman, J.W. (1982): Adjustment of connectivity in rat neocortex after destruction of precursor cells of layers II–IV. *Dev. Brain Res.* **2**, 425–431.

Jonsson, G. & Hallman, H. (1982): Effects of prenatal methylazoxymethanol treatment on the development of central monoamine neurons. *Dev. Brain Res.* **2**, 513–530.

Matsumoto, H., Spatz, M. & Laqueur, G.L. (1972): Quantitative changes with age in the DNA content of methylazoxymethanol-induced microcephalic rat brain. *J. Neurochem.* **19**, 297–306.

Matsutani, T.M.N., Tamaru, M. & Tsukada, Y. (1980): Elevated monoamine levels in the cerebral hemispheres of microencephalic rats treated prenatally with methylazoxymethanol or cytosine arabinoside. *J. Neurochem.* **34**, 950–956.

Mischel, P.S., Nguyen, L.P. & Vinters, H.V. (1995): Cerebral cortical malformation associated with pediatric epilepsy. Review of neuropathological features and proposal for a grading system. *J. Neuropathol. Exp. Neurol.* **54**, 137–153.

Palmini, A., Gambardella, A., Andermann, F., Dubeau, F., da Costa, J.C., Olivier, A., Tampieri, D., Gloor, P., Quesney, F., Anderman, E., Paglioti, E., Paglioti-Neto, E., Coutinho, C., Leblanc, R. & Kim, H.I. (1995): Intrinsic epileptogenicity of human dysplasic cortex as suggested by corticography and surgical results. *Ann. Neurol.* **37**, 467–487.

Rabe, A. & Haddad, R.K. (1972): Methylazoxymethanol-induced micrencephaly in rats: behavioral studies. *Fed. Proc.* **31**, 1536–1539.

Rafiki, A., Chevassus-au-Louis, N., Ben-Ari, Y., Khrestchatisky, M. & Represa, A. (1998): Glutamate receptors in rat with diffuse cortical malformation: an in situ hybridization and immunohistochemical study. *Brain Res.* **782**, 142–152.

Robain, O. (1996). Introduction to the pathology of cerebral cortical malformation. In: *Malformations of the cerebral cortex and epilepsy*, Guerrini, R. (ed.), pp. 1–9. Philadelphia: Lippincott-Raven.

Robertson, R.T., Gragnola, T.G. & Yu, J. (1990): Patterns of transiently expressed acetylcholinesterase activity in cerbral cortex and dorsal thalamus of developing rats with cytotoxin-induecd microencephaly. *Int. J. Devl. Neuroscience* **8**, 223–232.

Roper, S.N., Gilmore, R.L. & Houser, C.R. (1995): Experimentally induced disorders of neuronal migration produce an increased propensity for electrographic seizures in rats. *Epilepsy Res.* **21**, 205–219

Roper, S.N., King, M.A., Abraham, L.A. & Boillot, M.A. (1997): Disinhibited *in vitro* neocortical slices containing experimentally induced cortical malformation demonstrate hyperexcitability. *Epilepsy Res.* **26**, 443–449.

Tamaru, M., Yoneda, Y., Ogita, K., Shimizu, J., Matsutani, T. & Nagata, T. (1992): Excitatory amino acid receptors in brains of rats with methylazoxymethanol-induced microencephaly. *Neurosci. Res.* **14**, 13–25.

Taylor, D.C., Falconer, M.A., Bruton, C.J. & Corsellis, J.A.N. (1971): Focal malformation of the cerebral cortex in epilepsy. *J. Neurol. Neurosurg. Psych.* **34**, 369–387.

Trottier, S., Evrard, B., Biraben, A. & Chauvel, P. (1994): Altered patterns of catecholaminergic fibers in focal cortical malformation in two patients with partial seizures. *Epilepsy Res.* **19**, 161–179.

Trottier, S., Evrard, B., Vignal, J.-P., Scarabin, J.-M. & Chauvel, P. (1996): The serotoninergic innervation of the cerebral cortex in man and its changes in focal cortical malformation. *Epilepsy Res.* **25**, 79–106.

Vorhees, C., Fernandez, K. & Dumas, R. (1984): Pervasive hyperactivity and long-term learning impairments in rats with induced microcephaly from prenatal exposure to methylazoxymethanol. *Dev. Brain Res.* **15**, 1–10.

Watanabe, M., Kinuya, M., Mamiya, G., Tatsunuma, T., Nagayoshi, M., Matsutani, T. & Tsukada, Y. (1990): Increased uptake sites for serotonin and dopamine with decreased S2 serotonin receptors in microencephalic rat brain. *Neurochem. Res.* **15**, 1017–1022.

Watanabe, M., Kinuya, M., Ohtakeno, S., Watanabe, H. & Mamiya, G. (1992): Effects of foetal treatment with methylazoxymethanol on noradrenergic synapses in rat cerebral cortex. *Pharmacol. Toxicol.* **71**, 314–316.

Yurkewicz, L., Valentino, K.L., Floeter, M.K., Fleshman, J.W. & Jones, E.G. (1984): Effects of cytotoxic deletions of somatic sensory cortex in fetal rats. *Somatosens. Res.* **1**, 303–327.

Zhang, L.L., Collier, P.A. & Ashwell, K.W.S. (1995): Mechanisms in the induction of neuronal heterotopiae following prenatal cytotoxic brain damage. *Neurotoxicol. Teratol.* **17**, 297–311.

Zoli, M., Merlo Pich, E., Cimino, M., Lombardelli, G., Peruzzi, G., Fuxe, K., Agnati, L. & Cattabeni, F. (1990): Morphometrical and microdensitometrical studies on peptide and tyrosine hydroxylase-like immunoreactvities in the forebrain of rats prenatally exposed to methylazoxymethanol acetate. *Dev. Brain Res.* **51**, 45–61.

Part III
Age-specific syndromes

Chapter 8

Infantile spasms: a pathophysiological hypothesis

Olivier Dulac[1], Catherine Chiron[1,2], Olivier Robain[1], Perrine Plouin[1], Isabelle Jambaque[1], Jean-Marc Pinard[1,3]

[1]*Neuropaediatric Department and INSERM U29, Hospital Saint Vincent de Paul, Paris, France;* [2]*Serv. Hosp. F. Joliot, Department for Medical Research, Atomic Energy Commission, Orsay, France; and*[3]*Neuropaediatric Department, Hospital Poincaré, Garches, France*

Infantile spasms (IS) are one of the most frequent and devastating epileptogenic encephalopathies of childhood. Epidemiology studies suggest that 1500 to 2000 new cases occur each year in the United States, of which over three-quarters remain mentally retarded and/or with intractable epilepsy (Hurst, 1994). The syndrome is characterized by age-related onset, a very specific type of seizure contrasting with variable topography of associated brain lesion, a wide range of EEG tracings although hypsarrhythmia is the most characteristic, and various causes. One-third of cases called 'cryptogenic', have no identifiable cause. Rare cases, with no evidence of brain lesion, recover and are considered as 'idiopathic'. Control of spasms may be obtained with several medications including steroids (Sorel & Dusaucy-Bauloye, 1958), valproate (Siemes *et al.*, 1984), benzodiazepines (Farrell, 1986) and vigabatrin (Chiron *et al.*, 1990). Even though the seizure type (epileptic spasms) is the same, there appears to be some specificity of action of these medications related to the etiology (Chiron *et al.*, 1997). Cognitive disorders often persist, even in patients who are rendered seizure free by treatment and whose EEG becomes normal (Jambaqué *et al.*, 1993). Better knowledge of the basic mechanisms should improve treatment, care and outcome.

Because there is no animal model for this unusual disorder, investigation of the basic pathophysiologic mechanisms is a challenge. Hypothesis about potential mechanisms can only be based on speculations drawn from both clinical observations and a growing knowledge of maturational features in the normal human and animal brain. In this chapter several problems will be addressed separately. Is there a specific site from which the spasms originate? Which mechanisms are involved in the organization of hypsarrhythmia? Why is onset of the syndrome age-related? What produces spontaneous cessation of spasms in some cases and what features account for the variable outcomes of this type of epilepsy? Why does the type of cognitive disorder vary from patient to patient and often persist although the epilepsy is controlled or dies out?

Site of the brain generating the spasms

Spasms usually occur in clusters. On EEG, each spasm is associated with a high amplitude slow wave followed by the disappearance of interictal spikes for a variable period of time. These ictal electro-clinical characteristics are similar whether spasms are caused by a diffuse malformation such as agyria

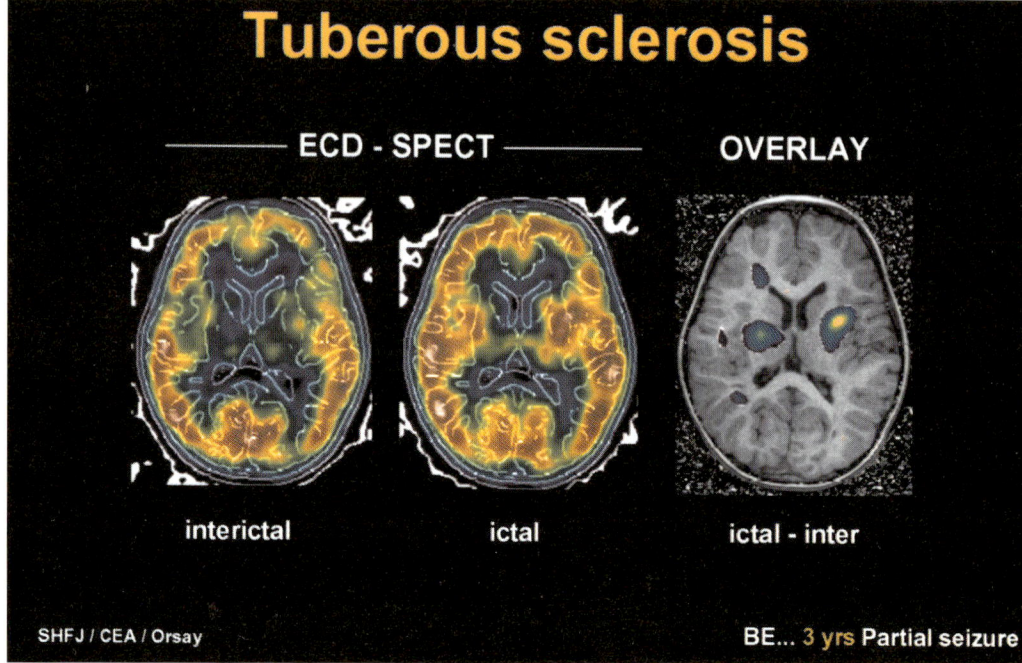

Fig. 1. Interictal (on the left) and ictal (in the middle) SPECT using 99mTc-ECD in a child with infantile spasms. The image of difference ictal–interictal coregistered on MRI shows a hyperperfusion in striata, bilaterally.

(Dulac *et al.*, 1983), multifocal cortical lesions such as in tuberous sclerosis (Dulac *et al.*, 1984) or single focal cortical lesions (Alvarez *et al.*, 1987). Spasms are frequent in hydranencephaly, a condition in which most of the cortical mantle has been destroyed (Neville, 1972). Therefore, there are several arguments supporting the idea that the spasms are not generated by the cortex but more likely by subcortical structures.

Increased metabolic activity and cerebral blood flow of the lenticulate nuclei have been observed in patients with infantile spasms interictally (Chugani *et al.*, 1992) and ictally (unpublished preliminary data) (Fig. 1). Other authors have suggested that the brainstem is more likely to be the site that generates the spasms because of the disorganization in the child's basic sleep–wake cycle (Hrachovy *et al.*, 1981). There is a decrease of rapid eye movement (REM) sleep and spasms tend to occur after arousal from sleep. However, other types of epilepsy, including partial epilepsy with definite cortical origin, may be associated with modification of sleep organization (Baldy-Moulinier, 1983). In addition, neuropathological studies show very minor or no changes in the brainstem of most children with infantile spasms (Vinters & Robain, 1994).

On the other hand, there has been growing evidence of cortical involvement in infantile spasms. When there is a cortical brain lesion, asymmetrical spasms with eyes or head deviation may be observed. This has been reported in Aicardi syndrome (Bour *et al.*, 1986), tuberous sclerosis (Dulac *et al.*, 1984) and focal cortical dysplasia (Chugani *et al.*, 1990). In addition, focal discharges combined with clusters of spasms have been recorded. In most instances these focal abnormalities precede the first spasm (Bour *et al.*, 1986), as if they were triggering and driving the whole cluster. Focal discharges occurring in the course of the cluster, and other focal discharges following the cluster, have also been reported (Donat & Wright, 1991). In such cases, the combination within the same ictal event of focal seizures and clusters of spasms suggests that two different sites are involved simultaneously. In symptomatic

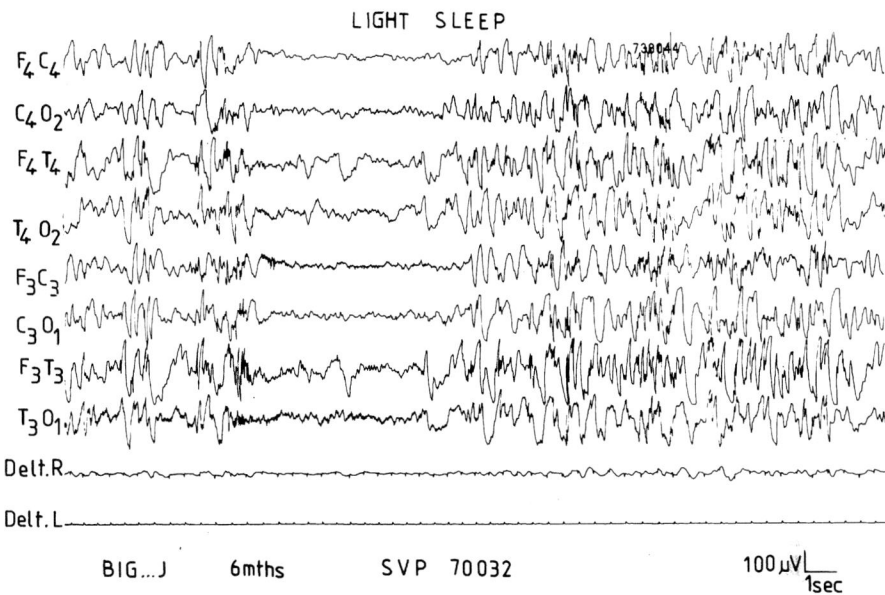

Fig. 2. Typical hypsarrhythmia (see text).

cases, between consecutive spasms of a cluster, the interictal spikes do not recur, and this pattern suggests that some focal discharge could also drive the whole cluster.

Some patients with infantile spasms but no cerebral lesion on MRI have recurrence of interictal spikes between consecutive spasms within a cluster, thus showing that each spasm is a single seizure. In addition, throughout an entire 24 h recording, the EEG abnormality exhibits no focal seizures (Plouin et al., 1993). We have found that these patients recover completely, which argues strongly against significant cortical lesions. Because the long-term evolution is favourable and cortical lesions cannot be shown, this constellation is appropriately called idiopathic West syndrome (Dulac et al., 1993).

Therefore, even though yet undetermined subcortical structures seem to be involved in the genesis of spasms, the triggering area(s) in most cases is probably localized in the cortex. In few instances, however, spasms may not be related to any cortical lesion.

Mechanisms involved in the organization of hypsarrhythmia

Hypsarrhythmia, the second major component of West syndrome, consists of non synchronous diffuse paroxysmal discharges involving a combination of spikes and slow waves, which may be intermingled, diffuse, continuous and asynchronous (Gibbs et al., 1954) (Fig. 2). This characteristic pattern is observed before 1 year of age. In older children, spike activity becomes more synchronous. Hypsarrhythmia has been said to be generated by subcortical structures because it is modified by the sleep–wake cycle (Hrachovy et al., 1981). However, in intractable patients, corpus callosotomy most often results in the disappearance of hypsarrhythmia (Pinard et al., 1993). This would not be the case if hypsarrhythmia was generated by subcortical structures projecting into the cortex. Moreover, the EEG pattern is modified by the type of cortical lesion or malformation such as that found in Aicardi syndrome, agyria-pachygyria, or tuberous sclerosis (Fariello et al., 1977; Dulac et al., 1984; Parmeggiani et al., 1990). We think that the specific EEG patterns are related to the anatomical organization of the cortex, not to functional epileptic features such as typical hypsarrhythmia.

The hypsarrhythmic pattern could be interpreted as the expression of three age-related characteristics

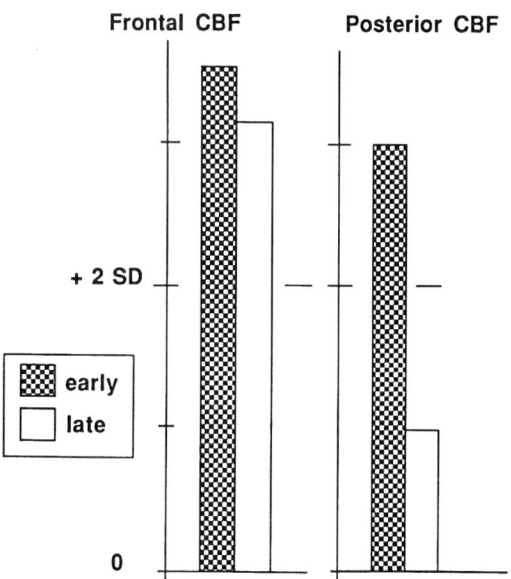

Fig. 3. Interictal regional cerebral blood flow (rCBF) measured in the non-lesioned cortex, expressed in standard deviations (SD) compared to normal population at the same age, in a population of patients with infantile spasms. Chequered columns represent CBF measured before the age of 1 year ('early') and white columns CBF measured after the age of 2 years ('late') in the same patients. The two columns on the left represent the CBF measured in frontal cortex, both on the right the CBF measured in posterior cortex. rCBF was increased in the entire cortex, frontal as well as posterior, since it is over 2 SD.

of the brain: (1) hyperexcitability; (2) high tendency of diffusion of paroxysmal activity throughout the brain; and (3) the inability to synchronize spike activity over both hemispheres. From animal studies, it is clear that the cortex shows transient hyperexcitability at the beginning of post-natal life. GABAergic synapses may be transiently depolarizing (Ben-Ari et al., 1990) and NMDA excitatory synapses are over-represented (Represa et al., 1988). Collateral axonal fibres are transiently increased, as shown by counting the number of axons that cross the midline in the corpus callosum in the cat and primate (Berbel & Innocenti, 1988; La Mantia & Racik, 1990). These features may combine to produce hyperexcitability and diffusion of epileptic phenomena.

In infants with infantile spasms, cerebral blood flow is increased throughout the brain, as a result of high metabolic activity. This high blood flow occurs even in regions, such as the frontal cortex, which normally have low values during the first year of life as a result of immaturity (Chiron et al., 1993) (Fig. 3). This immaturity is reflected by a lack of myelination, which can be shown by magnetic resonance imaging during the first year of life (Valk & Knaap, 1989). Even if paroxysmal activity involves the entire cortex, the poor myelination must result in slow interhemispheric conduction velocity, and therefore discharges are asynchronous in both hemispheres. After age 1 year, progressive myelination increases conduction velocity, and paroxysms become more synchronized.

Although hyperexcitability and diffusion both contribute to produce generalized interictal epileptic activity, one component could predominate over the other. Diffusion may be predominant in the cases with focal or multifocal cerebral lesions. Hypsarrhythmia would result from diffusion from these lesions, thereby corresponding to 'secondary generalization'. When there is no major cerebral lesion, hyperexcitability may predominate, and hypsarrhythmia would correspond to a 'primarily generalized' phenomenon. It is likely that optimal drug treatment with either steroids or conventional antiepileptic medications would vary according to the pattern of generalization. In addition, this hypothesis would explain the favourable outcome following cortical resection in those cases with focal cortical lesions (Chugani *et al.*, 1990), and the high efficacy of vigabatrin in spasms due to tuberous sclerosis (Chiron *et al.*, 1997) as well as in partial seizures (Nabbout *et al.*, 1997).

Relationship of age and the onset of the syndrome

The two major components of the syndrome (hypsarrhythmia and spasms) do not undergo similar maturational processes. Hypsarrhythmia occurs as an age-related phenomenon, beginning after the age of 3 months and mostly before 1 year. Only rarely does it appear for the first time during the second or third year. In a number of cases, it disappears as the patient grows older (Hrachovy *et al.*, 1991). In idiopathic cases, hypsarrhythmia begins in previously normal children between 3 and 12 months of age, and there is no evidence of a focal epileptogenic zone. In symptomatic cases, a number of patients exhibit partial seizures before the onset of infantile spasms, as shown with agyria (Dulac *et al.*, 1983), Aicardi syndrome (Bour *et al.*, 1986), tuberous sclerosis (Dulac *et al.*, 1984), hemimegalencephaly (Vigevano *et al.*, 1989) and focal cortical dysplasia (Chugani *et al.*, 1990). In the latter cases, spasms and hypsarrhythmia occur several weeks after the onset of focal seizures, as if the ability of the brain to produce 'secondary generalization' was age-related. Indeed, in hemimegalencephaly, diffusion of paroxysmal activity is an age-related phenomenon. It spreads to the normal hemisphere only several weeks or months after birth, together with an increase of cerebral blood flow (Chiron *et al.*, 1994). Focal cortical lesions combined with infantile spasms often involve parieto–occipito–temporal or mesial frontal areas (Cusmai *et al.*, 1988). This correlates well with the observation that the posterior areas of the cortex undergo rapid maturation between 3 and 7 months, the age at which the cortex reaches the highest tendency to produce hypsarrhythmia (Chugani *et al.*, 1987; Chiron *et al.*, 1992).

In contrast, clusters of spasms may begin at any age throughout infancy and childhood, from the neonatal period (Ohtahara, 1978) to the end of the first decade (Gobbi *et al.*, 1987). Spasms may persist into the second decade, particularly in patients with major cerebral malformations (Chevrie & Aicardi, 1986). This lack of a clear age relationship for the occurrence of spasms is probably related to different maturation of the various brain structures. Maturation of subcortical structures is mainly prenatal, and they are nearly mature by the time of birth (Chugani *et al.*, 1987) and do not undergo maturational processes postnatally as do cortical structures. Therefore, age relationships of the infantile spasms syndrome seem to be related to the maturation of cortical structures producing diffuse interictal paroxysmal activity, rather than to subcortical structures producing spasms.

Despite this, it seems that subcortical structures do generate spasms. This might occur when the cortex lacks normal inhibitory activity on subcortical structures, either as a consequence of major anatomical lesions or because continuous paroxysmal activity causes loss of normal function. In this setting, subcortical areas could be disinhibited by a lack of normal cortical activity. Spasms could then be triggered by the paroxysmal activity.

Variable outcome of epilepsy and spontaneous cessation of spasms

Patients with infantile spasms may exhibit various types of outcome according to the type of structural abnormalities involved. Diffuse malformations, such as Aicardi syndrome, holoprosencephaly and lissencephaly, produce a protracted course with persistence of spasms for many years (Chevrie & Aicardi, 1986). In multifocal cortical malformations, such as tuberous sclerosis with several epileptogenic tubers, the epilepsy more frequently turns to multifocal or secondarily generalized epilepsy (Cusmai *et al.*, 1990). Patients with a single epileptogenic focus progressively turn to focal epilepsy with ictal characteristics depending on the topography of the dysplastic area (Chugani *et al.*, 1990). Patients with single or multiple epileptogenic areas may also experience cessation of epilepsy.

From animal studies it appears that following the period of axonal and excitatory synaptic overgrowth, the latter are reduced as the different cortical areas undergo specification (Represa *et al.*, 1988). This decreases the tendency to produce epilepsy and generalization. These phenomena occur earlier in the posterior area of the brain than in the anterior portion. Human functional imaging studies have shown that the anterior areas also mature later than the posterior ones (Chugani *et al.*, 1987; Chiron *et al.*, 1992). On the other hand, epileptic discharges through an immature cortex have been proved to avoid the synaptic specification in rats (Grigonis & Murphy, 1994). Such a phenomenon could be the cause in the mechanisms of persistence of the epilepsy later on.

Based on the present understanding of maturation of the cortex, it is possible to suspect a potential mechanism underlying each type of outcome:

- In diffuse malformations such as Aicardi syndrome or agyria, the dysplastic cortex would not undergo the usual maturation process of area specification nor reduction of the excess of excitatory pathways. Spasms would therefore remain protracted. Indeed, a functional imaging study of agyria has shown that there is no antero–posterior differentiation in the first year of life and no modification of regional cerebral blood flow throughout the first decade (Chiron *et al.*, 1996).

- In multifocal cortical malformations, it is likely that the normal cortical areas intermingled with the malformed ones undergo normal maturation, progressively restricting the epileptogenic areas and modifying the expression of epilepsy. The seizures may be multifocal or secondarily generalized. Secondary generalization may be produced by several mechanisms. Paroxysmal discharges of epileptogenic malformed areas located in the posterior parts of the brain may project anteriorly through occipito–frontal and temporo–frontal pathways that are known to be very active, as shown in adults with epilepsy (Williamson *et al.*, 1992). As discussed above, maturation of frontal lobes is delayed in comparison with posterior ones. Once the frontal lobes mature, they may amplify paroxysmal features as these excitatory pathways become more functional (Dalla Bernardina & Watanabe, 1994). This may be particularly important when patients have additional frontal or temporal dysplasia. In addition, frontal lobes are known to be particularly prone to produce secondary bilateral synchrony, which could contribute to secondary generalized epilepsy with generalized tonic or tonic–clonic seizures (Cusmai *et al.*, 1990). The combination of bilateral slow spike waves and generalized seizures is often quoted as 'Lennox–Gastaut syndrome'. Some authorities have suggested that the EEG discharge in this disorder is the result of secondary bilateral synchrony (Gastaut & Zifkin, 1988).

- In patients with a single epileptogenic focus, diffusion of the paroxysmal features that characterize the beginning of the disease could die out as the major part of the cortex undergoes specification and reduction of 'excitatory pathways'. The remaining circumscribed epileptogenic zone could produce focal seizures.

- Cessation of epilepsy would of course be possible if the dysplastic area(s) is (are) not epileptogenic enough to produce paroxysmal events alone, as the cortex becomes less excitable. Spontaneous cessation of spasms without treatment has been reported (Hrachovy *et al.*, 1991), particularly in idiopathic cases (Bachman, 1981; Dulac *et al.*, 1986).

Cognitive disorders

Patients with cryptogenic West syndrome develop normally until they exhibit seizures. A sizable number of those with tuberous sclerosis also are cognitively normal until their seizures occur as the first manifestation of the syndrome. Patients with typical hypsarrhythmia then experience a deterioration of neurologic function. This most frequently involves axial hypotonia, visual agnosia and indifference to interpersonal contact (Jambaqué *et al.*, 1993). This corresponds to a relative rCBF decrease in posterior cortex associated with abnormal CBF increase in the whole brain (Chiron *et al.*, 1993; Jambaqué *et al.*, 1993).

Some children, particularly those with diffuse malformations, exhibit abnormal psychomotor devel-

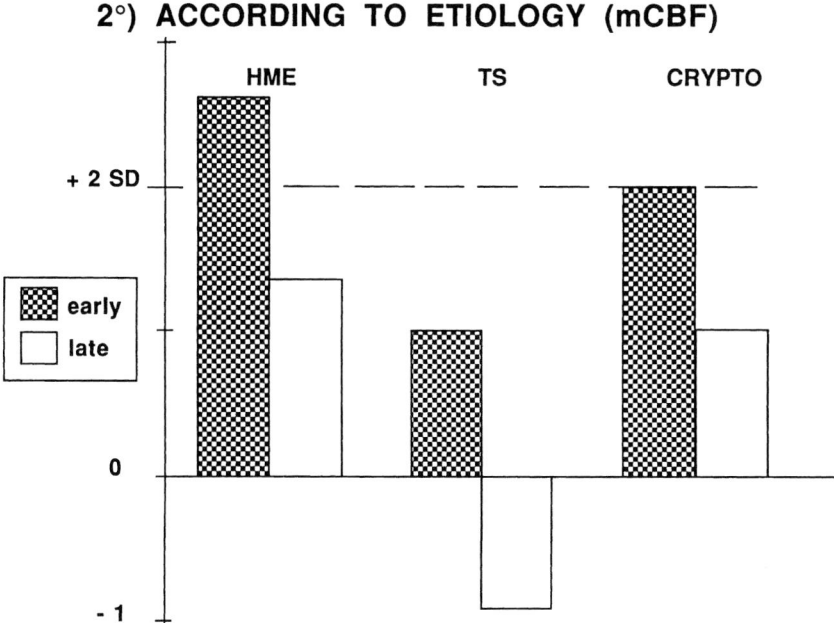

Fig. 4. Interictal cerebral blood flow (CBF) measured in the non-lesioned cortex, expressed in standard deviations (SD) in a population of patients with infantile spasms compared to normal population at the same age. Chequered columns represent CBF measured before the age of 1 year ('early') and white columns CBF measured after the age of 2 years ('late') in the same patients. On the left are CBF in hemimegalencephaly, in the middle CBF in tuberous sclerosis, and on the right CBF in cryptogenic cases. Note that interictal 'early' CBF is increased in hemimegalencephaly and cryptogenic cases whereas it is normal in tuberous sclerosis.

opment before the onset of seizures. Most cases are not investigated before the onset of epilepsy, and the first EEG already discloses diffuse abnormalities. Therefore, it is difficult to determine what contribution the epilepsy makes to psychomotor delay. In fact, patients with major dysplasia rarely exhibit a recent and clear-cut loss of abilities when hypsarrhythmia begins. Based on parents' observations, the onset of seizures appears to contribute only mildly to the initial psychomotor delay. Later, we suspect, the infantile spasm disorder adds to the delay produced by the original lesion.

During follow-up, cognitive functions are often severely affected, ranging from selective cognitive disorders to major mental retardation and autistic behaviour. Mental retardation characterizes patients with diffuse malformations or destructive brain lesions. Specific cognitive deficits mainly develop in patients with focal epileptogenic involvement:

- Patients with visual motor coordination dysfunction usually have evidence of focal epileptic involvement of occipito–parietal structures and rCBF decrease in the same areas (Jambaqué et al., 1993). At worst, these children are initially cortically blind with autistic behaviour. The contact with the surroundings becomes more appropriate as visual function becomes less impaired. Sophisticated communication is only possible if speech develops, giving to the child other means for effective communication (Jambaqué et al., 1993). These patients are often left with simultagnosia or other visual spatial disorders contrasting with the development of verbal abilities. Language is likely spared because the dysfunction predominates in the most posterior areas of the brain.

- Patients with speech delay usually suffer from mental retardation. In these patients, the focal

epileptic involvement is less selective, but still emphasizes posterior regions, especially the temporo–parietal areas (Jambaqué et al., 1993).
- A number of patients remain with autistic features combined with severe mental retardation. This is particularly the case in tuberous sclerosis where major epileptogenic tubers involve both posterior and anterior areas of the brain (Jambaqué et al., 1991). However, progress in drug treatment has considerably modified this pattern of evolution, particularly for those children with tuberous sclerosis (Chiron et al., 1997). This suggests that epilepsy plays a major role in the genesis of the autistic disorder.

At the time of onset of the spasms, the psychomotor delay could be related to the brain lesion. The epilepsy and especially major interictal EEG abnormalities and global CBF increase would account for the loss of skills. Continuous and diffuse slow wave activity could interfere with cognitive function, as occurs during an episode of non-convulsive status epilepticus. It is interesting to note that the loss of skills is usually less striking in tuberous sclerosis than in cryptogenic cases. Restriction of interictal abnormalities to a single focus with secondary generalization could account for this moderate impact on cognitive functions. This contrasts with the acute global reduction in cognitive function, which is often seen in patients with cryptogenic West syndrome associated with hypsarrhythmia where the disorder appears to be the result of diffuse cortical hyperexcitability. Conversely, the CBF increase in the non-lesioned cortex is moderate or absent in patients with tuberous sclerosis compared to cryptogenic cases (Fig. 4) (Chiron et al., 1995). The occurrence of paroxysmal electrical discharge in cortical areas undergoing rapid maturation is known to prevent fine tuning of the synaptic network which is so important for cognitive development (Pierson & Swann, 1991).

Psychomotor outcome is determined by the combination of the location and number of brain lesions and the later outcome of the epilepsy. The persistence of generalized epilepsy in patients with tuberous sclerosis with both posterior and anterior tubers could account for the presence of autistic behaviour (Jambaqué et al., 1991). Posterior epileptogenic tubers would disorganize communication abilities, whereas anterior lesions would account for stereotypic behaviour and indifference to surroundings which are so characteristic of autistic patients.

Conclusions

Neither the classical distinction of partial versus generalized epilepsy, nor that of cortical versus subcortical involvement applies to infantile spasms. There is often a combination of both focal and generalized features, as well as a combination of cortical and subcortical characteristics. Nevertheless, the topography of the cortical lesion may partly explain selective cognitive and behavioural disorders. Maturational changes suggest possible basic mechanisms of hypsarrhythmia, its age relationship and its evolution as the accompanying epilepsy changes. This approach does not exclude the potential contribution of some polypeptides acting as growth factors, i.e. the corticotrophin releasing hormone (CRF) (Baram, 1993).

References

Alvarez, L.A., Shinnar, S. & Moshé, S.L. (1987): Infantile spasms due to unilateral cerebral infarcts. *Pediatrics* **79**, 1024–1026.

Bachman, D. (1981): Spontaneous remission of infantile spasms with hypsarrhythmia. *Arch. Neurol.* **38**, 785.

Baldy-Moulinier, M. (1983): Temporal lobe epilepsy and sleep organization. In: *Sleep and epilepsy*, Sterman, M.B., Shouse, M.N. & Passouant, P. (eds), pp. 347–359. New York: Academic Press.

Baram, T.Z. (1993): Pathophysiology of massive infantile spasms. Perspective on the putative role of the brain adrenal axis. *Ann. Neurol.* **33**, 231–236.

Bednarek, N., Motte, J., Soufflet, C., Plouin, P. & Dulac, O. (1998): Evidence of late-onset infantile spasms. *Epilepsia* **39**, 55–60.

Ben-Ari, Y., Rovira, C., Gaiarsa, J.L., Corradetti, R., Robain, O. & Cherubini, E. (1990): GABAergic mechanisms in the CA3 hippocampal region during early postnatal life. In: Storm-Mathisen, I., Zimmer, J. & Ottersen, O.P. (eds) *Progr. Brain Res.* **83**, 313–321.

Berbel, P. & Innocenti, G.M. (1988): The development of the corpus callosum in cats: a light and electron microscopic study. *J. Comp. Neurol.* **276**, 132–156.

Bour, F., Chiron, C., Dulac, O. & Plouin, P. (1986): Caractères électrocliniques des crises dans le syndrome d'Aicardi. *Rev. EEG Neurophysiol. Clin.* **16**, 341–53.

Chevrie, J.J. & Aicardi, J. (1986): The Aicardi syndrome. In: *Recent advances in epilepsy, vol 3*, Pedley, T.A. & Meldrum, B.S. (eds), pp. 189–210. Edinburgh: Churchill, Livingstone.

Chiron, C., Dulac, O., Luna, D., Palacios, L., Mondragon, S., Beaumont, D. & Mumford, J.P. (1990): Vigabatrin in infantile spasms. *Lancet* **335**, 363–364.

Chiron, C., Raynaud, C., Mazière, B., Zilbovicius, M., Laflamme, L., Masure, M.C., Dulac, O., Bourguignon, M. & Syrota, A. (1992): Changes in regional cerebral blood flow during brain maturation in children and adolescents. *J. Nucl. Med.* **33**, 696–703.

Chiron, C., Dulac, O., Bulteau, C., Nuttin, C., Depas, G., Raynaud, C. & Syrota, A. (1993): Study of regional cerebral blood flow in West syndrome. *Epilepsia* **34**, 707–715.

Chiron, C., Delalande, O., Soufflet, C., Plouin, P. & Dulac, O. (1994): Longitudinal study of EEG and regional cerebral blood flow in hemimegalencephaly before and after surgery. *Epilepsia* **35** (Suppl. 8), 119.

Chiron, C., Pinton, F., Cusmai, R., Dulac, O. & Syrota, A. (1995): Longitudinal regional cerebral blood flow measurement in infantile spasms according to etiology. *Epilepsia* **36** (Suppl. 3), 137.

Chiron, C., Nabbout, R., Pinton, F., Nuttin, C., Dulac, O. & Syrota, A. (1996): Brain functional imaging SPECT in agyria–pachygyria. *Epilepsy Res.* **24**, 109–117.

Chiron, C., Dumas, C., Jambaqué, I., Dulac, O., et al. (1997): Randomized trial comparing vigabatrin and hydrocortisone in infantile spasms due to tuberous sclerosis. *Epilepsy Res.* **26**, 389–395.

Chugani, H.T., Shewmon, D.A., Sankar, R., Chen, B.C. & Phelps, M.F. (1992): Infantile spasms. II. Lenticular nuclei and brain stem activation on positron emission tomography. *Ann. Neurol.* **31**, 212–219.

Chugani, H., Phelps, M.E. & Mazziotta J.C. (1987): Positron emission tomography of human brain functional development. *Ann. Neurol.* **22**, 487–497.

Chugani, H.T., Shields, W.D., Shewmon, D.A., Olson, D.M., Phelps, M.E. & Peacock, W.J. (1990): Infantile spasms. I. PET identifies focal cortical dysgenesis in cryptogenic cases for surgical treatment. *Ann. Neurol.* **27**, 406–413.

Cusmai, R., Chiron, C., Curatolo, P., Dulac, O. & Tran-Dinh, S. (1990): Topographic comparative study of magnetic resonance imaging and electroencephalography in 34 children with tuberous sclerosis. *Epilepsia* **31**, 747–755.

Cusmai, R., Dulac, O. & Diebler, C. (1988): Lésions focales dans les spasmes infantiles. *Neurophysiol. Clin.* **18**, 235–241.

Dalla Bernardina, B. & Watanabe, K. (1994): Interictal EEG: variations and pittfalls. In: *Infantile spasms and West syndrome*. Dulac, O., Chugani, H. & Dalla Bernardin,a B.(eds). London: Saunders.

Donat, J.F. & Wright, F.S. (1991): Simultaneous infantile spasms and partial seizures. *J. Child Neurol.* **6**, 246–250.

Dulac, O., Plouin, P., Perulli, L. & Motte, J. (1983): L'épilepsie dans l'agyrie–pachygyrie classique. *Rev. EEG Neurophysiol. Clin.* **13**, 232–239.

Dulac, O., Lemaitre, A. & Plouin, P. (1984): The Bourneville syndrome: clinical and EEG features of epilepsy in the first year of life. *Boll. Lega. Ital. Epil.* **45/46**, 39–42.

Dulac, O., Plouin, P., Jambaqué, I. & Motte, J. (1986): Spasmes infantiles épileptiques bénins. *Rev. EEG Neurophysiol. Clin.* **16**, 371–382.

Dulac, O., Plouin, P. & Jambaqué, I. (1993): Predicting favorable outcome in idiopathic West syndrome. *Epilepsia* **34**, 747–756.

Fariello, R.G., Chun, R.W.M., Doro, J.M., Buncic, J.R. & Prichard, J.S. (1977): EEG recognition of Aicardi's syndrome. *Arch. Neurol.* **34**, 563–566.

Farrell, K. (1986): Benzodiazepines in the treatment of children with epilepsy. *Epilepsia* **27** (Suppl. 1), S45-S51.

Gastaut, H. & Zifkin, B. (1988): Secondary bilateral synchrony and Lennox–Gastaut syndrome. In: *The Lennox–Gastaut syndrome*. Niedermeyer, E. & Degen, R. (eds), pp. 221–242. New York: Alan Liss.

Gibbs, E.L., Fleming, M.M. & Gibbs, F.A.(1954): Diagnosis and prognosis of hypsarrhythmia and infantile spasms. *Pediatrics* **33**, 66–72.

Gobbi, G., Bruno, L., Pini, A., Rossi, P.G. & Tassinari, C.A.(1987): Periodic spasms: an unclassified type of epileptic seizure in childhood. *Dev. Med. Child Neurol.* **29**, 766–775.

Grigonis, A.M. & Murphy, E.H. (1994): The effects of epileptic cortical activity on the development of callosal projections. *Dev. Brain Res.* **77**, 251–255.

Hrachovy, R.A., Frost, J.D. & Kellaway, P. (1981): Sleep characteristics in infantile spasms. *Neurology* **31**, 688–694.

Hrachovy, R.A., Glaze, D.G. & Frost, J.P. (1991): A retrospective study of spontaneous remission and long-term outcome inpatients with infantile spasms. *Epilepsia* **32**, 212–214.

Hurst, D.L. (1994): The epidemiology of infantile spasms. In: *Infantile spasms and West syndrome*, Dulac, O., Chugani, H. & Dalla Bernardina, B. (eds). London: Saunders.

Jambaqué, I., Cusmai, R., Curatolo, P., Cortesi, F., Perrot, C. & Dulac, O. (1991): Neuropsychological aspects of tuberous sclerosis: relation to epilepsy and MRI findings. *Dev. Med. Child Neurol.* **33**, 698–705.

Jambaqué, I., Chiron, C., Dulac, O., Raynaud, C. & Syrota, P. (1993): Visual inattention in West syndrome: a neuropsychological and neurofunctional imaging study. *Epilepsia* **34**, 692–700.

La Mantia, A.S. & Rakic, P. (1990): Axon overproduction and elimination in the corpus callosum of the developing rhesus monkey. *J. Neurol. Sci.* **10**, 2156–2175.

Nabbout, R., Chiron, C., Mumford, J., Dumas, C. & Dulac, O. (1997): Vigabatrin in partial seizures in children. *J. Child Neurol.* **12**, 172–177

Neville, B.G.R. (1972): The origin of infantile spasms: Evidence from a case of hydranencephaly. *Dev. Med. Child Neurol.* **14**, 644–656.

Ohtahara, S. (1978): Clinico-electrical delineation of epileptic encephalopathies in childhood. *Asian Med. J.* **21**, 7–17.

Parmeggiani, A., Plouin, P. & Dulac, O. (1990): Quantification of diffuse and focal delta activity in hypsarrhythmia. *Brain Dev.* **12**, 310–315.

Pierson, M.G. & Swann, J.W. (1991): Ontogenetic features of audiogenic seizure susceptibility induced in immature rats by noise. *Epilepsia* **32**, 1–9.

Pinard, J.M., Delalande, O., Plouin, P. & Dulac, O. (1993): Callosotomy in West syndrome suggests a cortical origin of hypsarrhythmia. *Epilepsia* **34**, 780–787.

Plouin, P., Dulac, O., Jalin, C. & Chiron, C. (1993): Twenty-four-hour ambulatory EEG monitoring in infantile spasms. *Epilepsia* **34**, 686–691.

Represa, A., Tremblay, E. & Ben-Ari, Y. (1988): Transient increase of NMDA-binding sites in human hippocampus during development. *Neurosci. Lett.* **99**, 61–68.

Siemes, H., Siegert, M., Aksu, F., Emrich, R., Hanefeld, F. & Scheffner, D. (1984): CSF protein profile in infantile spasms. Influence of etiology and ACTH or dexamethasone treatment. *Epilepsia* **25**, 368–376.

Sorel, L. & Dusaucy-Bauloye, A. (1958): A propos de 21 cas d'hypsarythmie de Gibbs. Son traitement spectaculaire par l'ACTH. *Acta Neurol. Belg.* **58**, 130–141.

Valk, J. & Knaap, M.S. (1989): *Magnetic resonance of myelin, myelination and myelin disorders*. Berlin: Springer Verlag.

Vigevano, F., Bertini, E., Boldrini, R., Bosman, C., Claps, D., di Capua, M., di Rocco, C. & Rossi, G.F. (1989): Hemimegalencephaly and intractable epilepsy: Benefits of hemispheretomy. *Epilepsia* **30**, 833–843.

Vinters, H.V. & Robain, O. (1994): Neuropathology studies. In: *Infantile spasms and West syndrome*, Dulac, O., Chugani, H. & Dalla Bernardina, B. (eds). London: Saunders.

Williamson, P.D., Thadans, V.M., Darcey, T.M., Spencer, D.D., Spencer, S.S. & Mattson, R.H. (1992): Occipital lobe epilepsy: clinical characteristics, seizure spread pattern, and results of surgery. *Ann. Neurol.* **31**, 3–13.

Chapter 9

The Lennox–Gastaut syndrome: from baby to adolescent

Charlotte Dravet

Centre Saint-Paul, 300 Boulevard de Sainte Marguerite, 13009 Marseille, France

Summary

After a brief description of the classical Lennox–Gastaut syndrome (LGS), the author reviews the clinical and EEG features observed at different ages, in very young children and in adolescents. The semiological differences between these two age groups and the relationship between LGS and other types of epilepsy (West syndrome in infants, partial epilepsies and idiopathic generalized epilepsies in adolescents) are compared. Changes in the symptomatology that occur in the same patient during the course of the disease are described. These findings raise the question of the pathogenesis of this epilepsy, which seems to have the same underlying mechanisms but different clinical expressions according to age. LGS never occurs de novo after the age of 25 years and is in this respect age-dependent, but conversely to the West syndrome within wider limits.

Among childhood epilepsies, Lennox–Gastaut syndrome (LGS) is one of the most severe epileptic syndromes, considering seizure frequency, occurrence of sudden falls, marked pharmaco-resistance, and occurrence of mental and behavioural disturbances. The pathogenic mechanisms of LGS are not well understood and the borderlines with other types of severe epilepsies are not easy to define. Without a precise knowledge of the clinical and electroencephalographic characteristics of the patient concerned, it can be difficult to distinguish between LGS and other childhood epilepsies such as the Doose syndrome (myoclonic–astatic epilepsy), epilepsy with continuous spike-and-waves during slow sleep, and partial epilepsies with secondary bilateral synchrony.

In the International Classification of Epilepsies and Epileptic Syndromes (Commission, 1989) LGS is classified among the symptomatic or cryptogenic generalized epilepsies. It is defined by several criteria: (1) polymorphous epileptic seizures, mainly with atypical absences, axial tonic (Fig. 1), and atonic seizures; (2) EEG patterns consisting of diffuse slow spikes and waves (SSW) and bursts of fast rhythms at 10–12 Hz during sleep (Fig.1); (3) permanent psychological disturbances with psychomotor retardation or personality disorders or both. However, other types of seizures can be seen (myoclonic, partial, generalized tonic–clonic). Seizures are frequent and often repeat themselves in episodes of status. Focal and multifocal abnormalities can be associated with the diffuse SSW on the EEG. These electroclinical features can occur in a previously normal child, with no pathological antecedents or signs of brain lesion, usually between the ages of 1 and 8 years (constituting the *cryptogenic* form of LGS). They can also occur in a child with brain damage precedents, sometimes

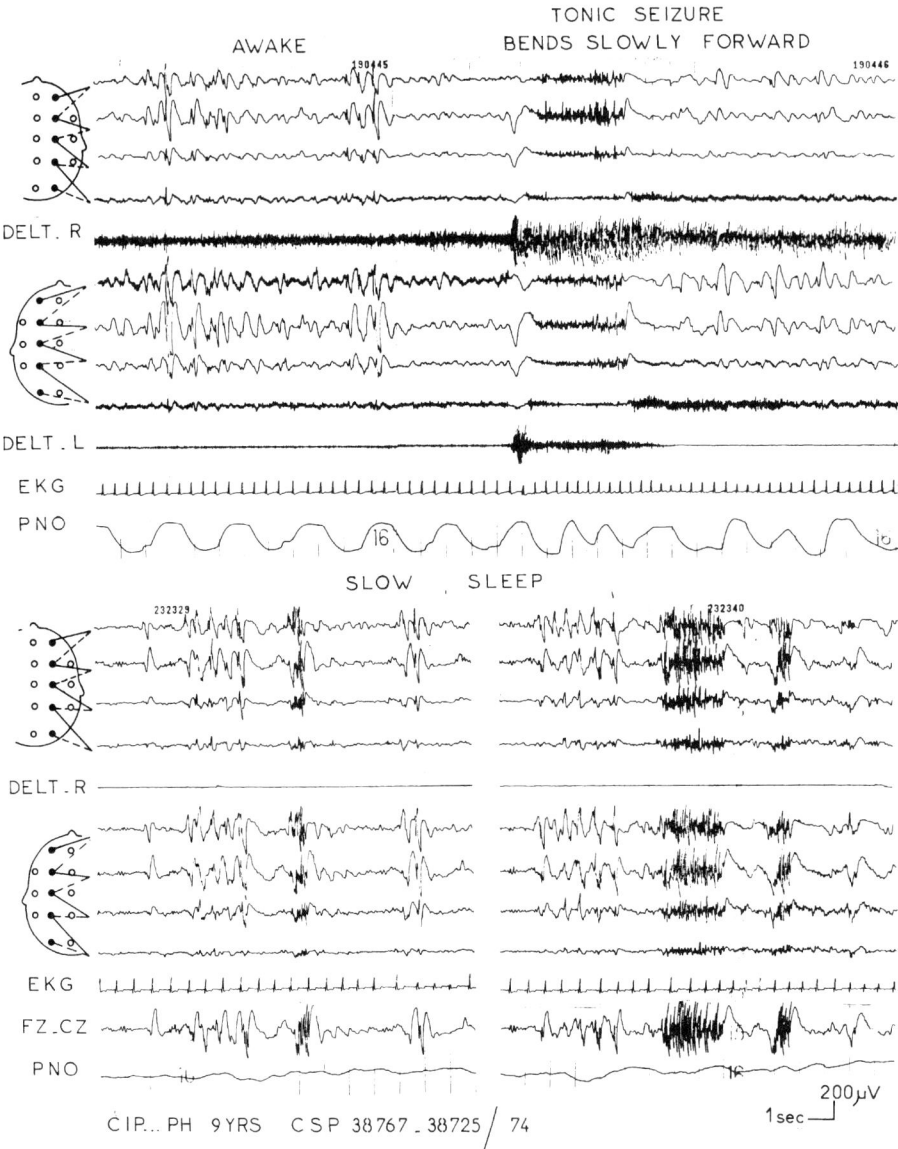

Fig. 1. Typical aspects of LGS in a boy of 9 years. Seizures started at the age of 4 years (adversive, tonic and atypical absences). Top: bursts of SSW more evident in the anterior regions and a tonic seizure accompanied by a slow wave, a flattening of the rhythms and slow waves. Bottom: diffuse SSW, polyspikes and burst of rapid rhythms with no clinical correlate. Note the decreased amplitude of the EEG recording. Delt. L. = left deltoid; Delt. R. = right deltoid ; PNO = pneumogram.

following another type of epilepsy, such as West syndrome or a focal epilepsy (*symptomatic* form). In the latter case, the age at onset can cover a wider range (between 1 and 15 years).

Aetiological circumstances are various, ante-, peri- or postnatal (anoxo–ischaemia, vascular accident, cerebral and cerebro–meningeal infection, HHE syndrome, brain malformation and migration disorders, tuberous sclerosis, Down syndrome, hydrocephalus, head trauma, brain tumour, radiotherapy

Chapter 9 The Lennox–Gastaut syndrome

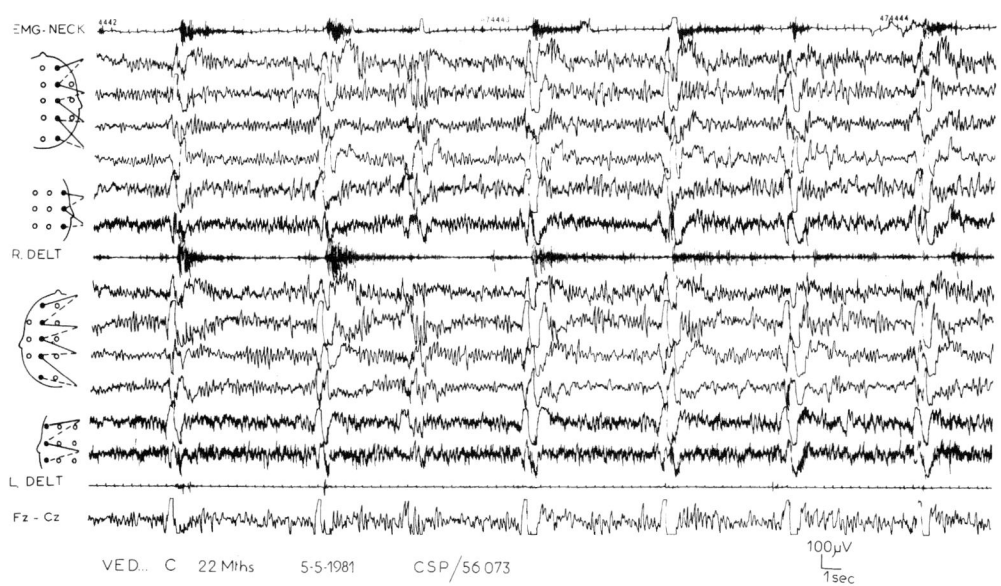

Fig. 2. A series of head drops in a boy of 22 months. Seizures started at the age of 11 months, consisting of head drops and atypical absences, associated with an arrest of psychomotor development. Polygraphic recording seems to show a brief tonic spasm on neck muscles and right deltoid, immediately preceded by a high voltage, large, diffuse slow wave. R. Delt = right deltoid; L. Delt. = left deltoid.

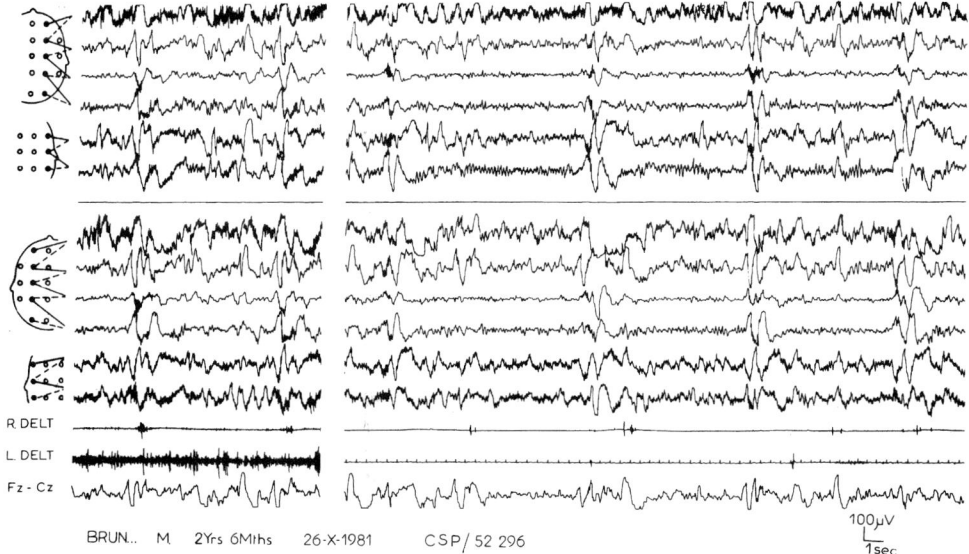

Fig. 3. A series of head drops in a girl of 2½ years. Seizures started at the age of 8 months, consisting of very sudden falls causing traumatisms. Polygraphic recording of the two deltoids does not show any change in muscular tone, but the neck muscles are not recorded. The EEG shows a concomitant diffuse, high voltage slow wave. R. Delt = right deltoid; L. Delt. = left deltoid.

for brain tumour etc.). Neuroimaging studies show abnormalities related to the aetiology. In some cases, in spite of psychomotor retardation before the onset of seizures, or of cerebral atrophy demonstrated by CT scan and MRI, there is no recognizable aetiology. When epilepsy starts in the first year of life, it is often in the form of West syndrome, followed by LGS. Otherwise the LGS can be preceded by focal seizures or immediately show complete symptomatology. It must also be underlined that, in some patients, the typical features of LGS can be observed only transiently. In the cryptogenic forms, there is no aetiology by definition.

The underlying mechanisms remain unknown. Even the neuro-physiological pathways leading to the expression of generalized SSW on the scalp are not explained. Common processes with idiopathic generalized epilepsies could be involved, but in LGS they would appear to be modified by other factors, either acquired or genetic. LGS is a specific age-dependent condition which looks like a diffuse encephalopathy. The reason why it appears in either normal or brain-damaged patients remains unresolved (Beaumanoir & Dravet, 1992).

Here we discuss the different aspects of the syndrome in relation to brain development, in other words according to age. Although described as 'a specific age-dependent condition', LGS starting during childhood may persist in adulthood; moreover, it may appear at various ages, affecting babies to adolescents and even adults.

LGS in babies with onset before the age of two

LGS is observed before the age of two in two circumstances: either de novo or after a West syndrome.

The de novo LGS is rarely described in babies. Cavazzuti (1972), reported 26 cryptogenic cases among which three started before the age of 1 year (5 months, 8 months) and seven between 12 and 24 months. Boniver *et al.* (1987) reported 23 'idiopathic' cases among which two started during the first year (8 months, 11 months) and three between 12 and 22 months. For these authors, head nodding is the characteristic seizure type at this age (Figs. 2 and 3). The mechanism of this head nodding is unclear: brief tonic spasm? brief loss of tone? Polygraphic recordings are not convincing. They were rarely similar to infantile spasms, as decribed by Ikeno *et al.* (1985) and Egli *et al.* (1985). These infantile spasm-like seizures are more often observed in patients with a post West LGS (Ikeno *et al.*, 1985). In the series of Boniver *et al.* (1987), all patients had *de novo* LGS. The interictal EEG traces are often unspecific, with rare SSW and no rapid sleep rhythms. However they become characteristic by the age of 2–3 years (Fig. 4).

LGS following a West syndrome is reported by all authors but without many details. Aicardi & Chevrie (1982) studied 80 cases with SSW in their EEGs. Twenty of these patients had had infantile spasms at onset, and 70 per cent continued to exhibit infantile spasms. Erba & Lombroso (1973) discussed the age factor in LGS, which appears less distinctive than in West syndrome. Superimposition of the two syndromes is not exceptional in infants and young children, with association of infantile spasms, tonic seizures and atypical absences. EEG features can also be associated on the same recording, or appear alternately from one recording to another. Dravet *et al.* (1973) reported the long-term evolution of 39 patients with a West syndrome. Fifty per cent evolved into LGS. In 14 patients there was no free interval between the occurrence of the two syndromes and their EEG continued to show more or less hypsarrhythmic patterns during several years. In these patients, seizures mainly consisted of brief tonic spasms associated with longer tonic seizures, but it was difficult to recognize atypical absences or myoclonic attacks. In the other four patients LGS followed West syndrome after a seizure-free interval of variable duration (from 45 months to 4 years). These children displayed a more typical LGS. In the study by Ohtahara (1978), among 116 LGSs, 42 (36.2 per cent) followed a West Syndrome, and, among 94 West syndromes, 51 (54.3 per cent) evolved into a LGS. The conversion between the two syndromes took place between the age of 1 and 2 years. During this transitory period it was frequently difficult to differentiate West syndrome from LGS as they often co-existed. Yamatogi

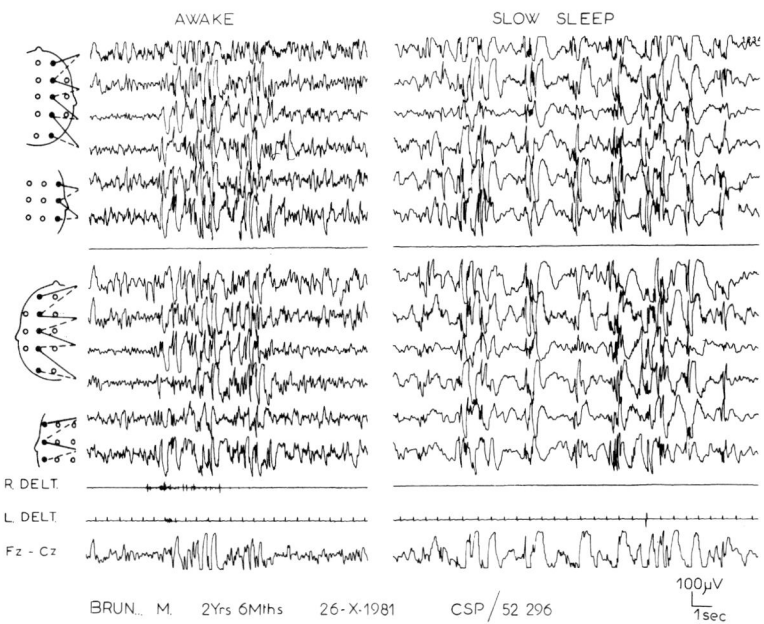

Fig. 4. Same girl as in Fig. 2, at the same age: on the left a burst of diffuse SSW, on the right SSW and rapid rhythms during slow sleep. R. Delt = right deltoid; L. Delt. = left deltoid.

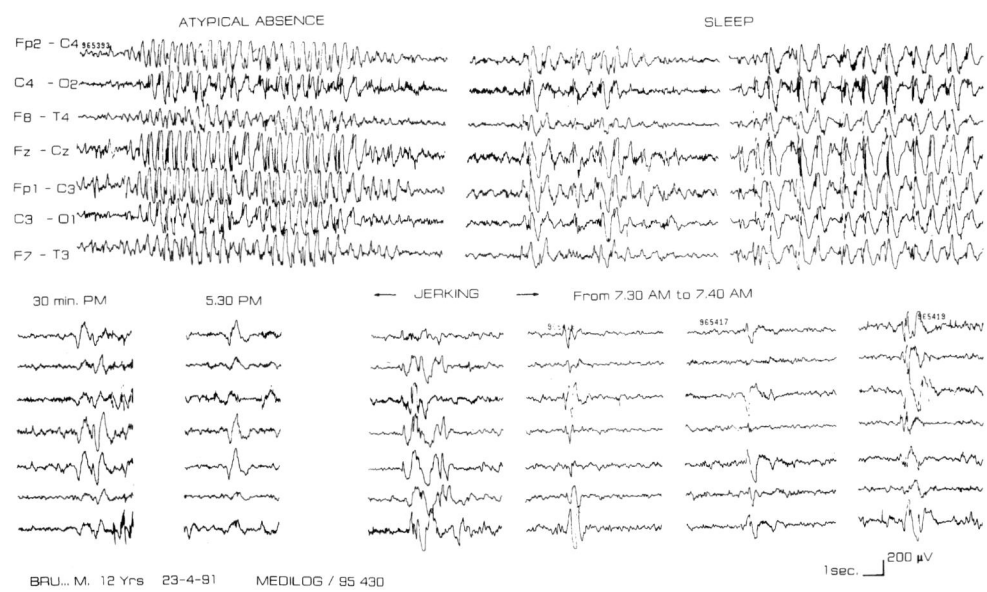

Fig. 5. Same girl as in Figs. 2 and 3, at the age of 12 years: an ambulatory EEG during 24 h allowed the recording of several types of events. Top left: atypical absence with diffuse SSW; top right: SSW and polySW during slow sleep. Bottom, from left to right, different ictal events described by the mother as sudden jerks of the head, accompanied by isolated or brief bursts of diffuse slow waves and SSW, sometimes asymmetical. Note the decreased amplitude of the EEG recording.

& Ohtahara (1981) confirmed these findings and observed that the EEG ictal expression was different, characterized rather by 'desynchronization' in West syndrome and by 'rapid synchronization' in LGS.

Weinmann (1988) described a series of 140 infants with West syndrome, followed for more than six years: in 41 of them (29.2 per cent) West syndrome progressed in LGS, 11 in continuation and 30 after a free interval (from 5 months to 5.8 years). He also studied 174 children with LGS, one-third with onset of epilepsy in their first year and 31 of them with infantile spasms. No differences could be found in the course of LGS with or without history of West syndrome, and aetiological disparities were sought. Reference was made to the work of Meencke & Gerhard (1985) who reported 24 autopsies of children suffering from symptomatic West syndrome, deceased between the ages of 6 months and 10 years. These authors found a relatively clear correlation between the occurrence of the lesions and the onset of symptoms. In the peri-postnatal group (eight cases), symptoms appeared later than for infants with embryo–foetal lesions (six cases). The time of intersection seemed to be the age of 6 months. A limited number of cases developed LGS. The authors suggest that the transition between West syndrome and LGS is more likely to occur in the group with late onset, i.e. with peri-postnatal lesions, than in the early onset group, with antenatal lesions.

LGS in adolescents, with onset after the age of ten

In adolescents, LGS can appear in three circumstances: *de novo*, after a partial epilepsy or after an idiopathic generalized epilepsy. However, in many cases the electro-clinical picture is incomplete and/or transitory. Several authors have studied this issue (Lipinski, 1977; Stenzel & Pantelli, 1983; Bladin, 1985; Roger *et al.*, 1987; Bauer *et al.*, 1988), but the data provided by these studies are heterogeneous because, in some of them, childhood LGS continuing in adolescence and adulthood is not dissociated from LGS starting in adolescence. For this reason, only the descriptions by Roger *et al.* (1987) and Bauer *et al.* (1988) are reported here.

In the 44 patients studied by Roger *et al.* (1987), the age at onset of LGS varies between 13 and 23 years in adolescents with no history of epilepsy. In 31 of them, a focal symptomatology was associated with the LGS features (either partial seizures or only localized, focal and multifocal, EEG abnormalities (Figs. 5–9)). In all patients, a mental deterioration occurred and epilepsy was extremely severe. In the other 13 patients, no sign of localization was present, and symptomatology and outcome were different according to age onset. When seizures started between the ages of 13 and 15 years, the syndrome was complete and the outcome very poor. When seizures started between the ages of 16 and 19 years, the syndrome was incomplete, without nocturnal tonic seizures and sometimes without drop attacks but with tonic–clonic seizures. The EEG did not show the specific rapid rhythms during sleep. Moreover mental deterioration was inconstant and five patients improved, the last one remaining severely handicapped. Bauer *et al.* (1988) reported somewhat different findings. However their study included patients with and without previous epilepsy. It is interesting to note that eight patients suffered from an apparently idiopathic generalized epilepsy with absences, generalized tonic–clonic seizures and generalized 3 Hz spike–waves. In seven of them, the electroclinical picture was incomplete. In one of them it was complete but transitory (6 months). In every patient, changes in symptomatology occurred after a status epilepticus due to withdrawal of antiepileptic drugs without medical advice. A similar evolution following an idiopathic generalized epilepsy (or an idiopathic partial epilepsy) has also been described by Beaumanoir (1982) and Aicardi & Chevrie (1982). These authors underlined the role of antiepileptic drugs in worsening of the syndrome which is usually transitory.

Other patients present with a cryptogenic or symptomatic partial epilepsy with onset in childhood and which is difficult to control. During the course of the disease and around adolescence, drop attacks occur. The EEG shows bilateral abnormalities, slow diffuse spike–waves, activated by sleep, but rarely runs of rapid rhythms during sleep. These EEG signs are usually not accompanied by true tonic seizures. In these patients a mechanism of secondary bilateral synchrony can be evoked (Gastaut & Zifkin, 1988).

Chapter 9 The Lennox–Gastaut syndrome

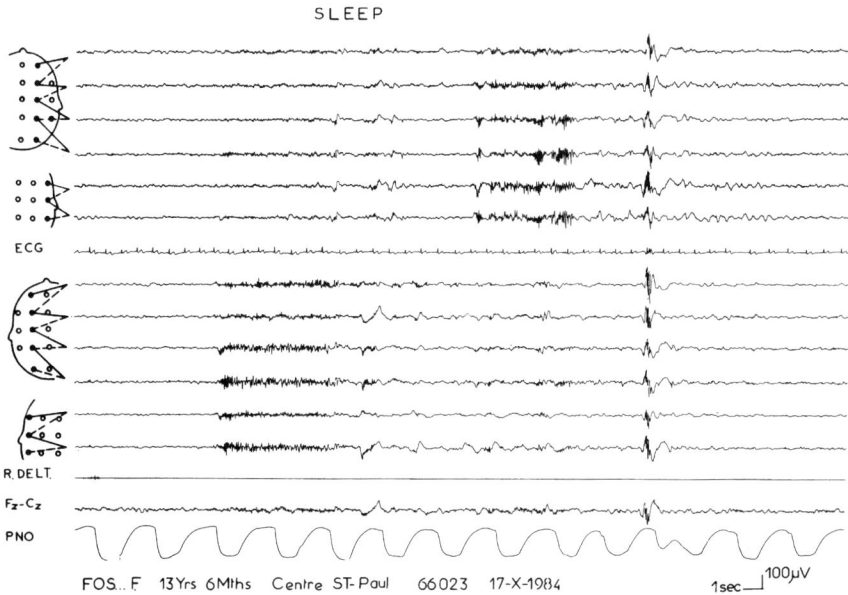

Fig. 6. Sleep recording in an adolescent of 13½ years. Seizures started at the age of 12 years (complex partial seizures at first, then atypical absences and nocturnal tonic seizures). From left to right: one left hemispheric discharge of low voltage rapid rhythms followed by slow waves, then one right hemispheric discharge of the same type, then one diffuse polySW. No appreciable clinical change. R. Delt. = right deltoid; PNO = pneumogram.

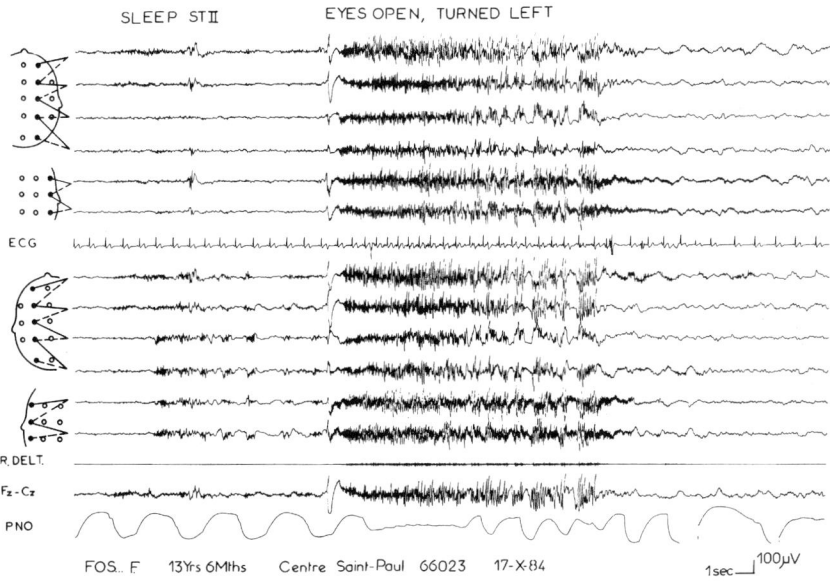

Fig. 7. For the same boy as in Fig. 6, at the same age, sleep recording with, from left to right: one left hemispheric discharge of rapid rhythms with no clinical correlate and one polySW on the right hemisphere; then a typical tonic seizure with a brief apnea, tachycardia, muscular contraction and eye deviation turning to the left. R. Delt. = right deltoid; PNO = pneumogram.

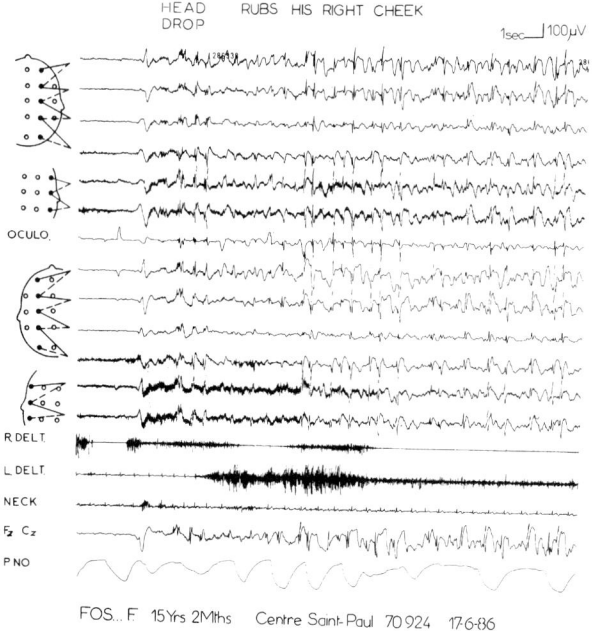

Fig. 8. For the same boy as in Figs. 6 and 7, at 15 years 2 months, one atypical absence starting by a head drop, followed by an automatism. EEG shows diffuse, irregular SSW and slow waves, more evident on the right side. R. Delt = right deltoid; L. Delt. = left deltoid ; PNO = pneumogram.

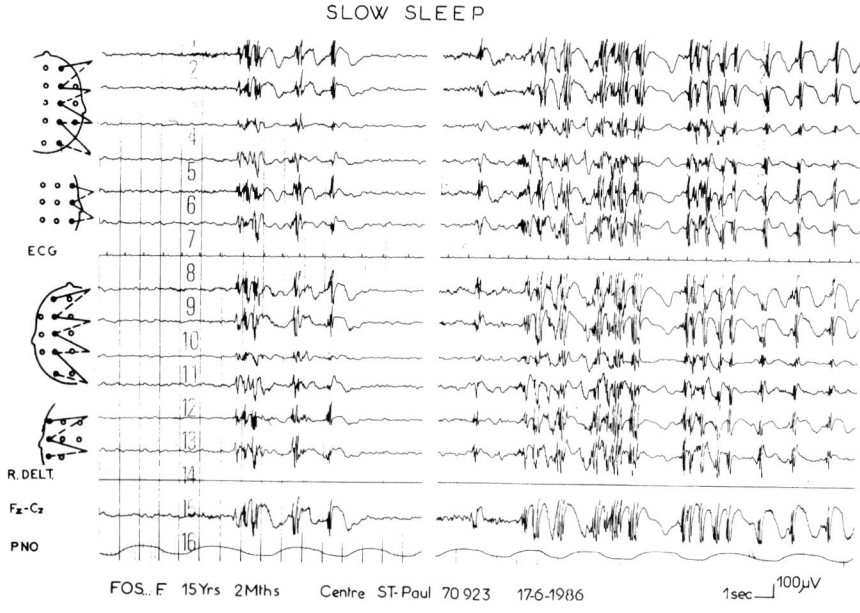

Fig. 9. For the same boy as in Figs. 6, 7 and 8, at the same age, typical aspects of LGS sleep: generalized poly SW and high voltage rapid rhythms. R. Delt = right deltoid; PNO = pneumogram.

Thus it appears that LGS exists in adolescence, typical and severe in *de novo* cases, incomplete and less severe in patients with a previous history of epilepsy. Conversely, no case of LGS starting after the age of 25 years has ever been published.

Changes in semiology at different ages in the same patient?

Most of the authors who have studied the long-term course of LGS (Osawa *et al.*, 1977; Beaumanoir, 1982; Oller-Daurella *et al.*, 1985) describe three situations: complete recovery with disappearance of all seizure types; persistence of the typical features of the syndrome; and disappearance of the specific seizures, such as atypical absences, myoclonic attacks, tonic seizures, but occurrence of partial seizures and/or generalized tonic–clonic seizures. Oller-Daurella (1970) emphasized a particular type of tonic seizure in which the classical tonic phase is followed by a phase of gestural automatisms, more or less intense, observed mainly in adolescents and older patients (72 per cent of late onset cases in this series). On the EEG, the diffuse rapid rhythms are replaced by diffuse slow spike–waves of variable duration. These phenomena were termed 'tonico-automatic seizures'.

We have observed different changes in semiology: the head noddings of the young children become true tonic spasms or disappear. Tonic seizures which are brief tonic spasms, often serially repeated in young children, become stronger and longer when patients grow older. Simultaneously, mild clonic components and asymmetry occur. In adolescents and adults, tonic–clonic and 'vibratory' seizures are sometimes observed in addition to classical tonic seizures. Atypical absences as well as myoclonic seizures have a tendency to decrease. Drop attacks persist, more often due to tonic contraction than to loss of tone. Even when the diurnal seizures become rare, the nocturnal ones persist, sometimes very mild and difficult to detect without polygraphic recording.

EEGs have been well studied by Ohtsuka *et al.* (1991). The diffuse SSW-waves tend to decrease gradually. They are replaced either by slow waves of the same frequency and lower voltage or by focal and multifocal spikes and spike–waves, but the bursts of diffuse rapid rhythms persist during sleep. Multiple independent spikes are observed mainly in patients with symptomatic LGS and severe mental deterioration. The authors named these cases 'severe epilepsy with multiple independent spike foci'. In these patients, atypical absences are no longer observed but other seizure types remain unchanged: diurnal drop attacks and nocturnal generalized tonic seizures.

Conclusion

LGS is actually an age-dependent syndrome since it appears only in the first two decades of life. It is much more common in childhood than in infancy or in adolescence. Clinical expression also varies according to age. It would be interesting to understand why a tonic phenomenon is extremely brief when produced by an immature brain and becomes longer and stronger when the brain is more mature. Moreover, what are the relationships between the pure tonic seizures in early childhood and the vibratory and tonic clonic seizures observed later in childhood and adolescence? For what reason do drop attacks and SSW occur in some patients at a variable stage of the course of an apparently idiopathic generalized epilepsy? The availability of an animal model would allow some of these questions to be approached. Progresses in genetics will probably also help to understand the various forms of this epilepsy.

Acknowledgements: I thank my friend Doctor Michelle Bureau for the images. I also thank the EEG technicians of the Centre Saint-Paul who made this work possible by recording the EEGs in patients who are not always co-operative.

References

Aicardi, J. & Chevrie, J.J. (1982): Atypical benign partial epilepsy of childhood. *Dev. Med. Child Neurol.* **24**, 281–292.

Bauer, G., Benke, T. & Bohr, K. (1988): The Lennox–Gastaut in adulthood. In: *The Lennox–Gastaut syndrome*, Niedermeyer, E. & Degen, R. (eds), pp. 317–327. New York: Alan Liss.

Beaumanoir, A. (1982): The Lennox–Gastaut syndrome: a personal study. In: *Henri Gastaut and the Marseilles school's contribution to the neurosciences* (EEG suppl no. 35), Broughton, R.J. (ed.), pp. 85–99. Amsterdam: Elsevier Biomedical Press.

Beaumanoir, A. & Dravet, C. (1992): The Lennox–Gastaut syndrome. In: *Epileptic syndromes in infancy, childhood and adolescence*, Roger, J., Bureau, M., Dravet, Ch., Dreifuss, F.E., Perret, A. & Wolf, P., pp. 115–132. London: John Libbey.

Bladin, B.F. (1985): Adult Lennox–Gastaut syndrome: features and diagnostic problems. *Clin. Exp. Neurol.* **21**, 93–104.

Boniver, C., Dravet, C., Bureau, M. & Roger, J. (1987): Idiopathic Lennox syndrome. In: *Advances in epileptology*, vol. 16, Wolf, P., Dam, M., Janz, D. & Dreifuss, F.E. (eds), pp. 195–200. New York: Raven Press.

Cavazzuti, G.B. (1972): The Lennox–Gastaut syndrome: childhood epileptic encephalopathy with diffuse slow spike waves (La sindrome di Lennox–Gastaut, encefalopatia epilettica infantile). *Clin. Pediat. (Bologna)* **54**, 237–292.

Chevrie, J.J. & Aicardi, J. (1972): Childhood epileptic encephalopathy with slow spike–wave. A statistical study of 80 cases. *Epilepsia* **13**, 259–271.

Commission on Classification and Terminology of the International League Against Epilepsy (1989): Proposal for revised classification of epilepsies and epileptic syndromes. *Epilepsia* **30**, 389–399.

Dravet, C., Munari, C. & Roger, J. (1973): Evolution de 39 cas de syndrome de West en relation avec l'épilepsie ultérieure. In: *Evolution and prognosis of epilepsies*, Lugaresi, E., Pazzaglia, P. & Tassinari, A. (eds), pp. 119–131. Milan: Itaselber.

Egli, M., Mothersill, J. & O'Kane, F. (1985): The axial spasm. The predominant type of drop seizure in patients with secondary generalized epilepsy. *Epilepsia* **26**, 401–415

Erba, G. & Lombroso, C. (1973): La sindrome di Lennox–Gastaut. *Prosp. Pediat.* **10**, 145–165.

Gastaut, H. & Zifkin, B.J. (1988): Secondary bilateral synchrony and Lennox–Gastaut syndrome. In: *The Lennox–Gastaut syndrome*, Niedermeyer, E. & Degen, R. (eds), pp. 221–242. New York: Alan Liss.

Ikeno, T., Shigematsu, H., Miyakoshi, M., Ohba, A., Yagi, K. & Seino, M. (1985): An analytic study of epileptic falls. *Epilepsia* **26**, 612–621.

Lipinski, G.G. (1977): Epilepsies with astatic seizures of late onset. *Epilepsia* **18**, 13–20.

Meencke, H.J. & Gerhard, C. (1985): Morphological aspects of aetiology and the course of infantile spasms (West syndrome). *Neuropediatrics* **16**, 59–66.

Ohtahara, S. (1978): Clinico-electrical delineation of epileptic encephalopathies in childhood. *Asian Med. J.* **21**, 7–17.

Ohtsuka, Y., Amano, R., Mizukawa, M., Maniwa, S. & Ohtahara, S. (1991): Long term prognosis of the Lennox–Gastaut syndrome: considerations in its evolutional changes. In: *Modern perspectives of child neurology*, Fukuyama, Y., Kamoshita, S., Ohtsuka, C. & Susuki, Y. (eds), pp. 215–222. Tokyo: The Japanese Society of Child Neurology.

Oller Daurella, L. (1970): Un type spécial de crises observées dans le syndrome de Lennox–Gastaut d'apparition tardive. *Rev. Neurol. (Paris)* **122**, 459–462

Oller Daurella, L., Oller Ferrer-Vidal, L. & Sanchez, M.E. (1985): Evolucion del sindrome de Lennox–Gastaut. *Rev. Neurol. (Barcelona)* XIII, **63**, 169–184.

Osawa, T., Sino, M., Miyokoshi, M., Yamamoto, K., Kagegawa, N., Yagi, K., Hirata, T., Morikawa, T. & Wada, T. (1977): Therapy resistant epilepsies with long term history. Slow spike and wave syndrome. In: *Epilepsy. The Eighth International Symposium*, Penry, K. (ed.), pp. 63–68. New York: Raven Press.

Roger, J., Rémy, C., Bureau, M., Oller-Daurella, L., Beaumanoir, A., Favel, P. & Dravet, C. (1987): Le syndrome de Lennox–Gastaut de l'adulte. *Rev. Neurol. (Paris)* **143**, 401–405

Stenzel, E. & Pantelli, C. (1983): Lennox–Gastaut syndrome des 2. Lebensjahrzehntes. In: *Epilepsie 1981*, Remschmidt, H., Rentz, R. & Jungmann, J. (eds), pp. 99–107. Stuttgart: Thieme.

Weinmann, H.M. (1988): Lennox–Gastaut syndrome and its relationship to infantile spasms (West syndrome). In: *The Lennox–Gastaut syndrome*, Niedermeyer, E. & Degen, R. (eds), pp. 301–316. New York: Alan Liss.

Yamatogi, Y. & Ohtahara, S. (1981): Age dependent epileptic encephalopathy: a longitudinal study. *Folia Psych. Neurol. Jpn.* **35**, 321–331.

Chapter 10

Developmental consequences of epilepsies in infancy

Thierry Deonna

Neuropaediatric Unit, CHUV, Lausanne, Switzerland

Introduction

In 1955, in a historical paper entitled 'Mental deterioration with convulsions in infancy', Illingworth made the following conclusions: '... The clinical picture of the cases does not in the least suggest that the fits are the cause of the mental deterioration ... it is far more likely that some change occurs in the brain which causes both the fits and the deterioration ...'. Reading the case histories clearly shows that these babies had sufffered from West syndrome (infantile spasms with hypsarrythmia) for which no effective therapy existed at the time. As an astute clinician, he had observed that some of these babies had developed normally initially and he documented in detail the stagnation, sometimes preceding the spasms, and the regression. However, he did not consider the possibility that the epilepsy in itself could be the cause of the deterioration, mainly because the mental symptoms preceded the seizures and because the seizures were brief and less severe than other types in this age group which did not have adverse developmental consequences. This opinion illustrates the difficulty of appreciating that stagnation or regression in development can reflect an ongoing epileptic activity without obvious clinical seizures, and a still current idea that seizures in infants are usually symptomatic of severe and diffuse brain pathologies which in themselves are the main or unique cause of the retardation.

Congenital focal brain lesions – Cognitive consequences and effects on the dynamics of development

Before examining the possible consequences of epilepsy with onset in infancy, one must first know what can be the effect of a cerebral pathology sustained prenatally or very early in developement.

It is increasingly recognized that major congenital structural lesions in one hemisphere (such as infarcts) may have remarkably few if any long-term cognitive effects. As a consequence, in a child with developmental retardation associated with symptomatic focal seizures, one cannot necessarily attribute this problem to the underlying brain pathology (Dall'Oglio *et al.*, 1994).

Retrospective studies of children with identical lesions with and without epilepsy can give a hint of the role of epilepsy. The careful study of Vargha-Khadem *et al.* (1992) of 40 children with hemiplegic cerebral palsy showed that intelligence and memory did not differ according to either side or size of the lesion, but were lower in the presence of epilepsy (or paroxysmal EEG activity). This of course is not a proof of a direct effect of epilepsy. Other factors such as drug effects could be responsible.

However, this study gave an important indication as to the potential detrimental effect of epilepsy and justifies further prospective studies to try to sort out the role of the different factors related to the epilepsy.

The results of prospective studies of early development of children with well documented focal cortical lesions sustained before birth or during the first 6 months of life using sophisticated methodologies now allow us to have a more precise knowledge of the range and type of developmental variations that can be observed in these circumstances (Bates *et al.*, 1992). For instance, temporary delays in language development, which are completely compensated for, can be observed in children with early focal brain lesions in various locations. These studies have also shown that the classical localizationist adult view does not apply in these situations.

However, there are so far only very limited data in this area and it remains very difficult in practice to sort out in an individual case what might be the direct effect of early epilepsy on development (Le Normand & Cohen, 1997).

At present we are able to recognize only the most obvious massive epileptic regressions and less commonly rapid recoveries associated with medical or surgical control of seizures.

Epilepsies and epileptic syndromes in infancy – variable effects on development

The immature brain has a greater seizure susceptibility, a tendency to status epilepticus, than the mature brain but possibly is more resistant to seizure-induced cellular damage (Holmes, 1997). The developmental consequences are not related only to severity or duration of seizures. The underlying pathophysiology of the seizures and its effects on brain development are probably very variable, depending on many factors. This is illustrated by the different epileptic syndromes in infancy whose clinical manifestations, mechanisms of seizures and modes of spread and prognosis vary. Mental development can be more or less affected or not at all. Table 1 summarizes some epileptic syndromes of infancy. The term 'benign' relates to the long-term good prognosis for seizures.

Table 1. Some epileptic syndromes of infancy: cognitive consequences

Syndrome	Seizures	Cognitive consequences
BNFC	Neonatal, multiform	None
BIFC	Partial (clusters)	None
BME	Myoclonic	None
West	Myoclonic spasms	Stagnation or regression ± reversible
SME	Focal febrile Myoclonic status	Normal development (→1½ years) Stagnation, marked retard
–	Partial with spasms*	Variable, regression (± autistic-like)
LKS & CSWS**	Simple partial & other	Acquired aphasia

BNFC: benign neonatal familial convulsions; BIFC: benign infantile familial convulsions; BME: benign myoclonic epilepsy of infancy; SME: severe myoclonic epilepsy of infancy; LKS: acquired epileptic aphasia (Lanau–Kleffner); CSWS: syndrome of 'continuous spike–waves during sleep'.

*'Late epileptic spasms' (after the first year, often between 2 and 4 years) are now reported to occur more frequently then previously recognized, usually along with other seizure types. These children may have a long recognized stagnation or regression before the diagnosis is made. (Bednarek *et al.*, 1997).
**Although these syndromes are typically recognized in older children, there are well documented cases of children with already well developed language or other cognitive functions who lost them before two years of age, together with major behavioural problems (Deonna, 1996).

West syndrome (infantile spasms with hypsarrythmia) is most often associated with developmental arrest or regression which can sometimes be reversed if epilepsy is controlled (Guzzetta *et al.*, 1993).

The later prognosis will then depend on the location and extent of the underlying pathology responsible for the epilepsy in the first place.

Severe myoclonic epilepsy of infancy (SME) is a very special situation in which one observes, after a period of normal development for about a year after onset of the seizures, a stagnation in development with ataxia correlating with increasing severity of the seizures and a permanent long-term mental retardation with autistic features (Perrot-Casse, 1994). No metabolic or degenerative disease can be demonstrated and the condition tends to stabilize with age (see case 3). There are genetic animal models of epilepsy which resemble SME, but they cannot be used as a general model of how epilepsy affects development (Burgess et al., 1997).

The effects of epileptic discharges on the developing brain, and the relationship between localization of epileptic lesion(s) and developmental consequences

Epileptic discharges in developing brain areas particularly implicated in cognitive functions and behaviour have important effects. The areas which support them have prolonged developmental periods, as opposed to those that mature more quickly, such as motor areas or primary sensory areas. If the brain systems involved are intermittently unavailable because of seizure activity, learning from experience and practice cannot take place. If the epileptic activity is maximal at the time of the normally occurring programmed development of these areas, the consequences will be greater because the stabilization of connections necessary for the consolidation of emerging cognitive functions cannot take place. Experimentally, it has been shown that local development and connectivity of the cortical zones affected by epileptic discharges in a developing animal can be significantly disturbed. Thus, in addition to the intermittent interruption of cognitive activity and learning during discharges, permanent structural brain changes can occur (Baumbach & Chow, 1981; Campbell et al., 1984; Grigonis & Murphy, 1994).

All these reasons explain why early epilepsy can be so detrimental to development, more so than even major fixed non-epileptic lesions. The cognitive and behavioural consequences of early epilepsy have been best documented in West syndrome. A cortical epileptogenic lesion can now be recognized with functional imaging studies in most cases of this syndrome and the pathology can be situated in any location. The onset of the epilepsy probably occurs at a younger age if the pathology affects cortical areas which have normally an early rate of maturation (i.e. occipital areas) (Koo & Hwang, 1996). The importance for cognitive development of the cortical zones implicated in the epileptic process, its age of onset and duration will, among other factors, determine the long-term cognitive and behavioural sequellae. Understandably, these are extremely variable and sometimes the infant can resume a normal development.

A particularly dramatic example of the influence of the location and spread of the epileptic focus on behaviour and development is seen in the syndrome of gelastic seizures with hypothalamic hamartomas. This dysplasia is intrinsically epileptogenic (Berkovic et al., 1997). The severe behavioural disturbances of young children with this syndrome and the progressive intellectual decline are very probably related to the strategic posture of this malformation and the spread of the epileptic discharges by hypothalamic–amygdala connexions.

The earlier the onset of epilepsy, the more restricted will be the repertoire of cognitive and behavioural performances that the baby will have achieved and the more difficult it is to evaluate the effect of epilepsy *per se* on development.

Clinical evaluation of the direct role of epilepsy during early developmental periods

Diagnosis of epilepsy in infancy

It is becoming increasingly clear that much or significant abnormal epileptic activity can occur in the infant's brain without evident clinical seizure activity. This is exemplified in some babies with West

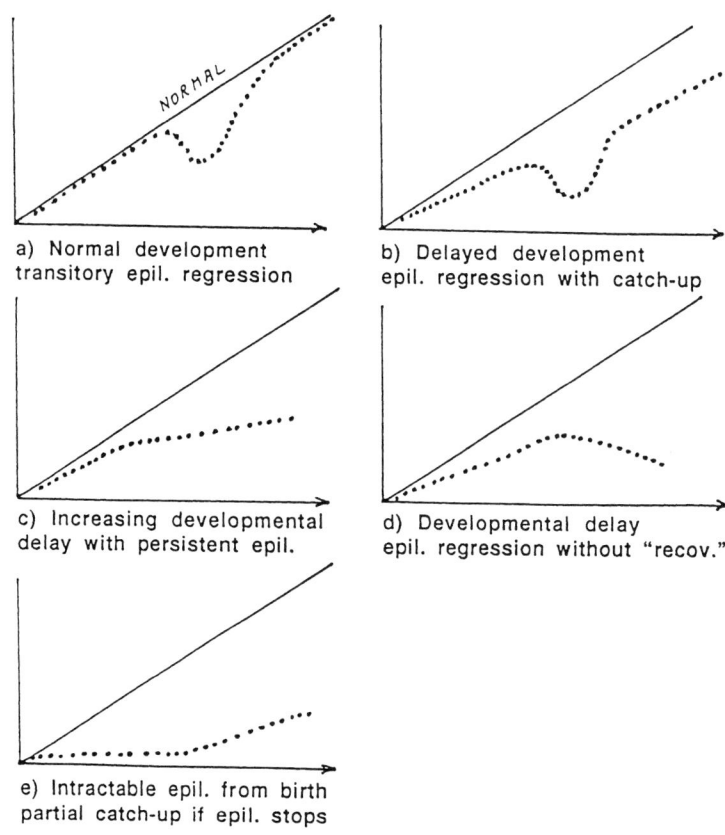

Fig. 1. Effects of early epilepsy (approx. 0–3 years) on development. Schematic representation.

syndrome who regress before clinical spasms are recognized. Also prolonged video EEG monitoring of these babies shows subtle clinically unrecognized motor seizures and lapses in vigilance corresponding to an epileptic discharge (Kellaway et al., 1979).

Partial complex seizures can easily escape diagnosis in young infants, specially those of frontal origin. Bizarre 'stereotypic' movements can be observed which are given various interpretations. In an ongoing study of seven such children, four were found to have long-standing unrecognized epilepsy, which was discovered during work-up for stagnation or regression in development. All had frontal foci (Deonna et al., 1995).

Surface EEGs can be silent in children with deep-situated foci (cingular, mesiofrontal, orbitofrontal, medial temporal) outside the actual seizure. In a recent study of babies with refractory partial epilepsy, four/18 recorded during several days with video EEG monitoring had no interictal discharges (Acharya et al., 1997).

The observation that seizures can directly lead to stagnation and regression in early development (independently of the underlying cause) has sometimes been shown in prospective studies where one observes that the deficit correlates with the onset of epileptic activity and is reversible when it is controlled.

Figure 1 shows how the dynamics of development can be altered by early epilepsy. (a) There is a transient regression in a child with a previously normal development and subsequent recovery. This occurs typically in some babies with idiopathic West syndrome. (b) The child shows some degree of developmental retardation from the onset, presumably due to an underlying congenital encephalopathy, but has a stagnation or a regression at the time when the epilepsy becomes active. If the epilepsy is controlled, the child may recover its previous development, but always with a lag. (c) If the epilepsy is unrecognized, persistent or uncontrolled, a progressively severe retardation will become evident. (d) If this is more severe, the child will show an increasing regression over time. These last situations may go long unrecognized, the more so if the child is significantly retarded and shows difficult behaviour. Subtle motor seizures may be mistaken as stereotypies, and variations in mood, vigilance or activity can be indistinguishable from other instances of abnormal paroxysmal behaviour.

As long as the child is making progress, even if the pace is very slow, the additional effect of ongoing seizures, the interruption of activities at crucial stages of learning, can pass unnoticed unless clear-cut episodic regressions with visible seizure activity are recognized.

Another possible but probably exceptional situation (e) is that of a baby with early intractable epilepsy from the first days or weeks of life who shows no or minimal development. If epilepsy stops spontaneously or finally becomes under control, some unexpected partial catch-up becomes possible even after a few months.

Prospective longitudinal studies of cases in which regression or catch-up in several areas of development (or only in a selective one) can be clearly correlated with the epileptic activity is the best demonstration of the direct role of epilepsy. It requires systematic and prolonged studies of babies even if they appear normal initially, and at the other extreme of severely retarded ones who may nevertheless significantly improve if the epilepsy is kept under control (Deonna *et al.*, 1993, 1995). Of course, such opportunities are rare, the more so because these epilepsies are often refractory to treatment, or improve only temporarily.

The best examples at present are the surgical cases. There are several reports of early surgery for young children with major dysplasias and intractable epilepsy who sometimes make rapid and remarkable progress after successful surgery (Pedespan *et al.*, 1995). However, these babies are rarely studied systematically with neuro-psychological methods and detailed behavioural observations (Caplan *et al.*, 1992; Gillberg *et al.*, 1996; Neville *et al.*, 1997).

We are now probably recognizing only those cases with early clinically evident epilepsy with major structural lesions on brain imaging. It is likely that very subtle seizures due to small but strategically located dysplasias (not visible on standard neuroimaging) might have a devastating effect on cognition and behaviour.

Illustrative cases

Case 1: Early multifocal partial epilepsy of unknown cause from infancy (Fig. 2)

This girl had severe intractable epilepsy from the third day of life with multiple seizure types. No specific aetiological diagnosis could be made. The pattern of electroclinical seizures did not conform to a particular syndrome, although it resembles a group of recently described babies reported as 'migrating seizures of infancy' (Coppola *et al.*, 1995). Several anticonvulsants were tried. She had practically no development until 11–13 months of life. At this time vigabatrin was given for newly occurring clusters of epileptic 'spasms' to which she was immediately responsive. From then on, she started to make regular and totally unexpected developmental progresses, although of course at a retarded level. We do not know the details of this developmental 'catch-up' because this had not been anticipated and no detailed prospective study had been done. It illustrates that, in spite of the major role of the underlying encephalopathy, epilepsy can play an additional important role with some residual potential for development despite months of uncontrolled epilepsy.

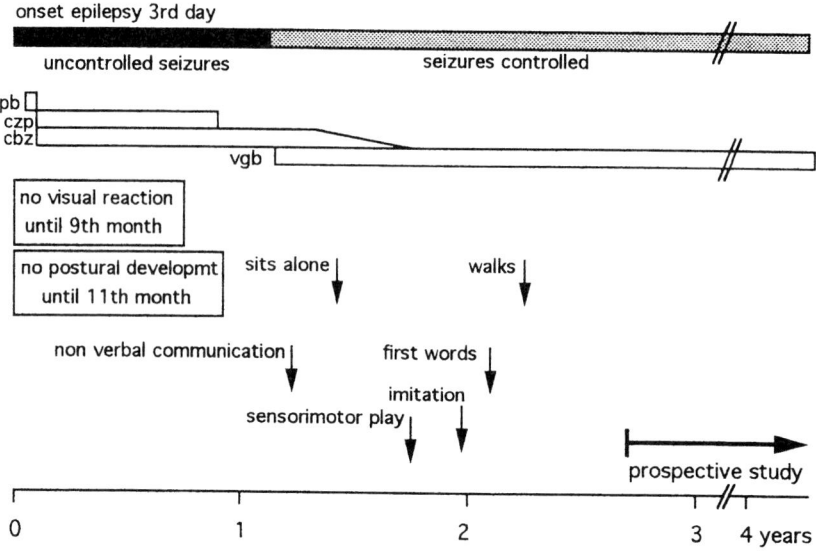

Fig. 2. Case 1 Early multifocal partial epilepsy of unknown cause from neonatal period.

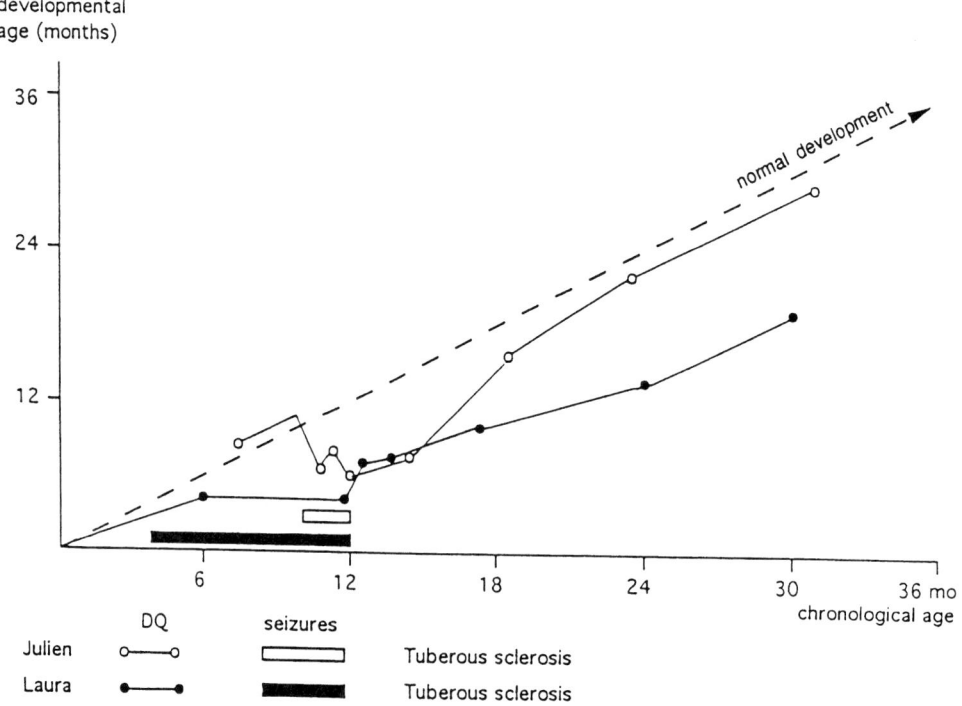

Fig. 3. Cases 2 and 3: infantile spasms with hypsarrythmia in tuberous sclerosis.

Cases 2 and 3: Infantile spasms with hypsarythmia in tuberous sclerosis (Fig. 3)

In these two children, a rapid cognitive improvement occurred with effective control of the seizures and EEG normalization. In one child the diagnosis had been delayed for several months and the child remains with severe retardation, whereas the other one who was rapidly treated and well controlled is developing normally at an age now of 6 years. Of course part of the variance can be explained by a difference in severity of the cerebral dysgenesis. However, the role of epilepsy is clearly demonstrated by the rapid progress from the beginning of anticonvulsant medication. It also shows that tuberous sclerosis presenting with symptomatic early West syndrome can be sometimes associated with normal development, if the epilepsy is controlled and if the cerebral malformation is limited.

Case 4: Severe myoclonic epilepsy of infancy (Fig. 4)

This child had a documented normal early development until 16–18 months of age, when a stagnation in cognitive development, unsteadiness of gait, became gradually apparent. Seizures were very frequent and refractory to all anticonvulsant drugs. The seizures have become less severe and somewhat responsive to therapy since 5 years of age. MRI of the brain at the age of 18 months and 5 years were normal with no visible cerebral or cerebellar atrophy after several years of uncontrolled epilepsy and severe mental retardation. There is no evidence of a known metabolic brain disorder. This case shows that epilepsy, ataxia and cognitive arrest are closely linked together. The mechanisms by which epilepsy affects development are probably very different from other early epilepsies in which development can proceed even if epilepsy is not fully controlled.

Case 5: Early partial epilepsy with complex partial seizures, epileptic spasms. Dynamics of development from 1 to 4 years (Fig. 5)

Figure 5 illustrates the dynamics of development observed from 1 to 4 years in this child followed prospectively in great detail with videofilms of development, questionaires, infant intelligence tests and frequent waking and sleep EEG. Discussions with parents and family videos showed that epilepsy started at least 3 months before it was first recognized. With initial control of the seizures and normalization of the EEG, the child pursued his development with a mild delay for a few months, until an insidious stagnation and development of autistic features became apparent with aggravation of the EEG (focal paroxysmal activity during waking state and diffuse dysrythmia with generalized spikes during sleep), followed by a catastrophic rapid deterioration within a week with epileptic 'stereotypies' and 'spasms during sleep' which could be controlled only with corticosteroids. He improved markedly after that, with a significant delay but a normal communication. In this child, the direct role of epilepsy could be clearly demonstrated. He probably has a highly epileptogenic focus (dysplasia) not visible on the MRI in the frontal region (site of his main EEG focus) whose activity became gradually very intense and refractory to conventional antiepileptic drugs during the second year of life.

Conclusion – the role of epilepsy in pervasive (PDD) and other developmental disorders

This last case illustrates a very important and presently major source of concern for clinicians dealing with children with so-called pervasive developmental disorders, particularly the children who show a regression in early development (autistic regression, disintegrative psychosis) (Tuchman & Rapin, 1997). Could epilepsy be a major causal factor in some of these children and, if so, how can we detect and evaluate it? The difficulty in recognizing partial complex seizures in infants and young children (especially in those with retarded or aberrant development), and the fact that surface EEG can be normal or show abnormalities only during some seizures, complicate the issue. It is possible that we are underestimating the number of children with PDD in whom a relatively 'hidden' epilepsy plays a direct role. Increasing awareness of this problem, improving clinical observation techniques (Caplan et al., 1992; Caplan, 1995), video EEG analysis of seizures and cerebral functional imaging, and study of privileged cases with electrocorticography who undergo epileptic surgery will improve our

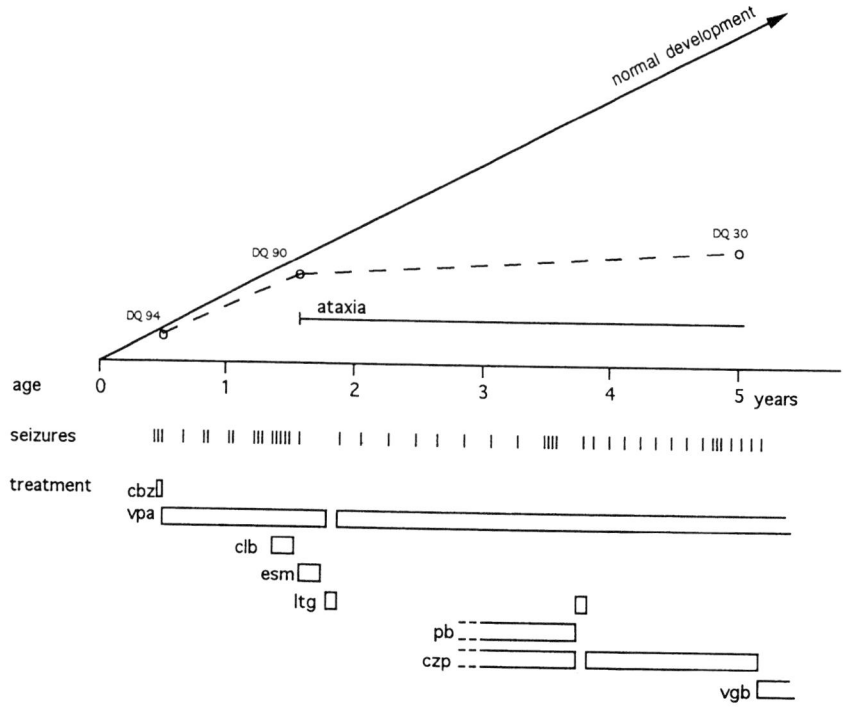

Fig. 4. Case 4: severe myoclonic epilepsy of infancy.

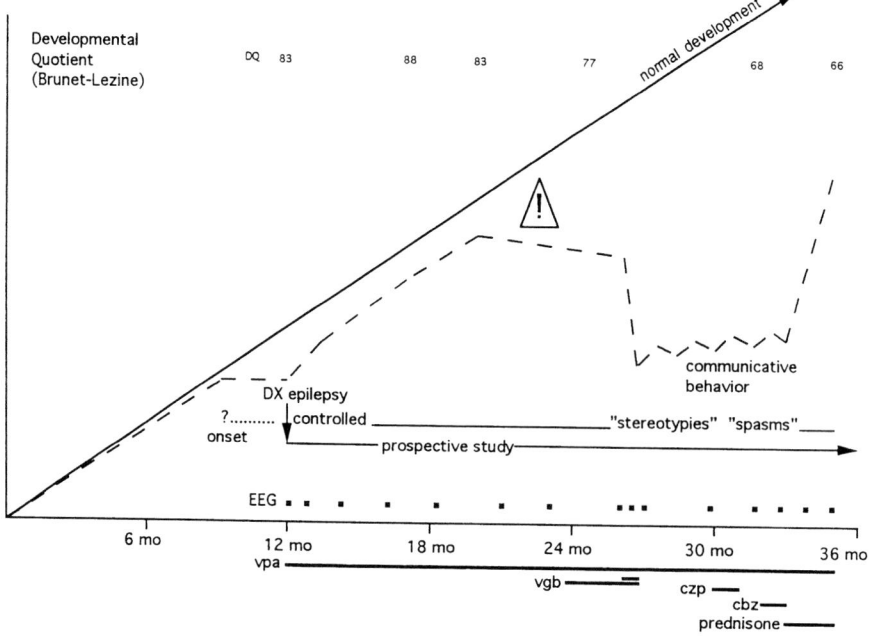

Fig. 5. Case 5: early partial epilepsy with complex partial seizures, epileptic spasms. Dynamics of development from 1 to 4 years (see text for EEG data).

knowledge in this area. It is probable that we are seeing only the tip of the iceberg, that is infants with severe, very early, clinically obvious seizures and findings on brain imaging. Neuropaediatricians and neuro-psychologists must move to study younger children in collaboration with child psychiatrists and people involved in early education of very young children with developmental retardation and autistic disorders.

References

Acharya, J.N., Wyllie, E., Luders, H.O., Kotagal, P., Lancman, M. & Coelho, M. (1997): Seizure symptomatology in infants with localization-related epilepsy. *Neurology* **48**, 189–196.

Bates, E., Thal, D. & Janowsky. J.J. (1992): Early language development and its neural correlates. In: *Handbook of neuropsychology*, vol 7, Segalowitz, J.J. & Rapin, I. (eds), pp. 69–110. New York: Elsevier.

Baumbach, H.D. & Chow, K.L. (1981): Visuocortical epileptiform discharges in rabbits: differential effects on neuronal development in the lateral geniculate nucleus and superior colliculus. *Brain Res.* **209**, 61–76.

Bednarek, N., Motte, J., Soufflet, C., Plouin, P. & Dulac, O. (1997): Evidence for late infantile spasms. *Epilepsia* (in press).

Berkovic, S.F., Kuzniecky, R.I. & Andermann, F. (1997): Human epileptogenesis and hypothalamic hamartomas: new lessons from an experiment of nature. *Epilepsia* **38**, 1–3.

Burgess, D.L., Jones, J., Meisler, M. & Noebels, J.L. (1997): Mutation of the Ca^{2+} channel β subunit gene Cchb4 is associated with ataxia and seizures in the lethargic (lh) mouse. *Cell* **88**, 385–392.

Campbell, B.G., Ostrach, L.H., Crabtree, J.W. & Chow, K.L. (1984): Characterization of penicillin- and bicuculline-induced epileptiform discharges during development of striate cortex in rabbits. *Dev. Brain Res.* **15**, 125–128.

Caplan, R. (1995): Epilepsy in early development: the lesson from surgery for early intractable seizures. *Sem. Pediatr. Neurol.* **2**, 238–245.

Caplan, R., Guthrie, D., Mundy, P., Sigman, M., Shields, D., Sherman, T. & Peakock, W. (1992): Nonverbal communication skills of surgically treated children with infantile spasms. *Dev. Med. Child Neurol.* **34**, 499–506.

Coppola, G., Plouin, P., Chiron, C., Robain, O. & Dulac, O. (1995): Migrating partial seizures in infancy: a malignant disorder with developmental arrest. *Epilepsia* **36**, 1017–1024.

Dall Oglio, A.M., Bates, E., Volterra, V. *et al.* (1994): Early cognition, communication and language in children with focal brain injury. *Dev. Med. Child Neurol.* **36**, 1076–1098.

Deonna, T. (1995): Cognitive and behavioral disturbances as epileptic manifestations in children: an overview. *Sem. Ped.Neurol.* **2**, 254–260.

Deonna, T. (1996): Troubles du langage et épilepsie chez l'enfant. In: *Le langage de l'enfant. Aspects normaux et pathologiques*, Chevrie-Muller, C. &. Narbona, J. (eds), pp. 386–398. Paris: Masson.

Deonna, T., Ziegler, A.L., Maeder, M.I., Ansermet, F. & Roulet, E. (1995): Reversible behavioural autistic-like regression: a manifestation of a special (new?) epileptic syndrome in a 28-month-old child. A 2-year longitudinal study. *Neurocase* **1**, 91–99.

Deonna, T.. Ziegler, A.L.. Moura-Serra, J. & Innocenti, G. (1993): Autistic regression in relation to limbic pathology and epilepsy: report of two cases. *Dev. Med. Child Neurol.* **35**, 166–176.

Gillberg, C., Uvebrant, P., Carlsson, G., Hedström, A. & Silfvenius, H. (1996): Autism and epilepsy (and tuberous sclerosis?) in two pre-adolescent boys: neuropsychiatric aspects before and after epilepsy surgery. *J. Intellect. Disab. Res.* **40**, 75–81.

Grigonis, A.M. & Murphy, E.H. (1994): The effects of epileptic cortical activity on the development of callosal projections. *Dev. Brain Res.* **77**, 251–255.

Guzzetta, F., Crisafulli, A. & Isaya Crine, M. (1993): Cognitive assessment of infants with West syndrome. How useful in diagnosis and prognosis? *Dev. Med. Child Neurol.* **35**, 379–387.

Holmes, G.L. (1997): Epilepsy in the developing brain: lessons from the laboratory and clinic. *Epilepsia* **38**, 12–30.

Illingworth, R.S. (1955): Sudden mental deterioration with convulsions in infancy. *Arch. Dis. Child.* **30**, 529–537.

Kellaway, P., Hrachovy, R.A., Frost, J.D. *et al.* (1979): Precise characterization and quantification of infantile spasms. *Ann. Neurol.* **6**, 214–218.

Koo, B. & Hwang, P. (1996): Localization of focal cortical lesions influences age of onset of infantile spasms. *Epilepsia* **37,** 1068–1071.

Le Normand, M.T. & Cohen, H. (1997): L'acquisition du langage chez l'enfant épileptique: retard de compréhension et déficit de production. In: *Perception auditive et compréhension du langage.* Lambert, J. & Nespoulous, J.L. (eds). Marseille: Solal.

Neville, B.G.R., Harkness, W.F.J., Cross, J.H., Cass, H.C., Burch, V.C., Lees, J.A. & Taylor, D.C. (1997): Surgical treatment of severe autistic regression in childhood epilepsy. *Pediatr. Neurol.* **16,** 137–140.

Pedespan, J.M., Loiseau, H., Vital, A., Marchal, C., Fontan, D. & Rougier, A. (1995): Surgical treatment of an early epileptic encephalopathy with suppression-bursts and focal cortical dysplasia. *Epilepsia* **36,** 37–40.

Perrot-Casse, C. (1994): Approche psychologique de l'épilepsie myoclonique sévère. In: *Neuropsychologie et Epilepsies.* Fondation Française pour la Recherche sur l'Epilepsie. Biarritz, 3–5 September.

Tuchman, R. & Rapin, I. (1997): Regression in pervasive developmental disorders: seizures and epileptiform electroencephalographic correlates. *Pediatrics* **99,** 560–566.

Vargha-Khadem, F., Isaacs, E., Van Der Werf, S. *et al.* (1992): Development of intelligence and memory in children with hemiplegic cerebral palsy. The deleterious consequences of early seizures. *Brain* **115,** 315–329

Chapter 11

Cognitive and behavioural consequences of epilepsies in childhood

Marie-Noëlle Metz-Lutz[1] and Rita Massa[1,2]

[1]*INSERM U398, Clinique Neurologique, Hôpitaux Universitaires de Strasbourg, Strasbourg, France;*
[2]*Istituto di Neurologia, Università degli Studi di Cagliari, Italy*

Summary

The relationship between epilepsy and impairment of neuro-psychological functioning in children has been observed for a very long time. Although specific cognitive impairments have been reported and their severity related to the type, frequency or age of onset of seizure, our understanding of the precise relationship between epilepsy and cognitive impairment is affected by a number of methodological issues. Thus, the consequences of epilepsy on cognitive functions should be studied in well-defined forms of childhood epilepsy occurring after a period of normal neuro-cognitive development and characterized by focal epileptic discharges occurring in the absence of lesions, rare epileptic seizures and spontaneous recovery at the end of childhood. At least two clinical entities of childhood epilepsy meet these precise criteria: the benign focal epilepsy of childhood (BFEC), one of the most frequent idiopathic childhood epilepsies, and the continuous spike waves during slow wave sleep (CSWS). These two forms of childhood epilepsy have common electro-clinical features, focal spike–wave discharges during wakefulness that are activated during sleep, but differ as regard to the severity of the cognitive consequences of epilepsy. From a review of recent longitudinal case studies of CSWS, we attempt to demonstrate that a variety of acquired neuro-psychological deficits are the direct consequences of the focal epileptic activity involving specific areas of the associative cortex. In BFEC, we examine the relationship between the immediate consequences of epileptic discharges on cognitive functioning and the learning and behavioural problems frequently attributed to the social incidence of seizures or to anti-epileptic medication. We also discuss the possible consequence of an active epileptogenic focus present during the functional differentiation of the associative cortex.

Many papers have discussed the impact of childhood epilepsies on cognitive development. A number of studies involving a large population of children with epilepsy and using well-known tests of intellectual ability such as the Wechsler Intelligence Scale for Children (WISC-R), (Wechsler, 1981) have shown lower mean IQ scores in epileptic children compared to controls (Ross *et al.*, 1980; Ellenberg *et al.*, 1985; Farwell *et al.*, 1985). Despite the large number of studies on this topic (Klein registered, in 1991, more than 250 papers) the proper effects of epileptic activity on cognitive functioning and development are not yet clearly defined. This situation results from two main methodological biases, the clinical heterogeneity inherent to the large population of epileptic children to be studied and the measurement of cognitive functioning. Indeed many studies are carried out with institutionalized epileptic patients with frequent seizures and/or epileptic syndromes associated with structural brain lesions. As for lower global IQ scores, they may result from a markedly deviant score in a single subtest indicating a specific neuro-psychological deficit rather than an overall intellectual impairment. Moreover, it has been demonstrated that epileptic children have a relatively high test–retest variability and show fluctuating performances from one testing period to another, even within a testing period depending on sub-clinical EEG changes (Kasteleijn-Nolst Trenité *et al.*, 1990b). Thus, the cognitive and behavioural deficits observed in epilepsy must be regarded as the result of complex interactions between biological, psychological and social factors. In addition, the anti-epileptic medications themselves have negative side-effects on cognitive processing which are difficult to distinguish from the direct effects of the epileptic activity. However, the direct consequences of epilepsy on cognitive functions may be studied in forms of childhood epilepsy occurring, in the absence of lesion, after a period of normal neuro-cognitive development. Due to the rarity of epileptic seizures and their spontaneous recovery at the beginning of adolescence, these epilepsies have limited psycho-social consequences. Among the various forms of childhood epilepsy two clinical entities of childhood epilepsy meet these precise criteria: the benign focal epilepsy of childhood (BFEC) and the syndrome of continuous spike waves during slow sleep (CSWS).

Definitions

Neuro-psychological impairments in idiopathic focal childhood epilepsies

The idiopathic partial epilepsies which are the most frequent epilepsies in childhood share several common clinical and electrophysiological features. The first epileptic seizure usually occurs after a period of normal neurological and psychomotor development, rarely before 2 years of age. In the daytime, epileptic seizures are rare, whereas waking EEG evidenced focal or generalized epileptiform EEG discharges, mostly spike–wave discharges. During sleep their frequency increases, particularly during non-REM sleep, becoming in some cases almost continuous. Recovery of idiopathic partial childhood epilesies typically occurs at the beginning of adolescence. In these epilepsies, concomitant cognitive and behavioural disorders appear correlated to the localization of focal discharges with their severity dependent on the extent of discharges during sleep. The BFEC and the CSWS are considered as two extreme manifestations of a common clinical spectrum (Doose & Baier, 1989; Roulet Perez, 1995).

Benign focal epilepsies of childhood: BFEC

The diagnostic criteria for benign focal epilepsies of childhood include the onset of stereotyped seizures after the age of two years in a child free of neurological or intellectual deficits (Holmes, 1993). The seizures occur more frequently during sleep. Typically, the EEG shows a normal background activity, epileptiform activity with a particular morphology activated during sleep but not during hyperventilation (Fejerman & Di Blasi, 1987). Three clinical variants of BFEC are recognized: the benign epilepsy with centro-temporal spikes or benign rolandic epilepsy, which represents the most frequent form, the childhood epilepsy with occipital paroxysms and the benign psychomotor epilepsy (Dalla Bernadina *et al.*, 1992).

In the benign rolandic epilepsy, seizures are characterized by peri–oral tonic or tonic–clonic activity with speech arrest and salivation but preserved consciousness. The facial motor phenomena may spread to the arms but rarely generalize during wakefulness. The frequency of seizures is typically low (Lerman & Kivity, 1975). The interictal EEG demonstrates typical centro-temporal spikes with a prominent following slow wave appearing on the mid-temporal and central region. The discharges are most often unilateral although bilateral foci are sometimes observed. The spike–waves are activated during sleep, but they may generalize and status epilepticus during sleep has been recorded in some cases (Fejerman & Di Blasi, 1987).

The benign occipital epilepsy, less common than benign rolandic epilepsy, is characterized by seizures beginning with visual symptoms and the presence of very distinct occipital spike–waves on a normal background activity. The discharges, unilateral or bilateral, are activated by darkness and inhibited by fixation (Panayiotopoulos, 1989). Their frequency is variable. Seizures are confined to childhood with a peaking from the age of 3 to 5 years and their prognosis is generally favourable (Gastaut, 1982).

In the benign psychomotor epilepsy, the major clinical features of seizures are variable manifestations of fear (Dalla Bernadina *et al.*, 1985). The EEG pattern includes normal background activity and interictal spike–waves in the fronto-temporal or parieto-temporal area of one or both hemispheres.

Epilepsy with continuous spike–waves during slow sleep (CSWS)

The sub-clinical electrical status epilepticus induced by sleep, described by Patry *et al.* (1971), was initially observed in six children who were all mentally retarded and two of them failed to develop speech. This EEG aspect now highlights a well-defined clinical entity: the CSWS. This EEG aspect is associated with mental and behavioural disturbances that improve with the recovery of epilepsy and EEG normalization (Tassinari *et al.*, 1992). More recent clinical case reports of epilepsy and CSWS emphasize the relationship between acquired neuro-psychological disorders and localized abnormalities on wake EEG (Deonna, 1993; Roulet Perez, 1995). Today, several authors consider the Landau and Kleffner Syndrome (LKS) and CSWS as a unique clinical entity characterized by a set of common clinical and EEG features (Roulet *et al.*, 1991; Hirsch *et al.*, 1995; Maquet *et al.*, 1995). In this conception, the aphasic disorders characteristic of the LKS would be the consequence of an abnormal epileptic activity originating in the temporal cortex most often in the left posterior one. Indeed, there are several electro-physiological arguments in favour of a focal epileptiform activity responsible for both, the localized epileptic discharges during wakefulness and the pattern of CSWS. The unilateral focal origin of the epileptogenic process has been convincingly evidenced by the methohexital suppression test in LKS (Morrell *et al.*, 1995) and intracarotid amobarbital injection in a case of CSWS (Park *et al.*, 1994) as well as by PET scan studies (Maquet *et al.*, 1995).

Acquired cognitive deficits concomitant to a persistent focal epileptic activity

In the syndrome of CSWS, the neuro-psychological deficits concomitant to epilepsy occur, in more than half of the cases reported in the literature (Tassinari *et al.*, 1992) after a period of normal neurological and mental development. The acquired neuro-psychological deficits have been initially described as global mental deterioration, but recent case studies involving detailed neuro-psychological investigation at the early stage of the disease demonstrated that the almost global deterioration is subsequent to an initial specific cognitive deficit (Maquet *et al.*, 1995; Roulet Perez, 1995). We will illustrate this point through four examples of CSWS with various acquired neuro-psychological deficits.

Acquired aphasia associated with CSWS (or LKS) typically differs from acquired aphasia due to brain structural lesions that mainly impairs verbal production with speech reduction, speech articulation and naming disorders and agrammatism, whereas verbal auditory comprehension is usually spared. In acquired epileptic aphasia, auditory comprehension is severely impaired and the auditory agnosia also involves non-verbal auditory stimuli.

GB (case no.1 in Maquet *et al.*, 1995), a normally developed French-speaking boy, experienced, at the age of 5 years and 5 months, a first partial motor seizure followed by a transient right upper limb paresis and language impairment. The waking EEG evidenced left side predominant rolandic spikes increasing during sleep. Then, the child had a full IQ of 116 with a verbal IQ of 106 and a performance IQ of 123 on the Wechsler Primary Preschool Scale of Intelligence (WPPSI, Wechsler, 1974). Seizures increased at the age of 6 years 4 months while auditory comprehension and oral language rapidly deteriorated. Then the detailed neuro-psychological testing showed severe auditory verbal comprehension deficit, word-finding difficulties, and reduced auditory verbal short-term memory with a digit span of two. While audiometry was within normal range, auditory recognition tests evidenced an auditory agnosia: GB recognized only seven out of 25 environmental sounds. Repetition of words and sentences was impossible without lip-reading. Psychometric measures evidenced a lowering of

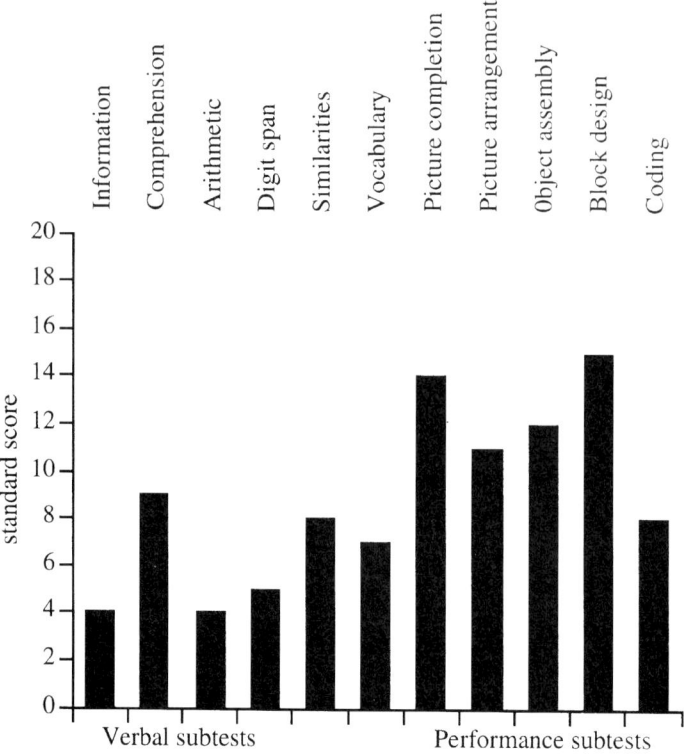

Fig. 1. Scores on verbal and performance subtests of the WISC-R in a case of acquired aphasia associated with CSWS.

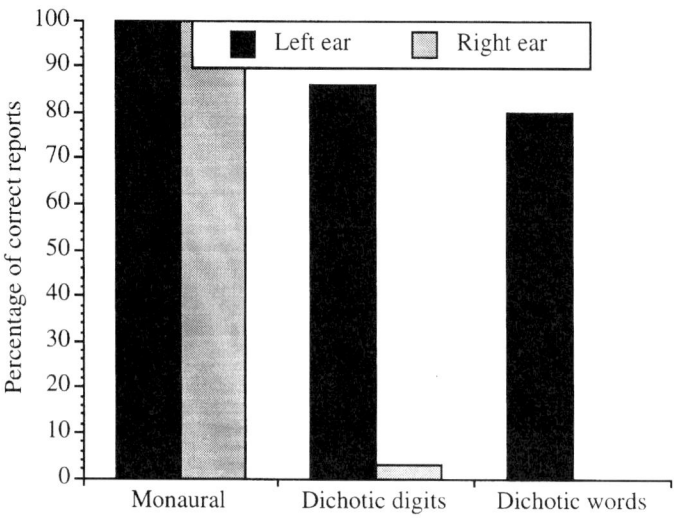

Fig. 2. Performances on monaural and dichotic listening tests in a case of acquired aphasia and CSWS.

Chapter 11 Cognitive and behavioural consequences of epilepsies in childhood

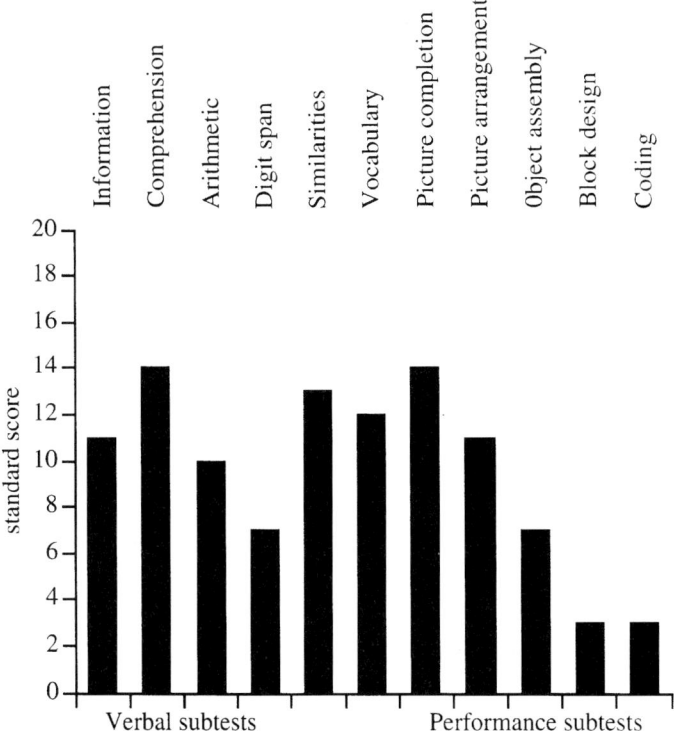

Fig. 3. Scores on verbal and performance subtests of the WISC-R in a case of acquired apraxia with CSWS.

intellectual efficiency, particularly in the verbal subtests. On the Wechsler Intelligence Scale for Children – Revised (WISC-R), the full IQ was 93, with a verbal IQ of 78 and a performance IQ of 112 (Fig. 1). The waking EEG showed left centro temporal spikes and spike–waves, and during sleep left sub-continuous spike–waves were recorded. NMR was normal, but a positron emission tomography scan, performed two weeks following the onset of aphasic disorders, showed a higher uptake of glucose over the left temporal cortex relative to the right one during sleep and wakefulness (Maquet et al., 1995). After two months under Clobazam, language transiently improved while EEG during sleep and wakefulness normalized. Neuro-psychological evaluation showed almost normal performance in naming, verbal fluency and real word repetition but auditory–verbal short term memory was still impaired. Dichotic listening tests showed complete right ear extinction for words and digits (Fig. 2).

Acquired apraxia with CSWS has been observed in one case of the series described by Maquet et al. (1995). SB, a bilingual (French–Arab) boy, had normal development and schooling until the occurrence of a first complex partial seizure at age 8 years 5 months. One month later, he evidenced severe apraxic agraphia. The apraxic disorders also involved dressing and usual object manipulation. They were predominant in the left hand movement while no motor impairment was noticed. Bilateral gestural activity revealed a left motor hemineglect. On memory tasks, SB had a normal auditory verbal but reduced visuo-spatial short-term memory span. Language performances were excellent despite attention deficit. Dichotic listening performances did not evidence any ear asymmetry. On WISC-R, he had severe difficulties on subtests involving visual praxic ability (Fig. 3). The full scale IQ was 99, with a verbal IQ of 111 and a performance IQ of 83. Waking EEG showed bilateral spike-and-wave discharges with a right frontal predominance. During sleep, generalized continuous spike–wave discharges were recorded. The PET scan study performed 3 months after the onset of epilepsy showed increased FDG uptake in the right middle and superior temporal regions, the inferior and superior parietal cortices.

Acquired frontal deficit associated with CSWS has been observed in three patients described by Roulet-Perez et al. (1995). One of our patients showed, over several months, severe frontal disorders leading to severe mental deterioration which progressively recovered after normalization of sleep EEG. SD, a right-handed young boy who had a normal psychomotor development and normal schooling, presented a first nocturnal generalized seizure at the age of 6 years 3 months. Then, neuro-psychological assessment did not show any impairment in verbal or visuo-spatial abilities. On WISC-R, he showed normal performances with a verbal and performance IQ of 102. Three months later, the boy experienced writing difficulties. Waking EEG evidenced frequent sub-clinical bilateral spikes and spike–waves over the frontal rolandic areas. He experienced several types of seizures while sleep EEG progressively showed increasing spike–wave discharges predominant alternately over the left or the right hemisphere. After a short period of improvement with Clobazam, seizures increased and, in one month, the child evidenced a psychomotor slowing down with severe learning impairment. Neuro-psychological testing performed two months after the onset of worsening evidenced apraxic disorders, visual and tactile agnosia, although auditory discrimination could not be evaluated. On WISC-R, the full IQ was 56 with a verbal IQ of 66 and performance IQ of 54 (Fig. 4). Verbal communication was preserved despite perseverative behaviour and reduced lexical fluency. Expressive language was slow but without disturbance in speech production, word finding or syntax. Auditory recognition was normal. Short-term memory span was three for both auditory verbal and visuo-spatial items. Visual constructive activity, such as drawing, writing, copying and block design, was severely disturbed. Thorough analysis of performances on Rey–Osterrieth complex figure copy and memory showed deficient graphomotor planning and perseverative tendencies (Fig. 5). Dichotic listening tests evidenced lower report for verbal items presented to the left ear but no complete extinction. Waking EEG evidenced bilateral frontal spike–waves predominant over the right side. During sleep, spike–wave discharges were continuous and covered 90 per cent of the sleep time. NMR was normal, but a positron emission tomography scan performed during sleep and wakefulness showed a higher glucose consumption over the right frontal and temporal areas relative to the left side.

After one month of treatment with Clonazepam added to valproic acid, the electro-clinical status improved. Sleep and waking EEG almost normalized. Only rare spikes predominant over the right frontal areas were recorded. Neuro-psychological assessment showed remarkable improvement of gesture and visual and tactile recognition but constructive abilities remained impaired. Whereas auditory verbal short-term memory span increased to five, for visuo-spatial items the span was still reduced at three.

Acquired behavioural disturbance in CSWS (ADHD and autistic-like syndrome). Among the various neuro-psychological and behavioural disturbances, hyperactivity with reduced attention span was present in all the 29 cases reviewed by Tassinari et al. (1992). In some cases the severe behavioural impairments suggested psychotic states (Tassinari et al., 1992).

In the early reports of LKS, hyperactivity and attention deficit were at first thought to be 'a regressive behavioural reaction to the loss of communication' (Landau & Kleffner, 1957). Distractibility and attention disorder were considered, afterwards, as a proper clinical feature of the syndrome and treated as such (Gascon et al., 1973). Without specific treatment, behavioural disorders and attention deficit usually disappear with the improvement of language and the complete abolition of seizures and EEG normalization.

One of our patients, FMC, a left-handed young girl, had a normal development and schooling when she developed, at the age of seven, behavioural disturbances with attention and auditory comprehension deficits. Neurological examination, CT scan, audiometry and brainstem auditory evoked potentials were normal.

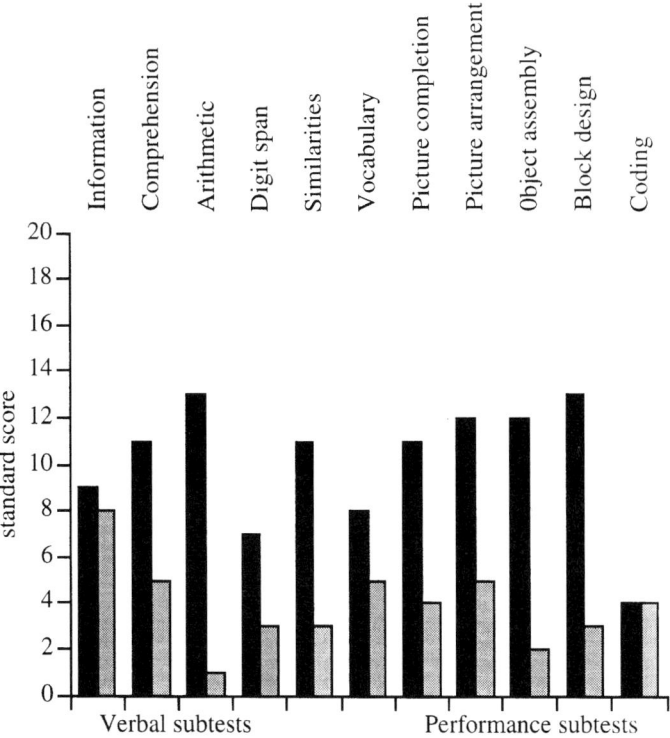

Fig. 4. Comparative scores on verbal and performance subtests of the WISC-R before (black columns) and during the active phase of a case of CSWS with acquired frontal deficit.

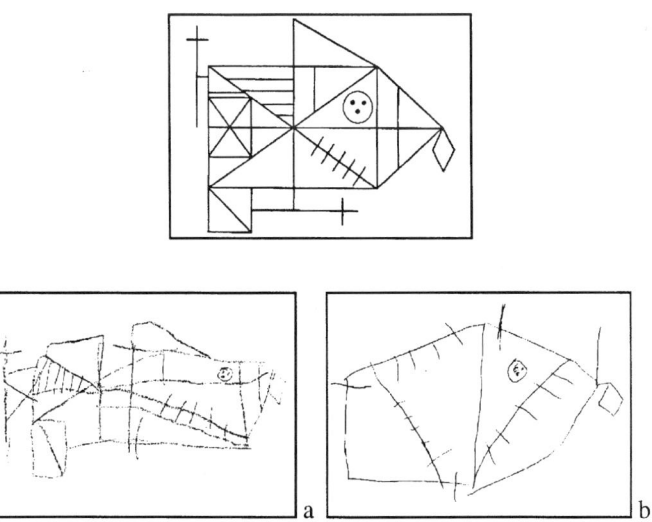

Fig. 5. Copy (a) and memory (b) of the Rey–Osterrieth complex figure showing deficient graphomotor planning and perseveration in CSWS with acquired frontal deficit.

At the age of 8, while behavioural impairments such as hyperactivity and impulsivity were increasing, she had a complex partial seizure. The EEG recordings showed right temporal spikes and waves with normal background activity. The high level of activity associated with irritability, disinhibition and inappropriate postures and talks suggested a childhood mania. According to the clinical state, she was treated with valproic acid, Clobazam and Pipamperon. The child had no more seizure but remained overactive and inattentive despite a mild behavioural improvement. Dichotic listening tests which require divided attention showed poor performances on both ears. After a transitory behavioural improvement under methylphenidate and valproic acid, the child remained inattentive. Spike–wave discharges became continuous during sleep two months later. On WISC-R, IQ was normal, but the lowest scores were recorded on coding and on digit span sub-tests which require sustained attention.

These four examples clearly show that in CSWS neuro-psychological deterioration involve as specific cognitive functions normally supported by the cortical area where the focal discharges originate. Other very specific neuro-psychological deficits like acquired visual agnosia have been described in children with CSWS (Martins *et al.*, 1993). Global deterioration reported in most cases of CSWS seems to result from progressive generalization of EEG abnormalities, as in the second case described above. Auditory agnosia and aphasic disorders are observed only in cases with right or left temporal spike–wave focus. When the focus is localized in a cortical area distant from the temporal cortex, verbal abilities are impaired only after a long period with generalized epileptiform discharges.

Transient cognitive impairments and learning deficits in benign focal epilepsies of childhood (BFEC)

In 1939, Schwab showed that clinically unnoticed epileptic discharges could be accompanied by subtle cognitive impairments. In a simple reaction task, the patient omitted to answer or answered with delay when spike–wave discharges occurred on EEG recording without any obvious clinical changes. Further studies confirmed the presence of transitory cognitive impairments concomitant to so-called 'subclinical' discharges (Tizard & Margerison, 1963; Porter *et al.*, 1973; Hutt & Gilbert, 1980; Aarts *et al.*, 1984; Binnie *et al.*, 1987; Kasteleijn-Nolst Trenité *et al.*, 1990b;). Aarts *et al.* (1984) labelled these cognitive deficits Transitory Cognitive Impairment (TCI).

TCI is observed in half of the patients having frequent subclinical discharges. Often neglected by clinicians, these subtle deficits can nevertheless disturb the daily life of epileptic patients. They may explain learning and academic problems in children. In this regard, they should be considered as clinical epileptic manifestations and, as such, evaluated in clinical practice.

Several studies showed the selectivity of cognitive deficit according to the focus and extent of epileptiform EEG activity (Aarts *et al.*, 1984; Binnie *et al.*, 1987; Kasteleijn-Nolst Trenité *et al.*, 1990a). Using two short-term memory tasks, one with verbal, the other with spatial items presented like a video game, they showed that focal discharges have dissociated effects on spatial and verbal tasks. The generalized discharges disturbed more readily spatial tasks, whereas verbal tasks were impaired only in one-third of occurrences. As regard to the timing of discharges during a task requiring a response to a stimulus, the effects are different depending on the modality of the task. When spike–wave discharges occur within a few seconds preceding the presentation of a critical stimulus, they interfere with both verbal and spatial tasks. The discharges occurring during stimulus presentation have the greatest effect on cognitive performance, suggesting that the stage of stimulus recognition is the most sensitive to discharges.

With the development of computerized assessment of cognitive function performed during Video EEG monitoring, the interferences of subclinical discharges with cognitive performance have excited considerable interest recently. They allow us to study in detail the relationship between discharges and cognitive performances in various types of cognitive tasks and at different times of the progress of a particular task.

The learning deficits of epileptic children might well be explained by TCI associated with the occurrence of sub-clinical discharges. Indeed, neuro-psychological findings indicate that academic problems arise from specific deficiencies rather than generalized cognitive dysfunction. Impairments mainly involve memory function and attention capacity. Recent studies showed a significant correlation between children's 'psycho-social' difficulties, such as attention deficits, behavioural disturbance, language impairment and dyslexia, and the frequency of subclinical discharges with cognitive impairments (Binnie *et al.*, 1987; Binnie, 1993).

Some studies evaluated the consequences of epileptic discharges on attention capacity. They showed that children with right-side or bilateral focus of rolandic paroxysmal discharges had impaired attention capacity, whereas the children with left-side rolandic discharges performed as well as the control group (Piccirilli *et al.*, 1994). The authors suggested that attentional deficits might be determined by two mechanisms: a focal dysfunction in the site of the epileptic focus and a disturbance of the functional balance between the two hemispheres.

Academic difficulties encountered by epileptic children may be related to disturbances at one of the various cognitive processes required for learning: perception, representation, sustained attention, strategy and retrieval. Tizard & Margerison (1963) suggested that the subclinical discharges decrease the capacity to process information. Later, Hutt & Fairweather (1975) introduced the concept of 'neural noise' to describe the interference of subclinical discharges with cognitive tasks.

In BFEC, the frequency of seizures is typically low but the interictal EEG shows frequent discharges during wakefulness. Therefore, it is important to measure their immediate cognitive consequences that may impair children's learning abilities. Indeed occurring in the critical period of academic achievement, these discharges may disturb the setting of specific cognitive processing routines like reading, counting, grammatical rules and orthographic lexicon.

Cognitive changes persisting after recovery of childhood epilepsy

Auditory verbal processing following acquired aphasia with epilepsy (LKS)

Almost all follow-up studies emphasized the very poor verbal outcome of LKS compared to acquired aphasia consecutive to brain lesion. Several years after complete recovery from epilepsy, language performances are still disturbed in various specific verbal tests, particularly those involving rapid word-finding and long and complex sentence comprehension. In four patients who recovered from LKS for several years we showed that persisting lower verbal IQ on WISC-R results from poor performances in sub-tests evaluating vocabulary or requiring auditory short-term memory, such as information sub-test, digit span and problem solving. In specific verbal memory tests, these patients showed reduced short-term memory span for auditory verbal items whereas it was within normal range for visual stimuli. Moreover in these patients the discrepancy of performances in repetition tasks with significantly lower performances while repeating non-words pointed to a deficit in the phonological memory system. This defect may account for impairments in lexical growth, acquisition of reading and writing, and comprehension of abstract words and syntax, usually observed following LKS (Metz-Lutz *et al.*, 1996).

Long-lasting dichotic listening extinction following LKS

An abnormal neural activity occurring within the critical period of brain maturation may disturb the structural and functional changes in the brain which contribute to the establishment of the neural substrate for language processing and its hemispheric lateralization. We examined this hypothesis in a long-term follow-up study of five children with LKS. During the active phase of epilepsy, PET scan studies showed in all five children an increase of glucose metabolism in either the left or right posterior temporal cortex correlated with the temporal focus of epileptic discharges. After recovery corresponding to complete normalization of the EEG, a mild but significant hypo-metabolism was present in the same areas. Repeated dichotic listening tests evidenced a unilateral ear extinction, contralateral to the temporal lobe involved by epileptic discharges during the active phase of epilepsy. This extinction persisted several years after the complete disappearance of epileptic discharges. In the absence of structural lesion, this long-lasting impairment suggests a permanent unilateral dysfunction in the auditory verbal system that correlates with the unilateral hypo-metabolism in the temporal cortex evidenced on PET scan performed in the late recovery period. It also demonstrates the deleterious effect of a focal epileptic activity in a neural network involved in a maturation process, as the functional differentiation of the temporal associative cortex (Metz-Lutz *et al.*, 1997).

Hemispheric asymmetries for language in BFEC

The possible relationship between the epileptic focus and hemispheric lateralization for language has been examined in a group study of children with benign rolandic childhood epilepsy (Piccirilli *et al.*, 1988). In this study, the individual cerebral organization for language of epileptic and normal children was investigated with a dual-task paradigm in which a verbal activity interferes with right- or left-hand movements. The interference between two tasks is particularly evident when the same hemisphere is involved in the two concurrent tasks. In verbal–manual tasks, the left ear dominance for language is evidenced by an increased decremental effect of verbal tasks on right-hand tapping performances compared to the left. In children with left epileptic focus no evident asymmetry between hands was observed. As for epileptic children with right hemisphere focus, they showed the same interference pattern as normal children. These results suggest that the presence of focal epileptic discharges may induce changes in the pattern of functional hemispheric representation, particularly for language. This functional alteration depends on the localization of the epileptogenic focus.

Conclusion

The behavioural and cognitive impairments observed in idiopathic childhood epilepsies appear clearly related to the focus and the extent of the abnormal neural activity represented by epileptiform discharges rather than to obvious epileptic seizures. However, as they are usually described and studied from the first occurrence of a clinical epileptic manifestation, it is difficult to assume that these impairments did not pre-exist. In that case, cognitive deficits and epilepsy would result from a common underlying brain dysfunction. Exceptional observations of benign partial epilepsy evolving after several months into CSWS with specific cognitive disorders provide strong argument in favour of the deleterious effect of epilepsy on cognitive ability. Furthermore, the persistent cognitive impairments following LKS as well as the changes in hemispheric lateralization for language in benign rolandic childhood epilepsy described above illustrate the interference between a focal epileptic activity and the development of specific cognitive functions of the corresponding cortical area.

References

Aarts, J.H.P., Binnie, C.D., Smit, A.M. & Wilkins, A.J. (1984): Selective cognitive impairment during focal and generalized epileptiform EEG activity. *Brain* **107**, 293–308.

Binnie, C.D. (1993): Significance and management of transitory cognitive impairment due to subclinical EEG discharges in children. *Brain Dev.* **15**, 23–30.

Binnie, C.D., Kasteleijn-Nolst Trenité, D.G.A., Smit, A.M. & Wilkins, A.J. (1987): Interactions of epileptiform EEG discharges and cognition. *Epil. Res.* **1**, 239–245.

Dalla Bernadina, B., Chiamenti, C., Capovilla, G., Trevisan, E. & Tassinari, C. (1985): Benign partial epilepsy with affective symptoms ('benign psychomotor epilepsy'). In: *Epileptic syndromes in infancy, childhood, and adolescence.* Roger J., Bureau, M., Dravet, C., Dreifuss, F. E. & Wolf, P. (eds), pp. 171–175. London: John Libbey.

Dalla Bernadina, B., Sgrò, V., Fontana, E., Colamaria, V. & La Selva, L. (1992): Idiopathic partial epilepsies in children. In: *Epileptic syndromes in infancy, childhood and adolescence (2nd edn)*, Roger, J., Bureau, M., Dravet, C., Dreifuss, F. E., Perret, A. & Wolf, P. (eds), pp. 239–244. London: John Libbey.

Deonna, T. (1993): Annotation: Cognitive and behavioural correlates of epileptic activity in children. *J. Child Psychol. Psychiatry* **34**, 611–620.

Doose, H. & Baier, W. (1989): Benign partial epilepsy and related condition: multifactorial pathogenesis with hereditary impairment of brain maturation. *Eur. J. Pediatry* **1989**, 152–158.

Ellenberg, J.H., Hirtz, D.G. & Nelson, K.B. (1985): Do seizures in children cause intellectual deterioration? *Ann. Neurol.* **18,** 389.

Farwell, J.R., Dodrill, C.B. & Batzel LW. (1985): Neuropsychological abilities of children with epilepsy. *Epilepsia* **26,** 395–400.

Fejerman, N. & Di Blasi, A. (1987): Status epilepticus in benign partial epilepsies in children: report of two cases. *Epilepsia* **28,** 351–355.

Gascon, G., Victor, D., Lombroso, C.T. & Goodglass, H. (1973): Language disorder, convulsive disorder and electroencephalographic abnormalities. *Arch. Neurol.* **28,** 156–162.

Gastaut, H. (1982): A new type of epilepsy: benign partial epilepsy of childhood with occipital spike waves. *Clin. Electroencephalogr.* **13,** 963–964.

Hirsch, E., Maquet, P., Metz-Lutz, M.N., Motte, J., Finck, S. & Marescaux, C. (1995): The eponym 'Landau–Kleffner Syndrome' should not be restricted to childhood acquired aphasia with epilepsy. In: *Continuous spikes and waves during slow sleep*, Beaumanoir, A., Deonna, T., Mira, L. & Tassinari, C.A. (eds), pp. 57–62. London: John Libbey.

Holmes, G. (1993): Benign focal epilepsies of childhood. *Epilepsia* **34,** S49-S61.

Hutt, S.J. & Fairweather, H. (1975): Information processing during two types of EEG activity. *Electroencephalogr. Clin. Neurophysiol.* **39,** 43–51.

Hutt, S.J. & Gilbert, S. (1980): Effect of evoked spike–wave discharges upon short-term memory in patients with epilepsy. *Cortex* **16,** 445–457.

Kasteleijn-Nolst Trenité, D.G.A., Siebelink, B.M., Berends, S.G.C., van Strien, J.W. & Meinardi, H. (1990a): Lateralized effects of subclinical epileptiform EEG discharges on scholastic performance in children. *Epilepsia* **31,** 740–746.

Kasteleijn-Nolst Trenité, D.G.A., Smit, A.M., Velis, D.N., Willemse, J. & van Emde Boas, W. (1990b): On-line detection of transient neuropsychological disturbances during EEG discharges in children with epilepsy. *Dev. Med. Child Neurol.* **32,** 46–50.

Klein, S.K. (1991): Cognitive factors and learning disabilities in children with epilepsy. In: *Epilepsy and behavior*, pp. 171–179. New York: Wiley-Liss.

Landau, W.M. & Kleffner, F.R. (1957): Syndrome of acquired aphasia with convulsive disorder in children. *Neurology* **7,** 523–530.

Lerman, P. & Kivity, S. (1975): Benign focal epilepsy of childhood. A follow-up study of 100 recovered patients. *Arch. Neurol.* **32,** 261–264.

Maquet, P., Hirsch, E., Metz-Lutz, M.N., Motte, J., Dive, D., Marescaux, C. et al. (1995): Regional cerebral glucose metabolism in children with deterioration of one or more cognitive functions and continuous spike-and-wave discharges during sleep. *Brain* **118,** 1492–1520.

Martins, I., Antunes, N. & Gomes, A. (1993): Acquired visual agnosia in a child: a neuropsychological study. *ANAE* **5,** 70–75.

Metz-Lutz, M.N., de Saint Martin, A., Hirsch, E., Maquet, P. & Marescaux, C. (1996): Auditory verbal processing following Landau and Kleffner syndrome. *Brain Lang.* **55,** 147–150.

Metz-Lutz, M.N., Hirsch, E., Maquet, P., de Saint Martin, A., Rudolf, G., Wioland, N. et al. (1997): Dichotic listening performances in the follow-up of Landau and Kleffner syndrome. *Child Neuropsychol.* **3,** 47–60.

Morrell, F., Whisler, W.W., Smith, M.C., Hoeppner, T.J., de Toledo-Morrell, L., Pierre-Louis, S.J.C. et al. (1995): Landau–Kleffner syndrome. Treatment with subpial intracortical transection. *Brain* **118,** 1529–1546.

Panayiotopoulos, C.P. (1989): Benign childhood epilepsy with occipital paroxysms: a 15-year prospective study. *Ann. Neurol.* **26,** 51–56.

Park, Y.D., Hoffman, J.M., Radtke, R.A. & DeLong, G.R. (1994): Focal cerebral metabolic abnormality in a patient with continuous spike waves during slow sleep. *J. Ped. Neurol.* **9,** 139–143.

Piccirilli, M., D'Alessandro, P., Tiacci, C. & Ferroni, A. (1988): Language Lateralization in Children with Benign Partial Epilepsy. *Epilepsia* **29,** 19–25.

Piccirilli, M., D'Alessandro, P., Sciarma, T., Cantoni, C., Dioguardi, M.S. et al. (1994): Attention problems in epilepsy: possible significance of the epileptogenic focus. *Epilepsia* **35,** 1091–1096.

Porter, R.J., Penry, J.K. & Dreifuss, F.E. (1973): Responsiveness at the onset of spike–wave bursts. *Electroencephalogr. Clin. Neurophysiol.* **34,** 239–245.

Ross, E.M., Peckham, C.S., West, P.B. & Butler, N.R. (1980): Epilepsy in childhood: Findings from the National Child Development Study. *Brit. Med. J.* **280**, 207–210.

Roulet, E., Deonna, T., Gaillard, F., Peter-Favre, C. & Despland, P. (1991): Acquired aphasia, dementia, and behavior disorder with epilepsy and continuous spike and waves during sleep in a child. *Epilepsia* **32**, 495–503.

Roulet Perez, E. (1995): Syndromes of acquired epileptic aphasia and epilepsy with continuous spike–waves discharges during sleep: models for prolonged cognitive impairment of epileptic origin. *Seminars in Pediatric Neurology* **2**, 269–277.

Schwab, R.S. (1939): A method of measuring consciousness in petit mal epilepsy. *J. Nerv. Mental Dis.* **89**, 690–691.

Tassinari, C.A., Bureau, M., Dravet, C., Dalla Bernadina, B. & Roger, J. (1992): Epilepsy with continuous spikes and waves during slow sleep. In: *Epileptic syndromes in infacy, childhood and adolescence (2nd edn)*, Roger, J., Bureau, M., Dravet, C., Dreifuss, F.E., Perret, A. & Wolf, P. (eds), pp. 245–256. London: John Libbey.

Tizard, B. & Margerison, J.H. (1963): The relationship between generalized paroxysmal EEG discharges and various test situations in two epileptic patients. *J. Neurol. Neurosurg. Psychiat.* **26**, 308–313.

Wechsler, D. (1974): *Echelle d'intelligence de Wechsler pour la période scolaire et primaire. WPPSI.* Paris: Les éditions du Centre de Psychologie Appliquée.

Wechsler, D. (1981): *Echelle d'intelligence de Wechsler pour enfants – Forme révisée. WISC-R.* Paris: Les éditions du Centre de Psychologie Appliquée.

Chapter 12

PET studies of Landau–Kleffner syndrome and related disorders

Pierre Maquet[1], Edouard Hirsch[2], Marie-Noëlle Metz-Lutz[2], Christian Marescaux[2] and Georges Franck[1]

[1]*Cyclotron Research Center and Department of Neurology, Liège, Belgium;*
[2]*INSERM U398 and Department of Neurology, Strasbourg, France*

Introduction

This chapter deals with the experimental efforts being made to explore the pathophysiology of the Landau–Kleffner syndrome and related disorders using positron emission tomography (PET). In the first part of the chapter, we will detail the pathological conditions concerned with this research. Emphasis will be put on the features that we feel are characteristic of the syndromes included in this study and that lead us to consider conjunctly the Landau–Kleffner syndrome (LKS) and the syndrome of continuous spike-and-wave discharges during slow sleep (CSWS). We also explain the reasons why we restricted our study to 'non-lesional' cases.

The second part of the chapter will summarize recent data from neuro-physiological and PET studies which suggest a focal origin for these syndromes. These data helped to establish a working hypothesis on the pathophysiological mechanisms of these syndromes. This hypothesis will be briefly presented in the third section of the chapter.

Finally, we recently looked for further experimental support for the hypothesis using PET and [^{11}C]flumazenil. A discussion of these preliminary results and directions for future research are outlined in the final section.

Landau–Kleffner syndrome and related disorders

The LKS (Landau & Kleffner, 1957) and the CSWS (Tassinari *et al.*, 1992) have been described separately. In many instances, they are still considered as two different nosological entities. However, they share so many basic features that it seemed warranted, at least in a first experimental step, to consider them together (Hirsch *et al.*, 1995). These characteristics can be summarized as follows:

1• Both syndromes appear in children between 3 and 10 years of age. They tend to regress before the end of adolescence.

2• Both are associated with a deterioration of one or several cognitive functions. This deterioration is most often acquired, i.e. the development of these higher cerebral functions had been normal before the outbreak of the disorder (Beaumanoir, 1992).

3• EEG recordings are always abnormal. The SWD are activated during slow sleep. By definition, they become continuous in CSWS patients. Although most of the LKS that we considered actually presented continuous spike-and-wave discharges (SWD) during slow sleep (at least at some point of their evolution), an increase in abundance of the discharges would have sufficed to include them in the study (Hirsch *et al.*, 1990).

4• The occurrence of epileptic seizures is frequently reported, although some patients may not present any seizures. Several types of seizures are observed but no tonic seizures are reported. Seizures are usually easily controlled by medical treatment (Hirsch *et al.*, 1990; Beaumanoir, 1992).

5• The pharmacological reactivity of the neuro-psychological deficits, of the EEG abnormalities and of the seizures is common to both affections: the symptoms are aggravated by phenobarbital, phenytoin and carbamazepine, whereas benzodiazepines, valproic acid (VPA) and ethosuximide alleviate the symptoms. Corticosteroids have a favourable influence on both syndromes (Marescaux *et al.*, 1990).

Finally, as it will appear in the following sections, the cerebral metabolic patterns of patients suffering from LKS or CSWS also share many characteristics. This lends support for the hypothesis of a common pathogenic mechanism.

The lumping of LKS and CSWS into a single nosological framework remains tentative. Future research will help to better understand their respective physiopathology and thus to evaluate this hypothesis. One advantage of this hypothesis is that it helps to categorize some rare patients who fit neither the LKS nor in the CSWS diagnostic criteria. This is the case of children with isolated deterioration of one cognitive function other than language (e.g. acquired apraxia) and EEG abnormalities similar to those observed in LKS.

Finally, many papers recently reported as cases of LKS or CSWS children presenting an acquired cognitive deterioration and EEG abnormalities concomitant with a macroscopic lesion, usually detected by CT or MRI scans (Otero *et al.*, 1989; Perniola *et al.*, 1993; Solomon *et al.*, 1993). At present, one cannot tell whether the pathological mechanisms involved in these patients are similar or dissimilar to LKS or CSWS cases. In consequence, in order to exclude a possible confounding factor in our studies, we adopted a restrictive attitude and only included in our population the patients with no detectable lesions on standard CT or MRI scans.

Experimental data

Experimental data gathered during the last 10 years leave little doubt that these syndromes are associated with a focal or regional cerebral dysfunction.

Neuro-physiological data

Standard EEG recordings (Rodriguez & Niedermeyer, 1982) most often show focal or multifocal spike-and-wave discharges (SWD). The topography of the discharges may vary with time. However, in the long term, a focus appears as the most frequent and leading source of the abnormalities. The focal origin of the SWD is more easily observed in LKS patients than in CSWS patients where the SWD are usually generalized. However, recent data showed, in three CSWS patients, small interhemispheric time differences in apparently synchronous SWD (Kobayashi *et al.*, 1994). The leading hemisphere preceded by 12 to 26 ms the SWD recorded contralaterally. Likewise, in LKS patients, during recovery from systemic injection of methohexital (during which EEG recordings are completely flat), the recurrence of SWD is first observed in the leading hemisphere (most often the left hemisphere) and the left-sided discharges lead by about 20 ms the contralateral discharges (Morrell *et al.*, 1995).

Magneto-encephalographic (MEG) recordings in a sleeping LKS patient (Morrell *et al.*, 1995) also showed that the dipole sources of epileptic spikes were concentrated in restricted cerebral areas localized in the posterior superior temporal gyrus (Wernicke's area) and inferior frontal cortex

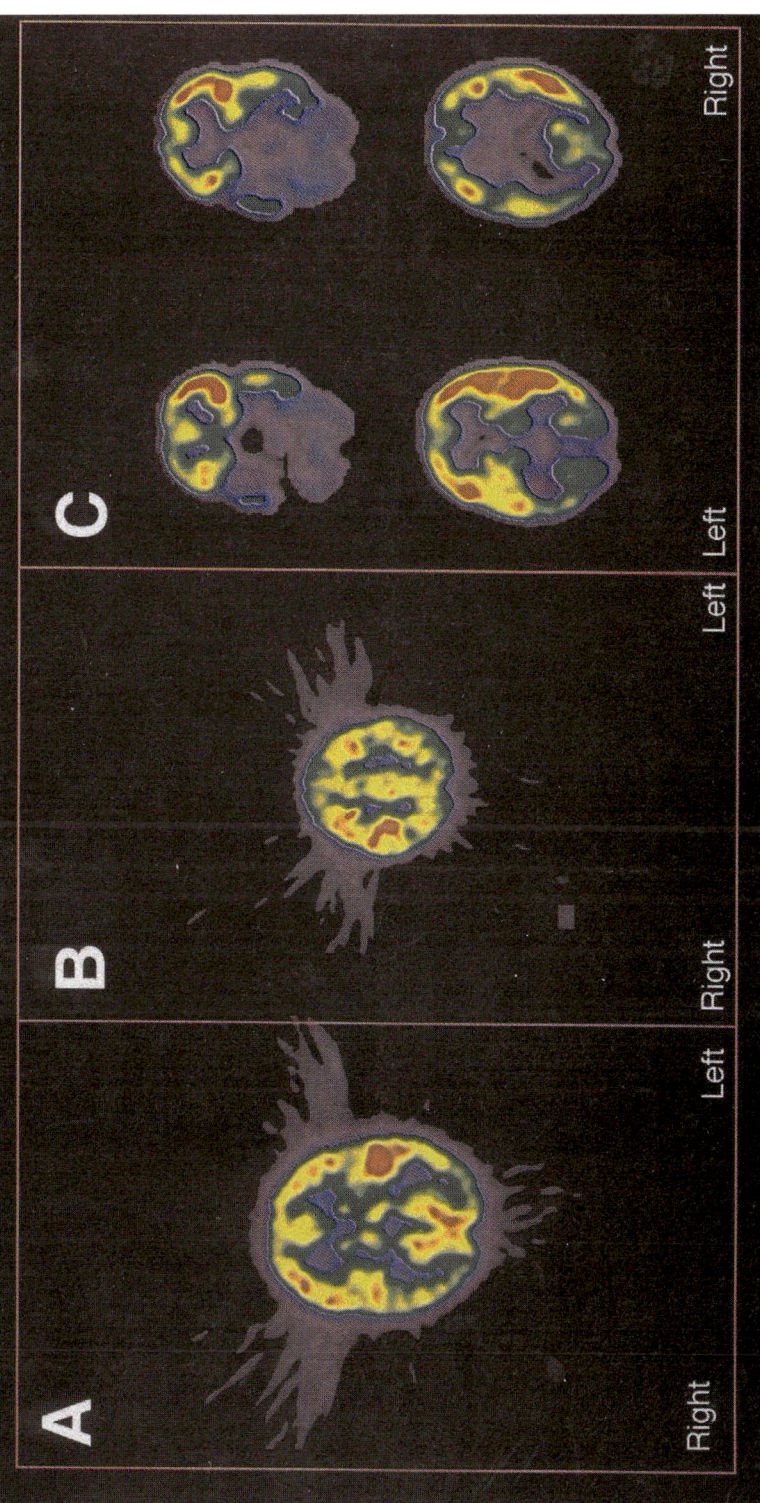

Fig. 1. Cerebral glucose metabolism observed in three patients, displayed at selected brain levels, demonstrating the variability of cerebral metabolic pattern in patients with deterioration of one or several cognitive functions and continuous spike-and-wave discharges during sleep. Panel A: acquired aphasia associated with left temporal hypermetabolism. Panel B: acquired left hand apraxia and left hemineglect associated with a right parietal hypermetabolism. Panel C: acquired global deterioration associated with a right hemispheric hypermetabolism.

(corresponding to Broca's area). These findings are in line with electrocorticographic (intraoperative) recordings in LKS demonstrating very localized discharges in the perisylvian cerebral cortex.

PET data

We had the opportunity to explore the cerebral glucose metabolism of seven patients, presenting CSWS associated with neuro-psychological deterioration. Three patients had an isolated aphasia; three patients had language disturbances with more widespread cognitive deterioration; one patient had isolated apraxia. For three of these seven patients, follow-up studies were obtained until recovery. A total of 21 studies were performed, 12 of which were done during sleep. The full description and discussion of these results can be found in Maquet *et al.* (1995).

Diversity of metabolic patterns

When examining the distribution of the cerebral glucose metabolism of these children, one is struck by the variability observed between patients and, in the same patient, with time. Metabolic abnormalities may appear as increases or decreases of glucose metabolism. Their extension may be quite limited or, in contrast, involve a large part of a hemisphere. They may be left- or right-sided.

Various factors may take this variability into account, not least being the nature of the neuro-psychological deficit, the SWD activity and the ongoing treatments.

The effects of treatments are beyond the scope of this paper. However, it appears unlikely that they could explain the marked cerebral metabolic deviations that we observed in the patients (for discussion, see Maquet *et al.*, 1995)).

The topography of the cortical metabolic abnormalities was in good agreement with the neuro-psychological findings. In Fig. 1, we present the PET data of three characteristic patients. Panel A shows the PET observed in a LKS patient who presented a deterioration of comprehension. This was related to a focal hypermetabolism in the left superior temporal area, a location including Wernicke's area. Panel B concerns a young boy who suffered acquired apraxia and left hemineglect. The clinical findings could be accounted for by the focal increase in glucose metabolism located in the right parietal lobe. As a rule, the more widespread the disturbances of cerebral glucose metabolism, the more severe the neuro-psychological deficit. For instance, in a severely affected patient presenting a dementia, the asymmetry involved a vast cortical area (Panel C). Bilateral dysfunction of the temporal lobes was found in three patients, at least once in their evolution.

The effects of discharges on the cerebral metabolism were difficult to ascertain. During the active phase of the disease (six patients during both sleep and wakefulness), we recorded continuous spike-and-wave discharges during sleep. In all but one of these patients, a regional increase in glucose utilization was observed both during sleep and during wakefulness. Most importantly, this regional hypermetabolism was still observed during wakefulness, although the EEG discharges were no longer continuous. Of course, one could argue that the continuous discharges recorded during sleep might explain the regional hypermetabolism. During wakefulness, SWD might also have been sustained sufficiently to cause the increase in glucose utilization. However, it should be stressed that such interictal hypermetabolism remains an exceptional observation in partial epilepsy (Chugani *et al.*, 1993), whereas it seems to be frequent in our patients. As a consequence, we cannot discard the possibility that some processes, possibly related to the disorder itself, cause both the focal increase in glucose metabolism and the outbreak of SWD. For instance, the focal hypermetabolism might represent an increased inhibitory drive controlling the outbreak of SWD.

Finally, during the recovery phase, no discharges were recorded either during sleep or during wakefulness, and the children were improving clinically. At this stage, the cerebral metabolic distribution was normal (one patient) or showed a regional decrease in glucose metabolism (three patients). The location of the residual hypometabolism was well correlated with the usual topography of the hypermetabolism and the EEG abnormalities observed during the active phase.

Common metabolic features

Despite the apparent disparity of the results, three basic features characterized the cerebral metabolic distributions in these children: a metabolic distribution suggestive of a immature brain, a focal or regional involvement of associative cortices and the absence of cortico–thalamic diaschisis.

Brain immaturity. We observed that the metabolic level was lower in subcortical structures than in the cortex. This feature was particularly constant in thalamic nuclei. This metabolic distribution was suggested by Chugani *et al.* (1987) to be the hallmark of the immature brain.

Focal or regional involvement of associative cortices. The metabolic abnormalities within the cortex spread mainly to associative cortices. The glucose metabolism in primary visual and sensori-motor areas was always normal in these children. The metabolism of the primary auditory cortex could not be selectively evaluated because of its small size and its anatomical position. However, it should be remembered that MEG data showed in a LKS patients during sleep that the primary auditory cortex was more medial than the source of the SWD (Morrell *et al.*, 1995).

As a consequence, the distribution of the metabolic disturbances within the cortex in our patients suggests that the pathogenic mechanisms responsible for LKS and CSWS predominantly interfere with the function of the associative cortices precisely at the time they are in an important maturational stage for the subsequent development of higher cerebral functions.

No thalamic diaschisis. As a rule, the thalamic glucose metabolism varies in parallel with the metabolism of the ipsilateral cortex: a hypometabolic cortical area is usually associated with a decrease in ispilateral thalamic metabolism (Feeney & Baron, 1986). Ictal PET studies usually show increased metabolism in the thalamic nuclei ipilateral to the discharging focus (Franck *et al.*, 1986; Chugani *et al.*, 1993). In contrast, in the LKS and CSWS patients, the cortical asymmetries were never associated with similar asymmetries in thalamic nuclei, even when the asymmetry involved a large cortical area. Because cerebral glucose utilization mainly labels the energy requirements of the synapse, increasing neuronal activity is reflected by an increase in glucose consumption of the downstream synapse (see review on this topic in Chadwick & Whelan, 1991). Our findings suggest that the cortico–thalamic neurones are not involved in the generation or support of SWD. In other words, it is likely that the pathological mechanisms do not involve all neuronal types present within the associative cortices. According to this hypothesis, the spike–wave activity would primarily involve other types of cortical neurones: local interneurones and cortico–cortical associative neurones. We cannot tell, on the basis of our PET studies, whether thalamo–cortical neurones participate in the generation of SWD or if these phenomena are purely intracortical.

Hypothesis

LKS and CSWS only appear in maturing brains when active maturational processes are still taking place in the brain and lead to the selective elimination of numerous axonal collaterals and synapses (O'Leary, 1992). The 'pruning' of the high connectivity reached earlier in the infant stage would be, in part, controlled by neuronal activity and would lead to refined, stable and more effective neuronal wiring (Katz & Callaway, 1992). It appears that neurotransmitters act as important molecular signals influencing the elaboration of neuritic morphology (Lipton & Kater, 1989). Moreover, the same neurotransmitter may have several actions, depending on its local concentration (Lipton & Kater, 1989), thereby precisely regulating the neuritic outgrowth and, in consequence, the neural plasticity. In this respect, the balance between excitatory (i.e. glutamatergic) and inhibitory (i.e. GABAergic) influences appears to play a critical role in modelling of the interneuronal circuitry.

Landau–Kleffner syndrome and CSWS might be due to an alteration of these maturational processes in one or several associative cortices, i.e. to an impairment of the pruning of synaptic contacts and collaterals in an otherwise normal cortex. These pathologic processes would lead to 'imperfect' neuronal wiring and in turn, to an imbalance between inhibitory and excitatory drives. A putative disequilibrium of these systems would impede the normal function of the affected associative areas, leading to the deterioration of higher cerebral functions that they usually subserve and hampering new acquisitions. The excitatory/inhibitory imbalance would also predispose to synchronous firing of local neuronal populations and thus would create conditions permissive to the development of discharges.

The physiological reinforced synchronization of neuronal firing characterizing non-REM sleep would further activate the SWD (Steriade *et al.*, 1993).

The putative involvement of interneurones or cortico–cortical neurones, characterized by their 'horizontal' collaterals, is consistent with the beneficial effects of subpial transections. Subpial transection would, among other effects, interrupt mechanically the deleterious intracortical circuitry by sectioning 'horizontal' intracortical connections, thus producing a new equilibrium state and resumption of more normal synaptization. Because of the persistent high connectivity at these ages, the formation of new, more appropriate, synaptic contacts is still possible, and would lead to the – occasionally swift – regression of the neuro-psychological deficit (Morrell *et al.*, 1995).

Final objective: testing the hypothesis

Many experimental strategies could be considered to explore this hypothesis. As a surgical approach is suggested by some authors, direct electrophysiological recordings of the discharging areas could be of some help. This procedure should be restricted to a small number of cases (see Morrell *et al.*'s (1995) selection criteria). Likewise, anatomical examination of cerebral biopsies has been reported and could provide invaluable findings. However, for ethical reasons, the procedure is not warranted, especially if the sample concerns the abnormal cortex, i.e. the left perisylvian cortex around the Wernicke's area.

More amenable to a prospective evaluation is the use of pharmacological trials, using new antiepileptic compounds with high specificity to a particular neurotransmitter system. However, these drugs are still under evaluation and are not readily available.

Finally, neuroimaging techniques (EEG, MEG, fMRI and PET), especially if coregistered, remain atraumatic ways of exploration that might provide new insights in the pathophysiology of these syndromes. Due to its high sensitivity and the use of highly selective compounds, PET might be useful to explore neurotranmitter systems *in vivo*. At present, no reliable marker of excitatory aminoacid neurotransmission is available. In contrast, GABAergic systems may be indirectly investigated, for instance with [^{11}C]flumazenil, which is an antagonist of the benzodiazepine binding site. As a first step in this direction, we recently evaluated the uptake of [^{11}C]flumazenil in five LKS/CSWS patients. Preliminary results show, in three of them, very localized increases of the uptake of flumazenil, precisely within the hypermetabolic areas. These regional modifications still have to be assessed quantitatively and confounding factors (such as a treatment by benzodiazepines, duration of the disorder etc.) have to be accounted for before any conclusions can be drawn from these data.

Conclusions

The cerebral metabolic pattern observed in the syndromes combining the deterioration of cognitive functions with CSWS in children is characterized by features of an immature brain, by focal or regional dysfunction of one or more associative cortices, and by the absence of significant thalamic diaschisis. A focal or multifocal dysfunction of associative cortical areas impeding normal synaptization is suggested, possibly in relation to an imbalance between inhibitory and excitatory intracortical neurones.

Further studies with different neuroimaging techniques should be used to confirm or contradict this working hypothesis and lead to better understanding of these disorders.

References

Beaumanoir, A. (1992): The Landau–Kleffner syndrome. In: *Epileptic syndromes in infancy, childhood and adolescence (2nd edition)*, Roger, J., Bureau, M., Dravet, C., Dreifuss, F. E., Perret, A. & Wolf, P. (eds), pp. 231–243. London: John Libbey.

Chadwick, D.J. & Whelan, J. (1991): *Exploring brain functional anatomy with positron emission tomography*. Chichester: John Wiley.

Chugani, H.T., Phelps, M.E. & Mazziotta, J.C. (1987): Positron emission tomography study of human brain functional development. *Ann. Neurol.* **22**, 487–497.

Chugani, H.T., Shewmon, D.A., Skhanna, S, & Phelps M.E. (1993): Interictal and postictal focal hypermetabolism on positron emission tomography. *Pediatr. Neurol.* **9**, 10–15.

Feeney, D.M. & Baron, J.C. (1986): Diaschisis. *Stroke* **17**, 817–830.

Franck, G., Sadzot, B., Salmon, E., Depresseux, J.C., Grisar, T., Peters, J.M. *et al.* (1986): Regional cerebral blood flow and metabolic rates in human focal epilepsy and status epilepticus. In: *Advances in Neurology, volume 44*. Delgado-Escueta, A.V., Ward, A., Woodbury, D.M. & Porter, R.J. (eds), pp. 935–948. New York: Raven Press.

Hirsch, E., Marescaux, C., Maquet, P., Metz-Lutz, M., Kiesmann, M., Salmon, E. *et al.* (1990): Landau–Kleffner syndrome: a clinical and EEG study of five cases. *Epilepsia* **21**, 756–767.

Hirsch, E., Maquet, P., Metz-Lutz, M., Motte, J., Finck, S. & Marescaux, C. (1995): The eponym 'Landau–Kleffner syndrome' should not be restricted to childhood-acquired aphasia with epilepsy. In: *Continuous Spikes and Waves during slow sleep electrical status epilepticus during slow sleep*, Volume 3. Beaumanoir, A., Bureau, M., Deonna, T., Mira, L. & Tassinari, C., pp. 57–62. London: John Libbey.

Katz, L.C. & Callaway, E.M. (1992): Development of local circuits in mammalian visual cortex. *Annu. Rev. Neurosci.* **15**, 31–56.

Kobayashi, K., Nishibayashi, N., Ohtsuka, Y., Okam E. & Ohtahara, S. (1994): Epilepsy with electrical status epilepticus during slow sleep and secondary bilateral synchrony. *Epilepsia* **35**, 1097–1103.

Landau, W.M. & Kleffnerm F.R. (1957): Syndrome of acquired aphasia with convulsive disorder in children. *Neurology* **7**, 523–530.

Lipton, S.A. & Kater, S.B. (1989): Neurotransmitter regulation of neuronal outgrowth, plasticity and survival. *Trends Neurosci.* **12**, 265–270.

Maquet, P., Hirsch, E., Metz-Lutz, M., Motte, J., Dive, D., Marescaux, C. *et al.* (1995): Regional cerebral glucose metabolism in children with deterioration of one or more cognitive functions and continuous spike-and-wave discharges during sleep. *Brain* **118**, 1497–1520.

Marescaux, C., Hirsch, E., Finck, S., Maquet, P., Schlumberger, E., Sellal, F. *et al.* (1990): Landau–Kleffner syndrome: a pharmacological study of five cases. *Epilepsia* **31**, 768–777.

Morrell, F., Whisler, W.W., Smith, M.C., Hoeppner, T.J., deToledo-Morrell, L., Pierre-Louis, S.J.C. *et al.* (1995): Landau–Kleffner syndrome. Treatment with subpial intracortical transection. *Brain* **118**, 1529–1546.

O'Leary, D.D.M. (1992): Development of connectional diversity and specificity in the mammalian brain by the pruning of collateral projections. *Curr. Opin. Neurobiol.* **2**, 70–77.

Otero, E., Cordova, S., Diaz, F., Garcia-Teruel, I. & Del Bruttom O.H. (1989): Acquired epileptic aphasia (the Landau–Kleffner syndrome) due to neurocysticercosis. *Epilepsia* **30**, 569–572.

Perniola, T., Margari, L., Buttiglione, M., Andreula, C., Simone, I.L. & Santostasi, R. (1993): A case of Landau–Kleffner syndrome secondary to inflammatory demyelinating disease. *Epilepsia* **39**, 551–556.

Rodriguez, I. & Niedermeyer, E. (1982): The aphasia-epilepsy syndrome in children: electroencephalographic aspects. *Clin. Electroencephalogr.* **13**, 23–35.

Solomon, G.E., Carson, D., Pavlakis, S., Fraser, R. & Labar, D. (1993): Intracranial EEG monitoring in Landau–Kleffner syndrome associated with left temporal lobe astrocytoma. *Epilepsia* **34**, 557–560.

Steriade, M., Contreras, D., Curro Dossi, R. & Nunez, A. (1993): The slow (1Hz) oscillation in reticular thalamic and thalamocortical neurons: scenario of sleep rhythm generation in interacting thalamic and cortical networks. *J. Neurosci.* **13**, 3284–3299.

Tassinari, C., Bureau, M., Dravet, C., Dalla Bernardina, B. & Roger, J. (1992): Epilepsie avec pointes-ondes continues pendant le sommeil lent – antérieurement décrite sous le nom d'ESES (épilepsie avec état de mal électroencéphalographique pendant le sommeil lent). In: *Les syndromes épileptiques de l'enfant et de l'adolescent (2ème édition)*. Roger J., Bureau, M., Dravet, C., Dreifuss, F. E. & Wolf, P. (eds), pp. 245–256. London: John Libbey.

Part IV

Non-genetic experimental models of childhood epilepsies

Chapter 13

Mechanisms of non-genetic, provoked seizures in the neonatal and infant brain

Tallie Z. Baram and Carolyn G. Hatalski

Departments of Paediatrics and Anatomy & Neurobiology, University of California at Irvine, CA, USA

Summary

The immature human, particularly during the neonatal and infancy periods, has a high propensity to develop seizures due to fever, trauma, hypoxia and other adverse circumstances. The mechanisms by which these instigators lead to enhanced neuronal excitability and seizures are not fully understood. We proposed that the common denominator of fever, trauma and other pro-convulsant 'stressors' was their activation of the peptide corticotropin releasing hormone (CRH), the key mediator of the limbic-neuroendocrine stress response.

We tested the hypothesis that CRH acts at specific limbic receptors to increase neuronal excitability, and that this effect is limited to the developing brain. In the infant rat, CRH was shown to be a potent convulsant: administration of picomolar doses caused limbic status epilepticus. CRH gene expression was found to increase after a variety of stressors in both the immature and adult rat, but the peptide's potency was maximal during infancy because hippocampal and amygdala CRH-receptors were present in maximal concentrations during this developmental period.

Thus, activation of the stress neurohormone CRH during fever, trauma and other stressors may increase limbic neuronal excitability and lead to seizures. The developmental regulation of the CRH receptor involved may determine convulsant potency of CRH, and limit the induction of 'reactive' seizures by proconvulsant stressful signals to specific developmental periods. The structure and regulation of CRH are highly conserved across species. Therefore, increased activity of this excitatory neuromodulator may contribute to the generation of age-specific seizures in the human neonate and infant.

Introduction

The immature brain is more excitable than the fully mature brain (see Holmes, 1997 for a recent review). This concept is manifest in the human by a much higher incidence of seizures in the infant and child, as compared with the adult (Hauser, 1995). Enhanced excitability and a higher propensity to develop seizures have also been demonstrated in immature experimental animals including rodents (primarily rats), cats (Purpura *et al.*, 1968) and monkeys (Kubova & Moshé, 1994). A number of characteristics of the developing neuronal circuitry which may account for this enhanced excitability have been documented, and are discussed in detail in other chapters of this book. For example, gamma-aminobutyric acid (GABA), the principal inhibitory neurotransmitter in the mature central nervous system (CNS), has depolarizing and excitatory properties during the first postnatal week in the rat (Ben-Ari *et al.*, 1994). In addition, excitatory amino acid receptors are both more abundant in the immature brain (Johnston, 1996) and possess a subunit-makeup which promotes neuronal depolarization (Monyer *et al.*, 1994). These factors are thought to promote an altered excitation–inhibition balance during development. At the circuit level, these properties may provide the mechanism for the increased neuronal interaction evident from the robust long-term potentiation observed during the second postnatal week in both hippocampal and cortical synapses (McDonald & Johnston, 1990; Crair & Malenka, 1995). Furthermore, the number of cortical and hippocampal excitatory synapses is increased during the second postnatal week (Swann *et al.*, 1993) and the regulation of the propagation of convulsant discharges by the substantia nigra is immature (Moshé *et al.*, 1994). All of these factors favour enhanced excitation and a susceptibility for seizure generation and propagation.

Despite its enhanced excitability and seizure susceptibility, the immature brain is mainly engaged in normal neuronal activity, and most immature humans and rodents do not have spontaneous seizures. Furthermore, the onset of spontaneous seizures which are determined by the presence of an abnormal genetic makeup, i.e. genetic epilepsies, typically occurs beyond the neonatal and infancy periods in both the human and rat (Noebels, 1996). During these early developmental periods, seizures are most commonly triggered, i.e. they are induced by abnormal alterations of either the internal or external environment. Thus, trauma, anoxia, fever or hypoglycemia are all stressful signals which rapidly lead to seizures during early postnatal development. In fact, in the case of fever (Baram *et al.*, 1997b) and anoxia (Jensen *et al.*, 1991), seizures are induced exclusively and uniquely during a restricted vulnerable period in the rat, limited to the second postnatal week. Human febrile convulsions, the most common type of seizures, are restricted to infancy and early childhood (Berg *et al.*, 1995). Anoxia-related seizures occur primarily in the full term neonate (Volpe, 1981) . Other non-genetic seizures such as infantile spasms, which have been linked to a large number of central nervous system injuries, malformations, infections and stressors, are highly age-specific and primarily restricted to the first year of life (Baram *et al.*, 1993; Dulac *et al.*, 1993).

Thus, although the immature brain is susceptible to seizures, the propensity to generate them is selective: spontaneous intrinsic and genetic seizures are relatively uncommon, while 'reactive' seizures induced by a large variety of adverse environmental events are prevalent. These facts raise several questions:

- How do abnormal excitation and seizures arise after external or internal perturbation of the normal neuronal environment?
- Why are many of these 'reactive' seizures limited to the early developmental periods?

The focus of this chapter is on the mechanisms by which adverse external stimuli are integrated to result in altered neuronal excitability. Specifically, this chapter describes studies of the neuronal and neuroendocrine modulators which are upregulated by stressful signals and alter neuronal excitability during the developmental period. The molecular events by which stress increases neurotransmission mediated by the stress neurohormone corticotropin releasing hormone (CRH) are discussed, as well as the excitatory effects of this neuropeptide on limbic neurons in the amygdala and hippocampus. Finally, the putative causes for the age-selectivity of CRH-mediated excitation are presented.

Methods

Animals

For the purpose of these studies in the rat, 'neonatal' denotes postnatal days 0–7, while 'infant' refers to postnatal days 7–14. The pertinent developmental correlations between human and rat brain are addressed in the discussion.

Pups were offsprings of time-pregnant Sprague–Dawley derived rats. Mothers were housed singly, kept on a 12 h light/dark schedule and given access to unlimited lab chow and water (Yi *et al.*, 1993; Yi & Baram, 1994). Time of birth of pups was determined every 12 h, and the day of birth was considered day 0. Litters were culled to 12 pups on the first postnatal day and kept in quiet, uncrowded AALAC-approved facilities at a room temperature of 21–22 °C.

Unless indicated otherwise, all determinations of CRH gene expression and of the peptide's receptors were performed on 'stress free' animals, sacrificed within 45 s of disturbance (Yi & Baram, 1994). Detailed discussion of these procedures, and of the standardized, age-appropriate stress, acute cold-separation, are found elsewhere (Yi & Baram, 1994; Avishai-Eliner et al., 1995).

Surgical procedures, CRH administration and EEG recordings

CRH and the CRH receptor antagonists were administered, using a micro-infusion pump, into the lateral cerebral ventricle via an indwelling cannula, while the pups were freely moving in a heated Plexiglas chamber (Baram & Schultz, 1991, 1995; Baram et al., 1992). Pups were implanted with cannulae 24 h prior to experiments, and the position of the cannulae was verified in all cases. Briefly, stainless steel cannulae were implanted into the lateral ventricles under halothane anaesthesia, using an infant-rat stereotaxic apparatus (Baram & Schultz, 1991; Yi & Baram, 1993). CRH doses were 22 to 750 pmoler, delivered in 0.5–1 µl. Subsequent to the infusion of CRH the latency to seizure onset and the duration of the resulting seizures were monitored for a minimum of 180 min. Animals were scored for behavioural limbic seizures every 5 min so that seizure duration is expressed in 5-min epochs (Baram & Schultz, 1991, 1995).

To establish the concordance of the limbic automatisms and motor behaviours that were induced by CRH with epileptic discharges, electroencephalographic (EEG) recording was obtained from relevant brain regions, i.e. dorsal and ventral hippocampus, the amygdala and frontal and parietal cortex (Baram et al., 1992). Separate groups of rats were implanted (in addition to cannulae) with bipolar electrodes directed to the amygdala, hippocampus, or both using coordinates established previously (Baram et al., 1992). EEGs were recorded using a GRASS 78E polygraph, connected via long, flexible wires to freely moving animals. All infusions were carried out at 8–10 a.m., to avoid the effects of circadian variability in endogenous CRH (Watts & Swanson, 1989).

Tissue processing and in situ hybridization histochemistry

For all experiments, brains were rapidly removed onto powdered dry ice and stored at –80 °C. Brains were cut into 20 µm coronal sections with a cryostat and mounted on gelatin-coated slides. Preparation of oligonucleotide probes for CRH and CRF_1, and details of the *in situ* hybridization histochemistry (ISH) and image analysis, have been described elsewhere (Yi et al., 1993, 1994). Briefly, sections were brought to room temperature, air-dried and fixed for 20 min in fresh 4 per cent buffered paraformaldehyde. After a graded ethanol treatment, sections were exposed to acetic anhydride–triethanolamine and dehydrated through 100 per cent ethanol. Sections were prehybridized for 1 h, then hybridized using 0.5×10^6 cpm of the appropriate probe for 20 h at 40 °C in a humidity chamber, using a buffer containing 50 per cent formamide (Yi et al., 1993). Sections were washed in 2 × saline–sodium-citrate buffer (SSC) for 15 min four times at 40 °C, followed by 1 × and 0.3 × SSC for 30 min each at room temperature. The sections were dehydrated through graded ethanol solutions, air-dried and apposed to film (Hyperfilm B-Max, Amersham, IL) for 5–7 days.

Quantitative image analysis of CRH and the CRF_1 receptor mRNAs was achieved using the MCID software image analysis system (Imaging Research, St. Catherine, Ontario, Canada). For CRH, optical density was determined over the hypothalamic paraventricular nucleus (PVN) and the central nucleus of the amygdala; for CRF_1, optical density was determined over the CA1 and CA3 hippocampal regions, the dentate gyrus, the frontal and piriform cortex and the lateral nucleus of the amygdala. Each point was derived from a minimum four sections from two or three individual rats. Brain-paste standardized values and the ratio of structure/background were both obtained for quantitation (Avishai-Eliner et al., 1996).

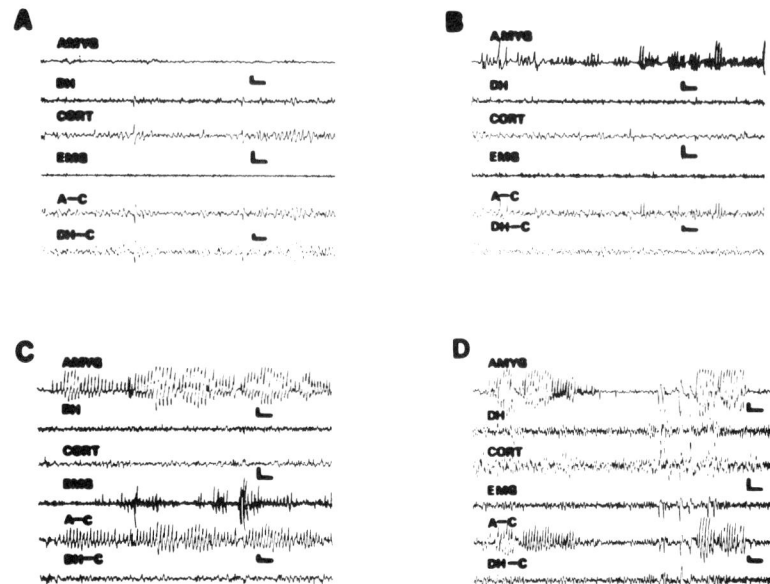

Fig. 1. EEG of a 13-day-old rat prior to (A) and 2, 35 and 174 min following administration of 150 picomole of CRH into the cerebral ventricle (B, C and D, respectively). Epileptic discharges are evident within 2 min in the bipolar amygdala lead (AMYG) and propagate to the amygdala-cortex (A-C) leads, but not, in this animal, to the contralateral dorsal hippocampus (DH). EMG is a motion-detecting electrode. Vertical bar = 50 µV; horizontal bar = 1 s (modified from Baram et al, (1992) and printed with permission).

Immunocytochemistry (ICC) for CRH

In the hippocampus, the anatomical relationships and synaptic interactions among neurons are critical for their functional integration (Freund & Buzsaki, 1996). Therefore, immuno-cytochemistry which permits visualization of individual neuronal cell bodies and their processes was used.

The ICC was a modification of the standard VECTOR ABC protocol, using a CRH antiserum generously provided by Dr W.W. Vale (Salk Inst., La Jolla, CA). Briefly, perfused, sucrose-cryoprotected 20 µm coronal sections were postfixed for 10 min in 4 per cent para-formaldehyde, rinsed twice in Tris-buffered saline and blocked using 0.5 per cent BSA. The sections were incubated overnight with the antiserum to CRH, rinsed and subjected to the appropriate biotinylated second antibody for 1 h. The signal was amplified (Vectastain ABC Elite, Vector), and CRH-immunoreactive cells were visualized using diamino-benzidine with Nickel ion enhancement (Yan et al., 1996).

Statistical analysis was performed using non-parametric tests (Mann–Whitney unpaired two tailed comparison, INSTAT software) without assumptions regarding the distribution of values.

Results

The neuro-excitatory effects of CRH are far more pronounced in the immature brain

In the neonatal and infant rat (first and second postnatal weeks, respectively), CRH given into the cerebral ventricles produced severe seizures. The latency to seizure onset depended on the dose of the peptide, but was as short as 1–2 min. Both the electrographic and behavioural seizures caused by CRH persisted for several hours (Baram & Schultz, 1991). The seizures occurred in the developing rats with doses 200-fold lower than those required for seizure generation in adults (7.5×10^{-12} mol). Furthermore, these doses of CRH did not result in neuroendocrine effects such as elevation of plasma corticosterone (Baram & Schultz, 1991). Once seizures commenced, however, the stress associated

Chapter 13 Mechanisms of non-genetic, provoked seizures in the neonatal and infant brain

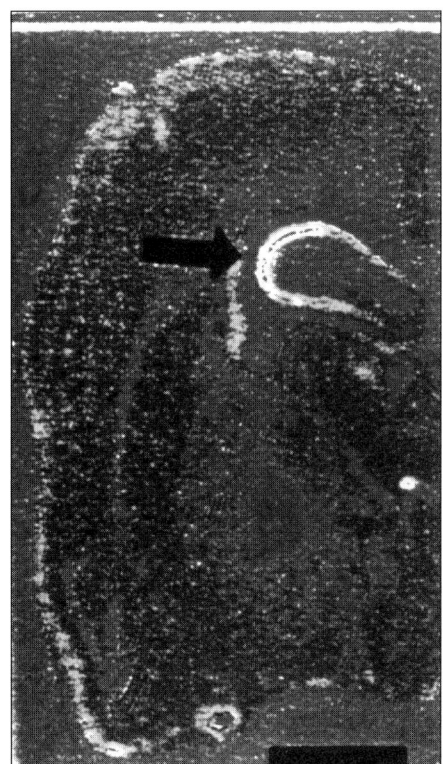

Fig. 2. A coronal hemi-section at the level of the diencephalon from a nine-day-old rat. The section was subjected to in situ hybridization using an ^{35}S-labelled deoxynucleotide probe complementary to the coding sequence of CRF_1-mRNA. This computer-generated false-colour image reveals high levels (pink-white) of the receptor-mRNA in the CA3 region of the dorsal hippocampus. Bar = 0.2 mm (from Avishai-Eliner et al. (1996), with permission).

with the ongoing electrographic and behavioural ictus led to marked elevations of plasma corticosterone (Baram & Schultz, 1991 and unpublished observations). The behavioural aspects of CRH-induced seizures conformed to the pattern observed in seizures with a limbic origin. The origin of CRH-induced epileptiform discharges was defined using multiple bipolar depth electrodes directed to limbic structures, i.e. the amygdala and the dorsal and ventral hippocampus, in addition to cortical electrodes. This approach permitted localization of the onset of CRH-induced epileptiform discharges to the amygdala (Fig. 1).

The mechanisms by which CRH activates limbic neurons have been investigated at a cellular level. In the *in vitro* hippocampal slice preparation, Smith & Dudek (1994) found an increase in the amplitude of population spikes in the CA1 region. Using single cell-patch clamp recording, Hollrigel et al. (1996, 1998) have demonstrated that CRH dramatically increased the frequency of spontaneous firing in CA3 pyramidal neurons.

The high potency of CRH in the developing amygdala and hippocampus may be due to the developmental profile of the CRH receptors

In situ hybridization histochemistry analysis demonstrated that mRNA levels of the first member of the CRH-receptor family, CRF_1, were high throughout development (Avishai-Eliner *et al.*, 1996). In the hippocampal CA3, CRF_1-mRNA levels peaked during the second postnatal week (Fig. 2). Since recent work has documented that the CRF_1 receptor mediates the excitatory effects of CRH (Baram *et al.*, 1997a), high levels of this receptor in target neurons in the hippocampus may predispose the developing brain to the proconvulsant actions of CRH.

Levels of CRF_1-mRNA in the amygdala were also maximal in the immature rat, consistent with our electrophysiological studies which localized the origin of the CRH-induced seizures to this region (Baram et al., 1992) (Fig. 3).

Age-specific stressors increase the levels of CRH in the hypothalamus and amygdala, and induce apparent release of the peptide in hippocampus

Cold exposure, a prototypical age-appropriate environmental stress, increases CRH synthesis in the hypothalamus

Cold-stress has been found to be a powerful, age-specific stimulus in the developing rat, due to the lack of fur and immature thermoregulation during the first two postnatal weeks (Yi & Baram, 1994). The paradigm was precisely defined and shown to result in significant augmentation of hypothalamic CRH-mediated neurotransmission in the hypothalamic–pituitary–adrenal axis (Yi & Baram, 1994). In the infant rat, i.e. during the second postnatal week, cold-stress caused a rapid secretion of CRH

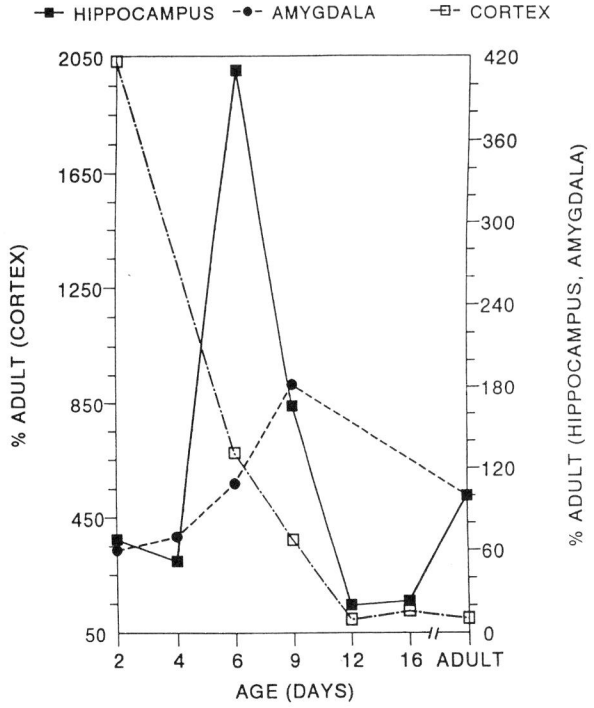

Fig. 3. Schematic quantitative representation of the developmental profile of CRF_1-mRNA in the hippocampus, amygdala and cortex of the rat. Values are described as per cent of adult levels. The dramatic peak of hippocampal and amygdala CRF_1-mRNA at the onset of the second postnatal week is evident (from Avishai-Eliner et al. (1996), with permission).

from peptidergic neurons, leading to elevation of plasma glucocorticoids. Within 4 h after the stress, an upregulation of CRH gene expression resulted in significantly increased CRH-mRNA levels in the hypothalamic PVN (Fig. 4).

A number of stressful conditions increase CRH production in the amygdala of infant rats

Synthetic CRH administered i.c.v. induces seizures which involve a limbic circuit including amygdala and hippocampus. The neuroanatomical origin of endogenous CRH which could mediate these limbic seizures has not been fully elucidated. The central nucleus of the amygdala (ACE) is a major site of CRH containing neurons and terminals (Sawchenko et al., 1993; Gray & Bingaman, 1996). About 1500 ACE neurons produce CRH, and many are interneurons impinging on cell bodies within the nucleus (Uryu et al., 1992; Gray & Bingaman, 1996). CRH receptors are found in the ACE and in the lateral/basolateral amygdaloid nucleus, which projects to the ACE (Chalmers et al., 1995; Avishai-Eliner et al., 1996). The preferential increase in CRH gene expression in the ACE after stress has been demonstrated in adult animals (Makino et al., 1994). Table 1 shows that CRH-mRNA levels in the ACE are increased under stressful conditions such as hypothermia in 9-day-old rats. A similar increase was documented after kainic acid-induced seizures (and stress) in the infant rat.

Table 1. Effect of the age-specific acute cold stress on steady-state messenger RNA for CRH in the central nucleus of the amygdala in nine-day old rats

Treatment group	(n)	CRH-mRNA in ACE	
Controls	(6)	0.316 ± 0.08	
Cold-stressed	(5)	0.546 ± 0.038	$p < 0.05$

CRH-mRNA was analysed in the central nucleus of the amygdala (ACE) of infant rats subjected to cold-separation stress, and sacrificed 4 h later. The experimental paradigm and methods of ISH have been published (Yi & Baram, 1994). N denotes the number of animals per group. One to three sections from each brain were analysed blindly using the MCID image analysis system. Results are expressed as of signal over ACE/background, to account for potential background variation (Baram & Lerner, 1991; Yi et al., 1993; Yi & Baram, 1994).

CRH is found in hippocampal interneurons and may be released by stress

No direct CRH-containing neuronal pathways between the amygdala or hypothalamus and the hippocampus have been documented. Therefore, we tested the hypothesis that CRH producing

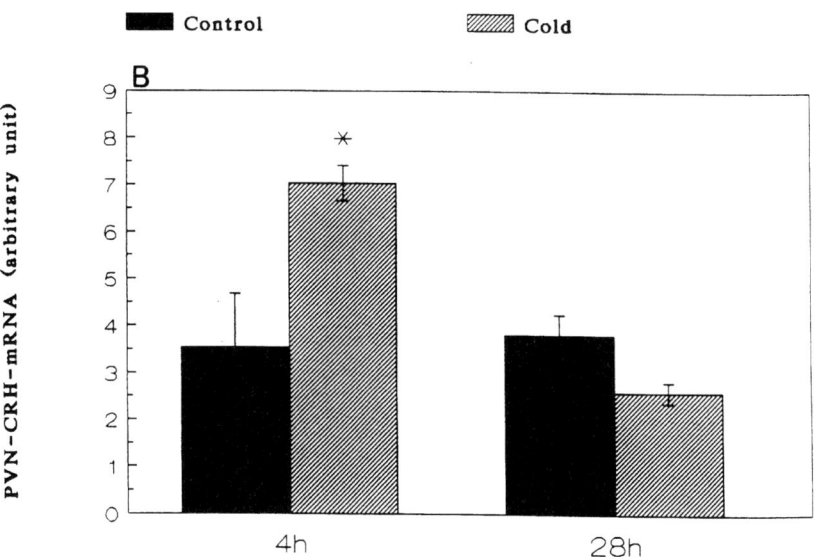

Fig. 4. Effect of cold-separation stress on CRH-mRNA in the paraventricular nucleus of the nine-day-old rat. Pups were subjected to age-appropriate maximal tolerated cold-stress (see text). CRH-mRNA was determined using in situ hybridization histochemistry. Values denote mean ± SEM and were derived as detailed in the Methods section. Asterisk denotes significantly different from control ($p < 0.05$). Modified from Yi & Baram (1994) and printed with permission.

neurons may be present in the hippocampal formation. Immunocytochemistry revealed a population of interneurons which contain CRH (Fig. 5). The CRH-immunoreactive cells possess the morphological features of interneurons and their distribution is similar to that of GABA neurons (Ribak et al., 1978). As described above, synthetic CRH causes excitation of CA3 hippocampal neurons. However, it is not clear whether seizure-inducing stressors, such as hyperthermia, result in a release of CRH from interneurons in the hippocampus. Studies are ongoing to investigate this issue.

Discussion

This chapter addresses the paradox that, despite enhanced excitability of the brain during development, the majority of seizures observed are not spontaneous but must be triggered by fever, anoxia, trauma and similar stressors. We focus on potential mechanisms by which proconvulsant stimuli lead to abnormal excitation in discrete brain regions and result in seizures. The specificity of some of these 'reactive' seizures to restricted developmental periods is also discussed. We propose a scenario in which mechanisms normally involved in the brain's response to threatening or injurious stimuli mediate these seizures. We hypothesize that, in the developing brain, adverse signals such as fever or trauma may result in seizures by up-regulating the release of the excitatory neuropeptide, CRH. This CRH activates specific receptors, leading to enhanced neuronal excitability in a number of limbic circuits (for example, increased firing of CA3 pyramidal neurons).

The strengths of the CRH hypothesis are that it offers a plausible mechanism for the important observation about seizure induction in the immature human and rat. Furthermore, the hypothesis offers discrete predictions which are amenable to experimental testing. For example, it predicts that CRH is a potent convulsant during development and that the peptide's effects decrease with age. The hypothesis further predicts that proconvulsant stressors increase the levels of CRH at sites which are relevant to the origin of reactive seizures and where CRH-receptor expressing neurons can respond by enhanced excitability.

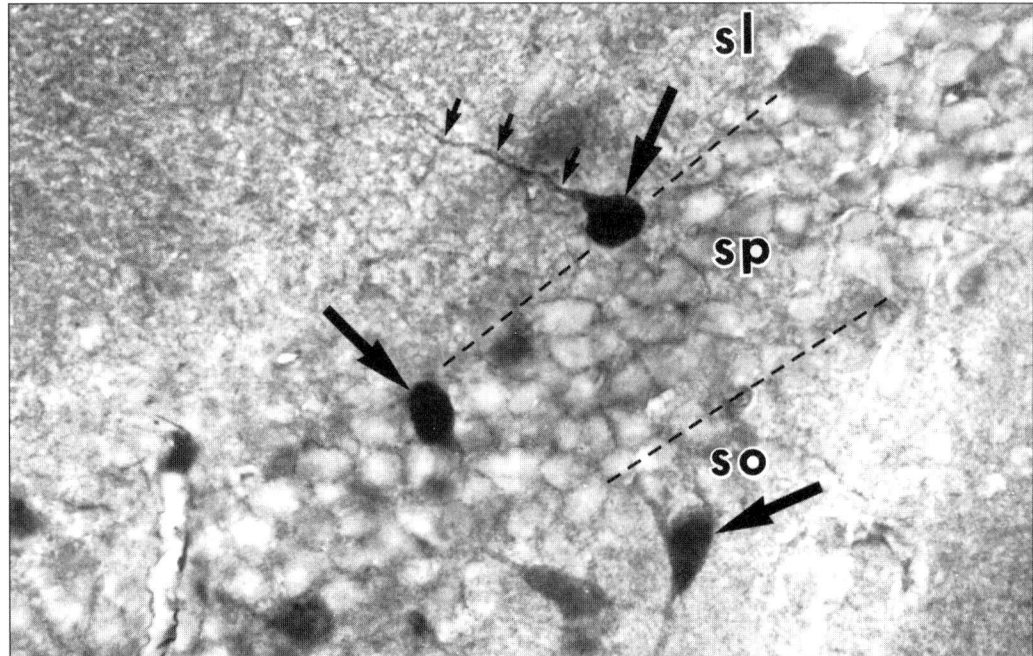

Fig. 5. A photomicrograph of the CA3 hippocampal region showing CRH-immunoreactive non-pyramidal neurons (large arrows). One of the cells, located at the border (dashed line) of strata pyramidale (sp) and lucidum (sl) extends a CRH-immunolabelled dendrite into sl (small arrows). The dendrite of the indicated CRH-labelled neuron in the stratum oriens (so) is located in the same layer, a feature of interneurons. (modified from Yan et al., 1998).

In support of the CRH hypothesis, the experimental findings described demonstrate that the neuropeptide excites neurons in the amygdala and hippocampus both *in vivo* and *in vitro*, leading to prolonged seizures in the immature brain. Studies of hippocampal neurons suggest that CRH enhances the firing of CA3 pyramidal cells (Hollrigel *et al.*, 1998). These effects of the peptide are mediated via activation of specific receptors and are maximal during the second postnatal week in the rat. This is considered to be at least partially due to the high abundance of these CRH receptors in the hippocampus and amygdala during this developmental period.

Clearly, the fundamental role of CRH in the central nervous system (CNS) is not seizure generation. A large body of literature has demonstrated that CRH is a neuropeptide with both neuroendocrine and neuro-transmitter properties (Vale *et al.*, 1981; Young, 1992). The peptide is the primary mediator of the neuroendocrine stress response (Lightman & Harbuz, 1993). The endocrine effects of CRH originate from clusters of peptidergic cells in the hypothalamic paraventricular nucleus (Herman & Cullinan, 1997). CRH is also a neuromodulator in a number of limbic and autonomic brain circuits (Fox & Gruol, 1993; Curtis *et al.*, 1995). CRH-producing neurons are widely but specifically distributed in the brain (Sawchenko *et al.*, 1993), including the central nucleus of the amygdala, which is considered a major source for non-endocrine CRH-mediated neurotransmission (Herman & Cullinan, 1997). Target neurons for the actions of this peptide, expressing specific receptors, are found in many brain regions including the hippocampus (Chalmers *et al.*, 1995; Avishai-Eliner *et al.*, 1996). Physiological effects of CRH on hippocampal neurons include facilitating memory retention and increasing protein-phosphorylation (Lee *et al.*, 1992; Behan *et al.*, 1995). Abnormalities of CRH-mediated neurotransmission may contribute to a number of adult neurological disorders such as depression (Nemeroff, 1992) or Alzheimer disease (Behan *et al.*, 1995).

In general, CRH is an excitatory neurotransmitter (Young, 1992; Curtis *et al.*, 1995). CRH-induced excitation has been demonstrated in the mature rat amygdala (Ehlers *et al.*, 1983; Rainnie *et al.*, 1992; Weiss *et al.*, 1993) and hippocampus (Marrosu *et al.*, 1988; Smith & Dudek, 1994). In the adult rat *in vivo*, the administration of CRH into the cerebral ventricles (i.c.v.) results in epileptiform discharges in the amygdala and the hippocampus, and in limbic seizures with a latency of 3–7 h (Ehlers *et al.*, 1983). There is indirect evidence suggesting that CRH may also be involved in excitotoxic neuronal death in the mature brain: increased levels of CRH have recently been reported in brain regions undergoing injury after kainic-acid-induced status epilepticus (Piekut *et al.*, 1996). Furthermore, the administration of CRH receptor blockers has been reported to decrease ischaemic neuronal injury (Lyons *et al.*, 1991; Maecker *et al.*, 1997).

The data presented in this chapter suggest that CRH may play a unique neuromodulatory role in the developing brain: both the proconvulsant potency of CRH (see above) and the peptide's excitotoxic actions are enhanced in the immature brain (Baram & Ribak, 1995; Ribak & Baram, 1996). These potent effects of CRH are probably due to the large number of limbic CRF_1 receptors which are available to be activated by synthetic CRH during *in vivo* and *in vitro* experiments. A likely cause for the marked reduction in the proconvulsant effects of CRH in the mature brain derives from the demonstration that the abundance of the receptors mediating the peptide's effects diminishes rapidly during the third postnatal week in the rat (Avishai-Eliner *et al.*, 1996).

It should be noted that the studies described above involve rats during the first and second postnatal weeks. Several issues regarding the species and the developmental age of this animal model require discussion. The infant rat was chosen because of the significant body of knowledge which confirms a developmental susceptibility to seizures in this species. Much of the information about brain excitability during development in general is derived from neuroanatomical, electrophysiological and molecular studies of the rat. The period of 'peak excitability' is generally considered to occur during the second postnatal week (Jensen *et al.*, 1991; Swann *et al.*, 1993; Kubova & Moshé, 1994). In addition, the rat and human CRH molecules are identical, and the CRH gene shows a 91 per cent homology in the coding region between these two species, suggesting a remarkable conservation of the function of this peptide across these two species. Furthermore, known regulatory mechanisms of CRH gene expression in the human CNS are considered very similar to those in the rat. The age of the rat which is comparable to infancy and early childhood in the human has not been addressed satisfactorily. Indirect species correlations, comparing corpus callosum development in the cat to both human and rat development constitute a rather imprecise approach (Berbel & Innocenti, 1988). Older evidence based on the rates of brain growth and myelination suggests that the 5–7-day-old rat may be 'equivalent' to the human newborn (Dobbing & Sands, 1973, 1979). Rat brain development during the period of 10–15 postnatal days thus best corresponds to the stage of brain development at which human infants are most susceptible to 'reactive' seizures such as febrile seizures (Hjeresen & Diaz, 1988; Baram *et al.*, 1997b).

If developmental, 'reactive' seizures involve CRH, then circumstances leading to them, such as fever, should result in elevated levels of the endogenous CRH in strategically located neurons in the hippocampus and amygdala. As illustrated above, a number of stresses, including those which are known to elicit age-specific seizures, result in augmented CRH production and release in specific CNS regions, including the amygdala and hypothalamus. The effect of hyperthermia on secretion of CRH from the newly described CRH-immunoreactive neurons in the hippocampus is currently under investigation.

Increased neuronal excitability by CRH is obviously only one of several potential mechanisms underlying the enhanced propensity of the immature human and rat to generate 'evoked' seizures. The CRH hypothesis does not propose a role for this peptide in mediating seizures arising in brain regions which are low in – or devoid of – CRH and its receptors. An additional weakness of the proposed CRH hypothesis is the need to account for the differential effects of stressors on seizures: certain stresses such as hyperthermia (fever), trauma or hypoglycemia, which increase CRH levels, also lead to seizures. In contrast, other stressors such as hypothermia, which also increase CRH production (Yi & Baram, 1994) are not proconvulsant.

The induction of seizures is determined in both the mature and developing brain by a complex balance of excitation and inhibition (Johnston, 1996). The components of the excitatory and inhibitory influences differ in immature brain as compared with the adult (Ben-Ari *et al.*, 1994; Holmes, 1997). The immature brain is considered more excitable, but this is manifested by enhanced sensitivity to seizure induction by a variety of manipulations, as opposed to increased prevalence of spontaneous seizures. A number of neuroanatomical and neurochemical characteristics of the immature developmental state probably combine to mediate this fact, and no one single mechanism may be singled out. Neuropeptides are emerging as important modulators of neuronal excitability in several limbic and cortical circuits (Schwarzer *et al.*, 1996). These compounds, such as somatostatin, cholecystokinin, NPY and CRH, co-exist and are co-secreted with classical neurotransmitters at presynaptic terminals (Schwarzer *et al.*, 1996). CRH is positioned to be a neuromodulator affecting neuronal excitability, which is regulated by environmental input. This neuropeptide is thus a likely contributor to the mechanisms by which signals such as fever or anoxia enhance excitation and lead to seizures in the developing brain. A better understanding of these mechanisms is of paramount importance to the design of effective anticonvulsants which are appropriate for reactive seizures in the developing brain.

Acknowledgements: We are indebted to Drs S. Shinnar, C.E. Ribak and I. Soltesz for their helpful comments. The studies reported have been supported by NIH NS01307, NS28912, NS 35439 and an award by the Epilepsy Foundation of America.

References

Avishai-Eliner, S., Yi, S.J., Newth, C.J. & Baram, T.Z. (1995): Effects of maternal and sibling deprivation on basal and stress induced hypothalamic–pituitary–adrenal components in the infant rat. *Neurosci. Lett.* **192**, 49–52.

Avishai-Eliner, S., Yi, S.J. & Baram, T.Z. (1996): Developmental profile of messenger RNA for the corticotropin-releasing hormone receptor in the rat limbic system. *Dev. Brain Res.* **91**, 159–163.

Baram, T.Z. & Lerner, S.P. (1991): Ontogeny of corticotropin releasing hormone gene expression in rat hypothalamus – comparison with somatostatin. *Int. J. Dev. Neurosci.* **9**, 473–478.

Baram, T.Z. & Ribak, C.E. (1995): Peptide-induced infant status epilepticus causes neuronal death and synaptic reorganization. *Neuroreport* **6**, 277–280.

Baram, T.Z. & Schultz, L. (1991): Corticotropin-releasing hormone is a rapid and potent convulsant in the infant rat. *Dev. Brain Res.* **61**, 97–101.

Baram, T.Z. & Schultz, L. (1995): ACTH does not control neonatal seizures induced by administration of exogenous corticotropin-releasing hormone. *Epilepsia* **36**, 174–178.

Baram, T.Z., Hirsch, E., Snead, O.C. & Schultz, L. (1992): Corticotropin-releasing hormone-induced seizures in infant rats originate in the amygdala. *Ann. Neurol.* **31**, 488–494.

Baram, T.Z., Hirsch, E. & Schultz, L. (1993): Short-interval amygdala kindling in neonatal rats. *Dev. Brain Res.* **73**, 79–83.

Baram, T.Z., Avishai-Eliner, S. & Schultz, L. (1995): Seizure threshold to kainic acid in infant rats is markedly decreased by corticotropin releasing hormone. *Epilepsia,* **36** (suppl). abst. B-05.

Baram, T.Z., Chalmers, D.T., Chen, C., Kotsoukos, Y. & De Souza E.B. (1997a): The CRF$_1$ receptor mediates the excitatory actions of corticotropin releasing factor in the developing rat brain. *Brain Res.* **770**, 89–95.

Baram, T.Z., Gerth, A. & Schultz, L. (1997b): Febrile seizures – an age appropriate model. *Dev. BrainRes.* **246,** 134–143.

Behan, D.P., Heinrichs, S.C., Troncoso, J.C., Liu, X.J., Kawas, C.H., Ling, N. & De Souza, E.B. (1995): Displacement of corticotropin releasing factor from its binding protein as a possible treatment for Alzheimer's disease [*see* comments]. *Nature* **378**, 284–287.

Ben-Ari, Y., Tseeb, V., Raggozzino, D., Khazipov, R. & Gaiarsa, J.L. (1994): gamma-Aminobutyric acid (GABA): a fast excitatory transmitter which may regulate the development of hippocampal neurones in early postnatal life. *Prog. Brain Res.* **102**, 261–273.

Berbel, P. & Innocenti, G.M. (1988): The development of the corpus callosum in cats: a light- and electron-microscopic study. *J. Comp. Neurol.* **276**, 132–156.

Berg, A.T., Shinnar, S., Shapiro, E.D., Salomon, M.E., Crain, E.F. & Hauser, W.A. (1995): Risk factors for a first febrile seizure: a matched case-control study. *Epilepsia* **36**, 334–341.

Chalmers, D.T., Lovenberg, T.W. & De Souza, E.B. (1995): Localization of novel corticotropin-releasing factor receptor (CRF2) mRNA expression to specific subcortical nuclei in rat brain: comparison with CRF1 receptor mRNA expression. *J. Neurosci.* **15**, 6340–6350.

Crair, M.C. & Malenka, R.C. (1995): A critical period for long-term potentiation at thalamocortical synapses [*see* comments]. *Nature* **375**, 325–328.

Curtis, A.L., Pavcovich, L.A., Grigoriadis, D.E. & Valentino, R.J. (1995): Previous stress alters corticotropin-releasing factor neurotransmission in the locus coeruleus. *Neuroscience* **65**, 541–550.

Dobbing, J. & Sands, J. (1973): Quantitative growth and development of human brain. *Arch. Dis. Child* **48**, 757–767.

Dobbing, J. & Sands, J. (1979): Comparative aspects of the brain growth spurt. *Early Hum. Dev.* **3**, 79–83.

Dulac, O., Plouin, P. & Jambaqué, I. (1993): Predicting favorable outcome in idiopathic West syndrome. *Epilepsia* **34**, 747–756.

Ehlers, C.L., Henriksen, S.J., Wang, M., Rivier, J., Vale, W. & Bloom, F.E. (1983): Corticotropin releasing factor produces increases in brain excitability and convulsive seizures in rats. *Brain Res.* **278**, 332–336.

Fox, E.A. & Gruol, D.L. (1993): Corticotropin-releasing factor suppresses the afterhyperpolarization in cerebellar Purkinje neurons. *Neurosci. Lett.* **149**, 103–107.

Freund, T.F. & Buzsaki, G. (1996): Interneurons of the hippocampus. *Hippocampus* **6**, 347–470.

Gray, T.S. & Bingaman, E.W. (1996): The amygdala: corticotropin-releasing factor, steroids, and stress. *Crit. Rev. Neurobiol.* **10**, 155–168.

Hauser, W.A. (1995): Epidemiology of epilepsy in children. *Neurosurg. Clin. N. Am.* **6**, 419–429.

Herman, J.P. & Cullinan, W.E. (1997): Neurocircuitry of stress: central control of the hypothalamo–pituitary–adrenocortical axis. *Trends. Neurosci.* **20**, 78–84.

Hjeresen, D.L. & Diaz, J. (1988): Ontogeny of susceptibility to experimental febrile seizures in rats. *Dev. Psychobiol.* **21**, 261–275.

Hollrigel, G., Baram, T.Z. & Soltesz, I. (1996): Corticotropin releasing hormone decreases inhibitory synaptic transmission in the hippocampus of infant rats. *Epilepsia* **37**, (suppl 5), 28.

Hollrigel, G., Baram, T.Z. & Soltesz, I. (1998): Corticotropin releasing hormone increases excitatory synaptic transmission in the hippocampus of infant rats. *Neuroscience* **84**, 71–79).

Holmes, G.L. (1997): Epilepsy in the developing brain: lessons from the laboratory and clinic. *Epilepsia* **38**, 12–30.

Jensen, F.E., Applegate, C.D., Holtzman, D., Belin, T.R. & Burchfiel, J.L. (1991): Epileptogenic effect of hypoxia in the immature rodent brain. *Ann. Neurol.* **29**, 629–637.

Johnston, M.V. (1996): Developmental aspects of epileptogenesis. *Epilepsia* **37** (Suppl 1), S2–S9.

Kubova, H. & Moshé, S.L. (1994): Experimental models of epilepsy in young animals. *J. Child Neurol.* **9** (Suppl 1), S3–S11.

Lee, E.H., Hung, H.C., Lu, K.T., Chen, W.H. & Chen, H.Y. (1992): Protein synthesis in the hippocampus associated with memory facilitation by corticotropin-releasing factor in rats. *Peptides* **13**, 927–937.

Lightman, S.L. & Harbuz, M.S. (1993): Expression of corticotropin-releasing factor mRNA in response to stress. *Ciba. Found. Symp.* **172**, 173–187; discussion 187–189.

Lyons, M.K., Anderson, R.E. & Meyer, F.B. (1991): Corticotropin releasing factor antagonist reduces ischemic hippocampal neuronal injury. *Brain Res.* **545**, 339–342.

Maecker, H., Desai, A., Dash, R., Rivier, J., Vale, W. & Sapolsky, R. (1997): Astressin, a novel and potent CRF antagonist, is neuroprotective in the hippocampus when administered after a seizure. *Brain Res.* **744**, 166–170.

Makino, S., Gold, P.W. & Schulkin, J. (1994): Corticosterone effects on corticotropin-releasing hormone mRNA in the central nucleus of the amygdala and the parvocellular region of the paraventricular nucleus of the hypothalamus. *Brain Res.* **640**, 105–112.

Marrosu, F., Fratta, W., Carcangiu, P., Giagheddu, M. & Gessa, G.L. (1988): Localized epileptiform activity induced by murine CRF in rats. *Epilepsia* **29**, 369–373.

McDonald, J.W. & Johnston, M.V. (1990): Physiological and pathophysiological roles of excitatory amino acids during central nervous system development. *Brain Res. Rev.* **15**, 41–70.

Monyer, H., Burnashev, N., Laurie, D.J., Sakmann, B. & Seeburg, P.H. (1994): Developmental and regional expression in the rat brain and functional properties of four NMDA receptors. *Neuron* **12**, 529–540.

Moshé, S.L., Brown, L.L., Kubova, H., Veliskova, J., Zukin, R.S. & Sperber, E.F. (1994): Maturation and segregation of brain networks that modify seizures. *Brain Res.* **665**, 141–146.

Nemeroff, C.B. (1992): New vistas in neuropeptide research in neuropsychiatry: focus on corticotropin-releasing factor. *Neuropsychopharmacology.* **6**, 69–75.

Noebels, J.L. (1996): Targeting epilepsy genes. *Neuron* **16**, 241–244.

Piekut, D., Phipps, B., Pretel, S. & Applegate, C. (1996): Effects of generalized convulsive seizures on corticotropin-releasing factor neuronal systems. *Brain Res.* **743**, 63–69.

Purpura, D.P., Prelevic, S. & Santini, M. (1968): Postsynaptic potentials and spike variations in the feline hippocampus during postnatal ontogenesis. *Exp. Neurol.* **22**, 408–422.

Rainnie, D.G., Fernhout, B.J. & Shinnick-Gallagher, P. (1992): Differential actions of corticotropin releasing factor on basolateral and central amygdaloid neurones, *in vitro. J. Pharmacol. Exp. Ther.* **263**, 846–858.

Ribak, C.E. & Baram, T.Z. (1996): Selective death of hippocampal CA3 pyramidal cells with mossy fiber afferents after CRH-induced status epilepticus in infant rats. *Dev. Brain Res.* **91**, 245–251.

Ribak, C.E., Vaughn, J.E. & Saito, K. (1978): Immunocytochemical localization of glutamic acid decarboxylase in neuronal somata following colchicine inhibition of axonal transport. *Brain Res.* **140**, 315–332.

Sawchenko, P.E., Imaki, T., Potter, E., Kovacs, K., Imaki, J. & Vale, W. (1993): The functional neuroanatomy of corticotropin-releasing factor. *Ciba Found. Symp.* **172**, 5–21; discussion 21–29.

Schwarzer, C., Sperk, G., Samanin, R., Rizzi, M., Gariboldi, M. & Vezzani, A. (1996): Neuropeptides – immunoreactivity and their mRNA expression in kindling: functional implications for limbic epileptogenesis. *Brain Res. Rev.* **22**, 27–50.

Smith, B.N. & Dudek, F.E. (1994): Age-related epileptogenic effects of corticotropin-releasing hormone in the isolated CA1 region of rat hippocampal slices. *J. Neurophysiol.* **72**, 2328–2333.

Swann, J.W., Smith, K.L. & Brady, R.J. (1993): Localized excitatory synaptic interactions mediate the sustained depolarization of electrographic seizures in developing hippocampus. *J. Neurosci.* **13**, 4680–4689.

Uryu, K., Okumura, T., Shibasaki, T. & Sakanaka, M. (1992): Fine structure and possible origins of nerve fibers with corticotropin-releasing factor-like immunoreactivity in the rat central amygdaloid nucleus. *Brain Res.* **577**, 175–179.

Vale, W., Spiess, J., Rivier, C. & Rivier, J. (1981): Characterization of a 41-residue ovine hypothalamic peptide that stimulates secretion of corticotropin and beta-endorphin. *Science* **213**, 1394–1397.

Volpe, J. J. (1981): *Neurology of the newborn*. Philadelphia: Saunders.

Watts, A.G. & Swanson, L.W. (1989): Diurnal variations in the content of preprocorticotropin-releasing hormone messenger ribonucleic acids in the hypothalamic paraventricular nucleus of rats of both sexes as measured by in situ hybridization. *Endocrinology* **125**, 1734–1738.

Weiss, G.K., Castillo, N. & Fernandez, M. (1993): Amygdala kindling rate is altered in rats with a deficit in the responsiveness of the hypothalamo-pituitary-adrenal axis. *Neurosci. Lett.* **157**, 91–94.

Yan, X.X., Toth, Z., Schultz, L., Ribak, C.E. & Baram, T.Z. (1998): A corticotropin releasing hormone (CRH) containing neurons in the hippocampal formation: Morphological and neurochemical characterization. *Hippocampus* **8**, 1–13.

Yi, S.J. & Baram, T.Z. (1993): Methods for implanting steroid-containing cannulae into the paraventricular nucleus of neonatal rats. *J. Pharmacol. Toxicol. Methods* **30**, 97–102.

Yi, S.J. & Baram, T.Z. (1994): Corticotropin-releasing hormone mediates the response to cold stress in the neonatal rat without compensatory enhancement of the peptide's gene expression. *Endocrinology* **135**, 2364–2368.

Yi, S.J., Masters, J.N. & Baram, T.Z. (1993): Effects of a specific glucocorticoid receptor antagonist on corticotropin releasing hormone gene expression in the paraventricular nucleus of the neonatal rat. *Dev. Brain Res.* **73**, 253–259.

Yi, S.J., Masters, J.N. & Baram, T.Z. (1994): Glucocorticoid receptor mRNA ontogeny in the fetal and postnatal rat forebrain. *Mol. Cell Neurosci.* **5**, 385–393.

Young, W.S. (1992): Regulation of gene expression in the hypothalamus: hybridization histochemical studies. *Ciba Found. Symp.* **168**, 127–138; discussion 138–144.

Chapter 14

Excitatory amino acids and epileptogenesis during ontogenesis

Pavel Mareš

Institute of Physiology, Academy of Sciences of the Czech Republic; Prague, Czech Republic

The involvement of excitatory amino acids in epileptogenesis has been repeatedly demonstrated (Schwarcz & Ben-Ari, 1986; Dingledine *et al.*, 1990). Administration of excitatory amino acids leads to seizures (e.g. Ben-Ari, 1985), their antagonists exhibit anticonvulsant action (Chapman, 1991). I shall focus only on the anticonvulsant action of antagonists of excitatory amino acid ionotropic receptors.

The majority of epileptic seizures (generalized convulsive tonic–clonic seizures, simple as well as complex partial seizures) are due to a predominance of excitation over inhibition (Engel, 1989; Heinemann & Jones, 1990). The dysbalance between excitation and inhibition in convulsive epileptic seizures may be normalized either by a potentiation of inhibitory systems or by suppression of excitatory systems. The first type of anticonvulsant action – facilitation of GABAergic inhibition – was demonstrated with many classical (phenobarbital, valproate, benzodiazepines) as well as new (vigabatrin, tiagabine) antiepileptic drugs (Meldrum, 1989; Rogawski & Porter, 1990). The second possibility may be realized by means of antagonists of the main excitatory transmitters, the amino acids glutamate and aspartate. There is a lot of data on the anticonvulsant action of antagonists of NMDA and AMPA/kainate receptors in adult animals (Rogawski & Porter, 1990; Chapman, 1991) but information about their actions in immature animals is scarce. In contrast to this lack of data, studies of the action of excitatory amino acids in the developing brain are progressively increasing in number. A higher sensitivity of immature neurons to excitatory amino acids was found when compared with mature nerve cells (Tsumoto *et al.*, 1987; Hamon & Heinemann, 1988), and the overexpression of excitatory amino acid receptors at certain stages of ontogenesis was demonstrated (Insel *et al.*, 1990; Miler *et al.*, 1990). Recently, molecular biology of excitatory amino acid receptors has started to discover developmental changes in the composition of these supramolecular complexes (Portera-Cailliau *et al.*, 1996). Therefore some years ago my laboratory started a programme in this field. Two epileptogenic agents are used to elicit seizures in developing rats: systemic administration of pentylenetetrazol and low-frequency electrical stimulation of cerebral cortex. These two paradigms have the ability to evaluate more than one parameter. An appropriate dose of pentylenetetrazol is able to elicit minimal, clonic seizures of facial and forelimb muscles (with preserved righting reflexes) and, after a longer latency, generalized tonic–clonic seizures characterized by a short initial phase of wild running, then tonic and the longest clonic phase. Righting ability is lost at the beginning of the tonic phase (Velíšek *et al.*, 1992). Epileptic afterdischarges evoked by rhythmic electrical stimulation of the sensorimotor cortical area are characterized by spike-and-wave rhythm on the electroencephalogram and clonic seizures of the head and forelimbs as far as behaviour is concerned. The duration of afterdischarges might progressively increase with repeated stimulations. In addition, during stimulation rhythmic movements of head and forelimbs synchronous with individual stimuli are present as a sign of the direct activation of the motor system (Kubová et al., 1990; Makal et al., 1993).

Motor seizures elicited by systemically administered pentylenetetrazol were used to test the action of N-methyl-D-aspartate receptor competitive antagonists: 2-amino-7-phosphonoheptanoic acid (Velíšek et al., 1990), CGP 39551 (Velíšek et al., 1997) and CGP 40116 (Haugvicová & Mareš, 1998), the non-competitive antagonists ketamine (Velíšek et al., 1989) and dizocilpine (Velíšek et al., 1991); drugs acting at the strychnine-insensitive glycine site, kynurenic acid (Velíšek et al., 1995b) and 5,7-dichlorokynurenic acid (Haugvicová & Mareš – personal data); AMPA receptor antagonists CNQX, DNQX and NBQX (Velíšek et al., 1995a); and a non-specific antagonist, glutamic acid diethylester (Velíšek et al., 1995b). Minimal, clonic seizures induced by pentylenetetrazol represent an age-bound phenomenon – they can be reliably elicited from the third postnatal week in rats (Mareš & Schickerová, 1980; Velíšek et al., 1992). This type of seizure was generally left intact by all the antagonists studied. Only extremely high doses could decrease the incidence of minimal seizures in some cases (e.g. a 2 mg/kg dose of dizocilpine). In contrast, kynurenic acid and glutamic acid diethylester increase the incidence of minimal seizures in such age groups where this type of seizures cannot be reliably elicited, i.e. 7- and 12-day-old rat pups. Similar effects were observed after the administration of some classical antiepileptic drugs (phenobarbital – Kubová & Mareš, 1991; ethosuximide, benzodiazepines – Mareš et al., 1981). Generalized tonic–clonic seizures are suppressed by NMDA receptor antagonists in all age groups, mostly in a dose-dependent manner. A higher effect in rat pups than in adult animals is observed with the majority of drugs. The only exception concerns 2-amino–7-phosphonoheptanoic acid which is more efficient in adult than in immature rats. Another exception concerns the competitive antagonist CGP 40116 which at lower doses restricts and suppresses the tonic phase and only at higher doses blocks generalized tonic–clonic seizures completely. Kynurenic acid suppresses tonic–clonic seizures only in adult rats without any effect in rat pups. AMPA/kainate receptor antagonists exhibited a specific action against the tonic phase of generalized tonic–clonic seizures not touching the clonic phase. Glutamic acid diethylester decreased the incidence of generalized tonic–clonic seizures in adult and 7-day-old rats only.

Cortical epileptic afterdischarges were used as a model for studies of the action of competitive (2-amino–7-phosphonoheptanoic acid. CGP 40116 – Šlamberová & Mareš – personal data) and non-competitive (ketamine – Kubová & Mareš, 1995; dizocilpine – Šlamberová & Mareš – personal data) NMDA receptor antagonists, and competitive (NBQX – Mareš et al., 1997) and non-competitive (GYKI 52466 – Kubová et al. 1997) AMPA receptor antagonists.

Movements directly related to stimulation were hardly affected by NMDA receptor antagonists, but CGP 40116 decreased the intensity of these movements in all age groups. Within the two AMPA receptor antagonists, NBQX changed movements of forelimbs into minute jerks of digits whereas the 20 mg/kg dose of GYKI 52466 led to lower severity of movements as scored according to Racine's five-point scale (Racine, 1972).

The duration of the afterdischarges was influenced by all antagonists studied but there were marked differences in efficacy and developmental profile. Practically all drugs were able to block progressive prolongation of afterdischarges with repeated stimulation (this phenomenon was best expressed in 12-day-old animals). The only exception was a higher dose of 2-amino–7-phosphonoheptanoic acid (60 mg/kg i.p.) which led to even more marked prolongation of seizures in 12-day-old rat pups. Among NMDA receptor antagonists, CGP 40116 was found to shorten markedly the duration of afterdischarges in all age groups, dizocilpine being effective in 18- and 25-day-old rats, 2-amino–7-phosphonoheptanoic acid only in 25-day-old animals, and ketamine in 25- and 12-day-old rats. NBQX and GYKI 52466 led to the shortening of afterdischarges in all age groups with minor quantitative changes during development.

The intensity of seizures was again influenced by all drugs tested. CGP 40116 exhibited this action in all age groups, dizocilpine in 18- and 25-day-old rats, 2-amino-7-phosphonoheptanoic acid in 25-day-old animals only and ketamine in 25- and 12-day-old rat pups – in these two age groups high doses of ketamine (20 and 40 mg/kg i.p.) were able to suppress completely clonic seizures so that short EEG afterdischarges appeared without any motor correlates. The same was true for NBQX which was efficient in all age groups. The action of GYKI 52466 was observed also in all age groups but its effect was only moderate.

There is a marked difference when the effects of excitatory amino acid antagonists in the two tests are compared. The NMDA receptor antagonists exhibit marked anticonvulsant action against generalized tonic–clonic seizures in all age groups, and the intensity of this effect is highest in youngest animals and decreases with age. In contrast, these antagonists are more efficient against cortical epileptic afterdischarges in 25-day-old rats than in younger animals, and there are marked differences in the efficacy of individual antagonists. The explanation might relate to the nature of the structures that are important for the generation of these two seizure types. Generalized tonic–clonic seizures are generated in the brainstem (Browning & Nelson, 1986) whereas cortical afterdischarges are probably of thalamocortical origin with a spread of activity into the motor system. The differences in NMDA receptors in the two generators might be hypothesized – developmental changes in the subunit composition of NMDA receptors are far from being simultaneous in the different brain structures (Portera-Cailliau et al., 1996; Wenzel et al., 1996). AMPA receptor antagonists are not markedly efficient in pentylenetetrazol-induced motor seizures whereas their action on cortical afterdischarges is much better expressed. Many cortical efferents are glutamatergic, e.g. the corticostriate pathway (Headley & Grillner, 1990) which may be responsible for the spread of epileptic activity into the motor system and also for a marked action of NBQX and GYKI 52466 on afterdischarges and their motor correlates.

References

Ben-Ari, Y. (1985): Limbic seizure and brain damage produced by kainic acid: mechanisms and relevance to human temporal lobe epilepsy. *Neuroscience* **14**, 375–403.

Browning, R.A. & Nelson, D.K. (1986): Modification of electroshock and pentylenetetrazol seizure patterns in rats after precollicular transections. *Exp. Neurol.* **93**, 546–556.

Chapman, A.G. (1991): Excitatory amino acid antagonists and therapy of epilepsy. In: *Excitatory amino acid antagonists*, Meldrum, B.S. (ed.), pp. 265–286. London: Blackwell Scientific Publications.

Dingledine, R., McBain, C.J. & McNamara, J.O. (1990): Excitatory amino acid receptors in epilepsy. *Trends Pharmacol. Sci.* **11**, 334–338.

Engel, J., Jr. (1989): *Seizures and epilepsy*, pp. 536, Boston, MA: F.A. Davis Co.

Hamon, B. & Heinemann, U. (1988): Developmental changes in neuronal sensitivity to excitatory amino acids in area CA1 of the rat hippocampus. *Dev. Brain Res.* **38**, 286–290.

Haugvicová, R. & Mareš, P. (1998) Anticonvulsant action of a NMDA receptor antagonist CGP 40116 varies only quantiatively during ontogency in rats. *Fundam. Clin. Pharmacol.* **12**, 521–525.

Headley, P.M. & Grillner, S. (1990): Excitatory amino acids and synaptic transmission: the evidence for a physiological function. *Trends Pharmacol. Sci.* **11**, 205–211.

Heinemann, U. & Jones, R.S.G. (1990): Neurophysiology. In: *Comprehensive epileptology,* Dam, M. & Gram, L. (eds), pp.17–42, New York: Raven Press.

Insel, T.R., Miller, L.P. & Gelhard, R.E. (1990): The ontogeny of excitatory amino acid receptors in rat forebrain – I. N-methyl-D-aspartate and quisqualate receptors. *Neuroscience* **35**, 31–43.

Kubová, H. & Mareš, P. (1991): Anticonvulsant effects of phenobarbital and primidone during ontogenesis in rats. *Epilepsy Res.* **10**, 148–155.

Kubová, H. & Mareš, P. (1995): Suppression of cortical epileptic afterdischarges by ketamine is not stable during ontogenesis in rats. *Pharmacol. Biochem. Behav.* **52**, 489–492.

(1990): Influence of clonazepam on cortical epileptic afterdischarfes in rats. *Arch. Int. Paracodyn* **307**, 49–59.

Kubová, H., Világy. I., Mikulecká, A. & Mareš, P. (1997): Non-NMDA receptor antagonist GYKI 52466 suppresses cortical afterdischarges in immature rates. *Eur. J. Pharmacol.* **333**, 17–26.

Makal, V., Miòová, M., Kubová, H. & Mareš, P. (1993): Developmental changes of thresholds for cortical epileptic afterdischarges. *Physiol. Res.* **42**, 49–52.

Mareš, P. & Schickerová, R. (1980): Seizures elicited by subcutaneous injection of metrazol during ontogenesis in rats. *Activ. Nerv. Super.* **22**, 264–268.

Mareš, P., Marešová, D. & Schickerová, R. (1981): Effect of antiepileptic drugs on metrazol convulsions during ontogenesis in the rat. *Physiol. Bohemoslov.* **30**, 113–121.

Mareš, P., Mikulecká, A. & Pometlová, M. (1997): Anticonvulsant action of NBQX in immature rats: Comparison with the effects on motor performance. *J. Pharmacol. Exp. Therap.* (in press)

Meldrum, B.S. (1989): GABAergic mechanisms in the pathogenesis and treatment of epilepsy. *Brit. J. Clin. Pharmacol.* **27** (Suppl.1), 3S–11S.

Miller, L.P., Johnson, A.E., Gelhard, R.E. & Insel, T.R. (1990): The ontogeny of excitatory amino acid receptors in the rat forebrain. II. Kainic acid receptors. *Neuroscience* **35**, 45–51.

Portera-Cailliau, C., Price, D.L. & Martin, L.J. (1996): N-Methyl-D-aspartate receptor proteins NR2A and NR2B are differently distributed in the developing rat central nervous system as revealed by subunit-specific antibodies. *J. Neurochem.* **66**, 692–700.

Racine, R.J. (1972): Modification of seizure activity by electrical stimulation: II. Motor seizures. *Electroenceph. Clin. Neurophysiol.* **32**, 281–294.

Rogawski, M.A. & Porter, R.J. (1990): Antiepileptic drugs: pharmacological mechanisms and clinical efficacy with consideration of promising developmental stage compounds. *Pharmacol. Rev.* **42**, 223–286.

Schwarcz, R. & Ben-Ari, Y. (eds) (1986): *Excitatory amino acids and epilepsy.* New York: Plenum Press.

Tsumoto, T., Hagihara, K., Sato, H. & Hata, Y. (1987): NMDA receptors in the visual cortex of young kittens are more effective than those of adult cats. *Nature* **327**, 513–514.

Velíšek, L., Mikolášová, R., Blanková-Vaòková, S. & Mareš, P. (1989): Effects of ketamine on metrazol-induced seizures during ontogenesis in rats. *Pharmacol. Biochem. Behav.* **32**, 405–410.

Velíšek, L., Kusá, R., Kulovaná, M. & Mareš, P. (1990): Excitatory amino acid antagonists and pentylenetetrazol-induced seizures during ontogenesis: 1. The effects of 2-amino-7-phosphonoheptanoate. *Life Sci.* **46**, 1349–1357.

Velíšek, L., Verešová, S., Pobišová, H. & Mareš, P. (1991): Excitatory amino acid antagonists and pentylenetetrazol-induced seizures during ontogenesis: 2. The effects of MK–801. *Psychopharmacology* **14**, 510–514.

Velíšek, L., Kubová, H., Pohl, M., Staòková, L., Mareš, P. & Schickerová, R. (1992): Pentylenetetrazol-induced seizures in rats: an ontogenetic study. *Naunyn-Schmiedeberg's Arch. Pharmacol.* **346**, 588–591.

Velíšek, L., Kubová, H., Mareš, P. & Vachová, D. (1995a): Kainate/AMPA receptor antagonists are anticonvulsant against the tonic hindlimb component of pentylenetetrazol-induced seizures in developing rats. *Pharmacol. Biochem. Behav.* **51**, 153–158.

Velíšek, L., Roztoèilová, L., Kusá, R. & Mareš, P. (1995b): Excitatory amino acid antagonists and pentylenetetrazol-induced seizures during ontogenesis: III. The action of kynuretic acid and glutamic acid diethylester. *Brain Res. Bull.* **38**, 525–529.

Velíšek, L., Vachová, D. & Mareš, P. (1997): Excitatory amino acid antagonists and pentylenetetrazol-induced seizures during ontogenesis. IV. Effects of CGP 39551. *Pharmacol. Biochem. Behav.* **56**, 493–498.

Wenzel, A., Villa, M., Mohler, H. & Benke, D. (1996): Developmental and regional expression of NMDA receptor subtypes containing NR2D subunit in rat brain. *J. Neurochem.* **66**, 1240–1248.

Chapter 15

Acute and chronic epileptogenic effects of hypoxia in the immature brain

Frances E. Jensen

Department of Neurology, Children's Hospital, and Program in Neuroscience, Harvard Medical School, Boston MA, USA

Hypoxic encephalopathy and neonatal seizures

Hypoxia is a leading cause of encephalopathy and seizures in the human newborn, occurring in a variety of conditions including birth asphyxia or respiratory distress associated with prematurity (Volpe, 1994). In the neonate, seizures can be prolonged and refractory to medical therapy, whereas in the adult hypoxia less frequently leads to severe seizures. A subset of infants with hypoxia-induced seizures develop chronic epilepsy (Bergamasco et al., 1984; Connell et al., 1989; Volpe, 1989; Holmes & Kull, 1990). The mechanisms underlying the heightened vulnerability of the immature brain to hypoxia-induced seizures are unknown. In addition, the relationship of the perinatal hypoxic insult and seizures to the later development of epilepsy is poorly understood.

Experimental model of hypoxia-induced seizures

We have previously developed an animal model of perinatal hypoxia which reproducibly demonstrates the age-dependent epileptogenicity of hypoxia. In this model, brief periods of moderate global hypoxia (3–4 per cent O_2) induce spontaneous tonic–clonic seizure activity in rats aged P10–12, but not at older or younger ages (Jensen *et al.*, 1991a) (Fig. 1). Furthermore, rat pups which are exposed to hypoxia during this time window show minimal to no histopathologic damage, but exhibit increased susceptibility to convulsant-induced seizures as adults (Jensen *et al.*, 1991b, 1992). In contrast, performance on neurobehavioural tests in later adulthood is not affected by brief global perinatal hypoxia (Jensen *et al.*, 1992). Hence, hypoxia may selectively alter seizure susceptibility, and both the acute and chronic epileptogenic effects of hypoxia appear to be age dependent. Depth electrode recordings demonstrate that this seizure activity is regionally specific. Both the hippocampus and neocortex show ictal activity during hypoxia, but other areas, such as the amygdala, did not (Jensen *et al.*, 1998) (Fig. 2).

In addition to regional specificity, hypoxic seizures exhibit pharmacological specificity. Both the acute seizures and the chronic hyperexcitable state can be prevented by systemic pretreatment with NBQX, an antagonist of the AMPA subtype of glutamate receptors (Jensen *et al.*, 1995).

These results suggest involvement of excitatory amino acid receptors in the epileptogenic effect of

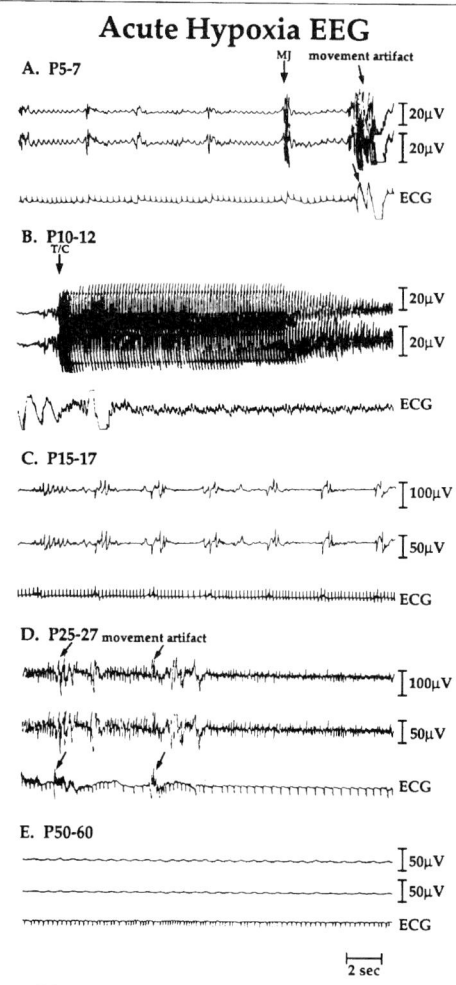

Fig. 1. EEG activity during hypoxia (3 per cent O_2) recorded with epidural electrodes in rats from different age groups and demonstrating that a hypoxia induces seizure activity in immature rats, but not adults, with peak seizure activity occurring at P10–12 (from Jensen et al., 1991a).

hypoxia in the immature brain, thus we evaluated excitatory synaptic transmission in hippocampal slices following hypoxia *in vivo*. Hippocampal slices prepared from P10 pups sacrificed at 10 min after recovery from hypoxia showed evidence of increased excitability. Extracellular field recordings revealed that the amplitude and duration of long-term potentiation (LTP) was significantly increased in area CA1 of hippocampal slices removed from hypoxic pups (Fig. 3). In addition, extracellular recordings within areas CA1 and CA3 showed significantly longer afterdischarge durations in response to kindling stimuli in slices from hypoxic pups compared to controls (Fig. 4). To evaluate whether there were also long-term changes in hippocampal excitability, hippocampal slices were prepared from adult rats which underwent hypoxia at P10 and compared with slices from adult litter mate controls. A Mg^{2+}-free medium was superfused to induce epileptiform activity within the slices. Extracellular recordings from stratum pyramidale of area CA1 showed that Mg^{2+}-free media induced significantly more frequent ictal discharges in slices from previously hypoxic rats compared to controls (Fig. 5).

These results provide evidence that the naturally occurring stimulus of hypoxia can result in both acute and chronic changes in the excitability of the CA1 neuronal network. These results parallel our previous *in vivo* studies demonstrating that global hypoxia acutely increases excitability in the immature brain, and that hypoxia during the age window around P10 results in long lasting increases in seizure susceptibility within hippocampus. Our results suggest that the age-dependent epileptogenic effects of hypoxia are in part mediated by a direct and permanent effect on neuronal excitability within hippocampal neuronal networks.

Maturational factors contributing to hyperexcitability of the imature brain

These studies demonstrate that a brief exposure to hypoxia during the second postnatal week in the rat is associated with both acute and chronic changes in hippocampal excitability. Clinically, the immature brain is more susceptible to seizures, with the highest incidence of seizures from all causes occurring in the first year of life (Aicardi & Chevrie, 1970). In our model of a common cause of neonatal seizures, hypoxia does not result in histologic changes in the hippocampus at the light microscopic level (Jensen *et al.*, 1991a), consistent with the recently reported findings of Owens *et al.* (1997) which also showed no dramatic acute or chronic morphologic changes using a similar

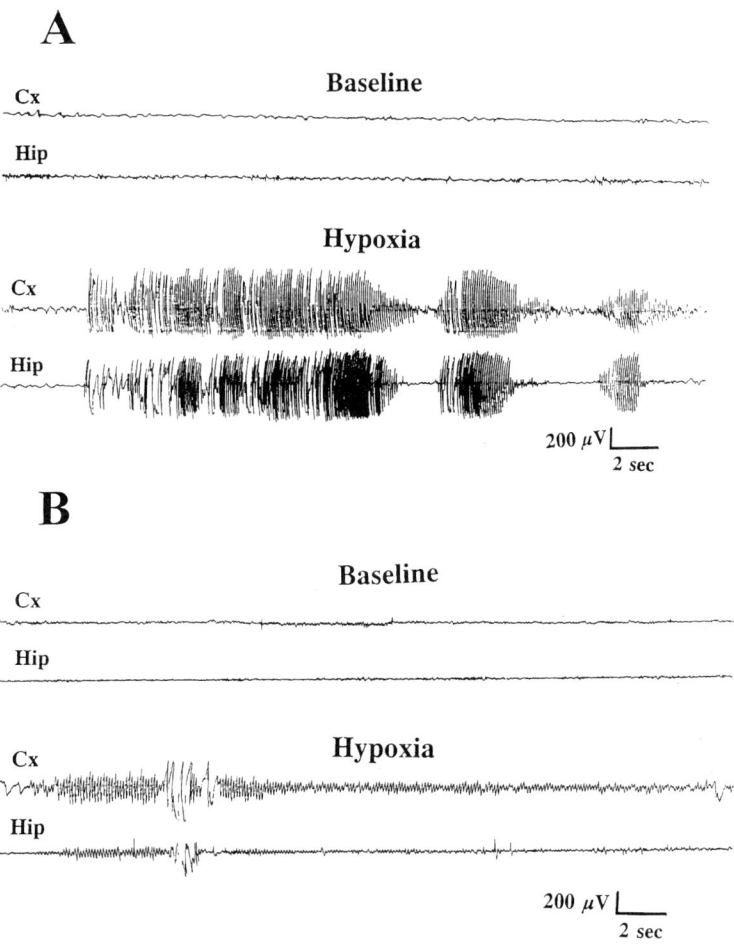

Fig. 2. Depth electrode EEG recordings from representative P10 pups at baseline and during exposure to 3–4 per cent O_2. (A) Simultaneous ictal activity in neocortex and hippocampus; (B) Activation of neocortex prior to recruitment of hippocampus (from Jensen et al., 1988).

model. Despite the lack of overt structural changes, we report here that significant increases in excitability occurred within the hippocampal network both in response to hypoxia acutely and as a long-term sequela.

Area CA1 of hippocampus is selectively vulnerable to hypoxia/ischaemia, and we now show that this region is also vulnerable to the epileptogenic effects of moderate global hypoxia. The selective vulnerability to hypoxic ischaemic injury is thought to be at least in part related to the extremely high density of glutamate receptors on these hippocampal pyramidal neurons (McDonald & Johnston, 1990). In our global hypoxia model, we have previously shown that the acute and chronic epileptogenic effects can be blocked by NBQX, an antagonist to the non-NMDA subtype of glutamate receptors (Jensen *et al.*, 1995). Hence alterations in excitatory transmission may play a critical role in the epileptogenic effects of perinatal hypoxia. Slices from hypoxic rats exhibited LTP which was of magnitude and duration comparable to adult animals, and never seen in control P10 hippocampal slices (Jackson *et al.*, 1993; Harris & Teyler, 1984). Hence, hypoxia appears to 'prime' the immature

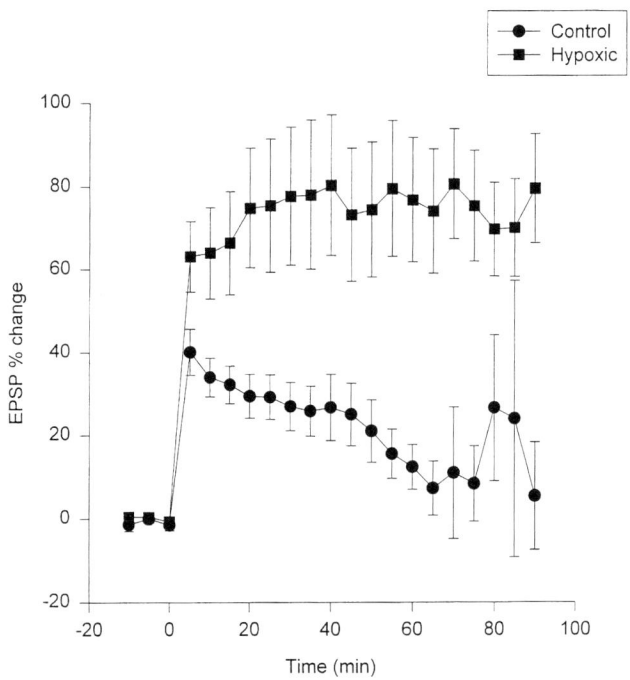

Fig. 3. Summary plot characterizing the amplitude and duration of LTP in slices removed from P10 pups after hypoxia-induced seizures (n =11) and control slices from P10 litter mates (n =10). The amplitude and duration of EPSP potentiation was significantly larger in the slices from hypoxic pups compared with controls ($p < 0.05$) (from Jensen et al., 1988).

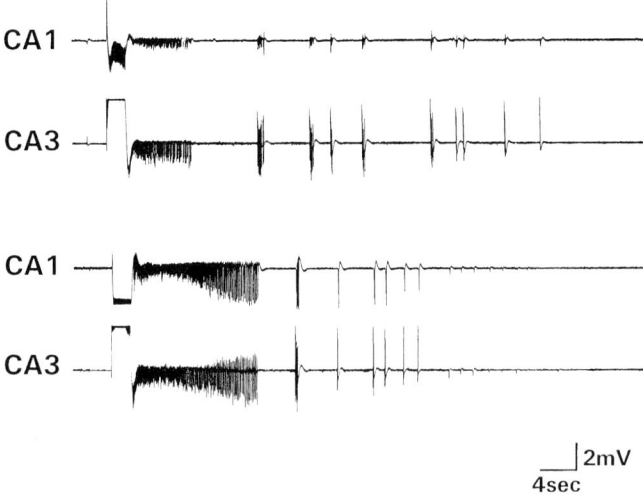

Fig. 4. Representative extracellular recordings in stratum pyramidale of CA1 and CA3 following kindling stimuli in hippocampal slices from P10 rat pups following hypoxia-induced seizures in vivo (A, top two traces) and from P10 rat pups in the control group (B, bottom two traces). Afterdischarges evoked by tetanic stimuli are shown from representative slices in each group. In both CA1 and CA3, the afterdischarge duration was significantly longer in slices removed from previously hypoxic pups (from Jensen et al., 1988).

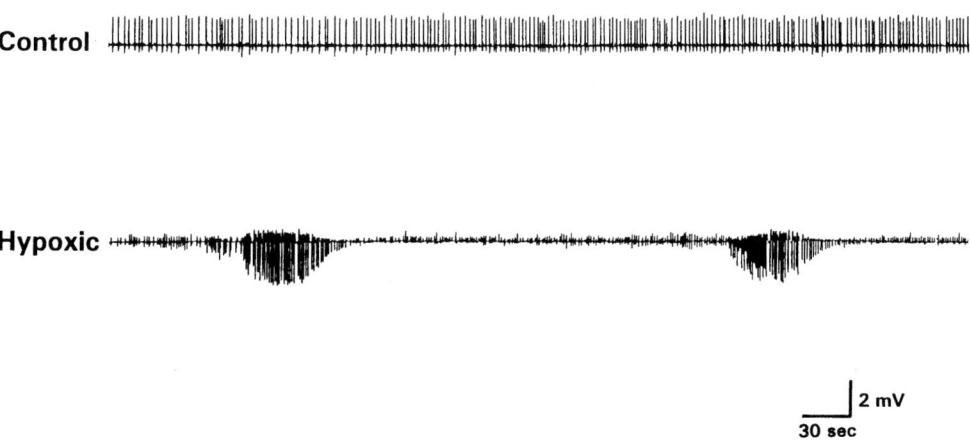

Fig. 5. Representative extracellular recordings of spontaneous activity in Mg^{2+}-free medium in area CA1 from hippocampal slices from control adult rats (top trace) and from slices from litter mate adult rats with previous hypoxia-induced seizures at P10 (bottom trace). Mg^{2+}-free media induced interictal spikes in all control adult rats (top trace). In contrast, ictal discharges were observed significantly more frequently in slices removed from adults with previous hypoxia-induced seizures at P10 (bottom trace) (from Jensen et al., 1988).

hippocampus for LTP. Similarly, *in vitro* kindling was enhanced in the slices prepared from P10 rats following hypoxia-induced seizures. Taken together, these observations from immature slices suggest that moderate hypoxia may acutely enhance excitatory synaptic transmission in the immature brain. As LTP and *in vitro* kindling both depend upon activation of EAA receptors (Harris & Taylor, 1984; Bliss & Collingridge, 1993; Stasheff et al., 1993a,b), we hypothesized that the enhanced seizure activity seen in the immature animal was at least in part mediated by maturational differences in EAA and significant neuronal death does not occur. The increased susceptibility to hypoxia-induced seizures is most likely due to a number of factors that are present during the second postnatal week which cause excitation to predominate over inhibition. Both NMDA and AMPA receptors are undergoing a transient overshoot in density before decreasing to adult level (Insel et al., 1990; McDonald & Johnston, 1990). This overshoot occurs at a developmental stage when maturation of synthetic enzymes and receptor number for the inhibitory neurotransmitter γ-amino-butyric acid (GABA) are incomplete (Palacios et al., 1979; Swann et al., 1989). We have previously shown that the acute and chronic effects of hypoxia are blocked by the AMPA receptor antagonist NBQX, while the NMDA antagonist MK–801 and the GABA agonist lorazepam have little effect on hypoxia-induced seizures at P10 (Jensen et al., 1995). The developmental window of susceptibility to these epileptogenic effects of hypoxia is not only occurring during a time of peak density of AMPA receptors in hippocampus and cortex, but also a period of enhanced sensitivity to AMPA toxicity (McDonald et al., 1992). Hence the efficacy of NBQX in suppressing hypoxia-induced seizures in P10 rats may be related to the maturational profile of the AMPA receptor.

The subunit composition of EAA receptors around P10 also enhances excitation. The NMDAR2c subunit, which confers lower Mg^{2+} sensitivity, is expressed to a greater degree in hippocampus during this developmental window than in adulthood (Pollard, 1993). The AMPA receptor is transiently permeable to Ca^{2+} because of a relative lack of expression of the GluR2 subunit compared to adulthood (Monyer et al., 1994), rendering the cell more excitable (Bowe & Nadler, 1990). During the same time period, it has been reported that levels of the Ca^{2+} binding protein calbindin D28K are lower than in adulthood (Wasterlain et al., 1991).

Possible mechanisms underlying the hyperexcitable phenomena observed in hippocampal slices following hypoxia-induced perinatal seizures

The mechanism whereby perinatal hypoxia-induced seizures permanently alter seizure susceptibility is unknown. Several possible mechanisms are discussed below. Hypoxia has been shown to disrupt Ca^{2+} homeostasis and mobilize intracellular Ca^{2+} stores in hippocampal neurons. Disordered Ca^{2+} homeostasis could be exaggerated in the immature hippocampus where Ca^{2+} binding proteins are below adult levels. Hence increased intracellular Ca^{2+} may provide a mechanism for the enhanced LTP and increased kindling seen in P10 hippocampus following hypoxia-induced seizures *in vivo*. Future studies are aimed at determining whether alterations in synaptic or intrinsic factors are altered by early life seizures. Hypoxia also may enhance subsequent LTP via hypoxia- or seizure-induced increases in neurotrophic factors. The immature brain has significantly higher levels of many neurotrophic factors compared to the adult and certain neurotrophic factors, such as brain-derived neurotrophic factor (BDNF), can be induced within hours after hypoxia/ischaemia episode or seizures *in vivo* (Tsubokawa *et al.*, 1992) and its application enhances potentiation in immature tissue (Figurov *et al.*, 1996). Hypoxia-induced increases in BDNF could contribute to the enhanced LTP seen in hippocampal slices removed from hypoxic pups.

Hypoxia-induced alteration in EAA receptor function may be a candidate mechanism for the chronic enhancement of excitability. The functional effect on EAA receptors could be due to structural alterations such as receptor phosphorylation or a change in subunit composition, as these have previously been reported following seizures or hypoxia/ischaemic injury (Pellegrini-Giampietro *et al.*, 1992; Friedman *et al.*, 1994; Perez-Velazquez & Zhang, 1994).

Conclusions

In summary, the second postnatal week is a period of heightened excitability and susceptibility to epileptogenic stimuli, which is associated with a high rate of synaptogenesis and plasticity. Concurrently, the immature brain at this stage is relatively resistant to seizure-induced neuronal injury. Our data suggest that hypoxia-induced seizures lead to acute and long lasting hyperexcitability within hippocampal neuronal networks. There are numerous maturational factors which may be contributing to this clinically relevant form of age-dependent seizure susceptibility. These *in vitro* observations parallel our previous *in vivo* results and suggest that hippocampal hyperexcitability in part underlies the acute and chronic epileptogenic effects of perinatal hypoxia in our rat model. The present model of perinatal hypoxia suggests that a single brief episode of hypoxia-induced seizures can 'prime' neuronal networks within minutes to hours for subsequent EAA receptor-mediated processes such as LTP and kindling. Furthermore, brief hypoxia results in permanent increases in seizure susceptibility within these neuronal networks. These results suggest that the age-dependent epileptogenic effects of hypoxia are in part mediated by a direct and permanent effect on neuronal excitability within hippocampus. Future use of this model should provide insight into the mechanism underlying the age-dependent susceptibility of the immature brain to the epileptogenic effects of hypoxia and to the cellular events resulting in a chronically seizure-susceptible state.

Acknowledgements: This work was supported by Public Health Service Grants NS31718 and by a NIH-NICHD Mental Retardation Research Center Grant (P30#HD18655). Additional support was provided by the Kaplan Foundation and the William Randolph Hearst Foundation.

References

Aicardi, J. & Chevrie, J.J. (1970): Convulsive status epilepticus in infants and children. A study of 239 cases. *Epilepsia* **11**, 187–197.

Bergamasco, B., Penna, P., Ferrero, P. & Gavinelli, R. (1984): Neonatal hypoxia and epileptic risk: A clinical prospective study. *Epilepsia* **25**, 131–146.

Bliss, T.V.P. & Collingridge, G.L. (1993): A synaptic model of memory: long term potentiation in the hippocampus. *Nature* **361**, 31–39.

Bowe, M.A. & Nadler, J.V. (1990): Developmental increase in the sensitivity to magnesium of NMDA receptors on CA1 hippocampal pyramidal cells. *Dev. Brain Res.* **36**, 33–61.

Connell, J., Oozeer, R. & De Vries, L. (1989): Continuous EEG monitoring of neonatal seizures: Diagnostic and prognostic considerations. *Arch. Dis. Child.* **64**, 459–464.

Figurov, A., Pozzo-Miller, L.D., Olafsson, P., Wang, T.& Lu, B. (1996): Regulation of synaptic responses to high-frequency stimulation and LTP by neurotrophins in the hippocampus. *Nature* **381**, 706–709.

Friedman, L.K., Pellegrini-Giampietro, D.E., Sperber, E.F., Bennet, M.V.L., Moshé, S.L. & Zukin, R.S. (1994): Kainate-induced status epilepticus alters glutamate and GABA$_A$ receptor gene expression in adult rat hippocampus: An *in situ* hybridization study. *J. Neurosci.* **14** (5), 2697–2707.

Harris, K.M. & Teyler, T.J. (1984): Developmental onset of LTP in area CA1 of the rat hippocampus. *J. Physiol.* **346**, 27–48.

Holmes, G.L. & Kull, L.L. (1990): Neonatal seizures. *Am. J. EEG Technol.* **30**, 281–308.

Insel, T.R., Miller, L. & Gelhard, R.E. (1990): The ontogeny of excitatory amino acid in the rat forebrain I: N-methyl-D-aspartate and quisqualate receptors. *Neurosci.* **35**, 31–43.

Jackson, P.S., Suppes, T. & Harris, K.M. (1993): Stereotypical changes in the pattern and duration of long term potentiation expressed at postnatal days 11 and 15 in the rat hippocampus. *J. Neurophysiol.* **70**, 1412–1419.

Jensen, F.E., Alvarado, S., Firkusny, I.R. & Geary, C. (1995): NBQX blocks the acute and late epileptogenic effects of perinatal hypoxia. *Epilepsia* **36** (10), 966–972.

Jensen, F.E., Applegate, C.D., Holtzman, D., Belin, T. & Burchfiel, J. (1991a): Epileptogenic effects of hypoxia on immature rodent brain. *Ann. Neurol.* **29** (6), 629–637.

Jensen, F.E., Applegate, C.D., Burchfiel, J.L. & Lombroso, C.T. (1991b): Differential effects of perinatal hypoxia and anoxia on long term seizure susceptibility in the rat. *Life Sci.* **49** (5), 399–407.

Jensen, F.E., Holmes, G.H., Lombroso, C.T., Blume, H. & Firkusny, I. (1992): Age dependent long term changes in seizure susceptibility and neurobehavior following hypoxia in the rat. *Epilepsia* **33** (6), 971–980.

Jensen, F.E., Wang, C., Staftstom, C.E., Liu. Z., Geary, C. & Stevens, M.C. (1998): Acute and chronic increases in excitability in rat hippocompal slices after perinatal hypoxia *in vivo*. *J. Neurophysiol* **79**, 73–81.

Liu, Z., Gatt, A., Werner, S.J., Mikati, M.A. & Holmes, G.L. (1994): Long term behavioral defects following pilocarpine seizures in immature rats. *Epilepsy Res.* **19**, 191–204.

McDonald, J.W. & Johnston, M.V. (1990): Physiological and pathophysiological roles of excitatory amino acids during central nervous system development. *Brain Res. Rev.* **15** (1), 41–70.

McDonald, J.W., Trescher, W.H. & Johnston, M.V. (1992): Susceptibility of brain to AMPA induced excitotoxicity transiently peaks during early postnatal development. *Brain Res.* **583** (1–2), 54–70.

Monyer, H., Burnashev, N., Laurie, D.J., Sakmann, B. & Seeburg, P.H.(1994): Developmental and regional expression in the rat brain and functional properties of four NMDA receptors. *Neuron* **12**, 529–540.

Owens, J., Robbins, C.A., Wenzel, J. & Schwartzkroin, P.A. (1997): Acute and chronic effects of hypoxia on the developing hippocampus. *Ann. Neurol.* **41**, 187–199.

Palacios, J.M., Niehoff, D.L. & Kuhar, M.J. (1979): Ontogeny of GABA and benzodiazepine receptors: effects of Triton X-100-bromide and muscimol. *Brain Res.* **179**, 390–395.

Pellegrini-Giampietro, D.E., Zukin, R.S., Bennett, M.V., Cho, S. & Pulsinelli, W.A. (1992): Switch in glutamate receptor subunit gene expression in CA1 subfield of hippocampus following global ischemia in rats. *Proc. Natl. Acad. Sci. USA* **89**, 10499–10503.

Perez-Velazquez, J.L. & Zhang, L. (1994): *In vitro* hypoxia induces expression of the NR2c subunit of the NMDA receptor in rat cortex and hippocampus. *J. Neurochem.* **63**, 1171–1173.

Petito, C.K., Feldmann, E., Pulsinelli, W.A. & Plum, F.A. (1987): Delayed hippocampal damage in humans following cardiopulmonary arrest. *Neurology* **37**, 1281–1286.

Pollard, H. (1993): Transient expression of the NR2C subunit of the NMDA receptor in the developing rat brain. *Neuroreport* **4**, 411–414.

Sherwood, N.M. & Timiras, P.S. (1970): *A stereotaxic atlas of the developing rat brain*. Berkeley: Univ. of California Press.

Stafstrom, C.E., Thompson, J.L. & Holmes, G.L. (1992): Kainic acid seizures in the developing brain: status epilepticus and spontaneous recurrent seizures. *Dev. Brain Res.* **65,** 227–236.

Stasheff, S.F., Bragdon, A.C. & Wilson, W.A. (1995): Induction of epileptiform activity in hippocampal slices by trains of electrical stimuli. *Brain Res.* **344,** 296–302.

Stasheff, S.F., Hines, M. & Wilson, W.A. (1993a): Axon terminal hyperexciatbility associated with epileptogenesis *in vitro*. I. Origin of ectopic spikes. *J. Neurophysiol.* **70,** 961–975.

Stasheff, S.F., Mott, D. & Wilson, W.A. (1993b): Axon terminal hyperexcitability associated with epileptogenesis *in vitro*. II. Pharmacological regulation by NMDA and GABAA receptors. *J. Neurophysiol.* **70,** 976–984.

Swann, J.W., Brady, R.J. & Martin, D.L. (1989): Postnatal development of GABA-mediated synaptic inhibition in rat hippocampus. *Neuroscience* **28** (3), 551–561.

Tsubokawa, H., Oguro, K., Robinson, H.P.C., Masuzawa, T., Kirino, T. & Kawai, N. (1992): Abnormal Ca^{2+} homeostasis before cell death revealed by whole cell recording of ischemic CA1 hippocampal neurons. *Neuroscience* **49** (4), 807–817.

Volpe, J.J. (1989): Neonatal seizures. *Pediatrics* **84,** 422–428.

Volpe, J.J. (1994): *Neurology of the newborn*. W.B.Saunders: Philadelphia.

Wang, C. & Jensen, F.E. (1996): NMDA involvment in age dependent differences in seizure susceptibility in hippocampal slices. *Epilepsy Res.* **23** (2), 105–113.

Wasterlain, C.G., Hattori, H., Yang, C., Schwartz, P.H., Rujikawa, D.G., Morin, A.M. & Dwyer, B.E. (1991): Selective vulnerability of neuronal subpopulations during ontogeny reflects discrete molecular events associated with normal brain development. In: *Neonatal seizures*, Wasterlain, C.G. & Vert, P. (eds). New York: Raven Press.

Part V
Consequences of seizures in the immature and mature brain

Chapter 16

Hippocampal neuropathology in children with severe epilepsy

Gary W. Mathern,[1,2,3] James K. Pretorius,[3] Joao P. Leite[4] and P. David Adelson[5]

[1]*Division of Neurosurgery,* [2]*The Mental Retardation Research Center, and* [3]*The Brain Research Institute, University of California, Los Angeles, Los Angeles, California, USA;* [4]*Department of Neurology, Ribeirão Preto School of Medicine, University of São Paulo, Ribeirão Preto, Brazil (SP); Department of Neurosurgery,* [5]*University of Pittsburgh, Pittsburgh, Pennsylvania, USA*

Summary

There is a long-standing controversy whether early childhood seizures cause hippocampal damage and subsequent complex-partial epilepsy. Our laboratory has addressed this pathogenic question by examining hippocampi of paediatric patients undergoing surgical treatment for their epilepsy. Results demonstrate that children with severe early-onset seizures from neocortical sources have: (1) decreased numbers of fascia dentata granule cells, while the Ammon's horn pyramids are not consistently less than expected; (2) no signs that longer seizure histories are associated with progressive reductions in hippocampal neuron densities; (3) neo-Timm stained mossy fibres in the supragranular molecular layer in about 75 per cent of cases; and (4) fascia dentata NCAM-H immunoreactivity (IR) that is maintained well into adulthood. These findings support the concept that seizures early in life are probably responsible for some hippocampal neuropathology, but not the generation of hippocampal sclerosis. Furthermore, certain seizure syndromes seem to be associated with persistent axon plasticity which may contribute to learning and other cognitive problems in children with early onset epilepsy.

Based mostly on clinical–pathological studies, for more than a century there has been a perception among physicians that early childhood seizures causes hippocampal damage and subsequent complex-partial epilepsy. For example, Bratz (1899) and Stauder (1936), using autopsy material, concluded that early childhood seizures may be one cause of hippocampal sclerosis and temporal lobe epilepsy. Margerison & Corsellis (1966) showed in adult autopsies that the mean age of first seizure for their 22 patients with hippocampal sclerosis was 6 years compared to 16 years in cases with minimal hippocampal pathology. In surgical specimens of mesial temporal lobe epilepsy (MTLE) patients the most common pathologic finding is hippocampal sclerosis, and MTLE patients have a frequent history of early childhood seizures (Falconer, 1970; Sagar & Oxbury, 1987; Bruton, 1988; French *et al.*, 1993). In addition, patients who die as a consequence of prolonged seizures show acute hippocampal damage reminiscent of sclerosis (Zimmerman, 1941; Ounsted *et al.*, 1966). However, epidemiological studies of children with many types of seizures indicate that the risk of subsequent adult epilepsy is very low (Aicardi & Chevrie, 1970; Nelson & Ellenberg, 1976; Verity *et al.*, 1993). For instance, children who experience generalized febrile convulsions or single unprovoked seizures have only a 2 to 7 per cent risk of developing epilepsy in subsequent years, and the later seizures are often generalized or partial rather than complex-partial (Nelson & Ellenberg,

1976; Annegers *et al.*, 1979; Cavazzuti *et al.*, 1984; Berg *et al.*, 1992; Verity *et al.*, 1993; Camfield *et al.*, 1994). Likewise, animal studies demonstrate that seizures early in development do not routinely damage the hippocampus (Moshé *et al.*, 1993; Wasterlain & Shirasaka, 1994; Schwartzkroin *et al.*, 1995; Holmes, 1997). Such observations support an alternative hypothesis that early human seizures do not routinely lead to temporal lobe epilepsy or adult hippocampal sclerosis. Hence, in humans an unresolved clinical–pathophysiologic issue is whether seizures during early childhood lead to hippocampal damage, and whether that injury evolves into adult hippocampal sclerosis and eventual complex partial temporal lobe epilepsy.

Over the last 5 years, our laboratory has started to address this pathogenic question by examining hippocampi of paediatric patients undergoing surgical treatment for catastrophic epilepsy (Mathern *et al.*, 1994, 1996). These children have severe repeated generalized seizures during the first few years of life, and many have histories of status epilepticus or infantile spasms. The clinical character of the seizures along with neuroimaging and electrophysiologic studies indicate that the primary epileptogenic regions are usually neocortical (i.e. non-hippocampal). Approximately two-thirds of the cases have cortical dysplasia and the other third regions of cerebral damage from ischaemic injuries or encephalitis (Jellinger, 1987; Vinters *et al.*, 1993). In other words, these children have severe symptomatic epilepsy with a low probability of seizure control or normal development (Cowan & Hudson, 1991). The seizures electrographically begin in the neocortex, the hippocampus is involved in the generalized seizure process, and if seizures during early human development produce hippocampal pathology then these children should show neuron loss and reactive synaptogenesis. Likewise, over time if repeated childhood seizures lead to greater amounts of hippocampal injury, then children with longer seizure histories should show greater hippocampal neuron loss evolving into hippocampal sclerosis.

The purpose of this chapter is to summarize the hippocampal pathologic findings in children with severe epilepsy. This will be accomplished by illustrative case histories and quantitative data. The reader will learn that repeated early childhood seizures are associated with hippocampal neuron loss and abnormal mossy fibre sprouting. However, the amount of damage and sprouting is much less than for patients with hippocampal sclerosis and MTLE.

Overview of clinical case material and histology methods

Children with intractable seizures were evaluated at several collaborating medical facilities using standard clinical protocols previously published; the protocols were approved by the institution's Human Subject Protection Committee, and informed consent was obtained for use of any data for research studies (Shewmon *et al.*, 1990; Engel *et al.*, 1991; Peacock *et al.*, 1993; Shields *et al.*, 1993; Mathern *et al.*, 1996). Surgical therapy was recommended if there was a confluence of clinical data which localized a structurally abnormal area for resection that was the probable source of the seizures; this region may be focal or involve the majority of one cerebral hemisphere, and the hippocampus was removed if the temporal lobe was part of the planned resection. Furthermore, patients did not respond to medical management, and showed signs of cognitive decline. If the surgical procedure was less than a hemispherectomy, then the resection was determined by neuroimaging and intraoperative electrocorticography (Peacock & Roper, 1994). Specimens collected from outside of UCLA were shipped via express mail, and the data for this chapter consist of hippocampi collected from July 1992 to February 1997 ($n = 48$).

In children with symptomatic surgical lesions, the main clinical syndromes and neuropathologic substrates are summarized in Tables 1 and 2. Most of our children had a clinical syndrome consisting of early onset seizures associated with neocortical abnormalities, such as cortical dysplasia or encephalomalacia (i.e. perinatal strokes). For these two groups, the seizures most often began in the first year (range 0 to 15 months), they were frequent (often multiple times per day), and the children often showed focal neurological deficits such as hemiparesis and/or visual field cuts. The age at surgery varied between 10 weeks to 12 years in the cortical dysplasia group, and 1 to 37 years in the encephalomalacia category. By comparison, children with Rasmussen's encephalitis or neoplasms were older and typically had a different clinical history. These children were normal and seizure-free before the onset of their epilepsy, the age at seizure onset varied from 1 to 10 years, the seizure frequency was one to two per week, and surgery occurred between 3 to 14 years. Finally, there were a small number of children with MTLE, which clinically were manifest by an initial precipitating injury, such as a complex febrile convulsion, followed by a silent or seizure-free latent period, and then the onset of complex partial seizures with temporal lobe features.

Table 1. Clinical-neuropathologic categories of pediatric epilepsy surgery cases

1	Early childhood seizures and neocortical lesions
	(A) Cortical dysplasia/dysgenesis (CD)
	(B) Encephalomalacia (i.e. perinatal anoxic-ischaemic)
2	Rasmussen's encephalitis
3	Neoplasm: (DNET; ganglioglioma)
4	Mesial temporal lobe epilepsy (MTLE)

Table 2. Clinical time course features of paediatric cases with hippocampal specimens (years ± SEM; summary of cases from 1992–1997)

Pathology category	Age seizure onset	Age at surgery	Duration of seizures
Cortical dysplasia $n = 23$	0.74 ± 0.44	2.78 ± 0.59	2.02 ± 0.33
Encephalomalacia $n = 10$	0.71 ± 0.27	9.04 ± 3.48	8.33 ± 3.55
Rasmussen's enceph. $n = 5$	$5.58 \pm 1.72^*$	6.60 ± 1.49	1.52 ± 0.43
Neoplasms $n = 6$	$4.60 \pm 1.37^*$	9.06 ± 1.85	4.47 ± 1.54
MTLE $n = 4$	2.39 ± 1.06	8.81 ± 3.57	6.42 ± 2.81
ANOVA	$P = 0.0002$	$P = 0.13$	$P = 0.055$

*Post-hoc tests (Games–Howell) indicate that these two groups are older than the cortical dysplasia and encephalomalacia categories.

For the purposes of this chapter, we will illustrate the hippocampal findings in children with early onset seizures from neocortical lesions (i.e. cortical dysplasia and encephalomalacia; $n=33$), those with MTLE and hippocampal sclerosis, and some unusual cases. By studying hippocampi from these individuals, the clinical syndrome can be incorporated into the experimental design. For example, in the neocortical groups the age at seizure onset was almost always less than age 1 year. Hence, the age at surgery and the duration of seizures can be used as variables to determine whether longer seizure histories were associated with greater amounts of hippocampal neuropathology. Likewise, the underlying neocortical pathologies were different. The cortical dysplasia group represents a prenatal congenital pathology and the encephalomalacia category a postnatal acquired lesion. Therefore, if the hippocampal neuropathology was similar between both categories, then our findings would most likely indicate that the damage must be the consequence of repeated seizures, and not from other causes such as genetic abnormalities.

Briefly, hippocampal specimens were collected in the operating room and 1 cm blocks immersed in neo-Timm's fixative to label zinc-rich mossy fibres (0.1 per cent sodium sulphide in Millonig's buffered 4 per cent glutaraldehyde), or freshly prepared buffered 4 per cent paraformaldehyde for immunocytochemistry (Mathern et al., 1994, 1996). As control comparisons, hippocampi from similarly aged autopsies were collected within a few hours after death. From the hippocampal blocks, sections cut transverse to the long axis were processed for Nissl stain, neo-Timm's histochemistry and immunocytochemistry using an antibody against the immature highly polysialylated form of the neural cell adhesion molecule (NCAM-H; Seki & Arai, 1991, 1993). NCAM-H is an embryonic form of the NCAMs transiently expressed on migrating neurons and new neurite processes, and is a marker of ongoing postnatal neuronal maturation especially in the fascia dentata (Doherty & Walsh, 1991). Neo-Timm's mossy fibre staining in the supragranular molecular layer was quantified on an image computer by measuring the gray value (GV) density, and comparing the inner and outer molecular layers (IML, OML). The IML – OML GV difference shows a high correlation with visual assessments of neo-Timm's staining (Mathern *et al.*, 1996). Adjacent sections from the same hippocampal block were also stained with cresylecht violet (CV) for histopathologic review (30 µm thick) and cell counts (10 µm; Babb *et al.*, 1984a, b; Mathern *et al.*, 1994; 1996). Counts were at 400 × using grid morphometric techniques with Abercrombie's (1946) corrections, and the hippocampal subfields counted were based on Lorente de Nó's (1934) classification. The subfields were the granule cells and hilar neurons of the fascia dentata, CA4, CA3, CA2, CA1 stratum pyramidale, prosubiculum, and subicular neurons.

Summary of anatomic results

We have identified several findings from our initial studies of hippocampi in children with neocortical seizures. First, the number of hippocampal neurons are fewer than age-matched autopsies, but the pattern is not typical for patients with hippocampal sclerosis and MTLE. In paediatric neocortical cases, the most uniform finding is decreased numbers of fascia dentata granule cells, while the Ammon's horn pyramids are not consistently less than expected (Fig. 7; Mathern *et al.*, 1997a). Second, about 75 per cent of paediatric hippocampal specimens show neo-Timm stained mossy fibres in the supragranular molecular layer, which is an aberrant location for these axons. The amount of supragranular neo-Timm's staining is less than that for children or adults with MTLE and hippocampal sclerosis. Third, longer seizure histories are not associated with progressive reductions in hippocampal neuron densities. Lastly, hippocampal NCAM-H immunoreactivity (IR) is maintained well into adulthood in patients whose repeated generalized seizures began in childhood. This contrasts with the NCAM-H findings in hippocampal sclerosis patients or those with histories of cerebral ischaemia where fascia dentata IR was normal or less than expected. The NCAM-H IR findings suggest that certain types of generalized childhood seizures may promote persistent neurite plasticity and perhaps neurogenesis beyond the normal postnatal neuronal and axonal developmental periods.

Illustrative cases

Perhaps the best way to illustrate these findings is through a series of clinical–pathological case presentations. Each of the following cases was chosen to illustrate some aspect of hippocampal neuron loss, mossy fibre sprouting and NCAM-H expression in patients of different ages, epileptic syndromes and duration of seizures.

The first case illustrates the typical hippocampal pathologic findings in a patient with a history of neocortical childhood epilepsy, and is the youngest surgical specimen in our collection (Fig. 1). This youngster was born with a severely malformed cerebral hemisphere and was observed to have clinical seizures within a few days after birth. In hindsight, the mother noted that during the last few weeks of her pregnancy the baby periodically and rhythmically thumped against her abdomen. After birth, the baby was repeatedly admitted to hospital with tonic seizures and 'jerking' episodes lasting many minutes, and scalp EEG confirmed repeated generalized seizures. Interictal EEG showed severe hemispheric slowing, nearly constant spikes and high-frequency background fast activity (PFA), and medications failed to control the events. Because of the severe repeated seizures and signs of developmental delay, the baby underwent a hemispherectomy at age 10 weeks, and pathologically the neocortex showed severe cortical dysplasia involving all resected lobes.

The hippocampus, by Nissl stain, showed that principal cells were located in their normal positions,

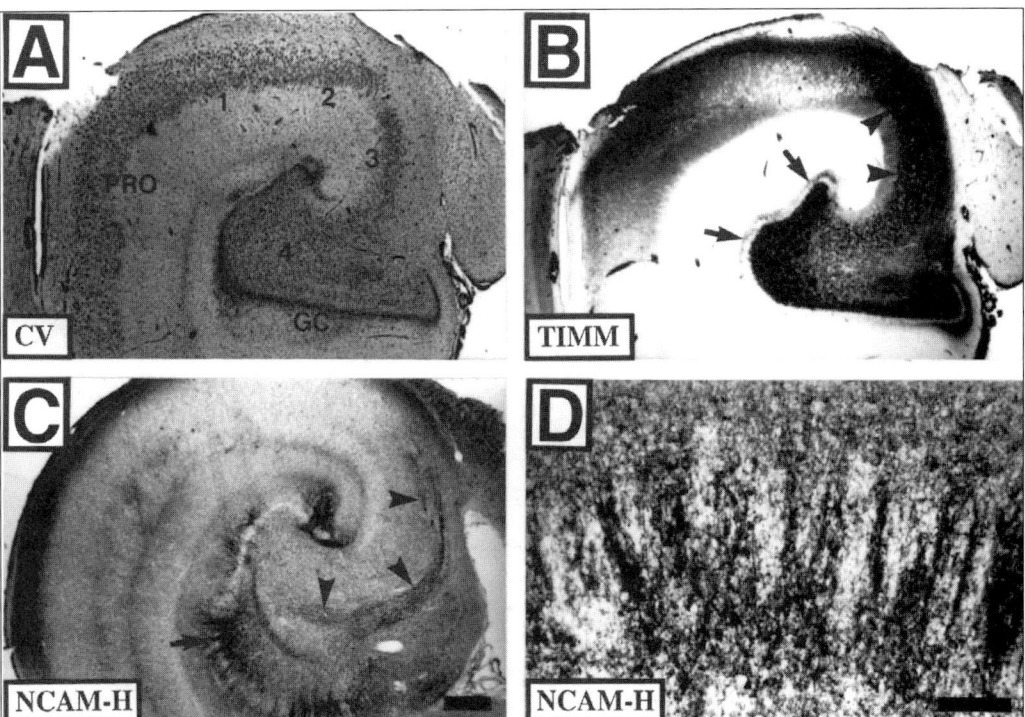

Fig. 1. Illustrative example of the hippocampal pathology from a child operated on at age 10 weeks with severe seizures from a hemispheric cortical dysplasia. This figure shows low magnified views of the Nissl (Panel A), neo-Timm's (Panel B) and NCAM-H (Panel C) staining. A higher magnified view of NCAM-H IR along the stratum granulosum is shown in Panel D. Panels A, B and C at equal magnification; calibration bar equals 500 µm. In Panel D the calibration bar equals 100 µm.

and qualitatively there is no obvious cell loss. By neuron density measurements, the fascia dentata granule cells (Fig. 1A, GC) were 16 per cent less than an age-matched autopsy, and the Ammon's horn pyramids (Fig. 1A, CA4 to CA1) were 17 per cent less. Normally, the neo-Timm's stains mossy fibres located within the hilus and CA3 stratum lucidum (Fig. 1B, arrowheads). However, in the supragranular molecular layer, there were neo-Timm's positive puncta indicating aberrant mossy fibres even at this young age (Fig. 1B, arrows). A typical age-matched autopsy case would show NCAM IR localized mostly to immature granule cells and mossy fibres, and this seizure case is similar in that cells within and just below the stratum granulosum were strongly NCAM-H IR (Fig. 1C, arrow). In addition, NCAM-H IR fibres were found in the hilus and stratum lucidum following the course of normal mossy fibres, (Fig. 1C, arrowheads), and in the stratum granulosum IR fibres coursed through the granule cells into the supragranular region (Fig. 1D). This case, therefore, illustrates that within a few weeks of life and in association with severe seizures from cortical dysplasia: (1) the density of hippocampal neurons was less than expected; (2) aberrant supragranular mossy fibre neo-Timm's staining can occur; and (3) aberrant axons appear at the same time as postnatal migration of new granule cells and neurite formation. Such findings, in the early postnatal period, suggest that seizures during axogenesis may promote aberrant axon circuit formation in the otherwise normally developing hippocampus.

Our second case shows what happens to the hippocampus after many years of repeated generalized seizures from neocortical sources (Fig. 2). This individual had a middle cerebral artery infarct discovered shortly at birth, and within weeks began to display clinical seizures. The seizures remained

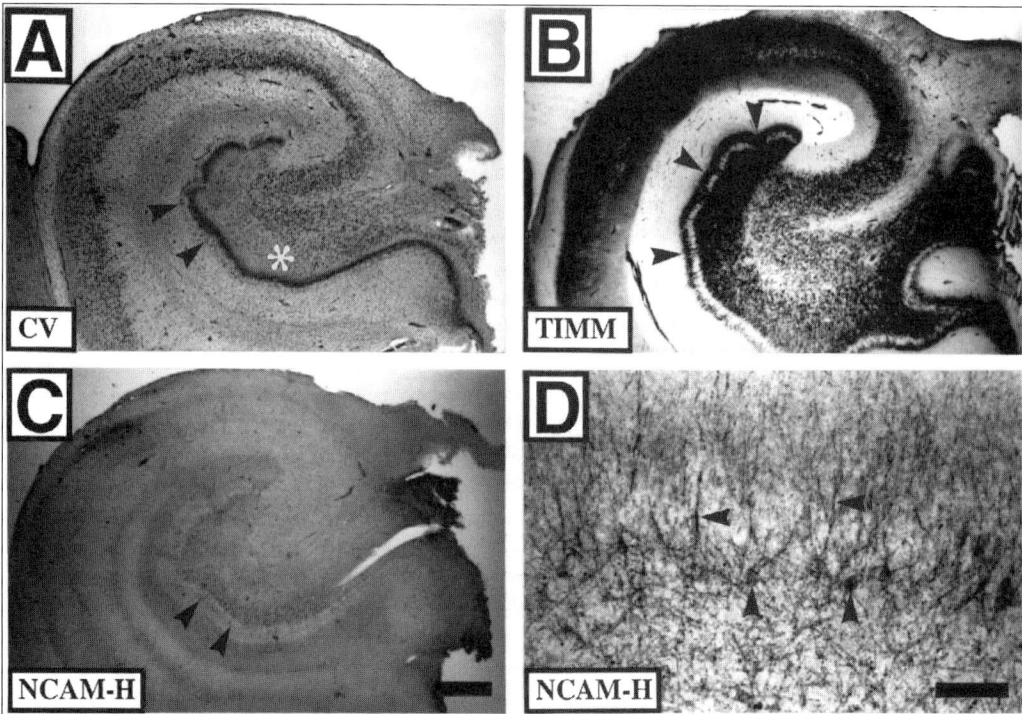

Fig. 2. Example of the hippocampal pathology from a patient with a 16 year history of repeated generalized seizures arranged in the same manner as Fig. 1. Panels A, B and C at equal magnification; calibration bar equals 1 mm. In Panel D the calibration bar equals 100 μm.

uncontrollable despite multiple anti-epilepsy medications, and on neuroimaging the mesial-basal temporal lobe and white-matter connections were anatomically intact. Clinically, the patient had a hemiparesis, was severely retarded with a three word vocabulary, was unable to perform activities of daily living, averaged 15 seizures per day even as an adult, and was in a chronic care facility. A hemispherectomy was performed at age 16 years for management of frequent status epilepticus episodes with secondary aspiration pneumonia. The Nissl stain shows that the hippocampus was nearly anatomically normal (Fig. 2A). The only area of visible neuron loss was within a portion of the hilus immediately beneath the stratum granulosum (Fig. 2A, white asterisk) with some secondary granule cell dispersion into the molecular layer (Fig. 2A, arrowheads; see Mathern et al., 1997a). The CA1 region (Sommer's sector) was not severely damaged as in a hippocampal sclerosis specimen (see Fig. 3). By neuron counts, the granule cells showed a 22 per cent decrease and the Ammon's horn a 12 per cent loss. Neo-Timm's histochemistry stained aberrant mossy fibres in the supragranular molecular layer (Fig. 2B, arrowheads). Furthermore, NCAM-H staining showed IR of individual cells within the infragranular region and fibres around granule cells (Fig. 2C and 2D, arrowheads). In an age-matched autopsy, NCAM-H showed scant to no hippocampal IR. Hence, repeated daily generalized seizures for 16 years was associated with hippocampal neuron loss, but mostly in the fascia dentata granule cells and a portion of the hilus. There was also a fair amount of aberrant supragranular mossy fibre staining. In addition, NCAM-H IR suggested that repeated seizures of non-hippocampal origin were associated with signs of persistent fascia dentata neurite formation and/or perhaps retained mitotic activity of fascia dentata precursor cells. This later finding may be similar to recent experimental findings in adult rats of increased granule cell neurogenesis after pilocarpine induced status epilepticus or perforant path stimulation (Parent et al., 1997).

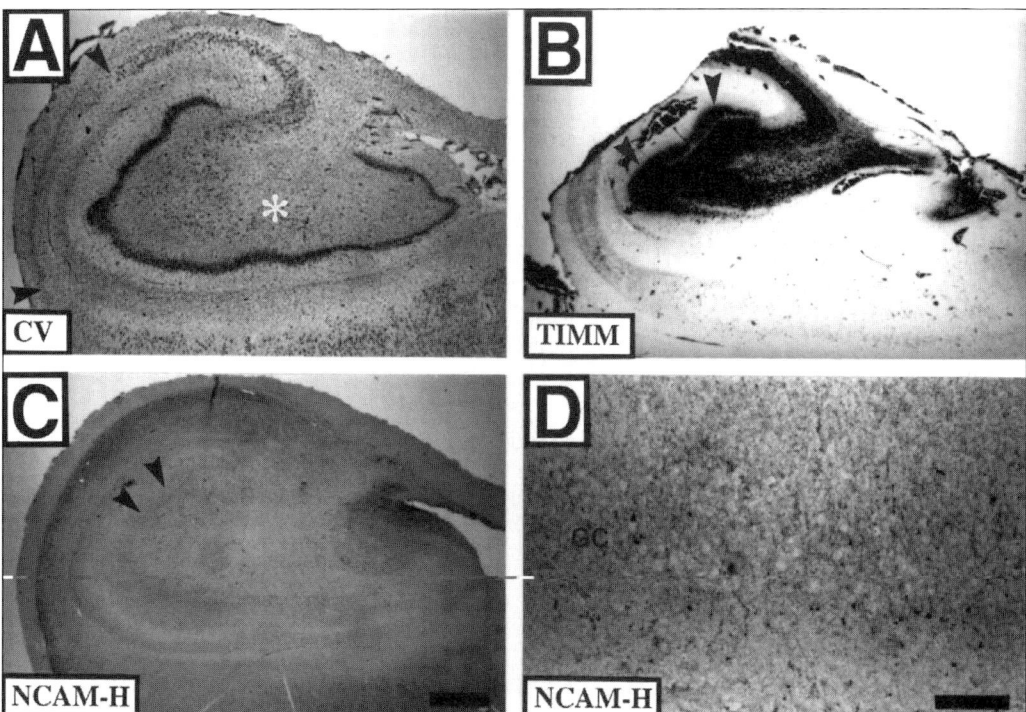

Fig. 3. A typical case of hippocampal sclerosis from a 17 year old patient with mesial temporal lobe epilepsy and hippocampal sclerosis. Panels A to D are arranged in a similar manner as Figs. 1 and 2. Panels A, B and C at equal magnification; calibration bar equals 1 mm. In Panel D the calibration bar equals 100 μm.

Figure 3 shows an example of a patient with MTLE and hippocampal sclerosis. This patient had a complex febrile convulsion at age 3 years, there was a seizure-free period until age 12 years when typical complex partial seizures developed, neuroimaging disclosed a small hippocampus, seizures averaged two to four per month, and surgery was performed at age 17 years. The Nissl section shows severe neuronal damage in a pattern typical for hippocampal sclerosis. There was diffuse hippocampal neuron damage with proportionally greater cell loss in the hilus/CA4 region (Fig. 3A, white asterisk) and Sommer's sector (Fig. 3A area between arrowheads). Moreover, even regions of relative cell preservation, such as the stratum granulosum and CA2 stratum pyramidale, show greater damage than the prior two cases (Figs. 1 and 2). By neuron counts, the granule cells showed a 44 per cent decrease, the hilus a 54 per cent decrease, and the averaged Ammon's horn a 55 per cent loss. The neo-Timm's stain showed dense supragranular mossy fibre sprouting (Fig. 3B, arrowheads). Furthermore, like autopsies of similar age there was minimal hippocampal NCAM-H IR, especially in the stratum granulosum (Figs. 3C and D). Hence, the pattern and amount of hippocampal neuron loss, mossy fibre sprouting and NCAM-H IR were different between two patients operated at similar ages (Figs. 2 and 3). The patient with a high frequency of neocortical generalized seizures since birth had less neuron loss and mossy fibre sprouting than the patient with a lower frequency of MTLE and hippocampal sclerosis. This indicates that the pathogenic mechanisms responsible for hippocampal injury are likely to be different in patients with various epileptic syndromes, and supports the concept that severe repeated childhood seizures by themselves do not necessarily generate hippocampal sclerosis even after many years of epilepsy. Furthermore, in young adults the NCAM-H IR suggests that repeated seizures affect axonal plasticity and neurogenesis depending on the type of epileptic syndrome.

In our children with early onset generalized seizures there are examples of severe hippocampal injury,

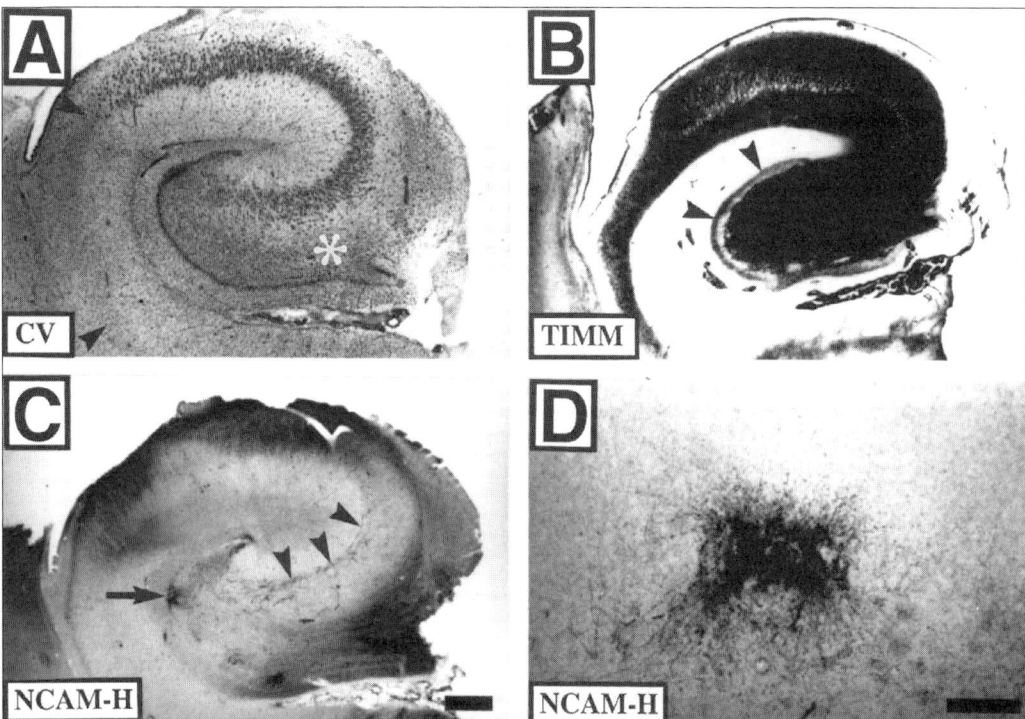

Fig. 4. Example of the hippocampal pathology seen in a 12 month old child with severe repeated generalized epilepsy from a region of cortical dysplasia and at least one well documented episode of status epilepticus and systemic hypotension. Panels A to D are arranged in a similar manner as Figs. 1 to 3. Panels A, B and C at equal magnification; calibration bar equals 500 μm. In Panel D the calibration bar equals 100 μm.

but so far these cases are few and have occurred in the clinical setting of secondary ischaemic or hypoxic injury. For example, the hippocampus in Fig. 4 is from a baby who had severe hemispheric cortical dysplasia with frequent daily seizures, much like the clinical history of our first case. However, at age 2 months the baby had a prolonged seizure that medical personnel felt required aggressive treatment. During a pharmacological coma the baby became hypotensive, and emergent surgery for bowel ischaemia was necessary. The child recovered, continued to seize, and a hemispherectomy was performed 10 months later at age 12 months. The Nissl section shows diffuse loss of hippocampal neurons, especially in the CA1 region (i.e. Sommer's sector; Fig. 4A, area between arrowheads), and the end folium (Fig. 4A, white asterisk). In addition, there was aberrant supragranular mossy fibre neo-Timm's staining (Fig. 4B, arrowheads). Both of these pathologic features were like the adult hippocampal sclerosis case (compare to Fig. 3). At age 1 year, there was also NCAM-H IR in the fascia dentata and regio inferior. However, unlike other paediatric cases (Figs. 1 and 5) and age-matched autopsies, NCAM-H IR was less than anticipated. NCAM-H IR was restricted to small islands of cells and fibres in the stratum granulosum (Fig. 4C arrow; Fig. 4D), and the stratum lucidum (Fig. 4C, arrowheads). In other words, clinically this case was similar to other children with neocortical epilepsy, but unlike those cases there was also a well-documented episode of systemic hypotension during a prolonged seizure. The hippocampal pathology showed more neuron loss than the other neocortical cases, and like that seen in patients with hippocampal sclerosis. Furthermore, there was less NCAM-H IR than expected suggesting that the ischaemic episode probably adversely affected the developing hippocampus by decreasing normal postnatal granule cell neurogenesis, migration and axogenesis.

Chapter 16 Hippocampal neuropathology in children with severe epilepsy

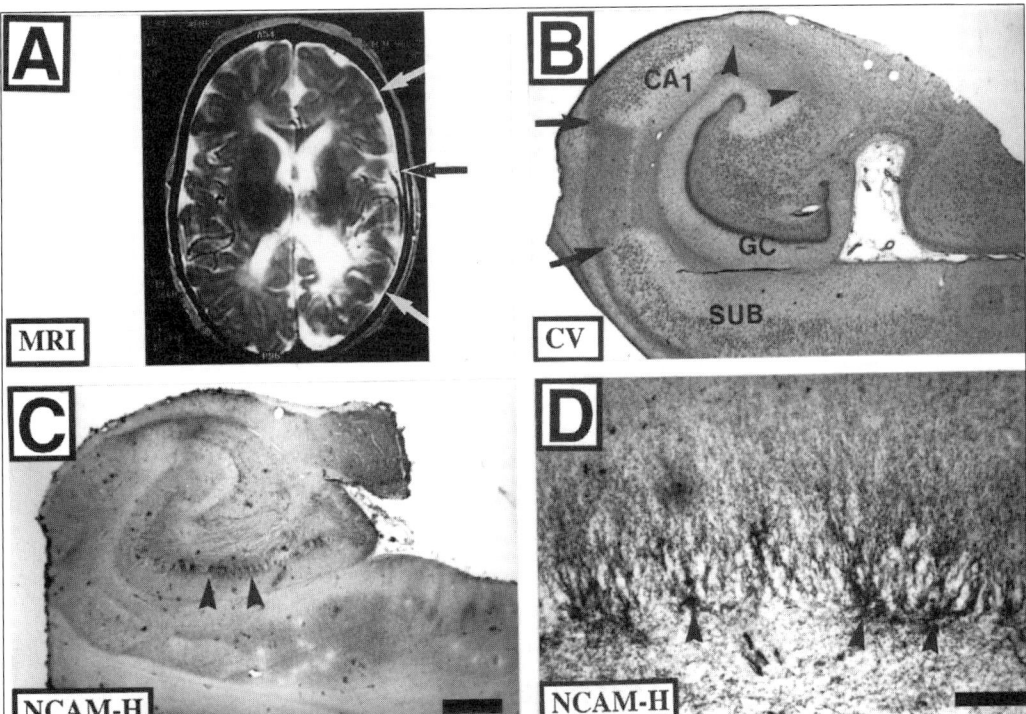

Fig. 5. Representative MRI (Panel A) and hippocampal pathology (Panels B to D) from a 15 month old child with severe seizures and hemispheric atrophy. Nissl section (Panel B) shows focal loss of CA2 and prosubicular neurons (areas between arrowheads and arrows). However, NCAM-H IR (Panels C and D) was similar to age-matched autopsy specimens. Panels B and C at equal magnification; calibration bar equals 1 mm. In Panel D the calibration bar equals 100 μm.

The next two cases were chosen to show interesting and unusual hippocampal findings in patients with severe seizures. The first child presented much like the others with neocortical epilepsy. The baby was noted to have repeated seizures within the first few days of life, the seizures averaged many per day, and there was severe developmental delay with a right-sided hemiparesis. However, the brain MRI showed left cerebral hemispheric atrophy (Fig. 5A, arrows); not hemimegencephaly or other focal or regional area of cerebral maldevelopment. A left hemispherectomy was performed at age 15 months, and pathologically the neocortex showed areas of laminar disorganization and neuronal heterotopias. The hippocampus showed that cells of the fascia dentata, CA1 and subiculum (Fig. 5B, GC, CA1 and SUB) were in their normal positions. However, there was focal neuronal loss in the CA2 (Fig. 5B, arrowheads) and prosubicular subfield (Fig. 5B, arrows). By neuron counts, the percentage loss, compared to an age-matched autopsy, was different for granule cells (56 per cent), CA4 (14 per cent), CA3 (49 per cent), CA2 (95 per cent), CA1 (41 per cent) pyramids, and prosubicular neurons (95 per cent). This is not the typical cell loss pattern in other children with cortical dysplasia, or those with hippocampal sclerosis (compare Fig. 5 to Figs. 1–3). Despite the focal CA2 cell loss, NCAM-H IR was evident in the infragranular region (Fig. 5C, arrowheads) with cells and fibres noted in the stratum granulosum (Fig. 5D, arrowheads), typical for autopsies of similar age. Based on the available clinical and pathologic information, we surmise that during the pregnancy some transient hemispheric ischaemic event or an infection damaged the left brain during some critical aspect of cortical and Ammon's horn neurogenesis and migration which disproportionately affected cortical cells, CA2 pyramids, and prosubicular neurons. By contrast, fascia dentata neurogenesis, which occurs

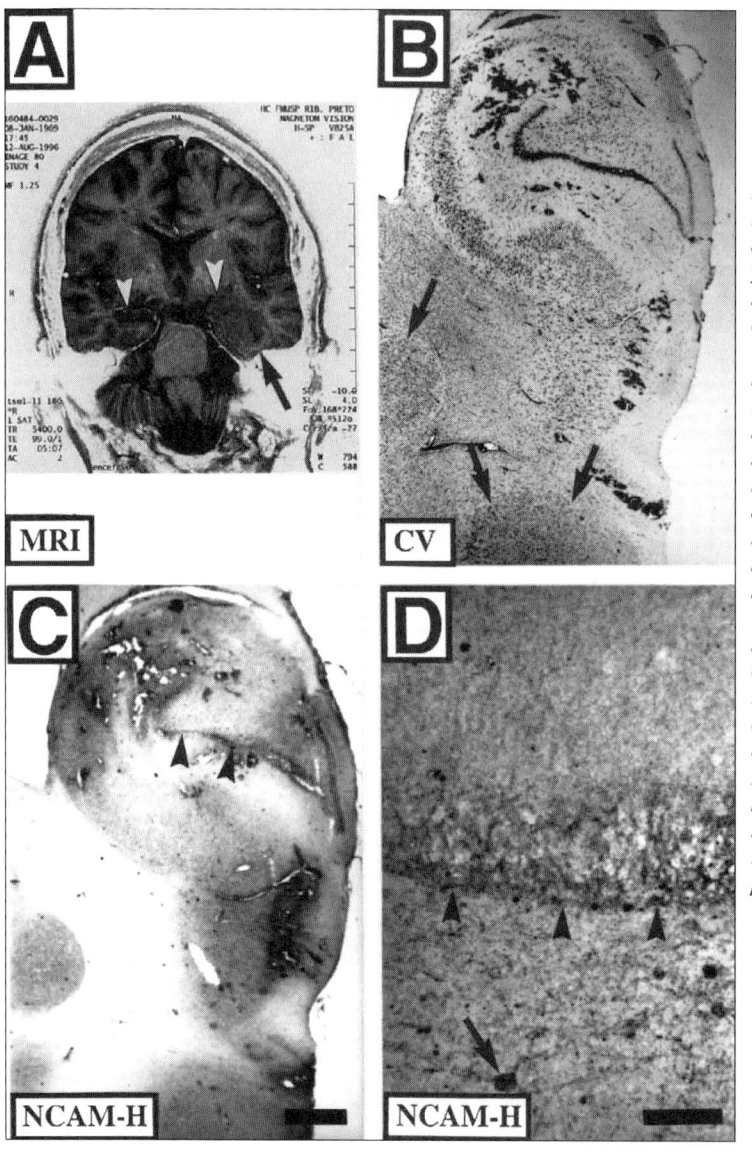

Fig. 6. A case of focal mesial temporal cortical dysplasia in a patient operated at age 28 years. The MRI (Panel A) shows the left-sided region of cortical malformation (arrow) with a small left sided hippocampus compared to the right (arrowheads). Nissl sections (Panel B) showed a small but normally formed hippocampus above a large areas of multiple nodular heterotopias (arrows). The magnification of Panel B is the same as Figs. 2A, 3A and 5B. There was NCAM-H IR in the small adult hippocampus (Panel C) localized mostly to the stratum granulosum (Panel D, arrowheads) and cells within the hilus (arrow). Panels B and C at equal magnification; calibration bar equals 1 mm. In panel D the calibration bar equals 100 μm.

after Ammon's horn development, was not similarly affected. Hence, the fascia dentata demonstrated more normal anatomic development, postnatal migration and axogenesis.

The final case illustrates that not all small hippocampi on neuroimaging are sclerotic on pathologic examination. This case involves an individual who began seizing at around age 1 year and continued until surgery at age 28 years. As an adult the individual lived in a board and care home, and could not handle a bank account or make change. A brain MRI disclosed a focal dysplastic region involving most of the left mesial temporal lobe (Fig. 6A, arrow), and the left hippocampus was smaller than the right (Fig. 6A, arrowheads). The Nissl sections showed a small normally formed hippocampus sitting on top of islands of heterotopic neurons (Fig. 6B, arrows). The principal cells of the left hippocampus were in their normal positions, and by neuron counts the granule cells were 50 per cent less than expected and the Ammon's horn pyramids 27 per cent less. At age 28 years, NCAM-H IR was noted

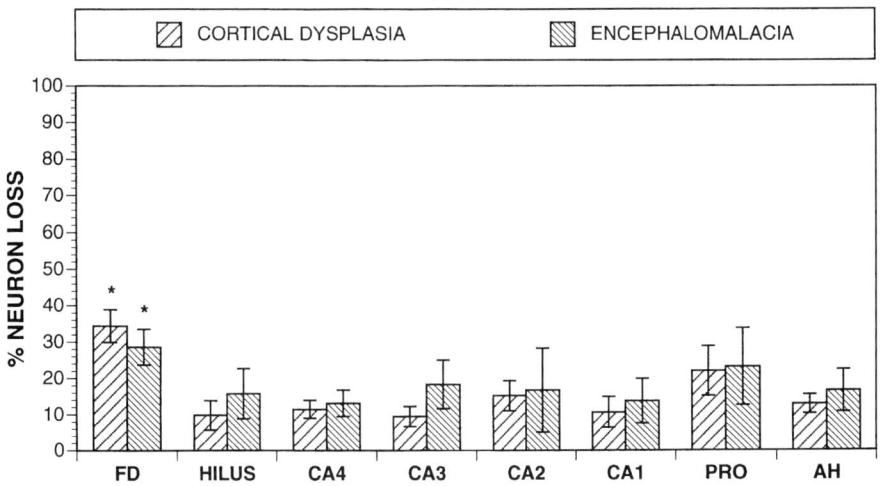

Fig. 7. Histogram showing the percentage mean (± SEM) neuron losses compared to age-matched autopsies for different hippocampal subfields in patients with early childhood seizures from areas of cortical dysplasia or encephalomalacia. The significant post-hoc results showing a difference to autopsies are indicated by asterisks (Games–Howell; $P < 0.05$).

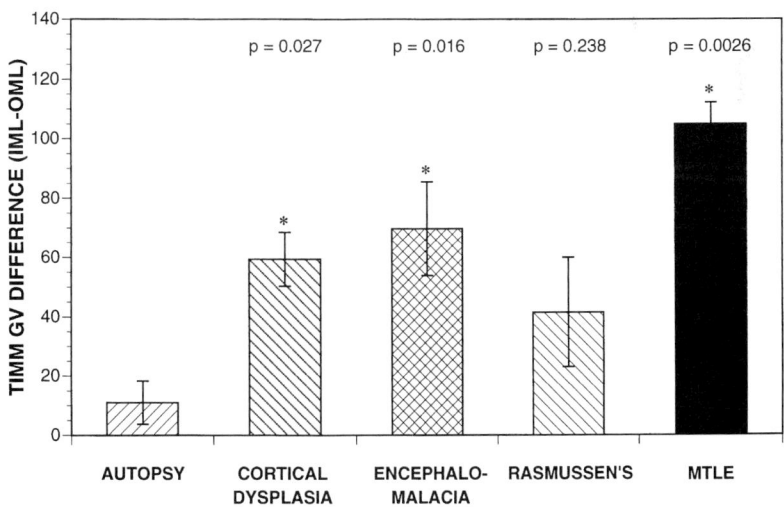

Fig. 8. Histogram showing the mean (± SEM) gray value (GV) differences between the inner and outer molecular layers (IML – OML) for different patient categories. A greater IML – OML GV difference indicates darker supragranular neo-Timm's staining. Significant differences compared to autopsies are shown above each bar.

along the stratum granulosum (Fig. 6C, arrowheads), and immunostained a few cells in the hilus (Fig. 6D, arrow). Hence, this case probably represents an example of hippocampal developmental arrest, and despite over 25 years of seizures from a very close epileptogenic focus the hippocampus was not sclerotic and still showed evidence of NCAM-H IR.

Hippocampal neuron densities and supragranular neo-Timm's staining

Collectively, our hippocampal pathologic findings in surgical paediatric cases show that the most consistent areas of cell loss were granule cells, and that supragranular mossy fibre staining was greater than autopsy controls but less than that for patients with hippocampal sclerosis. Figure 7 shows the mean (± SEM) percent neuron loss relative to age matched autopsies for the two neocortical pathology groups with seizures beginning early in life (i.e. cortical dysplasia and encephalomalacia). The only region that was significantly less than autopsies was the fascia dentata granule cells ($P < 0.001$), and other hippocampal subfields were not statistically less. Figure 8 illustrates the mean (± SEM) quantified gray value (GV) differences between the inner and outer molecular layers (IML – OML) as a measure of supragranular neo-Timm's staining. Greater GV differences indicate darker neo-Timm's staining. Compared to autopsies, children with cortical dysplasia and encephalomalacia demonstrated greater IML – OML GV differences ($P < 0.027$), patients with Rasmussen's encephalitis were not different ($P = 0.24$), and those with MTLE and hippocampal sclerosis showed the greatest GV differences ($P = 0.0026$). Hence, children with both prenatal and postnatal neocortical pathologies and seizures showed a similar pattern of hippocampal pathology with fewer than expected numbers of granule cells and supragranular neo-Timm's staining, but the amount of neuron loss and mossy fibre sprouting was less than that for children with hippocampal sclerosis and MTLE. Finally, regression analyses did not demonstrate significant negative correlations between neuron densities or supragranular neo-Timm's GV measurements with duration of seizures or age at surgery ($P < 0.11$).

Concluding remarks

The results of our hippocampal studies indicate that children with severe epilepsy do show signs of reduced neuron densities and aberrant locations of mossy fibres, but the pattern is not the same as that for patients with hippocampal sclerosis and MTLE. Furthermore, the duration of epilepsy was not associated with progressive declines in neuron densities. Based on these clinical–pathological correlations, we interpret these findings to support the notion that repeated severe seizures during the first few years of life are not routinely responsible for the generation of hippocampal sclerosis. Instead, severe hippocampal damage was associated with concomitant seizures and ischaemic injuries. Hence, there appears to be different pathogenic mechanisms of inducing hippocampal injury depending on the clinical epileptic syndrome.

While this addresses our initial purpose in studying these children, our studies also generated a number of unresolved issues. For example, it is unclear whether the reduced granule cell densities represents injury to existing neurons, a failure of normal granule cell development, or a combination of the two. Based on our NCAM-H data, it would appear that patients with prior histories of some severe ischaemic injuries may show a reduction in granule cell neurogenesis, and this may reduce postnatal granule cell numbers (Fig. 4). It is interesting to speculate that this could be an important mechanism in the generation of hippocampal sclerosis (Fig. 3). By comparison, patients with generalized seizures from neocortical sources demonstrated NCAM-H IR well into adulthood, and this suggests that repeated hippocampal activation may promote excessive axon plasticity well into adulthood (see Figs. 2 and 6). Whether this response is adaptive or maladaptive is also unclear.

There is also the question of whether there is a pathophysiologic relationship between persistent signs of axon plasticity and learning problems. Compared to those without seizures, children with epilepsy have lower averaged IQ scores, show progressive declines on serial intelligence tests, difficulty with school work and often have behavioural problems (Bourgeois *et al.*, 1983; Farwell *et al.*, 1985; Rodin *et al.*, 1986; Funakoshi *et al.*, 1988). While these cognitive problems may be from the underlying symptomatic pathology or anti-epileptic drug therapy, there is a strong suspicion among clinicians that the seizures themselves may contribute to this process (Holmes, 1997). Our studies found signs of persistent hippocampal NCAM-H IR in the same group of patients that is at risk for learning abnormalities and personality disorders (Jeavons & Bower, 1964; Hrachovy & Frost, 1988). Hence, another unresolved question is whether persistent axon plasticity associated with repeated generalized seizures may contribute to the disruption of normal neuronal functions and be partly responsible for the learning disabilities in these children. Consistent with our concept, initial studies indicate that surgical seizure control, which presumably would reduce NCAM-H expression, improves cognitive scores in symptomatic children with epilepsy (Asarnow et al., 1997).

These are just some of the interesting and important research questions that will require further study. In addition, experiments are necessary to further characterize the molecular neurobiology responsible for creating the aberrant axon circuits and neuron loss during postnatal cerebral development. For example, at the earliest stages NMDA receptors seem to be more influential than non-NMDA types in neuronal maturation and axogenesis (Bode-Greuel & Singer, 1989; Jackson et al., 1993; Durand et al., 1996). Furthermore, hippocampus activation of NMDA receptors in the immature brain frequently leads to ictal activity (Hablitz & Lee, 1992; Wang & Jensen, 1996). Hence, one possibility may be that seizures adversely affect the dynamics of NMDA receptor activation in a manner that promotes aberrant axon formation (Dailey & Smith, 1996). Alternatively, seizures could induce greater neurotrophic factor expression that secondarily induces abnormal axon growth (Mathern et al., 1997b). These and other possibilities will need to be explored in future clinical–pathological studies of children with severe seizures.

Acknowledgements: This work was supported by a Clinical Investigator Development Award to GWM (K08 NS 1603) and NS 02808. The UCLA paediatric Epilepsy Surgery Program was supported by NIH grant P01 NS 28383. JPL was supported by FAPESP 95/09248–5, CNPq and FAEPA. Delia Mendoza, Alana Lozada, Kristin M. Yeoman, and Paula A. Kuhlman provided technical support for tissue processing, and surgical material was provided with the additional collaborations of Warwick J. Peacock and Joao A. Assirati. Maria Melendez assisted in preparation of the manuscript. The authors thank W. Donald Shields, D. Alan Shewmon, Thomas L. Babb, Paul S. Mischel, Harley I. Kornblum, Leila Chimelli, Harry V. Vinters and others for their continued collaborations and constructive dialogues in the clinical–pathologic study of this unique group of children.

References

Abercrombie, M. (1946): Estimation of nuclear population from microtome sections. *Anat. Rec.* **94**, 239–247.

Aicardi, J. & Chevrie, J.J. (1970): Convulsive status epilepticus in infants and children. A study of 239 cases. *Epilepsia* **11**, 187–197.

Annegers, J.F., Hauser, W.A. & Elveback, L.R. (1979): Remission of seizures and relapse in patients with epilepsy. *Epilepsia* **20**, 729–737.

Asarnow, R.F., LoPresti, C., Guthrie, D., Elliott, T., Cynn, V., Shields, W.D., Shewmon, D.A., Sankar, R. & Peacock, W.J. (1997): Developmental outcomes in children receiving resection surgery for medically intractable infantile spasms. *Dev. Med. Child Neurol.* **39**, 430–440.

Babb, T.L., Lieb, J.P., Brown, W.J., Pretorius, J.K., & Crandall, P.H. (1984a): Distribution of pyramidal cell density and hyperexcitability in the epileptic human hippocampus. *Epilepsia* **25**, 721–728.

Babb, T.L., Brown, W.J., Pretorius, J.K., Davenport, C., Lieb, J.P. & Crandall, P.H. (1984b): Temporal lobe volumetric cell densities in temporal lobe epilepsy. *Epilepsia* **25**, 729–740.

Berg, A.T., Shinnar, S., Hauser, W.A., Alemany, M., Shapiro, E.D., Salomon, M.E. & Crain, E.F. (1992): A prospective study of recurrent febrile seizures. *N. Engl. J. Med.* **327**, 1122–1127.

Bode-Greuel, K.M. & Singer, W. (1989): The development of N-methyl-D-aspartate receptors in cat visual cortex. *Dev. Brain Res.* **46**, 197–204.

Bourgeois, B.F.D., Prensky, A.L., Palkes, H.S., Talent, B.K. & Busch, S.G. (1983): Intelligence in epilepsy: A prospective study in children. *Ann. Neurol.* **14**, 438–444.

Bratz, E. (1899): Ammonshornbefunde bei Epileptschen. *Arch. Psychiatr. Nervenkr.* **32**, 820–835.

Bruton, C.J. (1988): *The neuropathology of temporal lobe epilepsy*, p. 158. London: Oxford University Press.

Camfield, P., Camfield, C., Gordon, K. & Dooley, J. (1994): What types of epilepsy are preceded by febrile seizures? A population-based study of children. *Dev. Med. Child Neurol.* **36**, 887–892.

Cavazzuti, G.B, Ferrari, P. & Lalla, M. (1984): Follow-up study of 482 cases with convulsive disorders in the first year of life. *Med. Child Neurol.* **26**, 425–437.

Cowan, L.D. & Hudson, L.S. (1991): The epidemiology and natural history of infantile spasms. *J. Child Neurol.* **6**, 355–364.

Dailey, M.E. & Smith, S.J. (1996): The dynamics of dendritic structure in developing hippocampal slices. *J. Neurosci.* **16**, 2983–2994.

Doherty, P. & Walsh, F.S. (1991): The contrasting roles of N-CAM and N-cadherin as neurite outgrowth-promoting molecules. *J. Cell Sci.* **S15**, 13–21.

Durand, G.M., Kovalchuk, Y. & Konnerth, A. (1996): Long-term potentiation and functional synapse induction in developing hippocampus. *Nature* **381**, 71–75.

Engel, J. Jr., Lévesque, M.F., Crandall, P.H., Shewmon, A., Rausch, R. & Sutherling, W. (1991): The epilepsies. In: *Principals of neurosurgery*, Grossman, R.G. (ed.), pp. 319–358. New York: Raven Press.

Falconer, M.A. (1970): The pathological substrate of temporal lobe epilepsy. *Guy's Hosp. Rep.* **119**, 47–60.

Farwell, J.R., Dodrill, C.B. & Batzel, L.W. (1985): Neuropsychological abilities of children with epilepsy. *Epilepsia* **26**, 395–400.

French, J.A., Williamson, P.D., Thadani, V.M., Darcey, T.M., Mattson, R.H., Spencer, S.S. & Spencer, D.D. (1993): Characteristics of medial temporal lobe epilepsy: I. Results of history and physical examination. *Ann. Neurol.* **34**, 774–780.

Funakoshi, A., Morikawa, T., Muramatsu, R., Yagi, K. & Seino, M. (1988): A prospective WISC-R study in children with epilepsy. *Jpn. J. Psychiatry Neurol.* **42**, 562–564.

Hablitz, J.J. & Lee, W.-L. (1992): NMDA receptor involvement in epileptogeneis in immature neocortex. In: *Neurotransmitters in epilepsy*, Avanzini, G., Engel, J., Fariello, R. & Heinemann, U. (eds), pp. 139–146. Amsterdam: Elsevier.

Holmes, G.L. (1997): Epilepsy in the developing brain: Lessons from the laboratory and clinic. *Epilepsia* **38**, 12–30.

Hrachovy, R.A. & Frost, J.D. (1988): Infantile spasms. *Cleveland Clin. J. Med.* **56** (Suppl. 1), 10–16.

Jackson, P.S., Suppes, T. & Harris, K.M. (1993): Stereotypical changes in the pattern and duration of long-term potentiation expressed at postnatal days 11 and 15 in the rat hippocampus. *J. Neurophysiol.* **70**, 1412–1419.

Jeavons, P.M. & Bower, B.D. (1964): *Infantile spasms; a review of the literature and a study of 112 cases. Clinics in developmental medicine series*, no. 15, p. 82. London: The Spastics Society Medical Education and Information Unit, in association with William Heinemann Medical Books.

Jellinger, K. (1987): Neuropathological aspects of infantile spasms. *Brain Dev.* **9**, 349–357.

Lorente de Nó, R. (1934): Studies on the structure of the cerebral cortex. II. Continuation of the study of the ammonic system. *J. Psychol. Neurol.* **45**, 113–177.

Margerison, J.H. & Corsellis, J.A.N. (1966): Epilepsy and the temporal lobes. *Brain* **89**, 499–530.

Mathern, G.W., Leite, J.P., Pretorius, J.K., Quinn, B., Peacock, W.J. & Babb, T.L. (1994): Children with severe epilepsy: evidence of hippocampal neuron losses and aberrant mossy fiber sprouting during postnatal granule cell migration and differentiation. *Dev. Brain Res.* **78**, 70–80.

Mathern, G.W., Babb, T.L., Mischel, P.S., Vinters, H.V., Pretorius, J.K., Leite, J.P. & Peacock, W.J. (1996): Childhood generalized and mesial temporal epilepsies demonstrate different amounts and patterns of hippocampal neuron loss and mossy fiber synaptic reorganization. *Brain* **119**, 965–987.

Mathern, G.W., Kuhlman, P.A., Mendoza, D. & Pretorius, J.K. (1997a): Human fascia dentata stratum granulosum and hilar areas, and hippocampal neuron counts differ depending on the epileptic syndrome and age at first seizures. *J. Neuropathol. Exp. Neurol.* **56**, 199–212.

Mathern, G.W., Babb, T.L., Micevych, P.E., Blanco, C.E. & Pretorius, J.K. (1997b): Granule cell mRNA levels for BDNF, NGF, and NT–3 correlate with neuron losses or supragranular mossy fiber sprouting in the chronically damaged and epileptic human hippocampus. *Mol. Chem. Neuropath.* **30**, 53–76.

Moshé, S.L., Sperber, E.F. & Velisek, L. (1993): Critical issues of developmental seizure disorders [editorial]. *Physiol. Res.* **42**, 145–154.

Nelson, K.B. & Ellenberg, J.H. (1976): Predictors of epilepsy in children who have experienced febrile seizures, *N. Engl. J. Med.* **295**, 1029–1033.

Ounsted, C., Lindsay, J. & Norman, R. (1966): *Biological factors in temporal lobe epilepsy. Clinics in developmental medicine series*, no. 22, p. 135. London: The Spastics Society Medical Education and Information Unit, in association with William Heinemann Medical Books.

Parent, J.M, Yu, T.W., Leibowitz, R.T., Geschwind, D.H., Sloviter, R.S. & Lowenstein, D.H. (1997): Dentate granule cell neurogenesis is increased by seizures and contributes to aberrant network reorganization in the adult rat hippocampus. *J. Neurosci.* **17**, 3727–3738.

Peacock, W.J., Comair, Y., Hoffman, H.J., Montes, J.L. & Morrison, G. (1993): Special considerations for epilepsy surgery in childhood. In: *Surgical treatment of the epilepsies*, 2nd edn., Engel. J. Jr. (ed.), pp. 541–547. New York: Raven Press.

Peacock, W.J. & Roper, S.N. (1994): Surgical treatment of epilepsy. In: *Pediatric neurosurgery: surgery of the developing nervous system*, Cheek, W.R. (ed.), pp. 59–72. Philadelphia: W.B. Saunders.

Rodin, E.A., Schmaltz, S. & Twitty, G. (1986): Intellectual functions of patients with childhood-onset epilepsy. *Dev. Med. Child Neurol.* **28**, 25–33.

Sagar, H.J. & Oxbury, J.M. (1987): Hippocampal neuron loss in temporal lobe epilepsy: correlation with early childhood convulsions. *Ann. Neurol.* **22**, 334–340.

Schwartzkroin, P.A., Moshé, S.L., Noebels, J.L. & Swann, J.W. (1995): *Brain development and epilepsy*, p. 337. New York: Oxford University Press.

Seki, T. & Arai, Y. (1991): The persistent expression of a highly polysialylated NCAM in the dentate gyrus of the adult rat. *Neurosci. Res.* **12**, 503–513.

Seki, T. & Arai, Y. (1993): Highly polysialylated neural cell adhesion molecule (NCAM-H) is expressed by newly generated granule cells in the dentate gyrus of the adult rat. *J. Neurosci.* **13**, 2351–2358.

Shewmon, D.A., Shields, W.D., Chugani, H.T. & Peacock, W.J. (1990): Contrasts between pediatric and adult epilepsy surgery: rationale and strategy for focal resection. *J. Epilepsy* **3** (Suppl. 1), 141–155.

Shields, W.D., Peacock, W.J. & Roper, S.N. (1993): Surgery for epilepsy: Special pediatric considerations. *Neurosurg. Clin. N. Am.* **4**, 301–310.

Stauder, K.H. (1936): Epilepsie und Schläfenlappen. *Arch. Psychiat. Nervenkr.* **104**, 181–212.

Verity, C.M., Ross, E.M. & Golding, J. (1993): Outcome of childhood status epilepticus and lengthy febrile convulsions: findings of national cohort study. *Br. Med. J.* **307**, 225–228.

Vinters, H.V., Armstrong, D.L., Babb, T.L., Daumas-Duport, C., Robitaille, Y., Bruton, C.J. & Farrell, M.A. (1993): The neuropathology of human symptomatic epilepsy. In: *Surgical treatment of the epilepsies*, 2nd edn., Engel. J. Jr. (ed.), pp. 593–608. New York: Raven Press.

Wasterlain, C.G. & Shirasaka, Y. (1994): Seizures, brain damage and brain development. *Brain Dev.* **16**, 279–295.

Wang, C. & Jensen, F.E. (1996): Age dependence of NMDA receptor involvement in epileptiform activity in rat hippocampal slices. *Epilepsy Res.* **23**, 105–113.

Zimmerman, H.M. (1941): The histopathology of convulsive disorders in children. *J. Pediatr.* **13**, 859–890.

Chapter 17

GABA$_A$ receptor alterations in temporal lobe epilepsy

Douglas A. Coulter

Departments of Neurology, Physiology, Anatomy, and Pharmacology and Toxicology, Medical College of Virginia, Virginia Commonwealth University, and the MCV Comprehensive Epilepsy Center of Virginia Commonwealth University, Richmond, Virginia 23298-0599, USA

Introduction

Temporal lobe epilepsy (TLE) is a symptomatic condition. An asymptomatic patient experiences a precipitating event and after a latent period of months to years goes on to develop an epileptic condition. This means that an otherwise normal brain becomes permanently altered by a single event, with the end result being an underlying hyperexcitable state which leads to the induction of recurrent spontaneous seizures. Early hypotheses regarding possible epileptogenic mechanisms centred on the concept that there was an imbalance created between excitation and inhibition in the epileptic brain. One obvious mechanism which could create this type of imbalance would be reduced or damaged inhibitory efficacy in focal tissue. This concept was supported by experimental studies, which demonstrated that seizure activity could readily be elicited in disinhibited animals or in isolated cortical tissue (reviewed in Prince, 1985). Additional support for this 'GABA hypothesis' of epileptogenesis was provided by early studies which identified possible decreases in the numbers of inhibitory terminals in neocortical seizure foci (Ribak *et al.,* 1982). However, studies in epileptic human hippocampi demonstrated that, if anything, GABAergic neurons are selectively preserved in epileptic tissue, suggesting that mechanisms other than a widespread loss of GABAergic interneurons must be involved in epileptogenesis (Babb *et al.,* 1989). Although attention has remained focused on anatomical alterations which might contribute to disinhibition, many studies are now examining other aspects of inhibitory function which might also contribute to reduced inhibitory efficacy and epileptogenesis.

Several levels of inhibitory function must be studied in order to adequately assess whether this function is compromised. For inhibitory synaptic transmission to occur at the level of an individual GABAergic synapse, GABA must be synthesized and stored in vesicles in the presynaptic terminal. Upon synaptic activation, these vesicles then release their contents into the synaptic cleft, GABA diffuses to and activates postsynaptic GABA$_A$ receptors, opening chloride- and bicarbonate-permeable ion channels, and inducing an inhibitory postsynaptic potential. GABA also binds with pre- and postsynaptic GABA$_B$ receptors, which in turn modulate predominantly calcium and potassium channels through activation of intracellular intermediaries. GABA diffuses away from the synaptic cleft and is taken up by GABA transporter proteins in both neurons and glia. There are several potential sites for modifying synaptic strength even at this single synapse level. The levels of synthesis of GABA can be altered, or the amount of GABA contained within a single vesicle could be decreased. Postsynaptically, the numbers of subsynaptic GABA receptors could be altered, or the subunit composition of these receptors changed, which will alter their function and pharmacology, and the shape, conductance and pharmacological sensitivity of the synaptic response. GABA can remain in the synaptic cleft longer, due to alterations in the anatomy of the synapse or numbers or properties of GABA transporter proteins available to remove GABA. The transmembrane chloride gradient can be altered, changing the driving force for GABAergic inhibitory responses. $GABA_B$ receptor-mediated autoinhibition of GABA release could also be enhanced, reducing inhibitory efficacy. Looking beyond the individual inhibitory synapse, there are a number of circuit and tissue level alterations which could also impact inhibitory function. GABAergic neurons can die. GABAergic innervation can increase or decrease. Afferent excitatory drive onto GABAergic neurons can decrease or increase. Neuromodulatory receptors on GABAergic neurons can be altered, impacting their excitability.

Any or all of these changes, as well as many others not described in this overview, could combine to contribute to alterations in inhibitory efficacy in the epileptic hippocampus. Much attention has been focused on a thorough description of the patterns of cell loss and circuit rearrangements which occur in the brains of patients (and animals) with temporal lobe epilepsy. This is clearly warranted. Cell death certainly satisfies the condition of permanence required for a process to underlie a life-long alteration in excitability, as is evident in TLE. However, it must be recognized that the surviving cells of the hippocampus and dentate gyrus are triggering the seizures, and not the holes left by deceased cells. Accordingly, studies examining the excitability of surviving cells in the epileptic limbic system also have merit. The present chapter provides an overview of studies specifically examining possible alterations in $GABA_A$ receptors on surviving principal cells of the epileptic hippocampus. To that end, studies examining paired-pulse inhibition or other gross measures of inhibitory efficacy will for the most part not be reviewed. Although these types of experiments can certainly provide data pertinent to understanding the overall excitability state of epileptic tissue, the relevance of these types of measures specifically to $GABA_A$ receptor alterations is very difficult to determine, since distinct changes at so many other levels could also contribute to these types of responses.

$GABA_A$ receptors

$GABA_A$ receptors are highly specialized heterooligomeric protein aggregates which encompass both binding sites for GABA and a ligand-gated ionic pore within each receptor/ionophore complex. In addition to binding sites for GABA, there are several other binding sites contained within a $GABA_A$ receptor/ionophore, including sites which bind benzodiazepines, barbiturates, steroids, zinc and protons, among others (reviewed in Macdonald & Olsen, 1994). These substances can allosterically modulate the function of $GABA_A$ receptors. To date, seven families of subunit proteins have been identified which can come together to form a GABA receptor. Each of these families may have multiple members, with 6α, 4β, 3γ, 1δ, 1ϵ, 1π and 2ρ subunits identified to date. In addition, functionally distinct splice variants exist for several of these subunits, further contributing to the potentially bewildering complexity of these receptors. Assuming that $GABA_A$ receptors randomly assemble into pentamers (Chang et al., 1996; Tretter et al., 1997), over 500,000 possible distinct GABA receptors are possible. However, in the brain, as few as ten distinct preferred $GABA_A$ receptor conformations may exist (McKernan & Whiting, 1996). From cloning/expression studies examining the function and pharmacology of $GABA_A$ receptors with an identified composition, it is clear that altering the subunit conformation of a $GABA_A$ receptor can dramatically alter both the basic functional properties and the pharmacology of the receptor (reviewed in Macdonald & Olsen, 1994). Many of the subunits confer unique properties to the receptors containing them, which can be identified through a combination of physiological or pharmacological manipulations. For example, the presence of a γ subunit within a $GABA_A$ receptor is necessary for benzodiazepines to act (Pritchett et al., 1989a). Once a γ subunit is present, the nature of the α subunits contained within the receptor determines the nature and pharmacological properties of this benzodiazepine modulation (Pritchett *et al.*, 1989b). Presence of a δ subunit within a GABA$_A$ receptor can alter sensitivity to steroids (Zhu *et al.*, 1996), benzodiazepines (Saxena & Macdonald, 1996) and zinc (Saxena & Macdonald, 1994). The elucidation of unique properties associated with certain subunit conformations allows results derived from these cloning/expression studies to be applied to native receptors, to infer GABA$_A$ receptor subunit compositions present in various areas of the brain at varying developmental stages. These types of studies also allow one to begin to examine the issue of potential TLE-associated alterations in GABA$_A$ receptor subunit composition contributing to hyperexcitability within the limbic system.

Temporal lobe epilepsy models

There are a number of temporal lobe epilepsy models currently in wide experimental use. For the purposes of this chapter, these models will be divided into status epilepticus (SE) models and kindling models.

For the most part, SE models appear very similar in much of their behaviour, anatomy and method of induction. These models include the kainate model (see Franck *et al.*, 1988), the pilocarpine model (PILO) (see Mello *et al.*, 1993), and the self-sustaining limbic status epilepticus (SSLSE) model (cf, Mangan *et al.*, 1995). All involve inducing SE in animals (either by chemical or electrical means) and then allowing the animals to recover. The SE episode induces a pattern of cellular damage and circuit rearrangements in the limbic system and other areas of the brain, and, following a latent period, also results in recurrent spontaneous seizures of limbic origin. In these models, anatomical alterations within the limbic system are typical of mesial temporal sclerosis evident in patients with temporal lobe epilepsy (e.g. Mello *et al.*, 1993; Buckmaster & Dudek, 1997). The recurrent spontaneous seizures characteristic of these models are both a blessing and a curse for investigators studying epileptogenic mechanisms. Recurrent spontaneous seizures are the definition of epilepsy, so the models satisfy this requirement. However, since seizures are spontaneous, great care must be taken to determine when the last seizure has occurred relative to experimentation, to attempt to discriminate seizure-associated (acute) alterations from epilepsy-associated (chronic) changes associated with the underlying pathology.

Kindling

Kindling is probably the most widely studied temporal lobe epilepsy model. Animals are subjected to repeated, initially subthreshold stimuli which trigger afterdischarges. The stimulus site is usually associated with the limbic system, but can vary. Most models stimulate the amygdala, or various sites within the hippocampus. Stimulus-evoked afterdischarges grow in intensity and duration with repeated stimulation, until they trigger behavioural seizures, which also then progress in intensity and duration. Once this progression has occurred, it is permanent, and the induced hyperexcitability will persist even after long periods with no stimuli. Advantages of kindling are that the exact seizure focus is known and under experimental control, and that the time and frequency of seizures are also under experimental control, which is critical for distinguishing seizure-associated from epilepsy-associated (and possibly epileptogenic) changes. Disadvantages are that typical mesial temporal sclerosis (MTS) is not induced, and spontaneous seizures only appear after extensive overkindling. Both MTS and spontaneous seizures are typical of temporal lobe epilepsy.

Regionally selective GABA$_A$ receptor alterations in TLE models

Studies examining GABA$_A$ receptor alterations within the limbic system associated with development of TLE have clearly demonstrated distinct processes occurring in dentate granule cells and pyramidal cells within the limbic system.

Dentate granule cells

Dentate granule cells (DGCs) for the most part survive in sclerotic hippocampus, and exhibit a series of changes in inhibitory properties which appear to bridge both SE and kindling models. These neurons may act as gatekeepers regulating excitatory input into the hippocampus (reviewed in Lothman *et al.*, 1991). In addition, DGCs survive in the epileptic hippocampus, allowing them to generate seizure discharges in a sclerotic hippocampus which otherwise exhibits marked loss of principal cells. Therefore, DGCs are a primary cell type which have frequently been studied as candidate sites for epileptogenic alterations in TLE.

DGC $GABA_A$ receptor alterations in SE models

GABAergic function, immunohistochemistry and subunit mRNA expression patterns have been studied in DGCs in a number of SE models, including the PILO, kainate and SSLSE models (Table 1). Sperk and colleagues (Schwarzer *et al.*, 1997; Tsunashima *et al.*, 1997) have published a large set of studies examining the immunohistochemical distribution and mRNA expression patterns of $GABA_A$ receptor subunits in control and kainate-treated epileptic rat hippocampi. In the dentate gyrus, these investigators found increases in expression of $\alpha 1$-, $\alpha 2$-, $\alpha 4$-, $\alpha 5$-, $\beta 1$-, $\beta 3$-, $\gamma 2$- and δ-subunit immunoreactivity 7–30 days after kainate injection (Schwarzer *et al.*, 1997). Accompanying these changes in protein expression within the dentate gyrus, $GABA_A$ receptor subunit mRNA expression levels also showed marked increases, with $\alpha 1$, $\alpha 2$, $\beta 1$ and $\beta 2$ message showing marked elevations in expression between 7 and 30 days following kainate injection (Tsunashima *et al.*, 1997). In PILO animals, alterations in expression patterns for various $GABA_A$ receptor subunit mRNAs within the dentate gyrus have also been identified (Rice *et al.*, 1996; see Table 1). Mathern *et al.* (1997) also reported enhanced $GABA_A$ receptor immunoreactivity in the dentate gyrus inner molecular layer of spontaneously SSLSE rats, which is consistent with the findings above, and was accompanied by evidence of both excitatory and inhibitory axon sprouting, and other changes in excitatory amino acid receptors.

Table 1. Dentate granule cell $GABA_A$ receptor subunit expression alterations

Model	$\alpha 1$	$\alpha 2$	$\alpha 3$	$\alpha 4$	$\alpha 5$	$\beta 1$	$\beta 2$	$\beta 3$	$\gamma 2$	δ
PILO (1) mRNA (chronic)	NC	NC			+					
PILO (2) mRNA (chronic, single cell*)	−	NC	NC	+	NC	−	NC	+	NC	+
Kainate (30 d) mRNA+	NC	+	+	NC	+	+	NC	NC	−	
Immuno. (3)	+	+	NC	+	+	+	NC	+	+ total	+
Kindling (30 d) mRNA (4)	NC	NC	+	NC	NC	NC	NC	NC	(−γ2L)	NC

*Single-cell aRNA amplification study profiling mRNA expression levels semiquantitatively.

Abbreviations: Chronic, chronically epileptic stage; PILO, pilocarpine model; NC, no change; 30d, 30 days (roughly) after the last fully kindled seizure; mRNA, $GABA_A$ receptor subunit mRNA levels; Immuno., relative $GABA_A$ receptor subunit immunohistochemical staining levels.

References:
1: Rice *et al.* 1996; Houser & Esclapez (1996).
2: Brooks-Kayal *et al.* (1998).
3: Schwarzer *et al.* (1997); Tsunashima *et al.* (1997).
4: Kamphius *et al.* (1995).

However, anatomical studies like those described above suffer from the compromised cellular specificity of the findings. Principal cells and interneurons can express markedly different GABA receptors (see Schwarzer *et al.*, 1997), and are differentially sensitive to neurotoxicity associated with development of epilepsy (see Babb *et al.*, 1989; Obenaus *et al.*, 1993). Differences in expression patterns of GABA receptor subunits might therefore be due at least in part to differential cell death of certain populations of neurons, and not reflect alterations in GABA receptors in individual neurons. In addition, glia can express some GABAergic subunits (see Schwarzer et al., 1997) and therefore gliosis can also alter tissue level profiles of GABA receptor subunit expression, and confound analysis. To overcome some of these problems, we have recently undertaken a series of single-cell GABA$_A$ receptor subunit mRNA expression profile studies, to determine the relative levels of GABA subunit messages in individual epileptic (PILO) and control dentate granule cells, which we have anatomically and physiologically identified (Brooks-Kayal et al., 1998). Using semiquantitative aRNA amplification techniques, we found that α1 mRNA levels were decreased in epileptic DGCs, while α4 levels were increased in these same cells (Table 1). When considered in the light of the functional changes in the GABA$_A$ receptor properties evident in these same cells (Table 2), this strongly suggested that an α subunit switch in DGC GABA$_A$ receptors might be occurring accompanying the development of TLE. Furthermore, this data suggested that the functional alterations evident in epileptic DGC GABA$_A$ receptors might be under transcriptional control. This obviously has implications for the development of potentially novel therapies to control TLE. We are currently testing this hypothesis in additional studies.

Table 2. Dentate granule cell GABA$_A$ receptor functional alterations

Model	Efficacy	Zinc sensitivity	BZ modulation	Subunit alterations
PILO (1)	↑↑	↑↑	↑CNZ, ↓↓ZOL	Possible ↓α1
Kainate (2)	↑↑			
SSLSE (3)	↑↑			
Kindling (4)	↑↑	↑↑	↑Binding	Possible ↓α1
Human TLE (5)	↑	↑↑	↓Binding	Possible ↓α1

Abbreviations: PILO, pilocarpine model; SSLSE, self-sustaining limbic status epilepticus model; CNZ, clonazepam; ZOL, zolpidem.

Data is from:
(1) Gibbs et al. (1997).
(2) Sloviter (1992); Buckmaster & Dudek (1997).
(3) Mangan et al. (1995).
(4) Shin et al. (1985); Otis et al. (1994); Titulaer et al. (1995b); Buhl et al. (1996).
(5) Williamson et al. (1995); Hand et al. (1997); Shumate et al. (1998).

In addition to the anatomical changes described above, functional changes in inhibitory responses have also been identified in DGCs in SE models. Overall efficacy of GABA is significantly enhanced in DGCs acutely isolated from chronically epileptic PILO animals, probably reflecting an increase in GABA$_A$ receptor density on these neurons. In addition to the altered function of GABA$_A$ receptors evident in these cells, the pharmacology of these receptors was also quite different in epileptic animals. Sensitivity to block by zinc was enhanced by 190 per cent, while sensitivity to augmentation by the BZ1-selective benzodiazepine agonist, zolpidem, was decreased by 75 per cent (Table 2). Both sensitivity to zinc and zolpidem depend at least in part on the presence or absence of the α1 subunit within a GABA receptor (Macdonald and Olsen, 1994; White and Gurley, 1995). These pharmacological alterations led us to hypothesize that a subunit switch was occurring in epileptic DGCs in PILO animals, with reduced levels of expression of the α1 subunit (perhaps accompanied by increases in expression of other α subunits, see above and Brooks-Kayal et al., 1998) resulting in alterations in zinc and zolpidem sensitivity of GABA$_A$ receptors.

What could be the functional relevance of these GABA$_A$ receptor alterations in the epileptic hippocampus? Obviously, an enhanced density of GABA receptors is not consistent with disinhibition and hyperexcitability, and many studies in epileptic hippocampi have reported enhanced paired-pulse inhibition in the dentate gyrus. However, the augmented zinc sensitivity of these increased numbers of epileptic GABA$_A$ receptors may be critical, when viewed in the light of the circuit rearrangements present in the epileptic, but not in the control dentate gyrus. Mossy fibre terminals, in addition to their normal excitatory neurotransmitter vesicles, contain some of the highest concentrations of zinc present in the brain, also localized into vesicles. This zinc can be released upon repetitive synaptic stimulation (Howell *et al.*, 1984), and released zinc can achieve 100–300 μM concentrations in the extracellular space in hippocampus (Assaf & Chung, 1984). Control DGCs do not innervate themselves, and have GABA$_A$ receptors which are relatively zinc insensitive. Epileptic DGCs in sclerotic hippocampi send zinc-containing collaterals back onto the inner molecular layer, and reinnervate the proximal dendrites of DGCs (Tauck & Nadler, 1985; Mello *et al.*, 1993; Okazaki *et al.*, 1995; Mathern *et al.*, 1997). This provides a zinc release mechanism onto DGCs in the epileptic hippocampus, which, when considered in the light of the heightened zinc sensitivity of GABA$_A$ receptors identified in DGCs in these animals, provides the potential for a catastrophic failure of inhibition to occur. If this does happen, it will most likely occur in dentate gyrus of epileptic animals during repetitive activation (which will mobilize and release vesicular zinc; Howell *et al.*, 1984), as occurs during seizure initiation. The pharmacological alterations in the elevated density of GABA$_A$ receptors in epileptic DGCs can be thought of as an Achilles' heel, a critical weakness which can compromise inhibitory efficacy exactly at the times when it is most needed, under conditions which will release the zinc contained in sprouted mossy fibre collaterals.

DGC GABA$_A$ receptor alterations in kindled rats

Functional studies of inhibitory synaptic responses in DGCs from kindled animals have identified a similar series of GABA$_A$ receptor changes to those described above in DGCs of PILO animals (Table 2). These studies preceded the Gibbs *et al.* (1997) study described above, and examined synaptic responses rather than whole cell GABA responses. The amplitude of spontaneous miniature inhibitory synaptic currents (mIPSCs) was 80 per cent larger in kindled animals compared to controls, and non-stationary noise analysis provided support for the hypothesis that this was due to an increased number of subsynaptic GABA$_A$ receptors in epileptic animals (Otis *et al.*, 1994). In addition to the alterations in mIPSC amplitude evident in kindled animals, the pharmacological sensitivity of these events to blockade by zinc was significantly enhanced in DGCs from kindled animals (Buhl *et al.*, 1996). Control mIPSCs were completely zinc-insensitive, while mIPSCs recorded from kindled DGCs were sensitive to zinc, with a 30 per cent block on average. These findings are remarkably parallel to the studies in the PILO animals described above, and suggest that there may be some model-independent (and perhaps TLE-common) alterations in subunit composition of GABA$_A$ receptors in DGCs (Table 2). However, although there is a modest amount of sprouting present in kindled animals (Cavazos *et al.*, 1991), it is not nearly as robust as that evident in sclerotic hippocampi (e.g. Tauck & Nadler, 1985; Mello *et al.*, 1993; Gibbs *et al.*, 1997; Mathern *et al.*, 1997), and so the functional relevance of the changes in kindled rat DGCs to epileptic hyperexcitability may be somewhat less, given that there is less zinc released onto these cells.

CA1 and CA3 pyramidal cells

CA1 and CA3 pyramidal cells are damaged to varying degrees in epileptic hippocampus, and are critically important players in hippocampal function. For the most part, alterations in these cell populations are quite distinct from those evident in DGCs.

CA1 and CA3 GABA$_A$ receptor alterations in SE models

GABAergic function, immunohistochemistry and subunit mRNA expression patterns have been studied in hippocampal pyramidal neurons in a number of SE models, including the PILO, kainate, and SSLSE models (Table 3). In kainate-treated animals 30 days after injection, an extensive set of studies by Sperk and colleagues (Schwarzer *et al.*, 1997; Tsunashima *et al.*, 1997) have identified a series of alterations in subunit expression patterns in CA1 and CA3 neurons that are complicated by the large degree of cell loss evident in these areas in the kainate model (Table 3). Early (at 7 days post-injection) decreases in expression of virtually all subunits and messages was evident, which was followed at later times (30 days) by gradual increases in expression of the α2, α5, γ2 and δ subunits in CA3 neurons, as assessed immunohistochemically (Schwarzer et al., 1997). The early decreases in expression of all subunits was attributed to be entirely due to cell loss. In PILO animals, expression levels of the α2 and α5 GABA subunit message were significantly decreased (and remained decreased when cell loss was accounted for), with no significant changes in expression of the β2 or γ2 messages in the same animals (Rice et al., 1996; see also Houser & Esclapez, 1996) (Table 3).

Table 3. CA1 and CA3 GABA$_A$ receptor subunit expression alterations

Model	α1	α2	α3	α4	α5	β1	β2	β3	γ2	δ
PILO (1) mRNA (chronic)	NC	–			–		NC		NC	
Kainate (30 days; cell loss taken into account) mRNA	NC	NC	NC	NC	NC	NC	NC	NC	NC	NC
Subunits (2)	NC	+ (CA3)	NC	NC	+ (CA3)	NC	NC (CA3)	NC (CA3)	+	+
Kindling (30 d) (3)	NC	NC	NC	NC	NC	NC	NC	NC		–

Abbreviations: PILO, pilocarpine model; NC, no change; 30 days, 30 days (roughly) after the last fully-kindled seizure or kainate injection.

References:
(1) Rice et al. (1996); Houser & Esclapez (1996).
(2) Schwarzer et al. (1997); Tsunashima et al. (1997).
(3) Kamphius et al. (1995).

Table 4. CA1 and CA3 pyramidal cell functional GABA$_A$ receptor alterations

Model	Efficacy	BZ modulation	Subunit changes
PILO (2) (chronic)	↓↓	↓↓	possible ↓γ2
Kainate (2) (chronic)	↓↓	NC binding	
SSLSE (3) (chronic)	↓↓		
Kindling (4) (30 d)	↓↓	↓ binding	

Abbreviations: References: PILO, pilocarpine model; SSLSE, self-sustaining limbic status epilepticus model; Chronic, at a chronically epileptic stage; 30 days, 30 days (roughly) after the last fully kindled seizure; NC, no change.

References:
(1) Gibbs et al. (1997).
(2) Franck et al. (1988); Meier et al. (1992).
(3) Mangan et al. (1995); Mangan & Bertram (1997); Rempe et al. (1997).
(4) King et al. (1985); Zhao & Leung (1991); Titulaer et al. (1995a, b).

Functional changes accompanied the above-described anatomical changes in GABA$_A$ receptors. In the PILO model, CA1 pyramidal neurons exhibited an entirely distinct pattern of functional GABA$_A$ receptor changes from those we described in DGCs (Tables 2 and 4). The efficacy of GABA decreased by 50 per cent in CA1 pyramidal cells (in contrast to the 80 per cent increase in efficacy evident in DGCs), while the potency of GABA was significantly enhanced (Gibbs et al., 1997). This decreased efficacy could be due to a decreased density of GABA$_A$ receptors in the membrane of CA1 neurons, to a decreased single channel conductance of GABA$_A$ receptors in these cells, or both. Accompanying these alterations in efficacy of GABA were significant changes in the pharmacology of GABA$_A$ receptors on CA1 pyramidal neurons. Although there was no change in zinc sensitivity of the GABA$_A$ receptor responses, there was a dramatic decrease in sensitivity to augmentation by benzodiazepines

(Gibbs et al., 1997). Taken together, these data led us to hypothesize that there might be a decrease in expression of the γ2 subunit within GABA$_A$ receptors in these cells in epileptic animals, which could account for the decreased efficacy of GABA, the enhanced potency of GABA, and the loss of benzodiazepine sensitivity evident in these cells (reviewed in Gibbs et al., 1997). Decreased inhibitory synaptic efficacy in area CA1 has been described in studies in the kainate model of TLE (Franck et al., 1988; Meier et al., 1992), and in the SSLSE model of TLE (Mangan et al., 1995; Mangan & Bertram, 1997; Rempe et al., 1997), consistent with the above-described decreased efficacy of GABA in CA1 neurons of PILO animals. However, these changes in efficacy occurred without accompanying changes in flunitrazepam binding in kainate-treated rats (Franck et al., 1988), which does not support our hypothesis concerning decreased γ2 contribution to GABA$_A$ receptors in these cells (Table 4).

CA1 and CA3 GABA$_A$ receptor alterations in kindled animals

In a comprehensive study examining GABA$_A$ receptor subunit mRNA expression levels in pyramidal cells of kindled animals, Kamphius et al. (1995) found very few alterations in expression levels in CA1 pyramidal neurons 30 days after the last kindled seizure. The only change evident in CA1 neurons in these animals was a significant decrease in γ2 expression (Table 3).

Studies examining inhibitory function in CA1 and CA3 pyramidal neurons consistently have demonstrated decreased efficacy of these responses in kindled animals (King et al., 1985; Zhao & Leung, 1991; Titulaer et al., 1995a, b). Decreases in benzodiazepine binding have also been described in CA1 and CA3 areas of kindled animals accompanying this disinhibition (King et al., 1985) (Table 4). Therefore, decreases in inhibitory efficacy in hippocampal pyramidal cells appear to be a consistent finding across all of the above described epilepsy models, and this disinhibition is frequently accompanied by decreases in benzodiazepine binding or function (Table 4). This supports the concept that pyramidal cell disinhibition is a common phenomenon in many epilepsy models, and this lack of model-specific effects implicates this as a potentially epilepsy-specific mechanism which could contribute to epileptogenesis.

Relevance of experimental alterations in hippocampal GABA$_A$ receptors to epilepsy in humans

What relationship do all these studies in animal TLE models have to the human with TLE? Is there any evidence for similar disinhibitory mechanisms occurring in the human epileptic hippocampus? Physiological studies on resected epileptic human hippocampus have revealed similarities between the GABAergic inhibitory properties of DGCs from epileptic humans and epileptic rats (Table 2). Inhibition definitely remains operative in epileptic human dentate gyrus, and may even be augmented (Williamson et al., 1995; Shumate et al., 1998), as has been seen in epileptic rat dentate gyrus (De Jonge & Racine, 1987; Otis et al., 1994; Gibbs et al., 1997). In addition, DGCs isolated from human epileptic hippocampus exhibit similar high levels of GABA$_A$ receptor zinc sensitivity compared to epileptic (but not control) rat DGCs (Shumate et al., 1998). Since epileptic human hippocampus also exhibits the mossy fibre sprouting evident in epileptic rat hippocampus (Sutula et al., 1989; Houser et al., 1990; Babb et al., 1991; Shumate et al.,1998), this high zinc sensitivity of GABA$_A$ receptors on these epileptic human DGCs may prove to be equally responsible for functional disinhibition during repetitive activation, as we hypothesize for our rat studies (see above). However, despite this encouraging data, human studies suffer from a lack of adequate controls, and so must be viewed cautiously. Very few studies have been conducted on human CA1 or CA3 pyramidal neurons, since these areas tend to be severely damaged in the usual end stage epileptic tissue resected from epileptic patients. We have conducted similar studies on GABA receptor properties of neocortical pyramidal cells from human epileptic foci, comparing these responses to non-focal human neocortical pyramidal neurons (Gibbs et al., 1996, 1998). In these studies, we found a similar series of changes to those we found in GABA$_A$ receptor responses of rat epileptic CA1 neurons: a decreased efficacy and enhanced potency of GABA, and a loss of sensitivity to modulation by benzodiazepines. Once again, these findings provide encouraging support for the applicability of studies conducted in animal models of TLE to the human condition. As with other human studies, controls are an issue, and the data must be viewed with appropriate caveats in mind.

'Epileptic' GABA$_A$ receptors: implications for therapy

GABA$_A$ receptors are a major target for therapeutic drug development, not only in epilepsy, but also in other disease states. Currently, drugs are developed by testing for anticonvulsant efficacy using a number of different rapid throughput screens. These screens for the most part involve use of normal, non-epileptic animals, which are induced to have seizures through chemical or electrical means (White et al., 1998). Drugs are then tested against these seizures for efficacy. If the ion channels (including GABA receptors) of focal epileptic tissue are unique and differ from control animals, then these types of 'normal animal' screens will select for drugs which are only effective in non-focal tissue, in normal brain. Drugs developed using these tests might therefore be expected to be effective in controlling seizure spread, but are less likely to be effective in controlling seizure initiation in the focus, since the altered ion channels in focal tissue are not subjected to antiepileptic drug screening. Future therapeutic efforts designed to target drugs to the altered ion channels present in focal tissue have promise not only in increasing efficacy (stopping seizure initiation rather than spread), but also in decreasing toxicity, since drug design will focus on abnormal rather than normal brain.

References

Assaf, Y.S. & Chung, S.-H. (1984): Release of endogenous Zn^{2+} from brain tissue during activity. *Nature Lond.* **308**, 734–736.

Babb, T.L., Pretorius, J.K., Kupfer, W.R. & Crandall, P.H. (1989): Glutamate decarboxylase-immunoreactive neurons are preserved in human epileptic hippocampus. *J. Neurosci.* **9**, 2562–2574.

Babb, T.L., Kupfer, W.R., Pretorius, J.K., Crandall, P.H. & Levesque, M.F. (1991): Synaptic reorganization by mossy fibers in human epileptic fascia dentata. *Neuroscience* **42**, 351–363.

Brooks-Kayal, A., Shumate, M.D., Hong, Y., Rikhter, T.Y. & Coulter, D.A. (1998): Rapid and permanent epilepsy-associated alterations in GABAA receptor subunit expression and inhibitory function in hippocampal dentate granule neurons. *Soc. Neurosci. Abstr.* **24** (in press).

Brooks-Kayal, A., Shumate, M.D., Hong, Y., Rikhter, J.Y. & Coulter, D.A. (1998): Selective changes in single cell GABA$_A$ receptor subunit expression correlate with altered function in epileptic hippocampus. *Nature (Medicine)* **4** (10), 1166–1172.

Buhl, E.H., Otis, T.S. & Mody, I. (1996): Zinc-induced collapse of augmented inhibition by GABA in a temporal lobe epilepsy model. *Science Wash. DC* **271**, 369–373.

Cavazos, J.E., Golarai, G. & Sutula, T.P. (1991): Mossy fiber synaptic reorganization by kindling: time course of development, progression, and permanence. *J. Neurosci.* **11**, 2795–2803.

Chang, Y., Wang, R., Barot, S. & Weiss, D.S. (1996): Stoichiometry of a recombinant GABA$_A$ receptor. *J. Neurosci.* **16**, 5415–5424.

De Jonge, M. & Racine, R.J. (1987): The development and decay of kindling-induced increases in paired-pulse depression in the dentate gyrus. *Brain Res.* **412**, 318–328.

Franck, J.E., Kunkel, D.D., Baskin, D.G. & Schwartzkroin, P.A. (1988): Inhibition in kainate-lesioned hyperexcitable hippocampi: physiologic, autoradiographic, and immunocytochemical observations. *J. Neurosci.* **8**, 1991–2002.

Gibbs III, J.W., Zhang, Y.-F., Kao, C.-Q., Holloway, K.L., Oh, K.S. & Coulter, D.A. (1996): Characterization of GABA$_A$ receptor function in human temporal cortical neurons. *J. Neurophysiol.* **75**(4), 1458–1471.

Gibbs III, J.W., Shumate, M.D. & Coulter, D.A. (1997): Differential epilepsy-associated alterations in postsynaptic GABA$_A$ receptor function in dentate granule and CA1 neurons. *J. Neurophysiol.* **77** (4), 1924–1938.

Gibbs III, J.W., Morton, L., Amaker, B., Ward, J.D., Holloway, K.L. & Coulter, D.A. (1998): Physiological analysis of Rasmussen's encephalitis: Patch clamp recordings of altered inhibitory neurotransmitter function in resected frontal cortical tissue. *Epilepsy Res.* **31** (1), 13–27.

Hand, K.S., Baird, V.H., Van Paesschen, W., Koepp, M.J., Revesz, T., Thom, M., Harkness, W.F., Duncan, J.S. & Bowery, N.G. (1997): Central benzodiazepine receptor autoradiography in hippocampal sclerosis. *Br. J. Pharmacol.* **122**, 358–364.

Houser, C.R., Miyashiro, J.E., Swartz, B.E., Walsh, G.O., Rich, J.R. & Delgado-Escueta, A.V. (1990): Altered patterns of dynorphin immunoreactivity suggest mossy fiber reorganization in human hippocampal epilepsy. *J. Neurosci.* **10**, 267–282.

Houser, C.R. & Escaplez, M. (1996): Vulnerability and plasticity of the GABA system in the pilocarpine model of spontaneous recurrent seizures. *Epilepsy Res.* 26, 207–218.

Howell, G.A., Welch, M.G. & Frederickson, C.J. (1984): Stimulation-induced uptake and release of zinc in hippocampal slices. *Nature Lond.* **308**, 736–738.

Kamphius, W., De Rijk, T.C. & Lopes da Silva, F.H. (1995): Expression of $GABA_A$ receptor subunit mRNAs in hippocampal pyramidal and granular neurons in the kindling model of epileptogenesis: an in situ hybridization study. *Mol. Brain Res.* **31**, 33–47.

King, G.L., Dingledine, R., Giacchino, J.L. & McNamara, J.O. (1985): Abnormal neuronal excitability in hippocampal slices from kindled rats. *J. Neurophysiol.* **54**, 1295–1304.

Lothman, E.W., Bertram III, E.H. & Stringer, J.L. (1991): Functional anatomy of hippocampal seizures. *Prog. Neurobiol.* **37**, 1–82.

Macdonald, R.L. & Olsen, R. (1994): $GABA_A$ receptor channels. *Ann. Rev. Neurosci.* **17**, 569–602.

Mangan, P.S. & Bertram III, E.H.. (1997): Shortened-duration $GABA_A$ receptor-mediated synaptic potentials underlie enhanced CA1 excitability in a chronic model of temporal lobe epilepsy. *Neuroscience* **80**, 1101–1111.

Mangan, P.S., Rempe, D.A. & Lothman, E.W. (1995): Changes in inhibitory neurotransmission in the CA1 region and dentate gyrus in a chronic model of temporal lobe epilepsy. *J. Neurophysiol.* **74**, 829–840.

Mathern, G.W., Bertram III, E.H., Babb, T.L., Pretorius, J.K., Kuhlman, P.A., Spradlin, S. & Mendoza, D. (1997): In contrast to kindled seizures, the frequency of spontaneous epilepsy in the limbic status model correlates with greater aberrant fascia dentata excitatory and inhibitory axon sprouting, and increased staining for N-methyl-D-aspartate, AMPA, and $GABA_A$ receptors. *Neuroscience* **77**, 1003–1019.

McKernan, R.M. & Whiting, P.J. (1996): Which $GABA_A$ receptor subtypes really occur in the brain? *Trends Neurosci.* **19**, 139–143.

Meier, C.L., Obenaus, A. & Dudek, F.E. (1992): Persistent hyperexcitability in isolated hippocampal CA1 of kainate-lesioned rats. *J. Neurophysiol.* **68**, 2120–2127.

Mello, L.E.A.M., Cavalheiro, E.A., Tan, A.M., Kupfer, W.R., Pretorious, J.K., Babb, T.L. & Finch, D.M. (1993): Circuit mechanisms of seizures in the pilocarpine model of chronic epilepsy: cell loss and mossy fiber sprouting. *Epilepsia* **34**, 985–995.

Obenaus, A., Esclapez, M. & Houser, C.R. (1993): Loss of glutatmate decarboxylase mRNA-containing neurons in the rat dentate gyrus following pilocarpine-induced seizures. *J. Neurosci.* **13**, 4470–4485.

Okazaki, M.M., Evenson, D.A. & Nadler, J.V. (1995): Hippocampal mossy fiber sprouting and synapse formation after status epilepticus in rats: visualization after retrograde transport of biocytin. *J. Comp. Neurol.* **352**, 515–534.

Otis, T.S., De Konick, Y. & Mody, I. (1994): Lasting potentiation of inhibition is associated with an increased number of γ-aminobutyric acid type A receptors activated during miniature postsynaptic currents. *Proc. Natl. Acad. Sci. USA* **91**, 7698–7702.

Prince, D.A. (1985): Physiological mechanisms of focal epileptogenesis. *Epilepsia* **26** (S1), S3–S14.

Pritchett, D.B., Sontheimer, H., Shivers, B.D., Ymer, S., Kettenmann, H., Schofield, P.R. & Seeburg, P.H. (1989a): Importance of a novel $GABA_A$ receptor subunit for benzodiazepine pharmacology. *Nature* **338**, 582–585.

Pritchett, D.B., Luddens, H. & Seeburg, P.H. (1989b): Type I and type II $GABA_A$-benzodiazepine receptors produced in transfected cells. *Science* **245**, 1389–1392.

Rempe, D.A., Bertram, E.H., Williamson, J.H. & Lothman, E.W. (1997): Interneurons in area CA1 stratum radiatum and stratum oriens remain functionally connected to excitatory synaptic input in chronically epileptic animals. *J. Neurophysiol.* **78**, 1504–1515.

Ribak, C.E., Bradurne, R.M. & Harris, A.B. (1982): A preferential loss of GABAergic, symmetric synapses in epileptic foci: a quantitative ultrastructural analysis of monkey neocortex. *J. Neurosci.* **2, 1725–1735.**

Rice, A., Rafiq, A., Shapiro, S.M., Jakoi, E.M., Coulter, D.A. & DeLorenzo, R.J. (1996): Long-lasting reduction in inhibitory function and GABA$_A$ mRNA subunit expression in a model of temporal lobe epilepsy. *Proc. Natl. Acad. Sci. USA* **93**, 9665–9669.

Saxena, N.C. & Macdonald, R.L. (1994): Assembly of GABA$_A$ receptor subunits: role of the delta subunit. *J. Neurosci.* **14**, 7077–7086.

Saxena, N.C. & Macdonald, R.L. (1996): Properties of putative cerebellar gamma-aminobutyric acid A receptor isoforms. *Mol. Pharmacol.* **49**, 567–579.

Schwarzer, C., Tsunashima, K., Wanzenbock, C., Fuchs, K., Sieghart, W. & Sperk, G. (1997): GABA$_A$ receptor subunits in the hippocampus II: altered distribution in kainic acid-induced temporal lobe epilepsy. *Neuroscience* **80**, 1001–1017.

Shin, C., Pedersen, H.B. & McNamara, J.O. (1985): gamma-Aminobutyric acid and benzodiazepine receptors in the kindling model of epilepsy: a quantitative radiohistochemical study. *J. Neurosci.* **5**, 2696–2701.

Shumate, M.D., Lin, D.D., Gibbs III, J.W., Holloway, K.L. & Coulter, D.A. (1998): Physiological properties of GABA$_A$ receptors in epileptic human dentate granule cells: Comparison to epileptic and control rat. *Epilepsy Res.* 32 (1–2), 114–128.

Sloviter, R.S. (1992): Possible functional consequences of synaptic reorganization in the dentate gyrus of kainate-treated rats. *Neurosci. Lett.* **137**, 91–96.

Sutula, T., Cascino, G., Cavazos, J., Parada, I. & Ramirez, L. (1989): Mossy fiber synaptic reorganization in the epileptic human temporal lobe. *Ann. Neurol.* **26**, 321–330.

Tauck, D.L. & Nadler, J.V. (1985): Evidence of functional mossy fiber sprouting in hippocampal formation of kainic acid-treated rats. *J. Neurosci.* **5**, 1016–1022.

Titulaer, M.N., Kamphius, W. & Lopes da Silva, F.H. (1995a): Long-term and regional specific changes in [^{3}H] flunitrazepam binding in kindled rat hippocampus. *Neuroscience* **68**, 399–406.

Titulaer, M.N.G., Ghijsen, W.E.J.M., Kamphius, W., De Rijk, T.C. & Lopes da Silva, F.H. (1995b): Opposite changes in GABA$_A$ receptor function in the CA1–3 area and fascia dentata of kindled rat hippocampus. *J. Neurochem.* **64**, 2615–2621.

Tretter, V., Ehya, N., Fuchs, K. & Sieghart, W. (1997): Stoichiometry and assembly of a recombinant GABA$_A$ receptor subtype. *J. Neurosci.* **17**, 2728–2737.

Tsunashima, K., Schwarzer, C., Kirchmair, E., Sieghart, W. & Sperk, G. (1997): GABA$_A$ receptor subunits in the rat hippocampus III: altered messenger RNA expression in kainic acid-induced epilepsy. *Neuroscience* **80**, 1019–1032.

White, G. & Gurley, D.A. (1995): α Subunits influence Zn block of γ2 containing GABA$_A$ receptor currents. *Neuroreport* **6**, 461–464.

White, H.S., Wolf, H.H., Woodhead, J.H. & Kupferberg, H.J. (1998): The National Institutes of Health Anticonvulsant Drug Development Program: screening for efficacy. *Adv. Neurol.* **76**, 29–39.

Williamson, A., Telfeian, A.E. & Spencer, D.D. (1995): Prolonged GABA responses in dentate granule cells in slices isolated from patients with temporal lobe sclerosis. *J. Neurophysiol.* **74**, 378–387.

Zhao, D. & Leung, L.S. (1991): Effects of hippocampal kindling on paired-pulse response in CA1 *in vitro*. *Brain Res.* **564**, 220–229.

Zhu, W.J., Wang, J.F., Krueger, K.E. & Vicini, S. (1996): Delta subunit inhibits neurosteroid modulation of GABAA receptors. *J. Neurosci.* **16**, 6648–6656.

Chapter 18

Seizure-induced apoptosis and necrosis in the developing rat brain

Raman Sankar

Departments of Neurology and Paediatrics, UCLA School of Medicine, Los Angeles, CA 90095-1752, USA; and Epilepsy Research Laboratories, VA Medical Center, Sepulveda, CA 91343-2099, USA

Seizures cause selective neuronal death as a result of excessive neuronal activation, even in the absence of systemic complications (Meldrum *et al.*, 1973; Nevander *et al.*, 1985) in adult animals. In the developing brain, the effect of seizures on neuronal survival and brain growth has been controversial (Camfield, 1997; Wasterlain, 1997). Animal models suggest the existence in the young of both unique protective mechanisms as well as age-dependent vulnerability to specific types of experimental status epilepticus (SE) (Sankar *et al.*, 1995; see also Chapter 21 of this book). Our understanding of seizure-induced brain damage in immature animals remains patchy because available reports are based on a limited sampling of models and ages (Albala *et al.*, 1984; Okada *et al.*, 1984; Sperber *et al.*, 1991, 1992; Thompson *et al.*, 1998; Thompson & Wasterlain, 1997) or have examined specific aspects such as EEGs (Hirsch *et al.*, 1992) or behaviour (Liu *et al.*, 1994) without a detailed study of the histopathology.

Status epilepticus (SE) can produce neuronal damage by excessive activation of both *N*-methyl-D-aspartate (NMDA) and non-NMDA ionotropic glutamate receptors, and both NMDA and non-NMDA receptor antagonists have demonstrated neuroprotective properties in various seizure paradigms (Fujikawa *et al.*, 1994; Penix & Wasterlain, 1994; Fujikawa, 1995; Penix *et al.*, 1996). Different neuronal populations in the hippocampus have been shown to demonstrate selectively apoptotic or necrotic features of cell death in response to perforant path stimulation, a model of focal epilepsy (Sloviter *et al.*, 1996). Excitotoxic neuronal death is influenced by brain maturation (Portera-Cailliau *et al.*, 1997a,b). Since apoptosis plays an important role in early brain development it is possible that the immature brain displays a special vulnerability to undergo programmed cell death in response to seizures.

The kainic acid model of SE in developing animals

Seizures induced in adult rats by 10 mg/kg of kainic acid (KA), an excitatory neurotoxin, are severe, and produce a pattern of hippocampal damage similar to mesial temporal sclerosis. The damage is most severe in the pyramidal cells of CA3 and the hilus, followed by some damage to CA1; the CA2 pyramidal cells, the granule cells of the dentate gyrus and the fibres *en passage* are spared (Nadler *et al.*, 1978; Lothman & Collins, 1981). A KA dose of 3 mg/kg produces little damage but the SE produced by this dose is not severe in adults. Immature rats of age postnatal day 15 (P15) cannot survive 10 mg/kg of KA. Systemic KA (3 mg/kg) in P15 rats did not produce a similar pattern of damage (Albala *et al.*, 1984; Nitecka *et al.*, 1984; Sperber *et al.*, 1991), even though severe seizures occurred (Moshé *et al.*, 1983; Okada *et al.*, 1984). The drawback of this model is that kainate receptor expression in the developing brain lags that of AMPA and NMDA subtypes of glutamate receptors, and is present only in low levels in the P15 rat (Campochiaro & Coyle, 1978). The other drawback with this model is the high mortality (90 per cent) encountered in P15 rats (Albala *et al.*, 1984). Nevertheless, studies have shown that the 3-mg/kg dose of KA does produce very severe seizures in the P15 rats (Moshé *et al.*, 1983; Okada *et al.*, 1984) and that no discernible hilar or CA3 damage is seen in the survivors. It appears that the effect of KA-induced SE on the hippocampus is also species-dependent. In the P10 rabbit, systemic KA produces extensive lesions, predominantly in the CA1 (Franck & Schwartzkroin, 1984).

Administration of kainic acid (KA) by intra-amygdaloid (Pollard *et al.*, 1994), subcutaneous (Morrison *et al.*, 1996), or intraperitoneal (Filipkowski *et al.*, 1994) route has been shown to result in SE and apoptosis of select populations of neurons. In the intra-amygdaloid model co-administration of diazepam prevented the seizures and apoptosis of neurons in the CA3 region, but not in the amygdala suggesting that the apoptotic neurons reflect excitotoxic damage. Up-regulation of *bax* and down-regulation of *bcl–2* have been associated with KA-induced apoptosis of neurons (Gillardon *et al.*, 1995). Induction of p53 has been demonstrated in the brain following KA-induced seizures and mice deficient in p53 gene appeared to be protected from such KA-induced cell death (Morrison *et al.*, 1996). Data pertaining to the developmental aspects of KA-induced apoptosis are not available.

CRH-induced seizures

In infant rats (P10–P13) corticotropin releasing hormone (CRH) is a potent convulsant that induces limbic seizures at picomolar doses (Baram & Schultz, 1991). CRH-induced SE causes neuronal damage in the CA3b subfield of the hippocampus and mossy fibre reorganization in these rats (Baram & Ribak, 1995; Ribak & Baram, 1996). In adult rats, CRH produced seizures at much higher doses, but no neuronal degeneration. The possible relevance of CRH-induced seizures to infantile spasms, a catastrophic epilepsy of infancy, has been discussed (Baram, 1993). The consequences of CRH-induced SE in the immature rat suggest that the resistance of the immature rat brain to KA is a model-specific resistance. The limitation of this model may be that the long-term survival of the rat pups subjected to CRH-induced SE could be inadequate for demonstration of the development of chronic epilepsy following SE. Data from long-term monitoring of these animals for spontaneous seizures and observations in behavioural paradigms designed to test memory and learning are lacking.

Perforant path stimulation model of SE

The sustained intermittent stimulation of the perforant path model of SE has been described in detail by Sloviter (1983, 1991). In this model, analysis of the acute pathology (Sloviter *et al.*, 1996) caused by prolonged afferent stimulation of mature rats revealed that degenerating hilar neurons and pyramidal cells exhibited the morphological features of necrosis, characterized in part by early vacuolization of the cytoplasm. However, acutely degenerating granule cells exhibited the distinct morphological features of apoptosis, which included coalescence of nuclear chromatin into multiple nuclear bodies, compaction of the cytoplasm, cell shrinkage and budding-off of 'apoptotic bodies' engulfed by glia. The investigators also noted that while pyramidal cell debris persisted for months, granule cell debris decreased rapidly. The authors proposed that this observation might explain why significant granule cell vulnerability has not been described previously.

Another reason for previous studies describing the dentate granule cells to be relatively spared after SE may be the recent observation that seizures induce granule cell proliferation (Bengzon *et al.*, 1997; Parent *et al.*, 1997). Induction of hippocampal seizure activity by perforant path stimulation resulted in an increase in cell proliferation in the dentate subgranular proliferative zone, an area known to contain neuronal precursor cells. Newly generated dentate granule cells also appeared in ectopic locations in the hilus and inner molecular layer of the dentate gyrus. Furthermore, developing granule cells projected axons aberrantly to both the CA3 pyramidal cell region and the dentate inner molecular layer (Parent et al., 1997). These observations suggest that prolonged seizure discharges stimulate dentate granule cell neurogenesis, and that hippocampal network plasticity associated with epileptogenesis may arise from aberrant connections formed by newly born dentate granule cells.

Thompson et al. (1998) applied the perforant path model to rat pups of age P14-P16. *In situ* end-labelling performed 2 h after the end of 16 h of stimulation showed an intense band of positively-labelled eosinophilic cells with condensed profiles bilaterally in the dentate granule cell layer of stimulated animals (see also Chapter 21 of this book). Control animals showed no *in situ* end-labelling positivity in the dentate gyrus. These cells were not observed 24 h later, suggestive of rapidly scavenged apoptotic cells.

Pilocarpine (PC) and the lithium-pilocarpine (LiPC) models of SE

The cholinergic agent pilocarpine (PC) produces limbic and generalized SE in rodents accompanied by widespread brain damage in mature rats (Turski et al., 1983). The utility of PC-induced seizures as a model for studying SE, and SE-induced brain damage and epileptogenesis has been well described (Cavalheiro, 1995; Cavalheiro et al., 1996). Further, the susceptibility of rats to PC-induced seizures appeared to be age-dependent (Cavalheiro et al., 1987). Pre-treatment with lithium potentiates the epileptogenic action of PC, reduces mortality and avoids many of the peripheral cholinomimetic side effects of PC, while retaining all the salient electrophysiological and pathological features of PC-induced SE (Honchar et al., 1983; Jope et al., 1986; Clifford et al., 1987).

Thompson & Wasterlain (1997) have shown that P10 rabbits subjected to LiPC-induced SE show CA1 damage reminiscent of the pattern of damage reported by Franck & Schwartzkroin (1984) in immature rabbits treated with KA (see Chapter 21 of this book). Rat pups as young as two weeks demonstrate seizure-induced elevation in serum neuron-specific enolase (s-NSE) (Table 3) accompanied by histologic evidence of extrahippocampal (Table 2) and hippocampal damage (Table 1) as a result of SE (Sankar et al., 1997) induced by LiPC treatment. In the original study of Cavalheiro et al. (1987) 5 out of 14 rats between P11 and P21 sustained brain damage after high dose PC-induced SE. We have learned that there are substantial differences in the extent of brain damage between P7 and P21 rats and that the pattern seen in the P14 rat is different from that seen at P21, in the LiPC model of SE (Sankar et al., 1997).

Table 1. Percentage of neurons exhibiting eosinophilic cytoplasm in the rat hippocampus after lithium-pilocarpine SE

Age (weeks)	CA1	CA3	Hilus	Granule cells
2	36 ± 5	$1 \pm 0.2^{**}$	$1 \pm 0.5^{\S}$	5 ± 0.5
3	34 ± 10	25 ± 9	31 ± 2	$33 \pm 7^{\S}$
4	24 ± 8	21 ± 7	27 ± 2	7 ± 2
9–12	$9 \pm 3^{*}$	14 ± 3	28 ± 2	5 ± 1

$^{*}P < 0.05$ compared to 2- and 3-week old animals; $^{**}P < 0.05$ compared to 3- and 4-week old animals; $^{\S}P < 0.001$ compared to all other age groups.

In our experiments, Wistar rat pups of 1, 2, 3 and 4 weeks of age, and mature rats (12–16 weeks) were given 3 meq/kg lithium chloride (Sigma, St. Louis, MO) intraperitoneally on the day before the induction of SE. Seizures progressing to SE were induced by the injection of 60 mg/kg pilocarpine hydrochloride (Sigma, St. Louis, MO) subcutaneously (sc). Control animals ($n = 6$) were given 1 ml/kg saline sc. Rats were observed for behavioural evidence of seizures. Selected animals underwent blood gas monitoring and no hypoxia was encountered. After 24 h, a cardiac blood sample was drawn for the estimation of s-NSE under metofane anaesthesia. A commercially available kit (Pharmacia, Uppsala, Sweden) was used for the determination of s-NSE.

Table 2. Neuronal damage scores of extrahippocampal structures in rats after lithium-pilocarpine SE

Age (weeks)	Cortex	Caudate	Thalamus	Amygdala	Septum
1	0	0	0	0	0
2	0.9 ± 0.05	0.8 ± 0.17	$1.8 \pm 0.31^\S$	$1.0 \pm 0.26^\dagger$	$1.0 \pm 0.32^\dagger$
3	$2.5 \pm 0.32^*$	$2.0 \pm 0.26^*$	$1.3 \pm 0.33^\S$	$1.3 \pm 0.21^\S$	$1.7 \pm 0.33^\S$
4	$2.0 \pm 0.33^*$	$1.2 \pm 0.40^\S$	$1.0 \pm 0.00^\P$	$1.7 \pm 0.33^\S$	$2.0 \pm 0.26^\S$
Adult (12–16 weeks)	$2.0 \pm 0.11^*$	$1.3 \pm 0.21^\S$	$1.0 \pm 0.00^\P$	$2.5 \pm 0.34^\S$	$1.8 \pm 0.31^\S$

Scale: 0 = no damage; 1 = trace to 5 %; 2 = 6 to 10 %; 3 = 11–25 %; 4 = 26–50 %; 5 = >50 %.

$^*P < 0.001$ vs. 1 or 2-week old; $^\P P < 0.01$ vs. 1 or 2-week old; $^\S P < 0.002$ vs. 1-week old only; $^\dagger P < 0.05$ vs. 1-week old only.

Pattern of damage in the hippocampus

In the hippocampus, damage was determined by actual cell counts of the granule cells in the fascia dentata, the hilar interneurons, and the pyramidal cells in CA1 and CA3, using bilateral sections of the dorsal hippocampus approximating the region –3.8mm posterior to bregma (Paxinos & Watson, 1982). Neuronal damage in the CA1 subfield of the hippocampus as ascertained by the presence of Brown & Brierley's (1968) 'ischaemic cell change' with a pyknotic nucleus and an eosinophlic cytoplasm was maximal in the 2- (Fig. 1A) and 3-week-old rat pups (36 ± 5 per cent and 34 ± 10 per cent of CA1 neurons respectively). It decreased progressively with age to 25 ± 8 per cent in the 4 week-old animals and 9 ± 3 per cent ($P < 0.05$) in the adults (Fig. 1B and Table 1).

The neuronal damage seen maximally in the CA1 of our 2-week-old rats is attributable to the SE since hypoxia was not encountered in these animals. Further, hypoxia at p_aO_2 of 20 mmHg for 20 min without ischaemia did not result in cell loss, or even morphologic evidence of injury as evidenced by heat-shock protein expression (Pearigen et al., 1996).

The neuronal damage in the CA3 region of the 2-week-old rats (Table 1) was barely discernible at 1 per cent and no damage was seen in the 1-week-old pups. While the damage at 3, 4 and 12–16 weeks (20 ± 9 per cent, 18 ± 7 per cent and 14 ± 3 per cent respectively) did not differ significantly, a trend suggesting maximal vulnerability to SE-induced damage in this region followed by diminishing damage with further maturation can be seen.

The reason for the development-related vulnerabilities of the CA1 and CA3 neurons may be related to the following observations. In the rat, excitability comparable to that seen in fully mature animals could be demonstrated in the CA1 region after postnatal day 14, whereas the inhibitory processes did not reach an adult stage of maturation until several weeks later (Michelson & Lothman, 1989). Our observation of preferential CA1 damage at 2 weeks of age is consistent with the observations of the development of synaptic inhibition lagging in the CA1 compared to area CA3 (Swann et al., 1989) or the dentate gyrus (Bekenstein & Lothman, 1991).

Two-week-old pups were resistant to SE-induced hilar damage. The extent of damage in the 3-week-old rat pups (31 ± 2 per cent) was comparable to that in the 4-week-old (27 ± 2 per cent) and adult rats (28 ± 2 per cent) (Fig. 1C and D). Damage to the dentate granule cells is also shown in Figs. 3C and D. The 3-week-old pups demonstrated a special vulnerability to SE-induced damage in this cell population (33 ± 7 per cent) which is different from that seen in younger or older animals (5 ± 0.5 per cent, 7 ± 2 per cent, and 5 ± 1 per cent in 2, 4 and 9–12 week-old animals respectively).

Damage to the hilus and CA3 in this model of SE appears to be as severe in the 3-week-old rat pups as in mature rats. Previous studies demonstrating resistance to SE-induced hilar and CA3 damage in the developing brain have compared mature rats to only 2-week-old pups (Albala et al., 1984; Sperber et al., 1991, 1992) in the kainic acid model or have used groupings such as 15–21 day-old rats in the PC model of SE (Cavalheiro et al., 1987). In a detailed study of SE-induced damage in the KA model, Nitecka et al. (1984) documented progressive damage to limbic structures from postnatal day 18. The development of vulnerability to seizure-induced damage to the hilus and CA3 was attributed to the maturation of the mossy fibre terminals.

Extrahippocampal damage

For an estimation of extrahippocampal damage, brain regions were examined in three coronal planes. Damage scores for the cortex were obtained by averaging the scores from all three coronal planes that had been selected to achieve representations of the cingulate, piriform and entorhinal cortices. The neuronal damage seen in the thalamus decreased with development, while the opposite trend was encountered in the amygdala; on the other hand, the caudate was most vulnerable to SE-induced damage at 3 weeks (Table 2). We also observed that the substantia nigra shows severe damage in the adult as reported previously (Clifford et al., 1987), but not in the young pups, consistent with the observations of Moshé (1987) of lack of SE-induced activation of the substantia nigra in young animals as measured by 2-DG autoradiography.

Seizure-induced changes in s-NSE

The s-NSE concentrations from control animals and those that underwent and survived SE after lithium-pilocarpine treatment are shown in Table 3. The baseline serum concentrations of NSE decreased from 17.1 ng/ml in the 1-week-old pups to 5.4 ng/ml in the adults with maturation. The s-NSE level seen in adult rats was similar to that reported for adult humans. In the 1-week-old pups s-NSE was not elevated as a consequence of lithium pilocarpine seizures. All other ages showed elevations in s-NSE compared to their age-matched controls. Our data show that increases in s-NSE are accompanied by histologic evidence of neuronal damage and that such elevations of s-NSE appear to be roughly proportional to the extent of histologic damage.

Table 3. Serum neuron-specific enolase (ng/ml) in rats subjected to lithium-pilocarpine status epilepticus

Age (weeks)	Control[1]	LiPC SE[1]
1 week	17.1 ± 0.97*	14.8 ± 0.60
2 weeks	11.5 ± 0.45	18.9 ± 0.77**
3 weeks	12.1 ± 0.75	35.8 ± 2.06**
4 weeks	9.30 ± 0.46	34.9 ± 1.70**
Adults (> 12 weeks)	5.39 ± 0.37*	30.4 ± 1.25**

[1]Mean ± SEM ($n = 6$); *$P < 0.005$ compared to 2-, 3-, or 4-week old animals; **$P < 0.001$ compared to controls.

The baseline s-NSE level (control values) observed in the 1-week-old animals was significantly higher than all other ages, and there was a progressive decline in the baseline s-NSE with maturation. The programmed elimination of neurons during development is reported to be maximal around the first postnatal week in several structures studied, such as the cortex and thalamus (Spreafico et al., 1995), cerebellum (Wood et al., 1993) and the superior colliculus (Cunningham et al., 1981) in the rat. Our findings of a high baseline s-NSE in the 1-week-old pups and the decline in s-NSE with maturation probably reflect this phenomenon of apoptosis associated with early development.

Type of neuronal death

TUNEL stain-positive neurons were readily discernible only in the 2- and 3-week-old pups after SE. The distribution of these neurons was age-dependent, with the 2-week-olds demonstrating such injury predominantly in the CA1 region (Fig. 2A) in subiculum, and in thalamus, with lesser labelling of the inner dentate granule cells. In the 3-week-old animals, only the inner layer of the dentate granule cells (Fig. 2B) and a few thalamic neurons were TUNEL-positive. Fluorescence microscopy of ethidium bromide stained sections (Fig. 2C and D) revealed fragmented nuclei in the same areas that were TUNEL-stained. In the 3-week-old animals the neuronal injury delineated by the TUNEL and ethidium bromide methods (Fig 2B and D) in the inner layer of granule cells was different from that seen in outer granular neurons visualized by their eosinophilic cytoplasm (Fig. 1C). Two types of damage also appear to coexist in the CA1 subfield of 2-week-old pups subjected to SE.

Electron micrographs of CA1 in 2-week-old pups (Fig. 2E) and of the inner granule cell layer of the 3-week-olds (Fig. 2F) clearly demonstrated the presence of distinctive nuclear and cytoplasmic changes suggestive of necrosis in some neurons and of apoptosis in others. Twenty-four h after SE, many CA1 neurons displayed chromatin condensation coexisting with intact cytoplasmic and nuclear membranes and with relatively intact cytoplasmic organelles (Fig. 2E). In that same CA1 layer, however, were also seen swollen neurons with ruptured membranes, extensive cytoplasmic damage and all the hallmarks of necrosis (Fig.1A). It has been shown that both apoptosis and necrosis can result from qualitatively the same type of excitotoxic stimulus with the intensity of NMDA receptor activation deciding the process (Bonfoco *et al.*, 1995). In the 3-week-old dentate gyrus, inner granule cells with chromatin margination and nearly intact cytoplasms (Fig. 2F) were seen in close proximity to clearly necrotic hilar neurons (Fig. 1C).

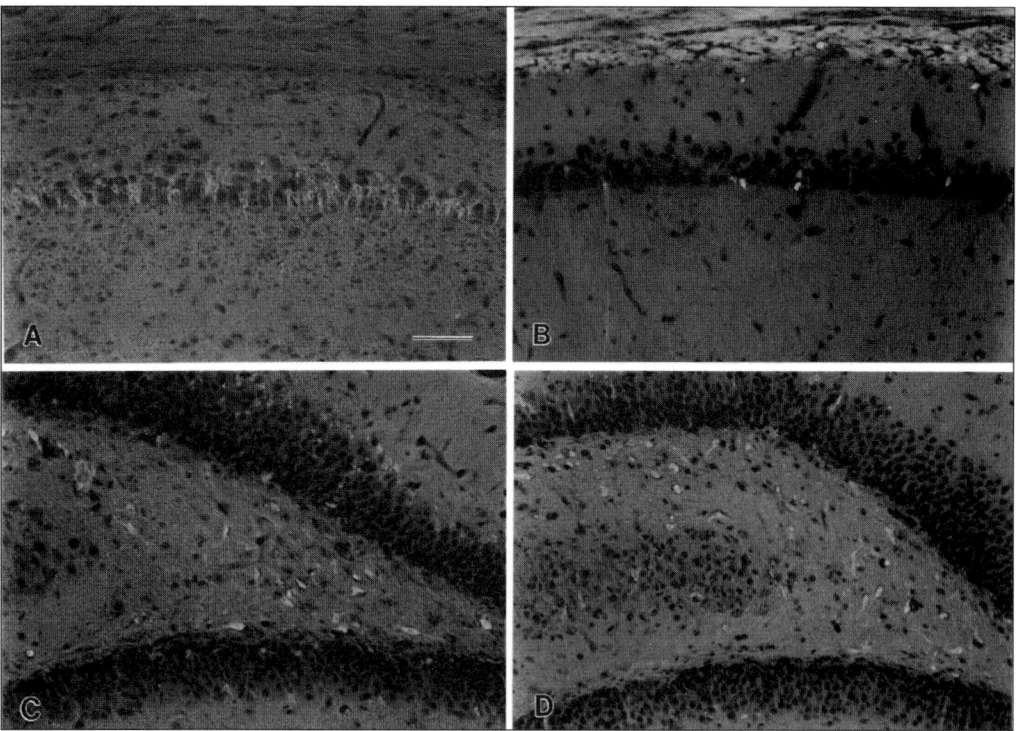

Fig. 1. Histological lesions in lithium pre-treated rats 24 h after SE from pilocarpine administration. CA1 of a 2-week-old pup (A) shows a large number of eosinophilic cells that fluoresce brightly under UV light, while the CA1 of a mature rat (B) is essentially devoid of injured cells. Several eosinophilic neurons are seen in the outer layers of the granule cells of the fascia dentata of a 3-week-old rat (C); much less granule cell injury is seen in the 4-week-old rat (D). Both 3- and 4-week-old rats show numerous damaged neurons in the hilus. Scale bar represents 75 μm.

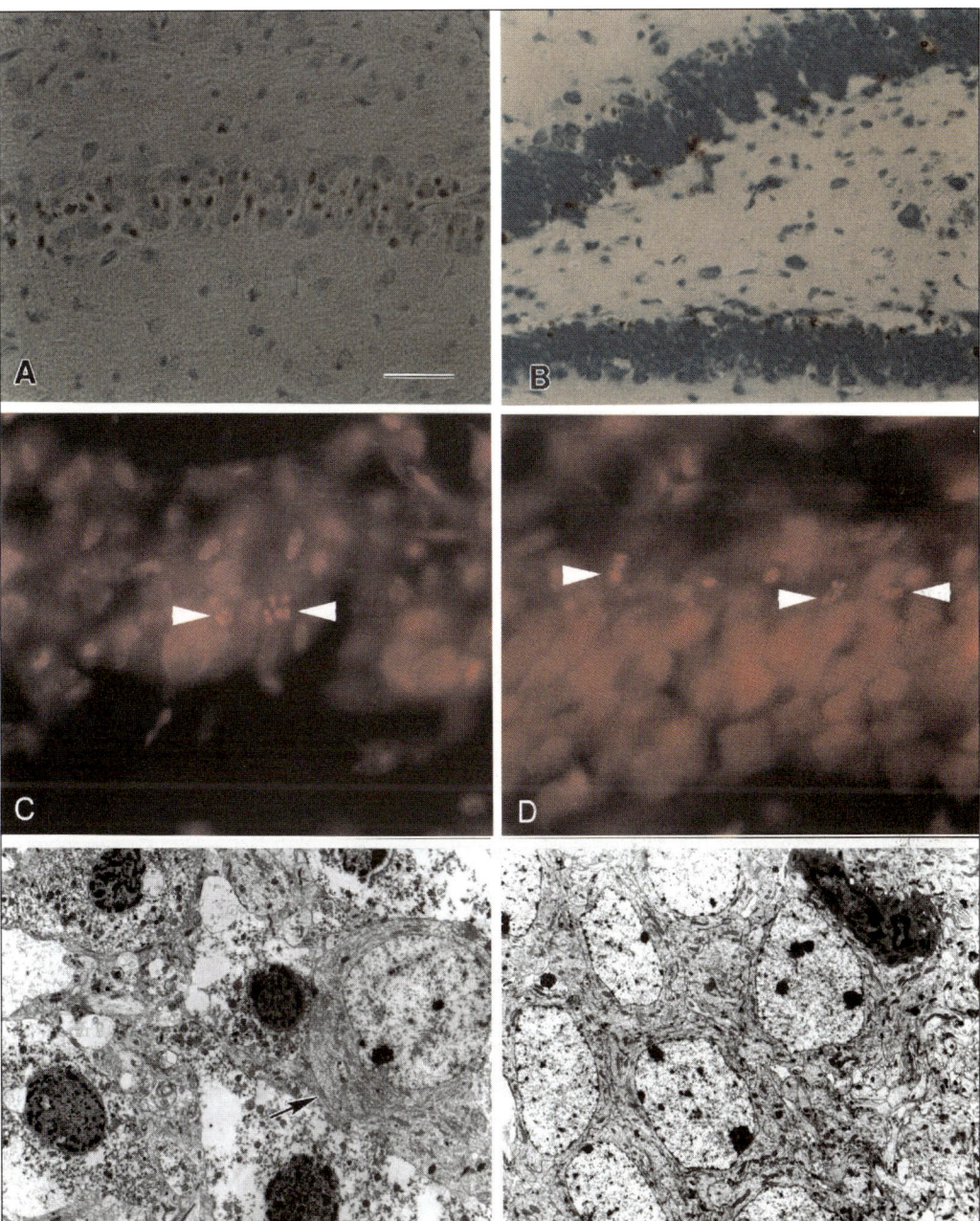

Fig. 2. TUNEL-stained section of the CA1 of a 2-week-old rat (A) and fascia dentata of a 3-week-old rat (B). Note that the distribution of TUNEL label is distinct in distribution from the fluorescent cells visualized under UV light. Ethidium bromide stained sections of the CA1 of a 2-week-old rat (C) and the granule cell layer of a 3-week-old rat (D) show cells displaying fragmented nuclei (arrowheads). Electron micrograph (EM) of the CA1 of a 2-week-old rat (E) shows an apoptotic cell with condensed cytoplasm (arrow) and several necrotic cells with shrunken nuclei and vacuolated cytoplasm. EM of the granule cells near the hilar border of a 3-week-old rat (F) shows apoptotic neurons. Scale bars represent 30 μm in (A and B), 18 μm (C and D) and 4 μm (E and F).

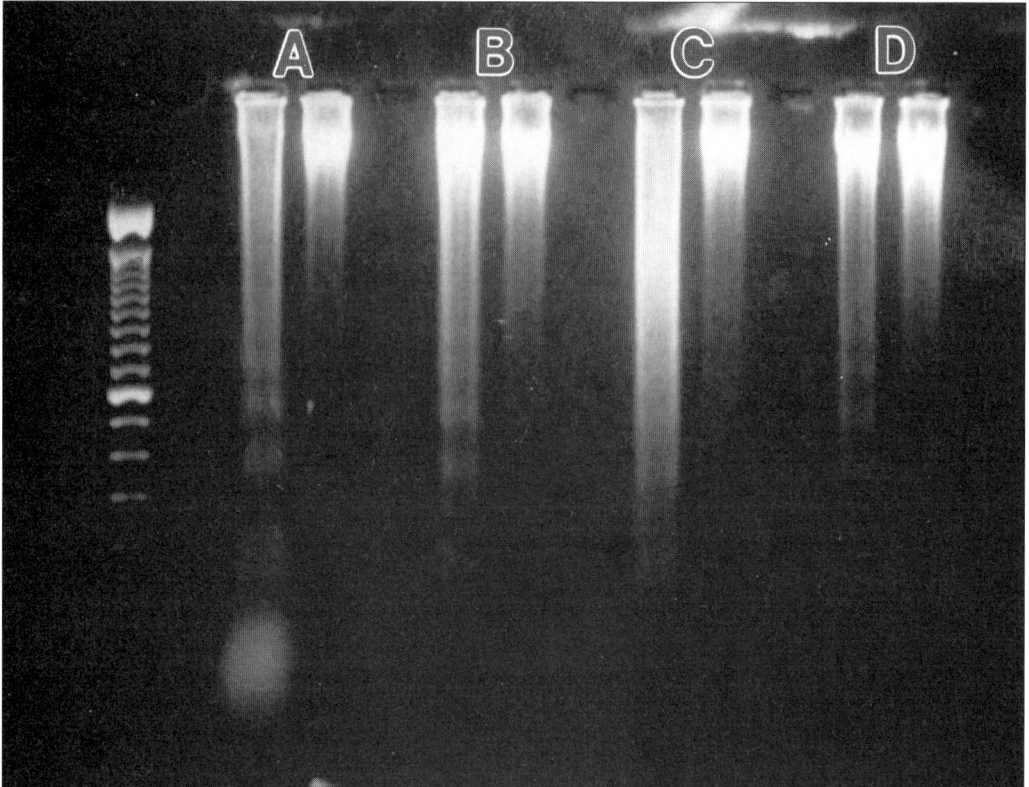

Fig. 3. Agarose gel (2 per cent) electrophoresis of DNA extracted from the hippocampi of rats 24 h after LiPC SE. DNA fragment standards are on the left extreme position. Paired lanes contain DNA from experimental and control rats of 2 weeks (A), 3 weeks (B), 4 weeks (C) and mature animals (D). Bands corresponding to oligonucleosomal breaks are seen in all four experimental groups even though morphological evidence supports apoptosis in the 2- and 3-week-old animals only.

The DNA extracted from the hippocampi of rats of various ages subjected to LiPC SE and of their age-matched controls was separated by agarose gel electrophoresis (Fig. 3). Laddering is not evident in the lanes in which DNA from control rats was placed. Discrete bands corresponding to fragments of DNA with a periodicity approximating 180 base pairs, suggesting oligonucleosomal breaks, are seen best in the hippocampal DNA from the 2- and 3-week-old rats that underwent SE. Laddering is also seen in the lanes containing DNA from the hippocampi and neocortices (the latter not shown) of 4-week-old and adult rats that underwent SE, even though we did not see significant numbers of TUNEL-positive neurons or apoptotic bodies in those animals.

In our experiments we saw evidence of damage to the granule cells of the dentate gyrus mainly in the 21 day-old rat pups. It is striking that eosinophilic neurons are seen mainly in the outermost layers of the granule cells, while scattered TUNEL-positive neurons are seen along the hilar border. The distribution of TUNEL-positive neurons in our experiments is reminiscent of the results reported by Bengzon *et al.* (1997) after kindling or KA administration. Apoptosis of granule cells has also been shown after repetitive perforant path stimulation (Sloviter *et al.*, 1996), and following adrenalectomy (Hu *et al.*, 1997), in mature rats. Under these circumstances apoptosis does not appear to be restricted to the granule cells along the hilar border. Weiss *et al.* (1996) have reported a significantly different pattern of DNA fragmentation in the hippocampus of rats subjected to KA-induced SE. It is likely that the pattern of DNA fragmentation detected by a particular technique is influenced by the timing after the excitotoxic insult as well as the variations in the technique. Didier *et al.* (1996) have suggested that the *in situ* nick translation method employing DNA polymerase 1 is very sensitive and labels single-strand breaks, and that such damage may be reversible, while the nick end labelling with terminal deoxynucleotidyl transferase identifies double-strand breaks.

Charriaut-Marlangue & Ben-Ari (1995) had cautioned on the use of the TUNEL stain as the sole criterion for the demonstration of apoptosis and had suggested that methods such as Hoechst 33258 staining be used to supplement the data. We have used ethidium bromide staining in such a manner. It is of interest that significant TUNEL labelling has not been seen in our experiments in regions where extensive eosinophilic neurons are encountered in animals older than the 3-week-old pups. This is consistent with the results of Fujikawa *et al.* (1997) who did not see significant evidence for apoptosis in mature rats subjected to LiPC SE. On the other hand, 'DNA laddering' on agarose gel is widely presented as evidence of apoptosis based on the suggestion that necrosis would lead to a 'smear' DNA pattern (Walker *et al.*, 1994). Our results show that laddering may be seen when there is extensive necrosis even though cells matching the morphologic criteria for apoptosis may be extremely rare. Hence, we would like to sound a cautionary note on the use of agarose gel electrophoresis of extracted DNA as a major criterion for apoptosis.

In summary, we have used different methods known to be sensitive to distinctive mechanisms that may lead to neuronal damage as a result of the recurrent excitation caused by SE during development. Previous studies by others (Albala *et al.*, 1984; Sperber *et al.*, 1991, 1992) have focused on specific aspects of hippocampal response to seizures such as hilar cell loss and mossy fibre sprouting and have remarked on the relative resiliency of the immature brain to seizures. Our results show enhanced vulnerability to CA1 neurons during early development at a stage when hilar injury and mossy fibre synaptic reorganization are not prominent. The damage seen at this age appears to involve both necrosis as evidenced by the eosinophilic cells, and apoptosis as demonstrated by a variety of techniques that included TUNEL staining, visualization of fragmented nuclei under fluorescence microscopy of EtBr-stained sections, electron microscopy and DNA electrophoresis.

Acknowledgements: Don Shin provided outstanding technical help. This work was supported by a Clinical Investigator Development Award NS01792 from NINDS, NIH.

References

Albala, B.J., Moshé, S.L. & Okada, R. (1984): Kainic-acid-induced seizures: a developmental study. *Brain Res.* **315**, 139–148.

Baram, T.Z. (1993): Pathophysiology of massive infantile spasms: perspective on the putative role of the brain adrenal axis. *Ann. Neurol.* **33**, 231–236.

Baram, T.Z. & Ribak, C.E. (1995): Peptide-induced infant status epilepticus causes neuronal death and synaptic reorganization. *Neuroreport* **6**, 277–280.

Baram, T.Z. & Schultz, L. (1991): Corticotropin-releasing hormone is a rapid and potent convulsant in the infant rat. *Dev. Brain Res.* **61**, 97–101.

Bekenstein, J.W. & Lothman, E.W. (1991): A comparison of the ontogeny of excitatory and inhibitory neurotransmission in the CA1 region and dentate gyrus of the rat hippocampal formation. *Dev. Brain Res.* **63**, 237–243.

Bengzon, J., Kokaia, Z., Elmer, E., Nanobashvili, A., Kokaia, M. & Lindvall, O. (1997): Apoptosis and proliferation of dentate gyrus neurons after single and intermittent limbic seizures. *Proc. Natl. Acad. Sci. USA* **94**, 10432–10437.

Bonfoco, E., Krainc, D., Ankarcrona, M., Nicotera, P. & Lipton, S.A. (1995): Apoptosis and necrosis: two distinct events induced, respectively, by mild and intense insults with N-methyl-D-aspartate or nitric oxide/superoxide in cortical cell cultures. *Proc. Natl. Acad. Sci. USA* **92**, 7162–7166.

Brown, A.W. & Brierley, J.B. (1968): The nature, distribution and earliest changes of anoxic-ischemic nerve cell damage in the rat brain as defined by the optical microscope. *Brit. J. Exp. Pathol.* **49**, 87–106.

Camfield, P.R. (1997): Recurrent seizures in the developing brain are not harmful. *Epilepsia* **38**, 735–737.

Campochiaro, P. & Coyle, J.T. (1978): Ontogenetic development of kainate neurotoxicity: correlates with glutamatergic innervation. *Proc. Natl. Acad. Sci. USA* **75**, 2025–2029.

Cavalheiro, E.A. (1995): The pilocarpine model of epilepsy. *Ital. J. Neurol. Sci.* **16**, 33–37.

Cavalheiro, E.A., Silva, D.F., Turski, W.A., Calderazzo, F.L., Bortolotto, Z.A. & Turski, L. (1987): The susceptibility of rats to pilocarpine-induced seizures is age-dependent. *Brain Res.* **465**, 43–58.

Cavalheiro, E.A., Santos, N.F. & Priel, M.R. (1996): The pilocarpine model of epilepsy in mice. *Epilepsia* **37**, 1015–1019.

Charriaut-Marlangue, C. & Ben-Ari, Y. (1995): A cautionary note on the use of the TUNEL stain to determine apoptosis. *Neuroreport* **7**, 61–64.

Clifford, D.B., Olney, J.W., Maniotis, A., Collins, R.C. & Zorumski, C.F. (1987): The functional anatomy and pathology of lithium-pilocarpine and high-dose pilocarpine seizures. *Neuroscience* **23**, 953–968.

Cunningham, T.J., Mohler, I.M. & Giordano, D.L. (1981): Naturally occurring neuron death in the ganglion cell layer of the neonatal rat: morphology and evidence for regional correspondence with neuron death in superior colliculus. *Brain Res.* **254**, 203–215.

Didier, M., Bursztajn, S., Adamec, E., Passani, L., Nixon, R.A., Coyle, J.T., Wei, J.Y. & Berman, S.A. (1996): DNA strand breaks induced by sustained glutamate excitotoxicity in primary neuronal cultures. *J. Neurosci.* **16**, 2238–2250.

Filipkowski, R.K., Hetman, M., Kaminska, B. & Kaczmarek, L. (1994): DNA fragmentation in rat brain after intraperitoneal administration of kainate. *Neuroreport* **5**, 1538–1540.

Franck, J.E. & Schwartzkroin, P.A. (1984): Immature rabbit hippocampus is damaged by systemic but not intraventricular kainic acid. *Brain Res.* **315**, 219–227.

Fujikawa, D.G. (1995): Neuroprotective effect of ketamine administered after status epilepticus onset. *Epilepsia* **36**, 186–195.

Fujikawa, D.G., Daniels, A.H. & Kim, J.S. (1994): The competitive NMDA receptor antagonist CGP 40116 protects against status epilepticus-induced neuronal damage. *Epilepsy Res.* **17**, 207–219.

Fujikawa, D.G., Cai, B.B., Shinmei, S.S. & Allen, S.G. (1997): Neuronal death induced by lithium-pilocarpine-induced seizures is necrotic, not apoptotic. *Soc. Neurosci. Abstr.* **23**, 1112.

Gillardon, F., Wickert, H. & Zimmermann, M. (1995): Up-regulation of bax and down-regulation of bcl–2 is associated with kainate-induced apoptosis in mouse brain. *Neurosci. Lett.* **192**, 85–88.

Hirsch, E., Baram, T.Z. & Snead III, O.C. (1992): Ontogenic study of lithium-pilocarpine-induced status epilepticus in rats. *Brain Res.* **583**, 120–126.

Honchar, M.P., Olney, J.W. & Sherman, W.R. (1983): Systemic cholinergic agents induce seizures and brain damage in lithium-treated rats. *Science* **220**, 323–325.

Hu, Z., Yuri, K., Ozawa, H., Lu, H. & Kawata, M. (1997): The in vivo time course for elimination of adrenalectomy-induced apoptotic profiles from the granule cell layer of the rat hippocampus. *J. Neurosci.* **17**, 3981–3989.

Jope, R.S., Morrisett, R.A. & Snead, O.C. (1986): Characterization of lithium potentiation of pilocarpine-induced status epilepticus in rats. *Exp. Neurol.* **91**, 471–480.

Liu, Z., Gatt, A., Werner, S.J., Mikati, M.A. & Holmes, G.L. (1994): Long-term behavioral deficits following pilocarpine seizures in immature rats. *Epilepsy Res.* **19**, 191–204.

Lothman, E.W. & Collins, R.C. (1981): Kainic acid induced limbic seizures: metabolic, behavioral, electroencephalographic and neuropathological correlates. *Brain Res.* **218**, 299–318.

Meldrum, B.S., Vigouroux, R.A. & Brierley, J.B. (1973): Systemic factors and epileptic brain damage. Prolonged seizures in paralyzed, artificially ventilated baboons. *Arch. Neurol.* **29**, 82–87.

Michelson, H.B. & Lothman, E.W. (1989): An in vivo electrophysiological study of the ontogeny of excitatory and inhibitory processes in the rat hippocampus. *Dev. Brain Res.* **47**, 113–122.

Morrison, R.S., Wenzel, H.J., Kinoshita, Y., Robbins, C.A., Donehower, L.A. & Schwartzkroin, P.A. (1996): Loss of the p53 tumor suppressor gene protects neurons from kainate-induced cell death. *J. Neurosci.* **16**, 1337–1345.

Moshé, S.L. (1987): Epileptogenesis and the immature brain. *Epilepsia* **28**, S3-S15.

Moshé, S.L., Albala, B.J., Ackermann, R.F. & Engel, Jr, J. (1983): Increased seizure susceptibility of the immature brain. *Brain Res.* **283**, 81–85.

Nadler, J.V., Perry, B.W. & Cotman, C.W. (1978): Intraventicular kainic acid preferentially destroys hippocampal pyramidal cells. *Nature* **271**, 676–677.

Nevander, G., Ingvar, M., Auer, R. & Siesjö, B.K. (1985): Status epilepticus in well-oxygenated rats causes neuronal necrosis. *Ann. Neurol.* **18**, 281–290.

Nitecka, L., Tremblay, E., Charton, G., Bouillot, J.P., Berger, M.L. & Ben-Ari, Y. (1984): Maturation of kainic acid seizure–brain damage syndrome in the rat. II. Histopathological sequelae. *Neuroscience* **13**, 1073–1094.

Okada, R., Moshé, S.L. & Albala, B.J. (1984): Infantile status epilepticus and future seizure susceptibility in the rat. *Brain Res.* **317**, 177–183.

Parent, J.M., Yu, T.W., Leibowitz, R.T., Geschwind, D.H., Sloviter, R.S. & Lowenstein, D.H. (1997): Dentate granule cell neurogenesis is increased by seizures and contributes to aberrant network reorganization in the adult rat hippocampus. *J. Neurosci.* **17**, 3727–3738.

Paxinos, G. & Watson, C. (1982): *The rat brain in stereotaxic coordinates.* Sydney: Academic Press.

Pearigen, P., Gwinn, R. & Simon, R.P. (1996): The effects *in vivo* of hypoxia on brain injury. *Brain Res.* **725**, 184–191.

Penix, L.P. & Wasterlain, C.G. (1994): Selective protection of neuropeptide containing dentate hilar interneurons by non-NMDA receptor blockade in an animal model of status epilepticus. *Brain Res.* **644**, 19–24.

Penix, L.P., Thompson, K.W. & Wasterlain, C.G. (1996): Selective vulnerability to perforant path stimulation: role of NMDA and non-NMDA receptors *Epilepsy Res. Suppl.* **12**, 63–73.

Pollard, H., Charriaut-Marlangue, C., Cantagrel, S., Represa, A., Robain, O., Moreau, J. & Ben-Ari, Y. (1994): Kainate-induced apoptotic cell death in hippocampal neurons. *Neuroscience* **63**, 7–18.

Portera-Cailliau, C., Price, D.L. & Martin, L.J. (1997a): Excitotoxic neuronal death in the immature brain is an apoptosis–necrosis morphological continuum. *J. Comp. Neurol.* **378**, 70–87.

Portera-Cailliau, C., Price, D.L. & Martin, L.J. (1997b): Non-NMDA and NMDA receptor-mediated excitotoxic neuronal deaths in adult brain are morphologically distinct: further evidence for an apoptosis–necrosis continuum. *J. Comp. Neurol.* **378**, 88–104.

Ribak, C.E. & Baram, T.Z. (1996): Selective death of hippocampal CA3 pyramidal cells with mossy fiber afferents after CRH-induced status epilepticus in infant rats. *Dev. Brain Res.* **91**, 245–251.

Sankar, R., Wasterlain, C.G. & Sperber, E.F. (1995): Seizure-induced changes in the immature brain. In: *Brain Development and Epilepsy,* Schwartzkroin, P.A., Moshé, S.L., Swann, J.W. & Noebels J.L. (eds), pp. 268–288. New York: Oxford University Press.

Sankar, R., Shin, D.H. & Wasterlain, C.G. (1997): Serum neuron-specific enolase is a marker for neuronal damage following status epilepticus in the rat. *Epilepsy Res.* **28**, 129–136.

Sloviter, R.S. (1983): 'Epileptic' brain damage in rats induced by sustained electrical stimulation of the perforant path. I. Acute electrophysiological and light microscopic studies. *Brain Res. Bull.* **10**, 675–697.

Sloviter, R.S. (1991): Permanently altered hippocampal structure, excitability, and inhibition after experimental status epilepticus in the rat: the 'dormant basket cell' hypothesis and its possible relevance to temporal lobe epilepsy. *Hippocampus* **1**, 41–66.

Sloviter, R.S., Dean, E., Sollas, A.L. & Goodman, J.H. (1996): Apoptosis and necrosis induced in different hippocampal neuron populations by repetitive perforant path stimulation in the rat. *J. Comp. Neurol.* **366**, 516–533.

Sperber, E.F., Haas, K.Z., Stanton, P.K. & Moshé, S.L. (1991): Resistance of the immature hippocampus to seizure-induced synaptic reorganization. *Dev. Brain Res.* **60**, 88–93.

Sperber, E.F., Haas, K.Z. & Moshé, S.L. (1992): Developmental aspects of status epilepticus. *Int. Pediatr.* **7**, 213–222.

Spreafico, R., Frassoni, C., Arcelli, P., Selvaggio, M. & De Biasi, S. (1995): *In situ* labeling of apoptotic cell death in the cerebral cortex and thalamus of rats during development. *J. Comp. Neurol.* **363**, 281–295.

Swann, J.W., Brady, R.J. & Martin, D.L. (1989): Postnatal development of GABA-mediated synaptic inhibition in rat hippocampus. *Neuroscience* **28**, 551–561.

Thompson, K. & Wasterlain, C. (1997): Lithium-pilocarpine status epilepticus in the immature rabbit. *Dev. Brain Res.* **100**, 1–4.

Thompson, K., Holm, A.M., Schousboe, A., Popper, P., Micevych, P. & Wasterlain, C. (1998): Hippocampal stimulation produces neuronal death in the immature brain. *Neuroscience* **82**, 337–348.

Turski, W.A., Cavalheiro, E.A., Schwarz, M., Czuczwar, S.-L.J., Kleinrok, Z. & Turski, L. (1983): Limbic seizures produced by pilocarpine in rats: behavioural, electroencephalographic and neuropathological study. *Behav. Brain Res.* **9**, 315–335.

Walker, P.R., Weaver, V.M., Lach, B., LeBlanc, J. & Sikorska, M. (1994): Endonuclease activities associated with high molecular weight and internucleosomal DNA fragmentation in apoptosis. *Exp. Cell Res.* **213**, 100–106.

Wasterlain, C.G. (1997): Recurrent seizures in the developing brain are harmful. *Epilepsia* **38**, 728–734.

Weiss, S., Cataltepe, O. & Cole, A.J. (1996): Anatomical studies of DNA fragmentation in rat brain after systemic kainate administration. *Neuroscience* **74**, 541–551.

Wood, K.A., Dipasquale, B. & Youle, R.J. (1993): In situ labeling of granule cells for apoptosis-associated DNA fragmentation reveals different mechanisms of cell loss in developing cerebellum. *Neuron* **11**, 621–632.

Chapter 19

Characterization of the pilocarpine model of epilepsy in developing rats

Esper A. Cavalheiro

Neurologia Experimental, Escola Paulista de Medicina/UNIFESP, Rua Botucatu, 862, 04023–900 Sao Paulo, SP, Brazil

The majority of cases of status epilepticus (SE) occur in young children, particularly in the first years of life (Aicardi & Chevrie, 1970; Dunn, 1988; Maytal *et al.*, 1989; Phillips & Suanahan, 1989). In these studies, the incidence of neurological sequelae after an episode of SE varies from 10 to 48 per cent, suggesting that the more immature brain is particularly susceptible to the effects of SE. The occurrence of SE without previous history of epilepsy is not rare and seems to be a function of age at the time of the SE (Maytal *et al.*, 1989). The occurrence of SE as the first ictal episode varies from 50 to 80 per cent in several studies of patients with SE (Aminoff & Simon, 1980; Aicardi & Chevrie, 1983; Maytal *et al.*, 1989; Phillips & Suanahan, 1989) and approximately 20 per cent of these patients develop epilepsy later in life (Aicardi & Chevrie, 1983; Maytal *et al.*, 1989). SE has also been a strong predictor of seizure intractability in patient with histories of anti-epileptic-drug-refractory epileptic seizures (Sillanpää, 1993).

In humans, the causal relation linking SE and the further development of epilepsy seems to be related to the aetiology of SE and has serious implications for the subsequent treatment of these patients (Gross-Tsur & Shinnar, 1993). Using a simplistic classification, taking together studies in both adults and children, idiopathic SE does not seem to increase the risk of epilepsy (Shinnar *et al.*, 1990, 1993) while symptomatic SE is able to facilitate the development of seizure disorders at some time in the future life (Hauser & Kurland, 1975; Nelson & Ellenberg, 1978; Annegers *et al.*, 1987, 1990; Hauser, 1990; Berg & Shinnar, 1991). Retrospective studies in patients with partial epilepsy subjected to surgery for temporal lobe epilepsy showed that approximately 50 per cent of the cases reported a history of 'severe' or 'prolonged' infantile convulsions (Falconer *et al.*, 1964; Margerison & Corsellis, 1966; Falconer, 1971). In a recent study in which only medial temporal lobe epileptics were evaluated (mass lesions excluded), 81 per cent of patients had histories of convulsions during early childhood or infancy. Complicated febrile seizures comprised 94 per cent of the patients in whom detailed descriptions of the febrile seizures were available (French *et al.*, 1993). On the other hand, prospective studies have shown that the risk for the development of epilepsy is similar for those presenting SE or an isolated seizure as the first unprovoked ictal event (Hauser *et al.*, 1982; Shinnar *et al.*, 1988, 1990, 1996; Hauser, 1990). Once again, the aetiology of SE seems to be determinant and substantial evidence indicates that febrile or symptomatic SE (Cendes *et al.*, 1993; Mathern *et al.*, 1995) are those with highest risk to induce later epilepsy.

A common problem for all clinical studies in addressing the issue of whether neurological sequelae and chronic epilepsy can be accounted for by a previous episode of SE is that of prior unrecognized brain dysfunction or damage that preceded both the SE and the presumed SE-induced neurological deficit (Lothman & Bertram, 1993). In temporal lobe epilepsy, for example, it has been suggested that mesial temporal sclerosis may represent a sequela of disturbed embryogenesis (Scheibel, 1991). Another limitation of human clinical–pathologic studies of refractory epileptic patients is the fact that surgically resected specimens always depict a frozen picture of an 'end-point' process of epileptogenesis. For these reasons, experimental preparations are particularly useful because they allow the study of SE-induced epileptogenesis starting from a 'non-pathologic' brain and the course of neuropathological changes can be assessed more dynamically.

During the last years we have developed an experimental model of chronic epilepsy using the cholinergic muscarinic agonist pilocarpine as the convulsant agent and that has been considered a good model for temporal lobe epilepsy in humans (for review, see Cavalheiro, 1995). Acute effects of pilocarpine administration to adult rodents are characterized by long-lasting limbic SE associated with sustained electrographic discharges in limbic structures. After a single application of pilocarpine, SE can last from 6 to 12 h. After spontaneous remission of SE, animals are comatose and both hippocampal and cortical recordings are depressed with high-voltage spiking activity (Turski *et al.*, 1983). These events have been called the 'acute period' of this model and metabolic studies performed during this period have revealed increased glucose utilization mainly in the hippocampus and other limbic structures, thalamus and substantia nigra (Scorza & Cavalheiro, 1996). The pattern of neuronal loss observed in these animals matches closely the areas that are metabolically activated during SE. Animals surviving the acute period of SE proceed to a latent 'seizure free' period with an apparently normal behaviour except for some aggressivity upon manipulation and towards other animals if they are maintained in groups (Cavalheiro *et al.*, 1991). This period lasts 1–8 weeks depending on animal strain and ends with the occurrence of the first spontaneous seizure. The recurrence of spontaneous seizures during the 'chronic period' ranges from 2 to 5 seizures per week (Cavalheiro *et al.*, 1991).

In accordance with these observations we performed a study in order to investigate whether pilocarpine-induced SE in developing rats would lead to the appearance of spontaneous seizures later in life.

Acute period in developing rats

The susceptibility of rats to pilocarpine-induced seizures have been shown to be clearly age-dependent (Cavalheiro *et al.*, 1987). Younger rats (post-natal day [PN] 3–9) resisted higher doses of pilocarpine when compared to adult rats. This higher threshold to the pilocarpine effects began to decrease in 10–14-day-old rats, reaching a completely inverse situation in 15–25-day-old animals. This increased susceptibility to the convulsant action of pilocarpine was characterized by a shortened latency for behavioural and electrographic signs, and increased severity to seizures and lethal toxicity relative to older and younger animals. The susceptibility to pilocarpine gradually decreased with age and reached the mature level in 35–45-day-old rats (Fig. 1).

Pilocarpine administered to developing rats induced a characteristic array of behavioural patterns. Hyper- or hypoactivity, tremor, loss of postural control, scratching, head bobbing and myoclonic movements of the limbs dominated the behaviour in 3–9-day-old rats. No overt motor seizures were observed in this age group. More intense behavioural signs evolving to limbic seizures and status epilepticus occurred when pilocarpine was administered in 10–12-day-old rats. The electrographic activity in these animals progressed from low-voltage spiking registered concurrently in the hippocampus and cortex during the first week of life (Fig. 2) into localized epileptic discharges in the hippocampus which spread to cortical leads during the second week of life (Fig. 3). No morphological alterations were observed in the brains of 3–12-day-old rats subjected to the action of pilocarpine.

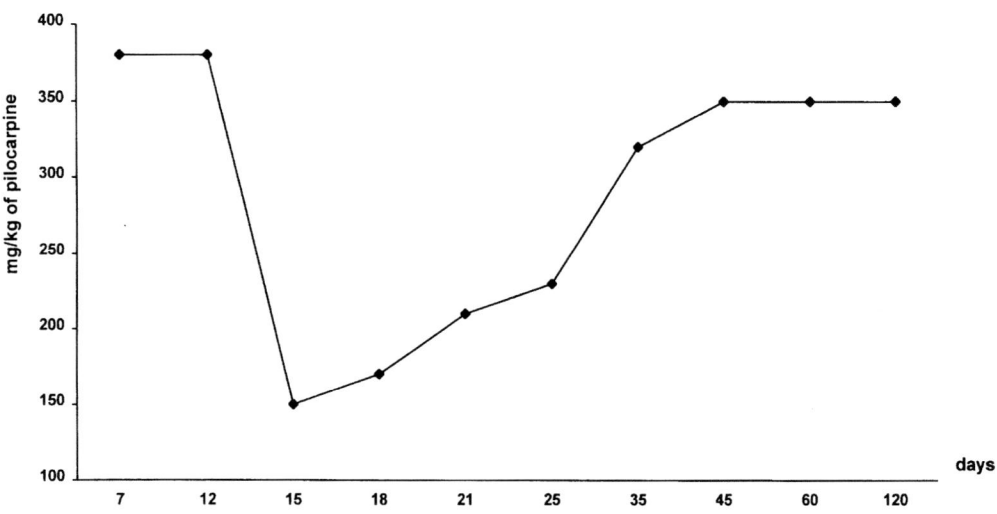

Fig. 1. Graphic representation of pilocarpine (PILO) doses needed to induce status epilepticus in rats according to age. Notice the increased susceptibility to pilocarpine in 15–25-day-old rats.

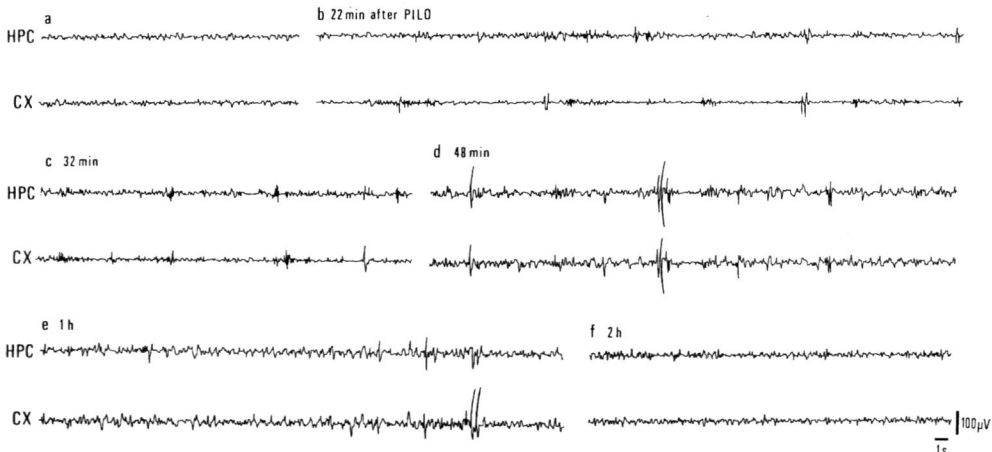

Fig. 2. Electrographic activity recorded after pilocarpine (380 mg/kg, i.p.) in a 6-day-old rat: (a) pre-drug recording; (b–f) recordings to illustrate changes observed following pilocarpine administration. HPC – hippocampus; CX – cortex.

The adult pattern of behavioural and electrographic changes after pilocarpine was encountered in 15–21-day-old rats. Akinesia, tremor and head bobbing progressed to motor limbic seizures and status epilepticus. High-voltage fast activity superposed over hippocampal tetha rhythm progressed into high-voltage spiking and spread to cortical records. The electrographic activity became well synchronized and then developed into seizures and status epilepticus (Fig. 4). Morphological analysis of frontal forebrain sections in 15–21-day-old rats which underwent status epilepticus after pilocarpine revealed an attenuated pattern of damage in hippocampus, amygdala, olfatory cortex, neocortex and certain thalamic nuclei. An adult pattern of damage to the brain, in terms of extent and topography, was present in 4–5-week-old rats.

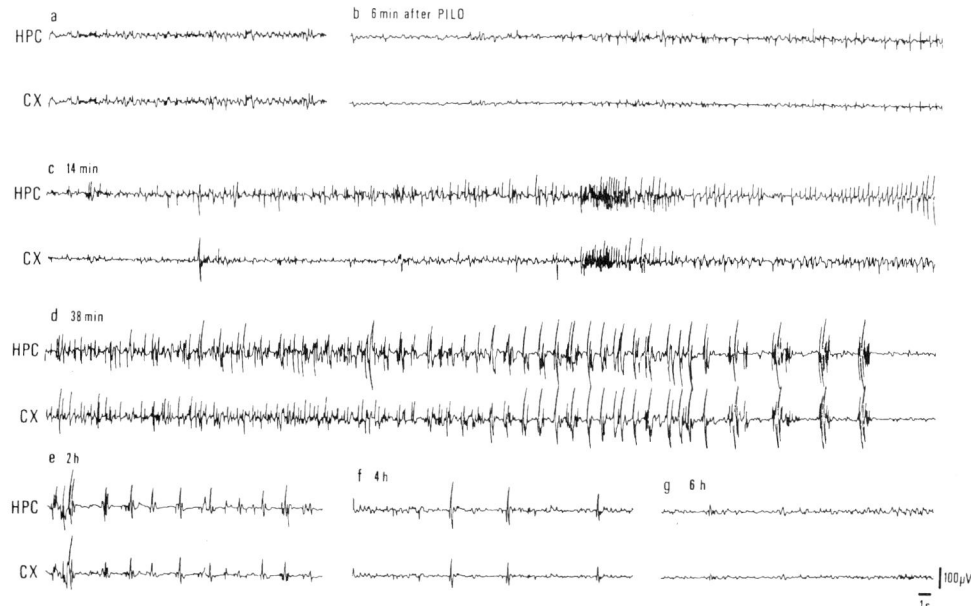

Fig. 3. Electrographic recordings demonstrating the effects of pilocarpine (100 mg/kg, i.p.) in a 15-day-old rat: (a) pre-drug recording; (b–g) recordings to illustrate electrographic correlates after pilocarpine injection. HPC – hippocampus; CX – cortex.

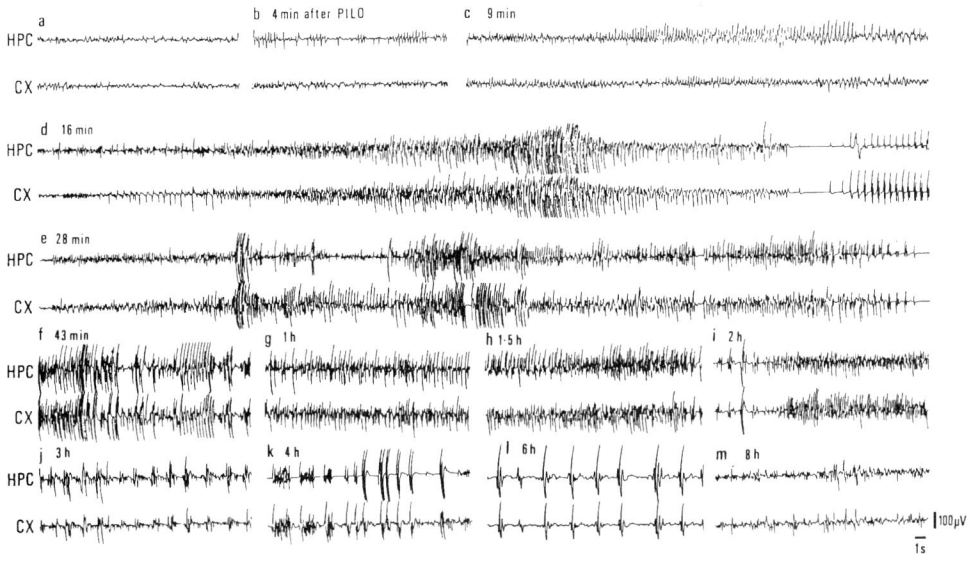

Fig. 4. Recordings to illustrate the effect of systemic administration of pilocarpine (200 mg/kg) in a 18-day-old rat: (a) pre-drug recording; (b–m) electrograhic recordings after pilocarpine. HPC – Hippocampus; CX – cortex.

Chapter 19 Characterization of the pilocarpine model of epilepsy in developing rats

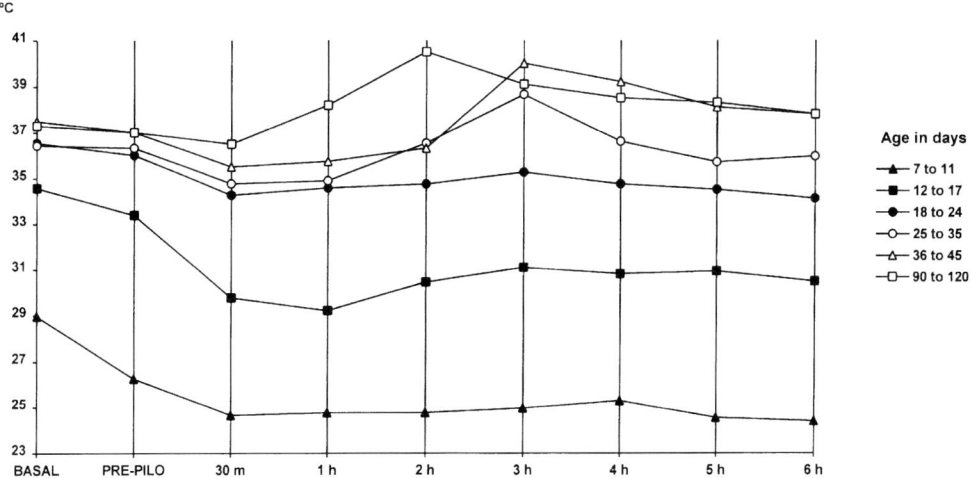

Fig. 5. Changes in rectal temperature during the development of pilocarpine-induced status epilepticus in rats according to age. The following is valid for this and Fig. 6: basal temperature was taken before the sc administration of scopolamine methylnitrate (1 mg/kg); pre-PILO temperature was measured immediately before the i.p. injection of pilocarpine.

More recently we have observed that, in contrast to adult rats, developing animals aged 7–17 days presented an evident hypothermia following pilocarpine administration and that could last up to 5 h (Fig. 5). When 7–11 day-old rats were maintained in a heating box at 35 °C following pilocarpine administration and during the whole period of status epilepticus, their body temperature was maintained at the same level as that of non-treated rats (Fig. 6a). In rats aged 12–17-days, in the same heating box, an increase in body temperature during pilocarpine-induced status epilepticus was observed, although this increase could not be considered as a sign of hyperthermia (Fig. 6b). A characteristic hyperthermia similar to that observed in adult rats during pilocarpine-induced status epilepticus was observed in rats older than 24 days, even if they are maintained at room temperature (Fig. 6c). Developing animals (7–24 days) that were maintained at 35 °C following pilocarpine administration presented more severe status epilepticus, with longer duration and increased mortality rate when compared with age-matched rats maintained at room temperature.

Chronic period in developing rats

Chronic seizures following pilocarpine-induced status epilepticus could be observed if the status was induced after the 18th day of life (Table 1), although some degree of brain damage could already be detected when status epilepticus was induced in earlier stages of life. In contrast to adult rats, the latency (silent period) for the appearance of the first spontaneous seizure was longer and seizure frequency in the chronic period was smaller in 18–24-day-old rats (Table 2). In addition, hilar cell loss and density of Timm staining were less prominent in these animals, suggesting a positive association between mossy fibre sprouting, de novo recurrent excitation of granule cells (Cronin et al., 1992) and the development of spontaneous seizures in this epilepsy model (Priel et al., 1996).

Although animals younger than 18 days of life did not develop spontaneous seizures as a consequence of pilocarpine-induced status epilepticus, they presented electrographic and behavioural alterations similar to those observed in rats with genetic absence epilepsy (Mauescaux & Vergnes, 1995) when studied 90–120 days later (Fig. 7). When the youngest group as submitted to three consecutive episodes of status epilepticus at PN days 7, 8 and 9, electrographic and behavioural changes observed

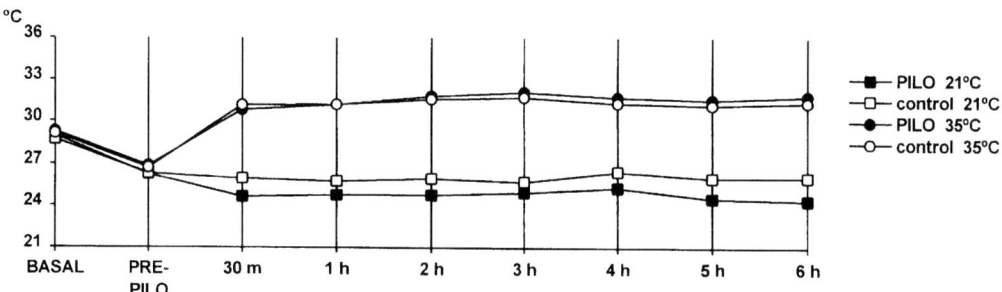

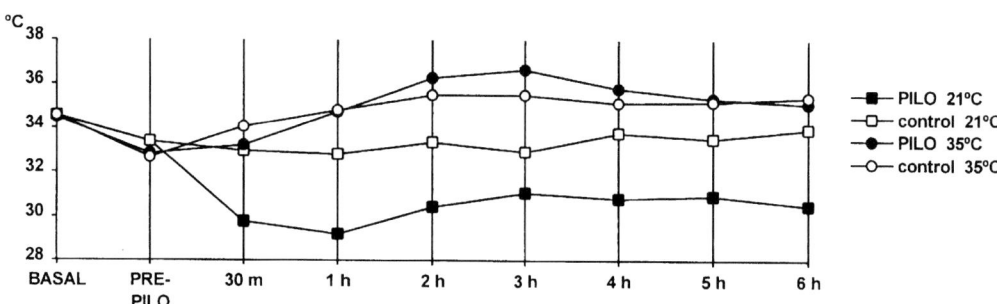

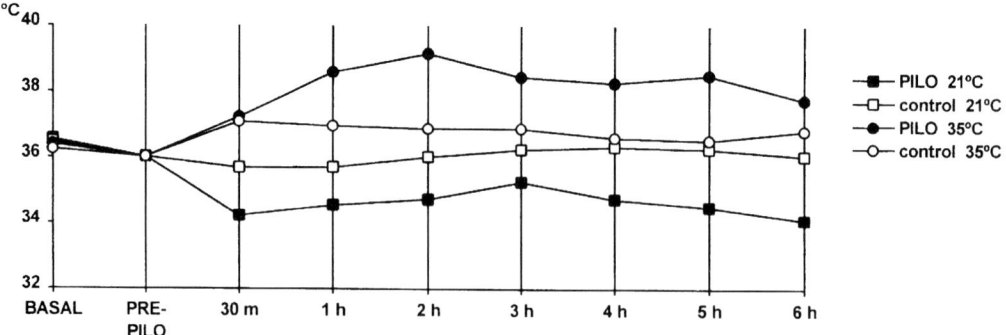

Fig. 6. Changes in rectal temperature in developing rats maintained at room temperature (21 °C) or in a heated box (35 °C) after systemic pilocarpine or saline administration. See also legend to Fig. 5.

Chapter 19 Characterization of the pilocarpine model of epilepsy in developing rats

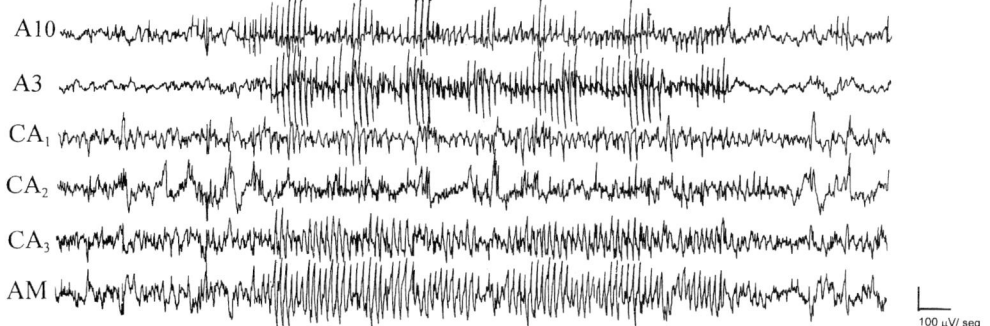

Fig. 7. Electrographic changes observed in an adult rat submitted to pilocarpine-induced status epilepticus 7 days after the birth. Notice the presence of spike and wave discharges in all recorded structures (A10, A3 – neocortical areas 10 and 3, respectively; CA1, CA2, CA3 – hippocampal fields; AM – amygdala).

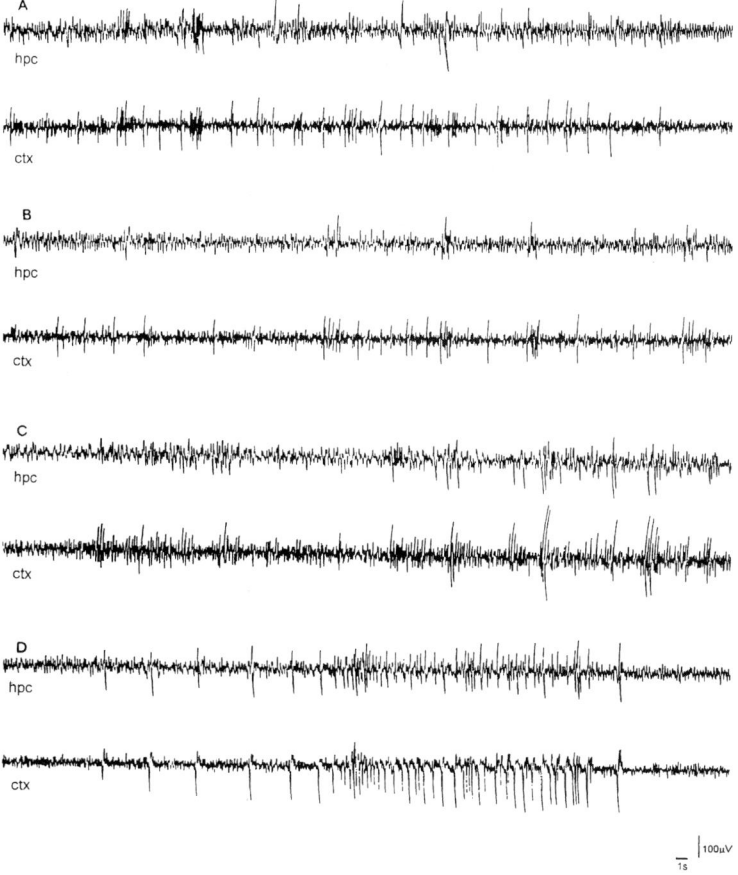

Fig. 8. Electrographic recordings of an adult rat that has been submitted to three consecutive episodes of pilocarpine-induced status epilepticus at post-natal days 7, 8 and 9. Notice the presence of complex spiking activity both in the hippocampal (HPC) and cortical (CX) leads.

in the adult life were much more severe, including episodes of continuous complex spiking activity (Fig. 8), and a small percentage (10–15 per cent) of these rats presented spontaneous seizures. The examination of the brains of these animals did not reveal any major pathological signs.

Table 1. Frequency of spontaneous recurrent seizures during 4 months of observation in rats subjected to pilocarpine-induced status epilepticus at different periods of postnatal development

Age (days)	1st month	2nd month	3rd month	4th month
7–11	–	–	–	–
12–17	–	–	–	–
18–24	0.5 ± 0.5	1.6 ± 0.7	1.8 ± 0.8	2.5 ± 1.3
25–35	1.3 ± 0.8	2.6 ± 1.3	3.5 ± 1.9	3.6 ± 2.0
36–45	2.7 ± 2.1	4.6 ± 3.1	7.3 ± 5.2	7.7 ± 4.1
50–60	4.5 ± 3.8	8.7 ± 4.1	9.2 ± 3.8	9.1 ± 4.2
90–120	6.6 ± 4.5	10.5 ± 8.3	12.3 ± 5.8	10.2 ± 6.2

Data are expressed as means ± SD.

Table 2. Number of rats that survived pilocarpine-induced status epilepticus over the number of injected animals, number of animals that developed spontaneous recurrent seizures later in life and the latency (in days) for the appearance of the first spontaneous seizure according to age

Age (days)	Surviving animals/total	Animals with SRS	Latency for the first seizure (days)*
7–11	29/35	0	0
12–17	61/70	0	0
18–24	36/95	8	36.5 ± 24.8
25–35	26/66	14	23.2 ± 10.3
36–45	42/74	39	19.1 ± 7.4
50–60	45/62	45	17.8 ± 6.4
90–120	32/41	32	14.2 ± 4.6

*Data are expressed as means ± SD.

The age-related differences in the susceptibility of young animals to develop chronic epilepsy following pilocarpine-induced status epilepticus reflect the complexity of seizure activity in immature brain and provide evidence for an apparent distinction between the epileptogenesis in mature and developing nervous system. Our observations show that developing rats subjected to pilocarpine-induced status epilepticus are able to develop typical manifestations of partial limbic epilepsy with secondary generalization later in life if status epilepticus occurs during or after the 3rd week of life, and thus is followed by morphological changes such as neuronal loss mainly in limbic structures and dentate mossy fibre sprouting. On the other hand, although pilocarpine-induced status epilepticus does not induce neuropathological changes in younger rats, it may lead to important plastic changes in critical periods of brain maturation which can become apparent through other types of epileptic features. The functional state of several pathways involving hippocampal and thalamic formation, substantia nigra, etc., key structures in the generation and spread of epileptic activity, should be taken into account in the interpretation of these age-related discrepancies.

Acknowledgements: The author wishes to thank M.R. Priel, N.F. Santos, B.L.C. Ferreira, C. Timo-Iaria and L. Turski for their participation in the experiments reported in this chapter. This work has been supported by research grants from FAPESP, CNPq, FINEP and PRONEX (Brazil).

References

Aicardi, J. & Chevrie, J.J. (1970): Convulsive status epilepticus in infantsand children: a study of 239 cases. Epilepsia 11, 187–197.

Aicardi, J. & Chevrie, J.J. (1983): Consequences of status epilepticus in infantsand children. In: *Status epilepticus*, Delgado-Escueta, A.V., Wasterlain, C.G., Treiman, D.W., Porter, R.J. (eds), pp. 115–125. New York: Raven Press.

Aminoff, M.J. & Simon, R.P. (1980): Status epilepticus. Causes, clinical features and consequences in 98 patients. *Am. J. Med.* **69**, 657–666.

Annegers, J.F., Hauser, W.A., Sirts, S.B. & Kurland, L.T. (1987): Factors prognostic of unprovoked seizures after febrile convulsions. *N. Engl. J. Med.* **316**, 493–498.

Annegers, J.F., Blakely, S.A., Hauser, W.A. & Kurland, L.T. (1990): Recurrence of febrile convulsions in a population-based cohort. *Epilepsy Res.* **5**, 209–216.

Berg, A.T. & Shinnar, S. (1991): The risk of seizure recurrence following a first unprovoked seizure: a quantitative review. *Neurology* **41**, 965–972.

Cavalheiro, E.A. (1995): The pilocarpine model of epilepsy. *Ital. J. Neurol. Sci.* **16**, 33–37.

Cavalheiro, E.A., Silva, D.F., Turski, W.A., Calderazzo-Filho, L.S., Bortolotto, Z.A. & Turski L. (1987): The susceptibility of rats to pilocarpine-induced seizures is age-dependent. *Dev. Brain Res.* **37**, 43–58.

Cavalheiro, E.A., Leite, J.P., Bortolotto, Z.A., Turski, W.A., Ikonomidou, C. & Turski, L. (1991): Long-term effects of pilocarpine in rats: structural damage of the brain triggers kindling and spontaneous recurrent seizures. *Epilepsia* **32**, 778–782.

Cendes, F., Andermann, F., Dubeau, F., Gloor, P., Evans, A., Jones-Gotman, M., Olivier, A., Andermann, E., Robitaille, Y., Lopes-Cendes, I., Peters, T. & Melanson, D. (1993): Early childhood prolonged febrile convulsions, atrophy and sclerosis of mesial structures, and temporal lobe epilepsy. *Neurology* **43**, 1083–1087.

Cronin, J., Obenaus, A., Houser, C.R. & Dudek, F.E. (1992): Electrophysiology of dentate granule cells after kainate-induced synaptic reorganization of mossy fiber. *Brain Res.* **573**, 305–310.

Dunn, D.W. (1988): Status epilepticus in children: etiology, clinical features and outcome. *J. Child Neurol.* **3**, 167–173.

Falconer, M.A. (1971): Genetic and related aetiological factors in temporal lobe epilepsy. A review. *Epilepsia* **12**, 13–21.

Falconer, M.A., Serafetinides, E.A. & Corsellis, J.A.N. (1964): Etiology and pathogenesis of temporal lobe epilepsy. *Arch. Neurol.* **10**, 233–248.

French, J.A., Williamson, P.D., Thadani, V.M., Darcey, T.M., Mattson, R.H., Spencer, S.S. & Spencer, D.D. (1993): Characteristics of medial temporal epilepsy: I. Results of history and physical examination. *Ann. Neurol.* **34**, 774–780.

Gross-Tsur, V. & Shinnar, S. (1993): Convulsive status epilepticus in children. *Epilepsia* **34**, S12–S20.

Hauser, W.A. (1990): Status epilepticus: epidemiological considerations. *Neurology* **40**, 13–22.

Hauser, W.A. & Kurland, L.T. (1975): The epidemiology of epilepsy in Rochester, Minnesota, 1935 through 1967. *Epilepsia* **16**, 1–66.

Hauser, W.A., Anderson, V.E. & Lowenson, R.B. (1982): Seizure recurrence after a first unprovoked seizure. *N. Engl. J. Med.* **307**, 522–528.

Lothman, E.W. & Bertram, E.H. (1993): Epileptogenic effects of status epilepticus. *Epilepsia* **34**, S59–S70.

Marescaux, C. & Vergnes, M. (1995): Genetic absence epilepsy in rats from Strasbourg (GAERS). *Ital. J. Neurol. Sci.* **16**, 113–118.

Margerison, J.H. & Corsellis, J.A.N. (1966): Epilepsy and the temporal lobes: a clinical, electroencephalographic and neuropathological study of the brain in epilepsy with particular reference to the temporal lobes. *Brain* **89**, 499–530.

Mathern, G.W., Pretorius, J.K. & Babb, T.L. (1995): Influence of the type of initial precipitating injury and at what age it occurs on course and outcome in patients with temporal lobe seizures. *J. Neurosurg.* **82**, 220–227.

Maytal, J., Shinnar, S., Moshé, S.L. & Alvarez, L.A. (1989): Low morbidity and mortality of status epilepticus in children. *Pediatrics* **83**, 323–331.

Nelson, K.B. & Ellenberg, J.H. (1978): Prognosis in children with febrile seizures. *Pediatrics* **61**, 720–727.

Phillips, S.A. & Suanahan, R.J. (1989): Etiology and mortality of status epilepticus in children. A recent update. *Arch. Neurol.* **46**, 74–76.

Priel, M.R., Santos, N.F. & Cavalheiro, E.A. (1996): Developmental aspects of the pilocarpine model of epilepsy. *Epilepsy Res.* 26, 115–121.

Scheibel, A.B. (1991): Are complex partial seizures a sequela of temporal lobe dysgenesis? *Adv. Neurol.* **55**, 59–77.

Scorza, F.A. & Cavalheiro, E.A. (1996): Metabolic study in the pilocarpine model of epilepsy. In: *Basic mechanisms of the epilepsies III*, Delgado-Escueta, A.V., Wilson, W., Olsen, R.W. & Porter, R.J. (eds), p. 568.

Shinnar, S., Berg, A.T. & Moshé, S.L. (1988): Recurrence risk after a first unprovoked seizure in childhood. *Ann. Neurol.* **24**, 315–317.

Shinnar, S., Berg, A.T. & Moshé, S.L. (1990): The risk of seizure recurrence following a first unprovoked seizure in childhood: a prospective study. *Pediatrics* **85**, 1076–1085.

Shinnar, S., Berg, A.T, Ptachewich, Y. & Alemany, M. (1993): Sleep state and the risk of seizure recurrence following a first unprovoked seizure in childhood. *Neurology* **43**, 701–706.

Shinnar, S., Berg, A.T., Moshé, S.L., O'Dell, C., Alemany, M., Newstein, D., Kang, H., Goldensohn, E.S. & Hauser, W.A. (1996): The risk of seizure recurrence after a first unprovoked afebrile seizure in childhood: an extended follow-up. *Pediatrics* **98**, 216–225.

Sillanpää, M. (1993): Remission of seizures and predictors of intractability in long-term follow-up. *Epilepsia* **34**, 930–936.

Turski, W.A., Cavalheiro, E.A., Schwarz, M., Czuczwar, S.J., Kleinrok, Z. & Turski, L. (1983): Limbic seizures produced by pilocarpine in rats: behavioral, electroencephalographic and neuropathological study. *Behav. Brain Res.* **9**, 315–335.

Chapter 20

Age-related metabolic and circulatory changes during seizures

Astrid Nehlig[1], Anne Pereira de Vasconcelos[1], Céline Dubé[1],
Maria José da Silva Fernandes[1,*] and Jacques Motte[1,2]

[1] *INSERM U398, Faculté de Médecine, Strasbourg, France;* [2] *American Memorial Hospital, Reims, France;*
*MJSF is a brazilian postdoctoral fellow sponsored by CNPq and FAPESP. Present address: Disciplina de Neurologia Experimental, Universidade Federal de Sao Paulo – Escola Paulista de Medicina, Rua Botucatu, 862, Sao Paulo, SP, Brazil

The immature brain is quite prone to develop seizures (for review, see Holmes, 1997). In humans, the incidence of seizures is highest during the first years of life (Hauser, 1992); in rats, there is an increased susceptibility to seizures induced by various convulsants and to kindling during the second and third postnatal week (Moshé *et al.*, 1983; Albala *et al.*, 1984; De Feo *et al.*, 1985; Cavalheiro *et al.*, 1987; Haas *et al.*, 1990; Michelson & Lothman, 1991; Velisek *et al.*, 1992; Priel *et al.*, 1996; Anderson *et al.*, 1997). Several features may underlie the high epileptogenicity of the developing brain. There is a temporary increase in excitability related to the overproduction of excitory synapses in the CA3 pyramidal neurons (Swann *et al.*, 1988, 1993) accompanied by a transient increased density of NMDA receptors in the immature brain (Tremblay *et al.*, 1988; Johnston, 1996). On the other hand, in the immature rat brain, seizures usually induce minimal brain damage (Cavalheiro *et al.*, 1987; Sperber *et al.*, 1991; Priel *et al.*, 1996, see also Chapters 18 & 21 in this book), probably because of the high plasticity and possibility of repair of the actively growing brain.

The metabolic and circulatory responses of the immature brain to various pathophysiological situations exhibit specific patterns that are quite different from those of mature individuals. This is particularly true during sustained seizures and status epilepticus (SE) which require metabolic and circulatory adaptations that are often close to or beyond the possible limits of the immature brain. In most physiological and pharmacological states, LCMRglcs and LCBF are tightly coupled in adult and immature animals and humans (Kuschinsky *et al.*, 1981; Baron *et al.*, 1984; Chugani & Phelps, 1986; Chugani *et al.*, 1986, 1987; Nehlig *et al.*, 1988, 1989; Chiron *et al.*, 1992; Kuschinsky, 1989 and 1989). Indeed, during the early phase of seizures induced in adult animals, LCBF rates and LCMRglcs usually increase to a similar degree. However, in vulnerable structures, such as hippocampus, cerebral cortex and thalamus, this early increase in LCMRglcs and LCBF rates is followed by a mismatch between flow and metabolism, i.e. a pronounced decrease in LCBF rates accompanied by still high LCMRglcs at 2 h of SE (Ingvar & Siesjö, 1983, 1990; Siesjö *et al.*, 1983; Ingvar, 1986). These prolonged hypermetabolism and hyperfusion for at least 25–30 min are also related to seizure-induced neuronal damage in adult animals (Meldrum, 1983; Ingvar, 1986; Ingvar *et al.*, 1987).

However, there are no data available on the relationship between LCBF and LCMRglcs during sustained seizures in immature animals. Therefore, in the present chapter we will focus on the effects of seizures on brain energy metabolism and blood flow during SE induced by pentylenetetrazol (PTZ) and lithium-pilocarpine (Li-PILO) in relation to potential neuronal damage in the immature brain. The metabolic changes induced by the seizures were measured by the quantitative autoradiographic [^{14}C]2-deoxyglucose technique of Sokoloff et al. (1977) adapted to the immature rat (Nehlig et al., 1988). Circulatory changes were assessed by the quantitative autoradiographic [^{14}C]iodoantipyrine technique of Sakurada et al. (1978) adapted to the immature rat (Nehlig et al., 1989).

Seizures induced by pentylenetetrazol in the immature rat

The PTZ model of seizures is a widely used model of generalized myoclonic, tonic and/or clonic seizures that originate in brainstem structures (Miller & Ferrendelli, 1991). This model has been commonly used for the screening of anticonvulsant drugs (Löscher & Schmidt, 1988; Löscher et al., 1991).

In the PTZ model, seizures were induced by the repetitive injection of subconvulsive doses of PTZ to rats, 10- (PN10) to 21-day-old (PN21). Briefly, the rats received a first i.p. injection of 40 mg/kg, followed by 20 mg/kg 10 min later. Thereafter, the animals received as many 10 mg/kg PTZ injections as necessary to reach SE which is characterized by the loss of postural control, the occurrence of a tonic seizure followed by long episodes of clonic seizures. The clinical and electroencephalographic characteristics of the seizures have been described in detail elsewhere (El Hamdi et al., 1992; André et al., 1998). This procedure allows the occurrence of seizures reproducible in intensity and features for a given age and lasting for 60–80 min. The long duration of the seizures allows the use of the fully quantitative [^{14}C]2-deoxyglucose technique which needs a 45-min steady state (Sokoloff et al., 1977). In this paradigm, the control animals received as many saline injections as their PTZ-exposed litter mates.

Acute metabolic and circulatory changes during pentylenetetrazol-induced seizures in the immature rat

During PTZ-induced SE in PN10 rats, LCMRglcs measured between 10 and 55 min after the onset of SE, i.e. over the first hour of SE, and increased by 100–400 per cent in almost all cerebral regions with the exception of most hippocampal areas, the inferior colliculus, cochlear nucleus and cerebellar cortex where LCMRglcs were similar to control levels (Figs. 1 and 3). Highest metabolic increases were recorded in brainstem regions involved in the circuitry of these seizures and in the control of autonomic functions essential for the survival of the animals (Pereira de Vasconcelos et al., 1992). Conversely, at PN21, PTZ seizures led to metabolic increases, decreases or no change compared to control levels. LCMRglcs remained increased (25–100 per cent) in most brainstem regions but were similar to control values in the anterior limbic areas, motor and some thalamic regions. LCMRglcs were lower than control rates at PN21 in the cerebral cortex, some thalamic nuclei, sensory regions and white matter fibre tracts as well as in the regions in which LCMRglcs were not increased by PTZ seizures at PN10, i.e. hippocampus, inferior colliculus and cerebellar cortex (Pereira de Vasconcelos et al., 1992 and Figs. 2 and 3).

During PTZ-induced SE in PN10 rats, rates of LCBF measured over 1 min at 30 min after the onset of SE showed a 32–184 per cent increase affecting all structures studied. Highest increases were recorded in the accumbens and septal nuclei, amygdala, reticular formation, and all thalamic and hypothalamic structures. Moderate increases occurred in sensory and limbic structures such as the hippocampus and piriform cortex (Figs. 1 and 3). At PN21, rates of LCBF increased (30–120 per cent) in two/three of the structures, including posterior limbic areas, substantia nigra and some thalamic nuclei, decreased by 29–43 per cent in most cortical areas, hippocampus and dentate gyrus of PTZ-treated rats, and were not affected by SE in one/three of the structures (Figs. 2 and 3). At both ages, as previously shown for LCMRglcs, highest increases in LCBF were recorded in posterior and

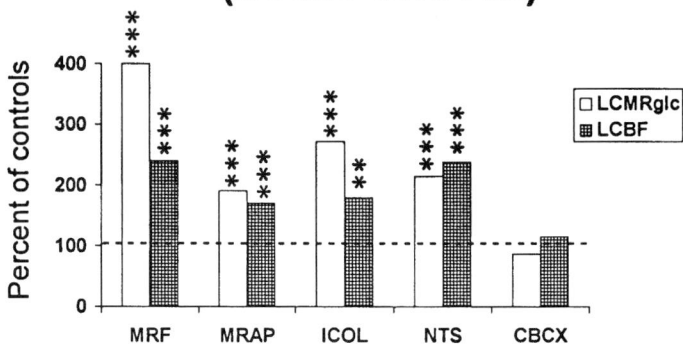

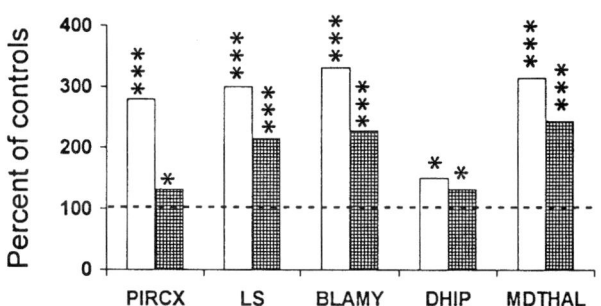

Fig. 1. Acute effects of PTZ-induced SE on LCMRglc and LCBF in PN10 rats (redrawn from Pereira de Vasconcelos et al., 1992, 1995). Values are expressed as percentage of control rates. Abbreviations: MRF: mesencephalic reticular formation; MRAP: median raphe; ICOL: inferior colliculus; NTS: nucleus of the tractus solitarius; CBCX: cerebellar cortex; PIRCX: piriform cortex; LS: lateral septum; BLAMY: basolateral amygdala; DHIP: dorsal hippocampus; MDTHAL: mediodorsal thalamus.
$*P < 0.05$, $**P < 0.01$, $***P < 0.001$, statistically significant differences from controls (Student's t test).

midbrain structures, and all thalamic and hypothalamic nuclei (Pereira de Vasconcelos et al., 1995 and Figs. 1–3).

When considering the coupling between LCMRglcs and LCBF during PTZ-induced seizures, it appears that at PN10, the adjustment between the metabolic demand and the blood supply was maintained only in a few regions, mostly posterior areas such as the medial raphe, nucleus of the solitary tract and the cerebellar cortex as well as in the hippocampus. In most other structures, there was a more or less pronounced hypoperfusion with a markedly lower increase in circulatory levels than in metabolic rates (Fig. 1). At PN21, LCMRglcs and LCBF rates appeared to be quite well coupled in most brain regions. When present, the lack of adjustment between the metabolic demand and blood

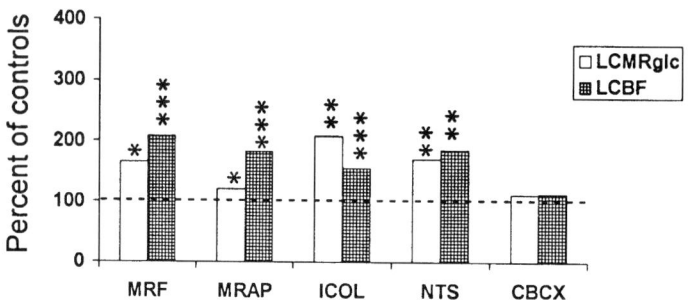
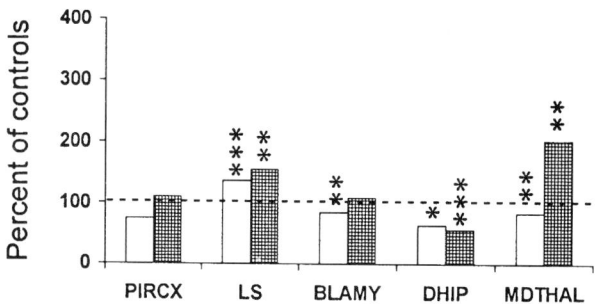

Fig. 2. *Acute effects of PTZ-induced SE on LCMRglc and LCBF in PN21 rats (redrawn from Pereira de Vasconcelos et al., 1992, 1995). Values are expressed as percentage of control rates. See legend to Fig. 1 for definition of abbreviations.*
*$P < 0.05$, **$P < 0.01$, ***$P < 0.001$, *statistically significant differences from controls (Student's t test).*

supply was rather moderate and in favour of a slight hyperperfusion, as can be seen in the medial raphe and the mediodorsal thalamus (Fig. 2). The only exception was the inferior colliculus in which the increase in LCMRglcs was larger than that in LCBF, leading to a slight hypoperfusion (Fig. 2).

Long-term metabolic consequences of pentylenetetrazol seizures induced in the immature rat

We also measured the long-term effects of PTZ seizures induced at PN10 or PN21 on LCMRglcs in young adult rats (PN60) (Hussenet *et al.*, 1995). At PN60, LCMRglcs were significantly reduced compared to control levels in 10 regions of rats exposed to PTZ at PN10 and in 29 structures out of 60 in rats subjected to PTZ at PN21. These regions were mainly sensory, cortical and hippocampal areas, and some thalamic and hypothalamic regions (Fig. 4). Thus, long-term metabolic consequences of early PTZ seizures were mainly prominent in forebrain and thalamic regions. In brainstem areas,

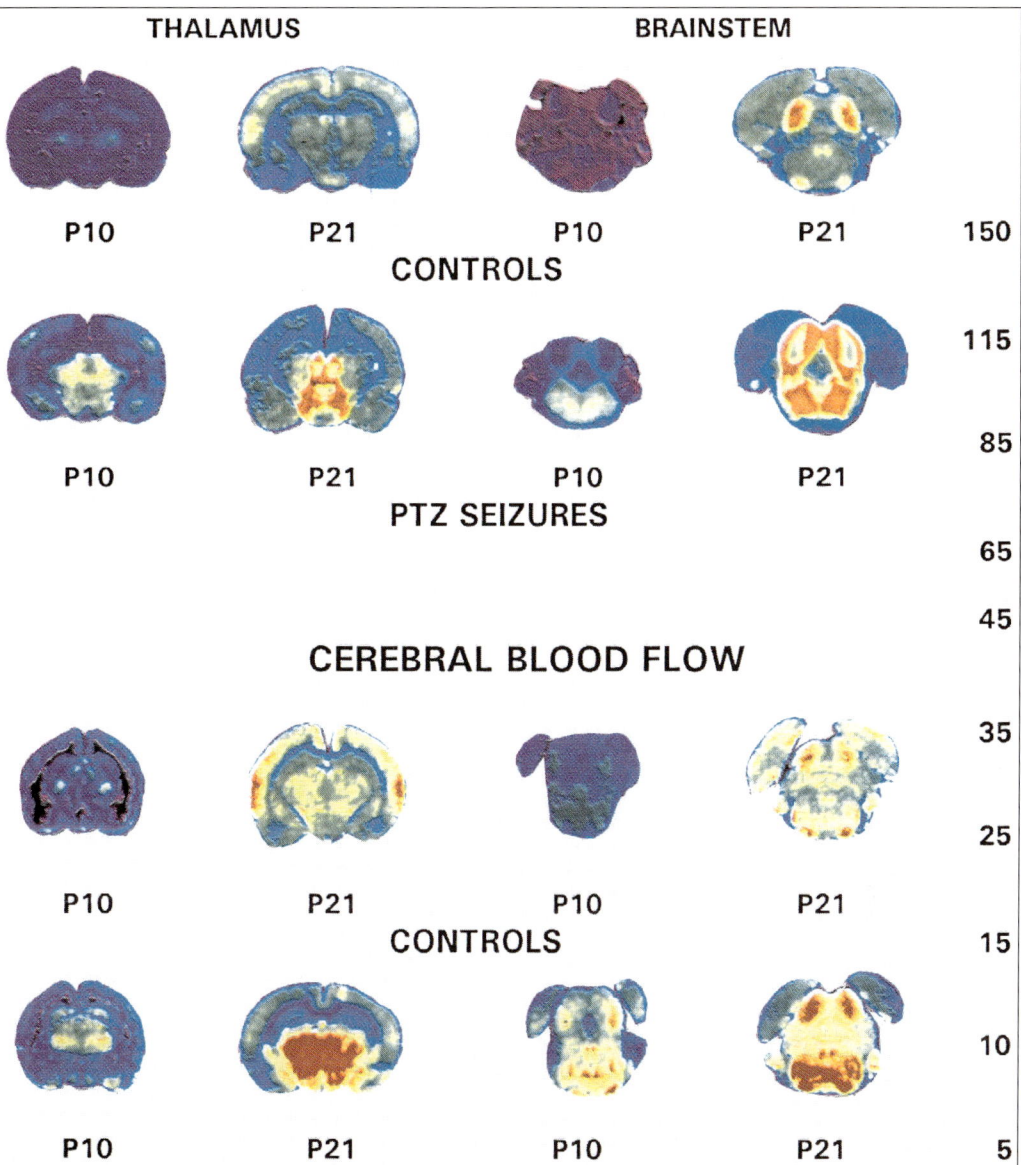

Fig. 3. [^{14}C]2-Deoxyglucose and [^{14}C]iodoantipyrine autoradiographs of rat brain sections taken at the level of the dorsal hippocampus and median thalamus, and the inferior colliculus (IC) in PN10 and PN21 control and PTZ-exposed rats. The scale bar on the right side of the figure represents μmol/100 g/min for LCMRglcs and ml/100 g/min for LCBF rates.

Note the low and homogeneous level of LCMRglcs and LCBF in control PN10 rats, except for slightly higher values in the ventromedian thalamus and hippocampus. In PN21 control rats, LCMRglcs and LCBF rates are more heterogeneous than at P10 and markedly higher than at PN10 in all brain areas. During PTZ-induced SE, LCMRglcs and LCBF rates are markedly increased over control levels in all subcortical areas and more moderately in cortical regions of PN10 rats. At PN21, PTZ seizures lead to large increases in LCMRglcs in the subcortical and mainly brainstem areas. Increases in LCMRglcs are strikingly heterogeneous in the thalamus and the inferior colliculus, while LCBF rates are homogeneously increased in these areas. Conversely, decreases in grain density can be seen in cortical regions and hippocampus.

PTZ seizures in PN10 and PN21 rats (long-term effects)

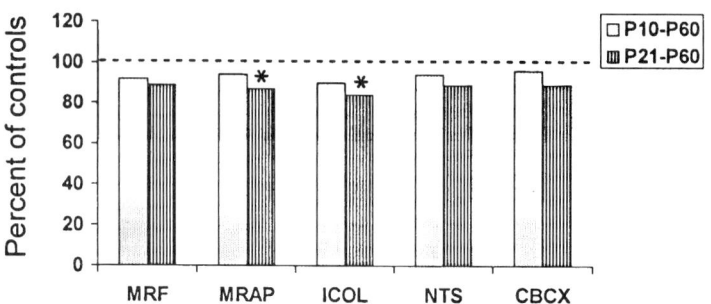

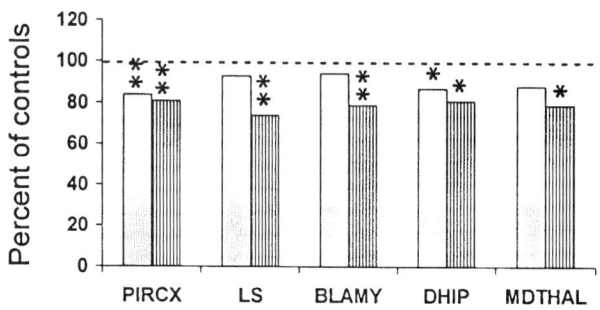

Fig. 4. Long-term effects of PTZ-induced SE at PN10 and PN21 on LCMRglcs measured in PN60 rats (redrawn from Hussenet et al., 1995). Values are expressed as percentage of control rates. See legend to Fig. 1 for definition of abbreviations.
$*P < 0.05$, $**P < 0.01$, statistically significant differences from controls (Student's t test).

PTZ seizures had no long-term metabolic consequences when induced at PN10 or led to functional decreases when induced at PN21. The long-term consequences of PTZ seizures induced at either PN10 or PN21 were independent of the presence or absence of mismatch between cerebral blood flow and metabolism during the acute phase of the seizures. Indeed, long-term metabolic decreases were recorded in structures that underwent hypoperfusion during the acute phase of the seizures as well as in structures in which the blood supply was adjusted to the metabolic demand (Figs. 1, 2 and 4).

Long-term neuropathological changes induced by pentylenetetrazol seizures occurring in the immature rat

Neuronal damage was assessed by the use of two markers, acid fuchsin staining and TUNEL staining in PN10 and PN21 rats subjected to PTZ seizures. Acid fuchsin staining is a reliable marker of dying neurons in adult rodents subjected to hypoglycemia (Auer *et al.*, 1984), seizures (Lowenstein, 1995; Shimosaka *et al.*, 1992; Motte *et al.*, 1998) or ischaemia (Tomioka *et al.*, 1993). In adult rats, acid fuchsin stains moribund neurons that have suffered irreversible injury and will subsequently die within a week (Auer *et al.*, 1984). TUNEL staining is a particularly convenient assay to describe DNA fragmentation at the cellular level with a high degree of reproducibility and resolution (Charriaut-Marlangue & Ben-Ari, 1995). In PN10 rats, acid fuchsin staining was limited to cortical regions at 1 and 4 h after the onset of PTZ-induced SE. The number of stained neurons was maximal at 24 h after the seizures and visible all over the brain. Staining was especially strong in the cerebral cortex and the different hippocampal subfields while being widespread but less intense in the midbrain, thalamic, hypothalamic and brainstem regions. By 72 h, acid fuchsin staining was only present in cerebral cortex and to a lesser degree in hippocampal subfields. At 144 h, acid fuchsin staining was virtually absent from all cerebral areas. Hematoxylin-eosin staining did not show a difference in the cell density between sections from saline- and PTZ-exposed animals. Moreover, there was no evidence of any DNA fragmentation at any time between 1 and 144 h after the onset of PTZ-induced SE in PN10 and PN21 rats, which is consistent with the absence of single and/or double-stranded DNA breaks (Pineau *et al.*, 1998).

The lack of neuronal damage in this model of seizures is also confirmed by the absence of the late wave of the c-Fos protein expression in PN10 or PN21 rats subjected to PTZ seizures (Motte *et al.*, 1997). Indeed, the prolonged expression of this transcription factor correlates with cell death occurring after severe seizures (Kaminska *et al.*, 1994a,b, 1997; Konopka *et al.*, 1995). Likewise, the expression of the 72 kDa heat-shock protein (HSP72) which represents a response to excitation-induced stress, potential brain cell injury and neuronal plasticity also occurs after seizures in adult rodents (Shimosaka *et al.*, 1992; Planas *et al.*, 1994; Lowenstein, 1995; Motte *et al.*, 1998). Similarly to what occurs with the late phase of c-Fos, HSP72 is not expressed after PTZ seizures induced in PN10 and PN21 rats (Motte *et al.*, 1997). The lack of expression of these two transcription factors correlates with the lack of neuronal damage in this model of seizures in the immature rat. However, the transient staining of the neurons by acid fuchsin reflects the occurrence of transient changes in the cell properties that allow the dye to enter the cells. The immature neurons subjected to sustained seizures appear to be able to recover and to survive the PTZ seizure insult, conversely to what occurs in most models of prolonged severe seizures in the adult rat (Meldrum, 1983; Nevander *et al.*, 1985; Ingvar *et al.*, 1987; Cavalheiro, 1995). Thus, the long-term metabolic decreases occurring in the PN60 rat as a consequence of PTZ seizures induced at PN10 or PN21 without any overt neuropathological damage, may reflect changes in the final synaptic organization and dendritic arborization in the brain of these animals (Hussenet *et al.*, 1995).

Seizures induced by lithium-pilocarpine in the immature rat

The pilocarpine (PILO) model of epilepsy shares many features with human temporal lobe epilepsy. This is especially true for the clinical evolution of the epilepsy, as for the type of the seizures and localization of the damage (Cavalheiro, 1995). Thus, the acute period of SE which lasts about 6–12 h in the rat, is followed by a seizure-free silent phase of a mean duration of 14 days in the adult and 37 days in the 18- to 24-day-old rat (Cavalheiro, 1995; Priel *et al.*, 1996). After that period, the onset of the chronic phase is characterized by the occurrence of recurrent seizures that last for the whole life of the animal. However, while 100 per cent of the adult and 22 per cent of PN21 rats become chronically epileptic, no animal subjected to seizures before PN18 is able to develop spontaneous recurrent seizures (Cavalheiro, 1995; Priel *et al.*, 1996). Many authors use lithium in addition to PILO instead of the PILO model originally described. The main differences between the two models are related, first to the dose of PILO necessary to induce seizures which is decreased by a factor of 10–12 when combined with lithium, and second to the better reproducibility of seizure induction after pretreatment with lithium.

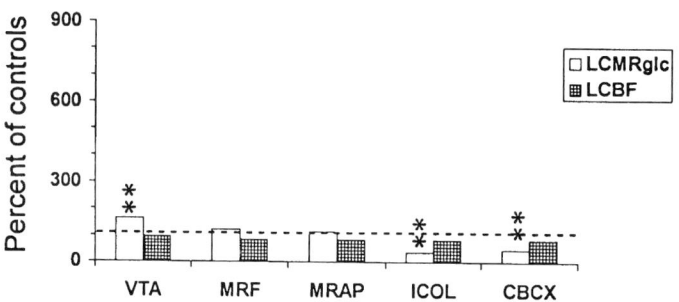

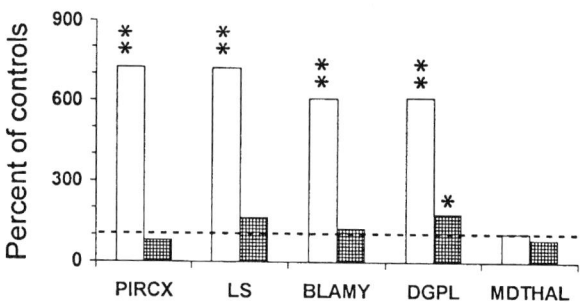

Fig. 5. Acute effects of Li-PILO-induced SE on LCMRglcs and LCBF rates in PN10 rats. Values are expressed as percentage of control values.
Abbreviations: VTA: ventral tegmental area; DGPL: polymorphic layer of the dentate gyrus: others, see legend to Fig. 1.
$*P < 0.05$, $** P < 0.01$, statistically significant differences from controls (Dunnett's t test).

Acute metabolic and circulatory changes during lithium-pilocarpine-induced seizures in the immature rat

Li-PILO seizures lead to generalized increases in LCMRglcs measured during the second hour of SE in both PN10 and PN21 rats. In PN10 animals, increases in LCMRglcs ranged from 63 to 625 per cent and were located in most cortices and forebrain areas. The largest increases (over 450 per cent) were recorded in the piriform cortex, the lateral septum, all parts of the amygdala, the hippocampal CA1 area and the hilus of the dentate gyrus. There were almost no seizure-induced metabolic changes in hypothalamic and thalamic areas. Significant decreases in LCMRglcs compared to the levels in control animals occurred in the inferior colliculus and cerebellar cortex (Fernandes *et al.*, 1998; Figs. 5 and 7). In PN21 rats, increases in LCMRglc were rather moderate (55–230 per cent) in most brainstem areas, cerebellar cortex, nuclei and white matter, i.e. in regions where no neuronal damage

Li-Pilo seizures in PN21 rats (acute phase)

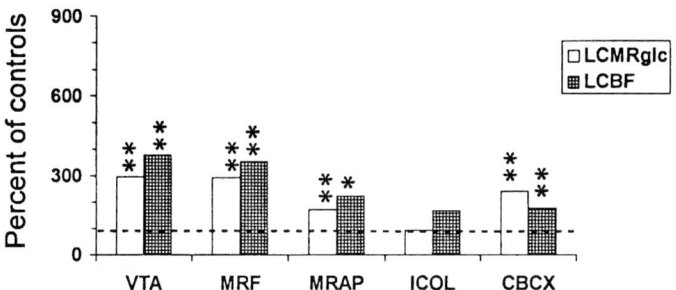

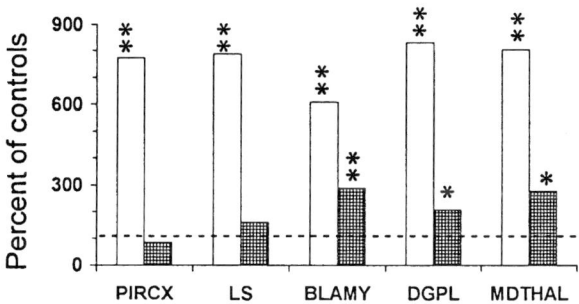

Fig. 6. *Acute effects of Li-PILO-induced SE on LCMRglcs and LCBF rates in PN21 rats. Values are expressed as percentage of control values. See legend to Figs. 1 and 5 for definitions of abbreviations.*
*$P < 0.05$, **$P < 0.01$, statistically significant differences from controls (Dunnett's t test).

was recorded. Conversely, dramatic increases in LCMRglcs (378–875 per cent) occurred in the cerebral cortex, hippocampus, amygdala, septum and thalamus (Figs. 6), i.e. in all brain regions in which neuronal damage later developed (Cavalheiro et al., 1987; Priel et al., 1996; Fernandes et al., 1998). The inferior colliculus was the only structure in which LCMRglc was similar in control and Li-PILO-treated PN21 rats (Fig. 6).

During Li-PILO-induced SE in PN10 rats, rates of LCBF measured over 1 min at 70 min after the onset of SE showed that the sustained seizures did not induce any significant change, except in the dentate gyrus hilus where rates of LCBF increased by 78 per cent (Fig. 5). In PN21 rats, Li-PILO-induced SE led to a 170–430 per cent increase in LCBF rates (Fig. 6). Highest increases (180 per cent) occurred in the ventral tegmental area, mesencephalic reticular formation, basolateral amygdala and mediodorsal thalamus. Moderate increases in LCBF values were seen in the dentate gyrus hilus, raphe nuclei and cerebellar cortex. No significant change in LCBF was recorded in the inferior colliculus, piriform cortex and lateral septum (Fig. 6).

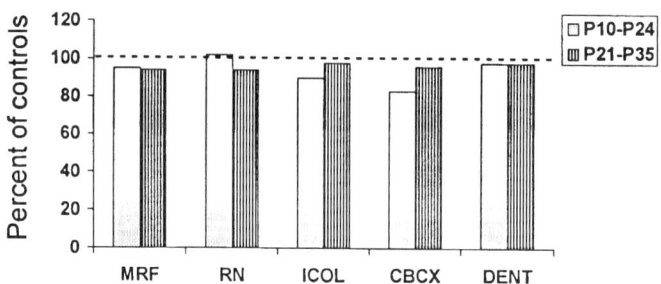
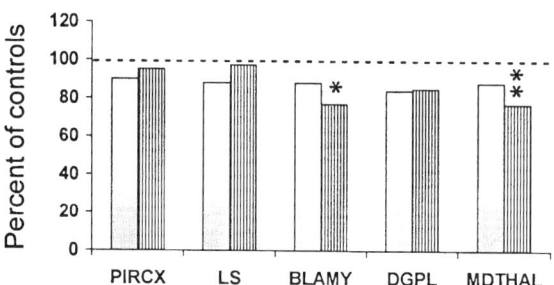

Fig. 7. LCMRglcs during the silent phase following Li-PILO-induced SE. Seizures were induced at PN10 or PN21 and LCMRglcs were measured 14 days later, i.e. at P24 and P35, respectively. Values are expressed as percentage of control values. See legend to Figs. 1 and 5 for definitions of abbreviations.
$*P < 0.05$, $**P < 0.01$, statistically significant differences from controls (Dunnett's t test).

When considering the coupling between LCMRglcs and LCBF during Li-PILO-induced seizures, it appears that at PN10, the adjustement between the metabolic demand and the blood supply was maintained only in the brainstem regions and the thalamic nuclei. In all anterior structures, a marked mismatch occurred between LCMRglcs and LCBF rates with metabolic rates increasing up to 600 per cent, while rates of LCBF remained identical to control rats or only slightly increased (about 80 per cent in the dentate gyrus hilus) (Fig. 5). The situation was identical at PN21 with a prominent hypoperfusion in all forebrain regions including the thalamic nuclei (Fig. 6).

Metabolic levels during the silent phase of lithium-pilocarpine seizures induced in the immature rat

We also measured LCMRglcs at 14 days after the acute Li-PILO treatment in PN10 or PN21 rats during which period the animals were returned to their normal environment. When rats were subjected to SE at PN10, LCMRglcs measured 14 days after the induction of seizures were similar in rats injected with Li-PILO and in saline-treated controls in all brain regions (Fig. 7). Conversely, when SE was induced at PN21, LCMRglcs were significantly reduced during the silent phase in Li-PILO-exposed rats compared to controls in cortical regions, such as the entorhinal cortex, in the basolateral amygdala, hippocampal CA3 area and most thalamic nuclei (Fig. 7). These metabolic decreases occurred in regions where LCMRglcs underwent the largest increases during the acute phase of SE (Fig. 6).

Neuropathological changes induced by lithium-pilocarpine seizures occurring in the immature rat

Silver staining performed at 6 h after the onset of Li-PILO-induced SE showed that the number of degenerating neurons was very limited in PN10 rats. In the latter age group, a few degenerating neurons could be seen in the piriform and entorhinal cortex and basolateral amygdala. Furthermore, the neuronal degeneration is not occurring in all animals. In PN21 rats undergoing Li-PILO SE, there was marked damage in the cerebral cortex, limbic forebrain and thalamic nuclei (Fig. 8). Lesions were present in all animals. As in the PTZ model of seizures, the late phase of c-Fos immunoreactivity as well as HSP72 expression were absent in PN10 rats subjected to Li-PILO seizures. Conversely, the expression of these two transcription factors was present at 24 h after the Li-PILO seizures in PN21 rats (Dubé et al., 1998).

Relationship between seizure-induced metabolic and circulatory changes, and neuronal damage in the immature rat

In adult animals subjected to sustained seizures, LCBF rates and LCMRglcs usually increase to a similar degree during the initial phase. However, in vulnerable structures, such as the hippocampus, cerebral cortex and thalamus, this early increase in LCMRglcs and LCBF rates is followed by a mismatch between flow and metabolism, i.e. a pronounced decrease in LCBF rates accompanied by largely elevated LCMRglcs (Ingvar & Siesjö, 1983; Siesjö et al., 1983; Ingvar, 1986). In a further phase, cerebral metabolism returns to normal levels and eventually decreases below the level recorded in the control situation. These very low LCMRglcs coincide with the occurrence of neuronal damage (Nevander et al., 1985).

In immature animals, the relationship between circulatory and metabolic changes during SE and subsequent cerebral damage is less clear. The immature rat brain is quite resistant to seizure-induced brain damage which is usually not seen until the age of PN20-P30 (Nitecka et al., 1984; Cavalheiro et al., 1987; Sperber et al., 1991; Wasterlain & Shirasaka, 1994). However, neuronal damage can be seen in younger animals in some models of severe seizures (see Chapters 18 and 21 in this book).

In PN21 rats subjected to Li-PILO SE, as seen in adult animals (Siesjö et al., 1983; Ingvar, 1986), there is a marked mismatch between LCBF and LCMRglcs restricted to the forebrain structures known to undergo neuronal damage at that age (Cavalheiro et al., 1987; Priel et al., 1996). In these structures, i.e. entorhinal and piriform cortices, hippocampus, amygdala, anterior olfactory nuclei and thalamus, there is abundant neuronal degeneration, as evidenced by silver staining (Fig. 9). Metabolic increases in PN21 rats subjected to Li-PILO-induced SE are very large in these structures (610–875 per cent) while LCBF rates increase much less, eventually not at all (0–265 per cent) (Fig. 6). In these structures, we also record metabolic decreases during the silent phase of the epilepsy (Fig. 7). On the other hand, at PN21, no mismatch between LCBF and LCMRglcs could be evidenced in structures where no damage occurred after Li-PILO seizures. The latter structures are mainly posterior and midbrain areas, cerebellar regions, and sensory areas such as superior and inferior colliculi (Pereira de Vasconcelos & Nehlig, unpublished data and Fig. 6). Thus, in the Li-PILO model of seizures, a marked hypoperfusion during the acute seizure phase seems to correlate with subsequent neuronal damage at PN21. Conversely, during PTZ-induced seizures that do not lead to neuronal damage in PN21 rats, there is only a moderate mismatch between LCBF and LCMRglcs in a limited number of structures which is rather in favour of a hyperperfusion. Moreover, in this age group, the metabolic levels are only slightly increased, and even decreased in a number of regions compared to controls (Fig. 2). Thus, in the PTZ model, the lack of damage could be partly related to the maintenance of the coupling between blood flow and metabolism during the seizures as well as to the reduced metabolic increase. Indeed, in adult

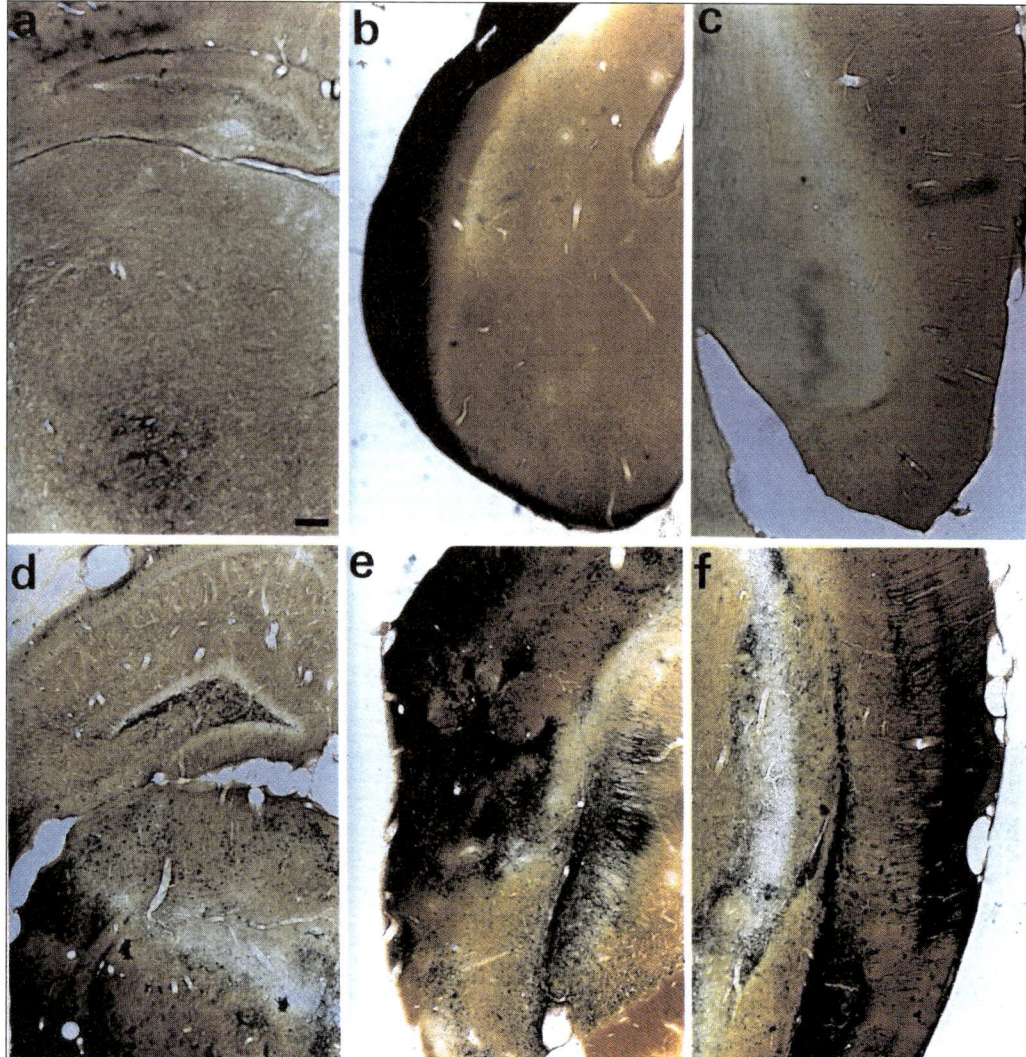

Fig. 8. *Silver staining of degenerating neurons in sections from PN10 and PN21 rats taken at the level of the hippocampus and the thalamus (a, d), the entorhinal cortex (b, c, e) and the lateral cortex (f).(a & b): PN10 rats; (d, e & f): PN21 rats subjected to lithium-pilocarpine SE and sacrificed at 6 h after the onset of seizures; (c): PN21 control animal.*

The control PN21 rat (c) was devoid of any dark cells. At PN10 (a, b), very few scattered dark cells were visible in the entorhinal cortex and the hippocampus while the thalamus was devoid of any dark cells. In the PN21 rat, dark cells were present in the polymorphic layer of the dentate gyrus and the dorsolateral thalamus (d). In the entorhinal (e) and lateral (f) cortex of the PN21 rat, there was abundant degeneration of cell bodies and fibres. Scale bar: 100 μm.

animals, prolonged hypermetabolism and hyperfusion are related to seizure-induced neuronal damage (Ingvar, 1986; Ingvar & Siesjö, 1990).

In PN10 rats, the relationship between circulatory and metabolic changes, and neuropathological consequences is much less obvious. In the two models of severe seizures studied, we recorded quite large increases in LCMRglcs not matched by similar increases in LCBF in PN10 rats. The mismatch between blood flow and metabolism was not paralleled by neuronal damage which was totally absent in the PTZ model and very discrete in the Li-PILO model. In addition to our studies, data in newborn marmoset monkeys subjected to bicuculline show a clear mismatch in vulnerable areas such as the cerebral cortex and the hippocampus, with relative LCMRglc increases higher than those of LCBF. By contrast, in the brainstem, blood flow and metabolism increased to a comparable degree, as in our study with Li-PILO seizures (Wasterlain & Dwyer, 1983; Wasterlain et al., 1984; Fujikawa et al., 1986, 1989, 1990; Wasterlain & Shirasaka, 1994). However, despite this flow-metabolism mismatch, no neuronal damage was seen in marmoset monkeys even after 4½ h of SE. Only minimal neuropathological changes such as potentially reversible perivascular edema and mitochondrial swelling in a few neurons of the cerebral cortex and hippocampus were reported (Söderfeldt et al., 1990). However, these studies were conducted under ketamine anaesthesia, which could have been neuroprotective, and survival was brief, so that delayed neuronal death would have been missed.

It appears from the present studies that the PN10 rat brain seems to be able to undergo large metabolic increases accompanied by pronounced mismatches between blood flow and metabolism without any subsequent overt damage. However, it must be noticed that PTZ seizures occurring in the PN10 rat induce long-term metabolic decreases (Hussenet et al., 1995 and Fig. 4) and Li-PILO seizures lead to discrete neuronal damage and to slight metabolic decreases, though not significant, in forebrain regions at 14 days after the SE at PN10 (Fig. 8). Thus, the resistance of the immature brain to the metabolic and circulatory consequences of seizures is by far greater than that of the more mature brain. The reasons for it are unknown. They might relate to the low basal metabolic levels of the very immature brain that reach only 15–20 per cent of the adult levels (Nehlig et al., 1988). At that age, the brain is also mostly dependent on anaerobic glycolysis since the enzymes of the oxidative breakdown of glucose mature only after PN14 and mostly between PN21 and PN35 (for review, see Nehlig & Pereira de Vasconcelos, 1993). Thus any activation will largely increase glucose breakdown since the energetic yield of glycolysis is 18 times lower than the oxidative breakdown of glucose. The ensuing production of lactate is much less toxic for the immature than for the mature brain because of the high permeability of the monocarboxylic acid transporter located at the blood-brain barrier (Cremer et al., 1976, 1979; Pardridge & Oldendorf, 1977). This allows the efflux of lactate from the brain and the equilibration between body and brain lactate avoiding an excessive build-up of toxic lactate levels in the brain, as we could record during both PTZ- and Li-PILO-induced seizures (Pereira de Vasconcelos et al., 1992; Fernandes et al., 1998). Finally, the metabolism of immature rat brain is also dependent on the supply of ketone bodies in addition to glucose (for review, see Nehlig & Pereira de Vasconcelos, 1993). All these factors may contribute to the relative resistance to seizure-induced metabolic increases and mismatches between blood flow and metabolism in the immature compared to the mature rat brain.

Conclusion

Thus, it appears that the PN21 rat has achieved a cerebral maturity that renders it sensitive to the neuropathological consequences of seizure-induced cerebral metabolism–blood flow mismatch, in other terms to marked hypermetabolism and relative hypoperfusion during SE. This is the case in the vulnerable areas of the forebrain in the Li-PILO model of SE. Conversely, in younger animals, such as PN10 rats or newborn marmoset monkeys, mismatches between LCBF and LCMRglcs take place without having clear neuropathological consequences. The reasons underlying the age-related difference and the resistance to the very immature brain to seizure-induced neuronal damage require further clarification. However, the data obtained in the PTZ model of SE show that although there is no overt damage, the neurons undergo transient changes in their membrane properties which seem to have functional changes that could reflect changes in synaptic organization and dendritic arborization of the neurons. Although subtle, these changes could lead to functional changes that should not be neglected.

References

Albala, B.J., Moshé, S.L. & Okada, R. (1984): Kainic acid-induced seizures: a developmental study. *Dev. Brain Res.* **13**, 139–148.

Anderson, A.E., Hrachovy, R.A. & Swann, J.W. (1997): Increased susceptibility to tetanus toxin-induced seizures in immature rats. *Epilepsy Res.* **26**, 433–442.

André, V., Pineau, N., Motte, J., Marescaux, C. & Nehlig, A. (1998): Mapping of neuronal networks underlying generalized seizures induced by increasing doses of pentylenetetrazol in the immature and adult rat. *Eur. J. Neurosci.* **10**, 2094–2106.

Auer, R.N., Wieloch, T., Olsson, Y. & Siesjö, B.K. (1984): The distribution of hypoglycemic brain damage. *Acta Neuropathol.* **64**, 177–191.

Cavalheiro, E.A. (1995): The pilocarpine model of epilepsy. *Ital. J. Neurosci.* **16**, 33–37.

Cavalheiro, E.A., Silva, D.F., Turski, W.A., Calderazzo-Filho, L.S., Bortolotto, A. & Turski, L. (1987): The susceptibility of rats to pilocarpine-induced seizures is age-dependent. *Dev. Brain Res.* **37**, 43–58.

Charriaut-Marlangue, C. & Ben-Ari, Y. (1995): A cautionary note on the use of the TUNEL stain to determine apoptosis. *NeuroReport* **7**, 61–64.

Chiron, C., Raynaud, C., Mazière, B., Zilbovicius, M., Laflamme, L., Masure, M.C., Dulac, O., Bourguignon, M. & Syrota, A. (1992): Changes in regional cerebral blood flow during brain maturation in children and adolescents. *J. Nucl. Med.* **33**, 696–703.

Chugani, H.T. & Phelps, M.E. (1986): Maturational changes in cerebral function in infants determined by 18FDG positron emission tomography. *Science* **231**, 840–843.

Chugani, H.T., Phelps, M.E. & Mazziotta, J.C. (1987): Positron emission tomography study of human brain functional development. *Ann. Neurol.* **22**, 487–497.

Cremer, J.E., Braun, L.D. & Oldendorf, W.H. (1976): Changes during development in transport processes of the blood–brain barrier. *Biochim. Biophys. Acta* **448**, 633–637.

Cremer, J.E., Cunningham, V.J., Pardridge, W.M., Braun, L.D. & Oldendorf, W.H. (1979): Kinetics of blood–brain barrier transport of pyruvate, lactate and glucose in suckling, weanling and adult rats. *J. Neurochem.* **33**, 439–445.

De Feo, M., Mecarello, O. & Ricci, G. (1985): Bicuculline- and allylglycine-induced epilepsy in developing rats. *Exp. Neurol.* **90**, 411–421.

Dubé, C., André, V., Covolan, L., Ferrandon, A. Marescaux, C. & Nehlig, A. (1998): c-Fos, JunD and HSP72 immunoreactivity, and neuronal injury following lithium–pilocarpine induced status epilepticus in immature and adult rats. *Mol. Brain Res.* (in press).

El Hamdi, G., Pereira de Vasconcelos, A., Vert, P. & Nehlig, A. (1992): An experimental model of generalized seizures for the measurement of local cereral glucose utilization in the immature rat. I. Behavioral characterization and determination of lumped constant. *Dev. Brain Res.* **69**, 233–242.

Fernandes, M.J.S., Boyet, S., Marescaux, C. & Nehlig, A. (1998): Correlation between hypermetabolism and neuronal damage during status epilepticus induced by lithium-pilocarpine in immature and adult rats. *J. Cereb. Blood Flow Metab.* **18** (in press).

Fujikawa, D.G., Dwyer, B.E. & Wasterlain, C.G. (1986): Preferential blood flow to brainstem during generalized seizures in the newborn marmoset monkey. *Brain Res.* **397**, 61–72.

Fujikawa, D.G., Dwyer, B.E., Lake, R.R. & Wasterlain, C.G. (1989): Local cerebral glucose utilization during status epilepticus in newborn primates. *Amer. J. Physiol.* **256** (*Cell Physiol.* **25**), C1160-C1167.

Fujikawa, D.G., Dwyer, B.E., Lake, R.R. & Wasterlain C.G. (1990): Cerebral blood flow and metabolism during neonatal seizures. In: *Neonatal seizures, pathophysiology and pharmacological management,* Wasterlain, C.G. & Vert, C.G. (eds), pp. 143–158. New York: Raven Press.

Haas, K.Z., Sperber, E.F. & Moshé, S.L. (1990): Kindling in developing animals: expression of severe seizures and enhanced development of bilateral foci. *Dev. Brain Res.* **56**, 275–280.

Hauser, W.A. (1992): Seizure disorders: the changes with age. *Epilepsia* **33** (Suppl. 4), S6-S14.

Holmes, G.L. (1997): Epilepsy in the developing brain: lessons from the laboratory and clinic. *Epilepsia* **38**, 12–30.

Hussenet, F., Boyet, S. & Nehlig, A. (1995): Long-term metabolic effects of pentylenetetrazol-induced status epilepticus in the immature rat. *Neuroscience* **67**, 455–461.

Ingvar, M. (1986): Cerebral blood flow and metabolic rate during seizures. Relationship to epileptic brain damage. *Ann. N.Y. Acad. Sci.* **462**, 194–206.

Ingvar, M. & Siesjö, B.K. (1983): Local blood flow and glucose consumption in the rat brain during sustained bicuculline-induced seizures. *Acta Neurol. Scand.* **68**, 129–144.

Ingvar, M. & Siesjö, B.K. (1990): Pathophysiology of epileptic brain damage. In: *Neonatal seizures. pathophysiology and pharmacological management,* Wasterlain, C.G. & Vert, C.G. (eds), pp. 113–122. New York: Raven Press.

Ingvar, M., Folbergrova, J. & Siesjö, B.K. (1987): Metabolic alterations underlying the development of hypermeatbolic necrosis in the substantia nigra in status epilepticus. *J. Cereb. Blood Flow Metab.* **7**, 103–108.

Johnston, M.V. (1996): Developmental aspects of epileptogenesis. *Epilepsia* **37** (Suppl. 1), S2-S9.

Kaminska, B., Filipowski, R.K., Zurkowska, G., Lason, W., Przewlocki, R. & Kaczmarek, L. (1994a): Dynamic changes in the composition of the AP-1 transcription factor DNA-binding activity in rat brain following kainate-induced seizures and cell death. *Eur. J. Neurosci.* **6**, 1558–1564.

Kaminska, B., Lukasiuk, K. & Kaczmarek, L. (1994b): Seizures-evoked activation of transcription factors. *Acta Neurobiol. Exp.* **54**, 65–72.

Kaminska, B., Filipowski, R.K., Biedermann, I.W., Konopka, D., Nowicka, D., Hetman, M., Dabrowski, M., Gorecki, D.C., Lukasiuk, K., Szklarczyck, A.W. & Kaczmarek, L. (1997): Kainate-evoked modulation of gene expression in rat brain. *Acta Bioch. Pol.* **44**, 781–790.

Konopka, D., Nowicka, D., Filipowski, R.K. & Kaczmarek, L. (1995): Kainate-evoked secondary gene expression in the rat hippocampus. *Neurosci. Lett.* **185**, 167–170.

Kuschinski, W. (1996): Regulation of cerebral blood flow: an overview. In: *Neurophysiological basis of cerebral blood flow control: an introduction,* Mraovitch, S. & Sercombe, R. (eds), pp. 245–262. London: John Libbey.

Löscher, W. & Schmidt, D. (1988): Which animal models should be used in the search for new antiepileptic drugs? A proposal based on experimental and clinical considerations. *Epilepsy Res.* **2**, 145–181.

Löscher, W., Honack, D., Fassbender, C.P. & Nolting, B. (1991): The role of technical, biological and pharmacological factors in the laboratory evaluation of anticonvulsant drugs. III. Pentylenetetrazole seizure models. *Epilepsy Res.* **8**, 171–189.

Lowenstein, D.H. (1995): The stress protein response and its potential relationship to prolonged seizure activity. *Clin. Neuropharmacol.* **18**, 148–158.

Meldrum, B.S. (1983): Metabolic factors during prolonged seizures and their relation to nerve cell death. In: *Advances in neurology, Vol 34: Status epilepticus,* Delgado-Escueta, A.V., Wasterlain, C.G., Treiman, D.M. & Porter, R.J. (eds), pp. 261–270. New York: Raven Press.

Michelson, H. & Lothman, E. (1991): An ontogenetic study of kindling using rapidly recurring hippocampal seizures. *Dev. Brain Res.* **61**, 79–85.

Miller, J.W. & Ferrendelli, J.A. (1991): Brain stem and diencephalic structures regulating experimental generalized (pentylentetrazol) seizures in rodents. In: *Anatomy of epileptogenesis,* Meldrum, B.S., Ferrendelli, J.A. & Wieser, H.G. (eds), pp. 57–69. London: John Libbey.

Moshé, S.L., Albala, B.J., Ackerman, R.F. & Engel, J., Jr. (1983): Increased seizure susceptibility of the immature brain. *Dev. Brain Res.* **7**, 81–85.

Motte, J., Fernandes, M.J.S., Marescaux, C. & Nehlig, A. (1997): Effects of pentylenetetrazol-induced status epilepticus on c-Fos and HSP72 immunoreactivity in the immature rat brain. *Mol. Brain Res.* **50**, 79–84.

Motte, J., Fernandes, M.J.S., Baram, T.Z. & Nehlig, A. (1998): Spatial and temporal evolution of neuronal activation, stress and injury in lithium-pilocarpine seizures in adult rats. *Brain Res.*793; 61–72.

Nehlig, A. & Pereira de Vasconcelos, A. (1993): Glucose and ketone body metabolism in the neonatal rat brain. *Prog. Neurobiol.* **40**, 163–221.

Nehlig, A., Pereira de Vasconcelos, A. & Boyet, S. (1988): Quantitative autoradiographic measurement of local cerebral glucose utilization in freely moving rats during postnatal development. *J. Neurosci.* **8**, 2321–2333.

Nehlig, A., Pereira de Vasconcelos, A. & Boyet, S. (1989): Postnatal changes in local cerebral blood flow measured by the quantitative autoradiographic [^{14}C]iodoantipyrine technique in freely moving rats. *J. Cereb. Blood Flow Metab.* **9**, 579–588.

Nevander, G., Ingvar, M., Auer, R.N. & Siesjö, B.K. (1985): Status epilepticus in well-oxygenated rats causes neuronal necrosis. *Ann. Neurol.* **18**, 281–290.

Nitecka, L., Tremblay, E., Charton, G., Bouillot, J.P., Berger, M.L. & Ben-Ari, Y. (1984): Maturation of kainic acid seizure–brain damage syndrome in the rat. II. Histopathological sequelae. *Neuroscience* **13**, 1073–1094.

Pardridge, W.M. & Oldendorf, W.H. (1977): Transport of metabolic substrates through the blood–brain barrier. *J. Neurochem.* **28**, 5–12.

Pereira de Vasconcelos, A., El Hamdi, G., Vert, P. & Nehlig, A. (1992): An experimental model of generalized seizures for the measurement of local cereral glucose utilization in the immature rat. II. Mapping of brain metabolism using the quantitative [14C]2-deoxyglucose technique. *Dev. Brain Res.* **69**, 243–259.

Pereira de Vasconcelos, A., Boyet, S., Koziel, V. & Nehlig, A. (1995): Effects of pentylenetetrazol-induced status epilepticus on local cerebral blood flow in the developing rat. *J. Cereb. Blood Flow Metabol.* **15**, 270–283.

Pineau, N., Charriaut-Marlangue, C., Motte, J. & Nehlig, A. (1998): Pentylenetetrazol seizures induce cell suffering but not death in the immature rat brain. *Dev. Brain Res.* (in press).

Planas, A.M., Soriano, M.A., Ferrer, I. & Farré, E.R. (1994): Regional expression of inducible heat shock protein–70 mRNA in the rat brain following administration of convulsant drugs. *Mol. Brain Res.* **27**, 127–137.

Priel, M.R., Ferreira dos Santos, N. & Cavalheiro, E.A. (1996): Developmental aspects of the pilocarpine model of epilepsy. *Epilepsy Res.* **26**, 115–121.

Raichle, M.E. (1981): Measurement of local cerebral blood flow and metabolism in man with positron emission tomography. *Fed. Proc.* **40**, 2331–2334.

Sakurada, O., Kennedy, C., Jehle, J., Brown, J.D. & Sokoloff, L. (1978): Measurement of local cerebral blood flow with [14C]iodoantipyrine. *Amer. J. Physiol.* **234**, H59–H66.

Shimosaka, S., Yuen, T.S. & Simon, R.P. (1992): Distribution of HSP72 induction and neuronal death following limbic seizures. *Neurosci. Lett.* **138**, 202–206.

Siesjö, B.K., Ingvar, M., Folbergrova, J. & Chapman, A.G. (1983): Local cerebral circulation and metabolism in bicuculline-induced status epilepticus: relevance for development of cell damage. In: *Advances in Neurology, Vol 34: Status epilepticus,* Delgado-Escueta, A.V., Wasterlain, C.G., Treiman, D.M. & Porter, R.J. (eds), pp. 217–231. New York: Raven Press.

Söderfeldt, B., Fujikawa, D.G. & Wasterlain, C.G. (1990): Neuropathology of status epilepticus in the neonatal marmoset monkey. In: *Neonatal seizures. pathophysiology and pharmacological management,* Wasterlain, C.G. & Vert, P., pp. 91–98. New York: Raven Press.

Sokoloff, L., Reivich, M., Kennedy, C., Desrosiers, M.H., Patlak, C.S., Pettigrew, K.D., Sakurada, O. & Shinohara, M. (1977): The [14C]deoxyglucose method for the measurement of local cerebral glucose utilization: Theory, procedure, and normal values in the conscious and anesthetized albino rat. *J. Neurochem.* **28**, 897–916.

Sperber, E.F., Haas, K.Z., Stanton, P.K. & Moshé, S.L. (1991): Resistance of the immature brain to seizure-induced synaptic reorganization. *Dev. Brain Res.* **60**, 88–93.

Swann, J.W., Brady, R.J. & Martin, D.L. (1988): Posnatal development of GABA-mediated synaptic inhibition in rat hippocampus. *Neuroscience* **28**, 551–562.

Swann, J.W., Smith, K.L. & Brady, R.J. (1993): Localized excitatory synaptic interactions mediate the sustained depolarization of electrographic seizures in developing hippocampus. *J. Neurosci.* **13**, 4680–4689.

Tomioka, C., Nishioka, K. & Kogure, K. (1993): A comparison of induced heat shock protein in neurons destined to survive and those destined to die after transient ischemia in rats. *Brain Res.* **612**, 216–220.

Tremblay, E., Roisin, M.P., Represa, A., Charriaut-Marlangue, C. & Ben-Ari, Y. (1988): Transient increase density of NMDA binding sites in the developing rat hippocampus. *Brain Res.* **461**, 393–396.

Velisek, L., Kubova, H., Pohl, M., Stankova, L., Mares, P. & Schickerova, R. (1992): Pentylenetetrazol-induced seizures in rats: an ontogenetic study. *Naunyn-Schmiedeberg's Arch. Pharmacol.* **346**, 588–591.

Wasterlain, C.G. & Shirasaka, Y. (1994): Seizures, brain damage and brain development. *Brain Dev.* **16**, 279–295.

Wasterlain, C.G. & Dwyer, B.E. (1983): Brain metabolism during prolonged seizures in neonates. In: *Advances in neurology, Vol 34: Status epilepticus,* Delgado-Escueta, A.V., Wasterlain, C.G., Treiman, D.M. & Porter, R.J. (eds), pp. 241–260. New York: Raven Press.

Wasterlain, C.G., Dwyer, B.E. & Fujikawa, D. (1984): Metabolic studies of neonatal seizures in newborn marmoset monkeys: a possible role in the pathogenesis of brain damage for mismatch between flow and metabolism. In: *Cerebral blood flow, metabolism and epilepsy,* Baldy-Moulinier, M., Ingvar, D.H. & Meldrum, B.S. (eds), pp. 121–129. London: John Libbey.

Chapter 21

Long-term effects of recurrent seizures on the developing brain

Claude G. Wasterlain, Kerry W. Thompson, Harley Kornblum,
Andrey M. Mazarati, Yukiyoshi Shirasaka, Hiroshi Katsumori, Hantao Liu and
Raman Sankar

VA Medical Center, Sepulveda, CA 91343–2099, Department of Neurology and Brain Research Institute, UCLA School of Medicine, Los Angeles, CA 90095, USA

Introduction

Epilepsy is very common in infancy and childhood; status epilepticus (SE) is more common in children than in adults (infants 156/100,000/year; children 38/100,000/year; adults 27/100,000/year; De Lorenzo, 1998), and experimental evidence suggests that the propensity to develop SE is greater in immature than in mature animals (Moshé *et al.*, 1983; Okada *et al.*, 1984; Sperber *et al.*, 1992; Swann *et al.*, 1992). However, mortality from SE is lower in children than in adults (children 3 per cent, young adults 14 per cent, elderly 38 per cent in the Richmond study) and the controversy regarding the long-term consequences of seizures on the immature brain has never been resolved. Human evidence is equivocal, and traditional animal models show little damage from seizures in the immature brain (Wasterlain 1976; Albala *et al.*, 1984; Nitecka *et al.*, 1984), but recently developed models strongly dispute that result. The effects of severe, recurrent seizures which stay short of SE are even more hotly debated. However, given the frequent occurrence of severe seizures in the young, and the unquestionable risk of vigorous medical treatment, the question of vulnerability (or lack of it) of the developing brain to seizure-induced damage acquires great importance. If in neonates, in infants, or in children, epileptic seizures in the absence of any medical complications are incapable of producing brain damage and neuronal loss, there is no justification for running the risk of intravenous medications (in the case of SE) or of chronic drug administration (for less acute situations). On the other hand, if seizures themselves, when sufficiently severe and prolonged, cause neuronal loss in a particular age group, the risk of treatment must be balanced against the risk of brain damage from seizures to reach a reasonable therapeutic philosophy. Since the complexity of human clinical situations is such that definite evidence is rarely forthcoming, we must rely on experimental models to establish the basic principles of vulnerability. The human brain differs from that of lower mammals more in size and organization than in its basic cell biology, and the latter is the main determinant of neuronal injury. Experimental studies of neuronal injury have the advantage of being considerably more sensitive than human studies. Investigations into Parkinson's and Huntington's diseases have shown that for most cell groups in the brain, clinical symptoms do not appear until 80 per cent of the cells are lost. Furthermore, infants and children have a tremendous potential for recovery from even severe insults, so that a good outcome does not guarantee that no damage occurred. However, in animals, we can count injured neurons easily, and our control of experimental situations guarantees that clear answers can be obtained to basic biological questions. Of course, one could argue that only permanent damage should be of concern, so that even severe insults from which recovery is complete do not need to be treated. In this chapter, we will not examine the therapeutic implications but only the long-term consequences of seizures in the immature brain, with emphasis on cell survival and brain growth.

The consequences of status epilepticus in childhood: an unresolved clinical problem

Status epilepticus

Neuropathologists frequently find damage in the brains of children who died in SE (Corsellis & Bruton, 1983; Sagar & Oxbury, 1987; Margerison & Corsellis, 1996), but it is generally believed that 'it is not the status epilepticus that produces the damage but rather the underlying insult to the brain that causes both status epilepticus and damage' (Freeman, 1989). Margerison & Corsellis (1996) found hippocampal lesions in all cases of childhood SE that they autopsied, but the clinical details available to them were not sufficient to rule out a transient fall in blood pressure, or a period of hypoxemia, which might be contributing to or even be the only cause of the damage they found. Aicardi and collaborators (Aicardi & Chevrie, 1970; Aicardi & Baraton, 1971; Aicardi, 1986) studied childhood SE of over 1 h duration in community hospitals, and reported that one-third of their patients had acquired deficits acutely at the time of their seizures. They documented the development of atrophy after SE (Aicardi & Baraton, 1971; Aicardi, 1986). These studies show that some episodes of SE in children have bad outcomes, but they were retrospective and subject to all the limitations and pitfalls of retrospective studies. Maytal *et al.* (1989) studied 137 children with SE lasting over 30 min and treated in a teaching hospital, and found a much lower mortality and a much lower incidence of severe complications. Patients without pre-existing brain damage were few, but their incidence of newly acquired severe damage was only 2 per cent. Maytal *et al.* (1989) attributed the difference in outcome between the two studies to the retrospective nature of Aicardi's investigations, and on the selection factor which brings sicker patients to the attention of investigators. However, they did not rule out an alternative explanation, namely that better treatment in more sophisticated hospitals was the reason for the better outcome of the more recent study.

Febrile SE and severe febrile seizures

These seizures are very common, relatively benign and highly controversial. The definition of febrile SE is very much debated. Episodes of seizures lasting over 30 min, and apparently triggered by fever, are common, but many paediatricians do not consider them to be SE. The usual definition of febrile seizures precludes complications, and their outcome is uniformly good, but when severe seizures triggered by fever are examined, some bad outcomes are reported. Van Esch *et al.* (1996) reported a 24 per cent incidence of sequelae involving the nervous system after febrile SE. Maher & McLachlan (1995) found that, in families with febrile convulsions, the best predictor of medial temporal sclerosis was febrile seizures of long duration. Sagar & Oxbury (1987) found a correlation between neuronal loss in the temporal lobe and early childhood convulsions. Verity *et al.* (1993) reported neuronal deficits in 8 per cent of patients after seizures of long duration or SE. Schiottz-Christiansen & Bruhn (1973) found mild deficits in intellectual performance in monozygotic twins with febrile seizures compared with their monozygotic seizure-free twins raised in the same environment.

The catastrophic epilepsies of childhood

In West or Lennox–Gastaut syndromes, frequent EEG seizures are associated with mild convulsive activity and often with progressive intellectual and behavioural impairment. Behavioural regression (e.g. in West syndrome) is strikingly associated temporally with seizure activity, and anecdotal reports

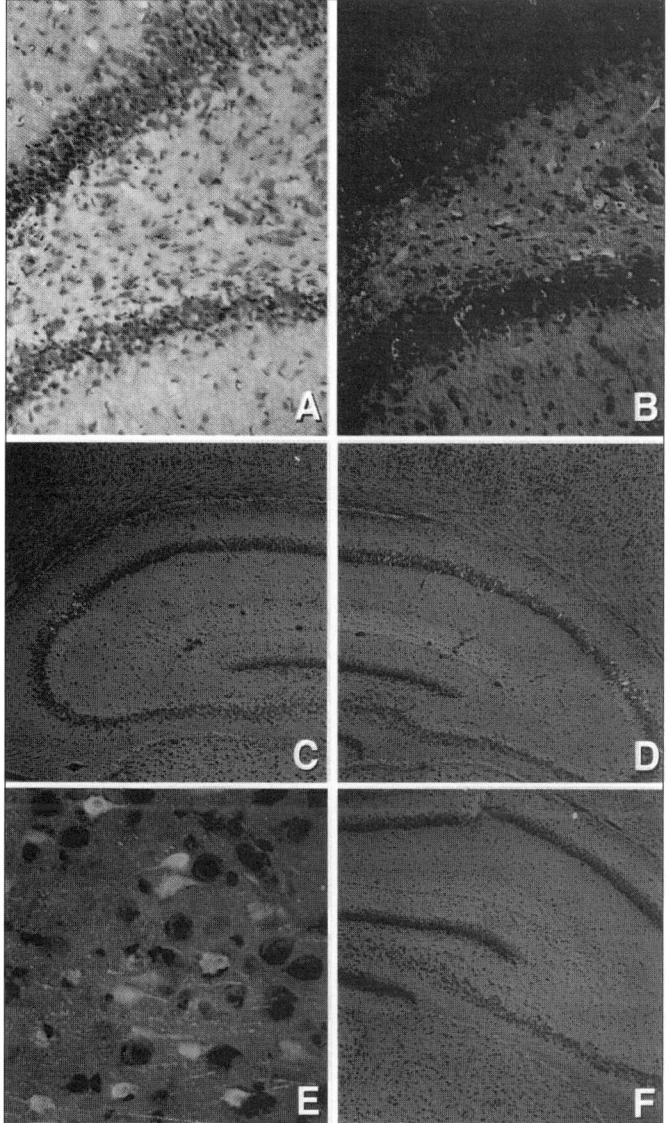

Fig. 1. Histological lesions 24 h after the end of perforant path stimulation. At 24 h, sections were processed for a standard H&E stain. In the stimulated hilus, cells viewed under light microscopy showed shrunken and pyknotic nuclei and eosinophilic cytoplasm (A), while under ultraviolet light necrotic cells showed bright yellow eosin fluorescence (B). This pattern of damage was seen in all stimulated animals. Many animals had additional damage in areas CA3, CA1 and subiculum (C, D & E). Control animals showed no hippocampal lesions. A fluorescent view of one unstimulated control animals (F) shows the electrode track through the pyramidal cell layer but no hilar or pyramidal cell damage resembling that seen in stimulated animals.

Reproduced from Thompson et al. (1998) with permission.

of improved developmental outcome after surgery to remove the epileptic zone (Asarnow et al., 1997) may suggest that this is brought about by protecting the rest of the brain from the spread of seizures. In the Landau–Kleffner syndrome, there is no good correlation between acquired neurological deficits and clinical seizures, and recent studies suggest that impairment is progressive when electrographic seizure activity occupies over 80 per cent of slow wave sleep for over two years (Ohtahara et al., 1998). Again, this might suggest that behavioural impairment is a result of ongoing seizure activity, but these studies are not sufficiently controlled to satisfactorily resolve these questions, and this very brief review does not cover the many studies in which developmental outcome is only correlated with seizure aetiology. Undoubtedly, with the advent of rapid MR which is available to be used in children, most of our questions regarding the long-term consequences of SE in humans will be resolved over the next few years, and until that happens we have to rely on experimental evidence.

Long-term effect of seizures in the young: experimental data

Some of the mechanisms for excitotoxic neuronal death are fully developed at an early age, while others appear late during development. During childhood, many brain regions in both rats and humans have a paucity of kainate receptors, but also show transient overexpression of brain NMDA and AMPA receptors, a transient overabundance of synaptic connections, and a metabolic rate higher than that of the adult (Chugani & Phelps, 1986; McDonald *et al.*, 1988). The result is that immature rats show enhanced vulnerability to injected excitotoxins in both cortex and hippocampus. Hypoxia–ischaemia also appears to very effectively kill neurons through excitotoxic mechanisms in immature animals (Hattori & Wasterlain, 1990). Seizures kill neurons in adults by excitotoxic mechanisms, which many neurons in the immature brain are able to respond to, therefore the question is whether seizures are able to activate those mechanisms in the immature brain.

Animal models of status epilepticus

We will examine four groups of studies: kainic acid SE; SE induced by flurothyl; SE induced by electrical stimulation; and SE induced by pilocarpine. Many of these models have only been examined in the rat, and predominantly around the age of postnatal day 15 (P15). In only a few of them is full ontogenic information available. This is a significant limitation, since neonates with a low metabolic rate and poorly connected neuronal circuitry are probably quite different from animals in the 'childhood' period, with very high metabolic rates, and a highly plastic and exuberant neural circuitry. The tendency to generalize conclusions by applying them to 'the immature brain' can at times overlook these vast biological differences.

Kainic acid SE

Kainic acid easily damages the hippocampus of adult rats, but fails to damage the hippocampus of rats aged P15 or younger (Albala *et al.*, 1984; Nitecka *et al.*, 1984). This clearly shows that not all seizures cause damage. However, this model has several serious drawbacks. In contrast to AMPA and NMDA receptors which are overexpressed in the immature brain, kainate receptors are not fully expressed until relatively late in life (Campochiaro & Coyle, 1978), and display low levels of expression in the hippocampus of P15 rats. This could be a significant factor in the paucity of damage induced by kainic acid SE in these animals. In fact, the resistance of the hippocampus to kainic acid SE could be species-specific: the P10 rabbit, which is at least as immature as P15 rats, shows extensive damage in response to kainic acid SE (Franck & Schwartzkroin, 1984). The high mortality induced by kainic acid SE is another problem in interpreting those results. Albala *et al.* (1984) reported no brain damage in 15-day-old survivors of kainic acid SE, but mortality was 90 per cent. While the brain of survivors showed no lesions, the brain of the 90 per cent of animals that died was not examined. The dose of 10 mg/kg of kainic acid used to produce damage in the adult rats was 100 per cent fatal to rat pups, and could not be studied. The dose used in pups (3 mg/kg) also fails to produce histological lesions in most adult rats. However, these experiments did establish the fact that 3 mg/kg of kainic acid induced repetitive seizures/SE in the pups, and therefore that even SE in young animals can have a benign outcome.

Flurothyl SE

The flurothyl model of SE was initially developed in our laboratory, and even after 2 h of SE in P4 rats, no histological damage is seen (Wasterlain, 1976). However, we developed this model specifically to stay short of inducing histological lesions, since our goal was to study the effect of seizures on brain growth. It is not clear what additional studies have been made to push this model to more severe levels of seizure activity. In other words, this model does show that 2 h of repetitive seizures induced by flurothyl do not produce histological lesions in P4 rats, but it does not show that flurothyl SE is incapable of producing lesions in immature rats.

SE induced by electrical stimulation

We stimulated the large glutamatergic projection from entorhinal cortex to hippocampus intermittently, in seizure-like fashion, in free-running P14-P16 rat pups (Thompson & Wasterlain, 1998, 1997a). The position of the electrode was optimized by recording the population spike from the recording electrode in the granule cell layer, and adjusting the position of the perforant path electrode to elicit a population spike with maximal amplitude. Stimulation used 10-s trains of a 20 Hz stimulus delivered once per minute to the perforant path (biphasic square wave stimuli, 30–40 V) with continuous 2 Hz. Several animals lost their population spike response to each train during the first hour of stimulation and were eliminated from the study. Two of 26 animals lost their population spike late during stimulation and were also discarded. We used two kind of controls: implanted unstimulated controls, and stimulated controls in which the stimulating electrode was raised until no population spike was elicited from the dentate gyrus electrode, so that they received the same amount of current but not the same amount of granule cell activation.

During stimulation, the rats showed frequent wet dog shakes and stereotyped hind limb scratching movements similar to those observed in kainic acid SE in immature rats (Albala *et al.*, 1984; Okada *et al.*, 1984). Of the 24 animals, only two displayed brief periods of clonic seizure-like activity of both forelimbs with occasional rearing. In the two animals which were sampled hourly during the 16 h of stimulation, granule cell population spikes decreased considerably in amplitude by 12 h. Response to paired pulses was tested immediately after the end of stimulation, and then daily until 72 h when most of the animals were perfused for histological studies. The remaining rats were tested once a week and sacrificed at one month.

Neuronal injury

The stimulated hilus showed extensive neuronal injury which predominated in the polymorph layer, and was less severe in the subgranular layer, together with milder CA3c pyramidal cell injury (Fig. 1). These lesions, which were strictly ipsilateral to the stimulus, were accompanied by bilateral damage to CA3 pyramidal cells (10 of 12 rats), which were considerably more severe on the side of stimulation. There was bilateral damage greater on the stimulated side in CA1 pyramids (six of 12 animals, bilateral in five) and subiculum (five of 12, all bilateral) and in granule cells. There was also extrahippocampal damage which was completely symmetrical in pyriform cortex (10 of 12 animals, sections loss in processing for one). No damage was seen in untreated controls or in implanted controls, but one of the stimulated controls showed injured neurons in pyriform cortex, similar in number and intensity to the damage seen in experimental animals, but occurring in the total absence of any hippocampal injury. This particular animal had frequent wet dog shakes during stimulation, and the possibility of seizure activity mediated by non-hippocampal circuits cannot be ruled out.

Hilar neurons showed classical 'ischaemic cell change' (Brown & Brierley, 1967) with a highly eosinophilic cytoplasm which was brightly fluorescent under ultraviolet light. The cytoplasmic fluorescence of hilar cells was already maximal 2 h after the end of stimulation, and did not evolve further. By contrast, injured granule cells and pyriform cortex neurons showed delayed development of fluorescence which was minimal (granule cells) or absent (pyriform neurons) at less than 24 h, and developed later but was never as marked as that seen in the cytoplasm of hilar neurons. This result documents the occurrence of neuronal death triggered by seizures only on the stimulated side, making it extremely unlikely that they are the result of a systemic change such as hypoxemia or hypotension, and very likely that they are the result of the seizure activity itself. These lesions are similar to those found in the brain of children dying in SE, and in the hippocampi of intractable epileptics who come to surgery after experiencing seizures early in life (Norman, 1964; Margerison & Corsellis, 1966; Corsellis & Bruton, 1983; Sagar & Oxbury, 1987). They clearly show that the resistance of the immature brain to seizure-induced damage is not absolute, and that seizures that are severe and prolonged enough can cause neuronal death.

The NMDA channel blocker MK801 significantly reduced seizure-associated cell loss, supporting the concept that, in the immature hippocampus, seizures kill neurons by excitotoxic mechanisms involving the activation of glutamate receptors (Thompson & Wasterlain, 1997b).

Dentate inhibitory circuits

Together with these histological changes, physiological changes were seen in response to perforant

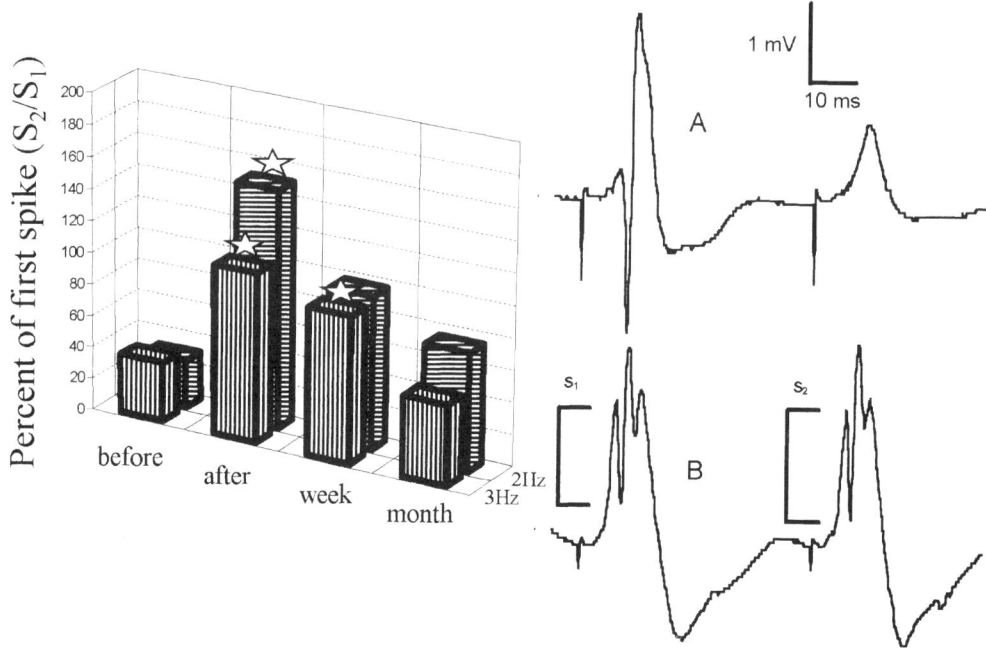

Fig. 2. Losses in frequency-dependent paired pulse inhibition following perforant path stimulation in 14–15-day-old rats. Paired pulses were delivered 50 ms apart, at 2 Hz (dark bars), and 3 Hz (open bars). Paired-pulse test responses were recorded before, immediately after (n = 12), one week (n = 7), and one month (n = 5) after stimulation. The results are expressed as the ratio of second spike (S2)/first spike (S1) × 100 (left side). Statistical significance was demonstrated using a one-way ANOVA. Symbols indicate significance (P < 0.05). The right side of the figure shows an example of the 2 Hz paired-pulse inhibition test. Before stimulation (A) the first spike activates inhibitory mechanisms which suppress the second granule cell spike. Immediately after stimulaton (B) the first spike (S1) no longer inhibits the second spike (S2). Black circles indicate the stimulus artifact. Reproduced from Thompson et al. (1998) with permission.

path stimulation. Immediately after stimulation, all animals showed a significant loss of frequency-dependent $GABA_A$-mediated inhibition at 2 and 3 Hz. At 2 Hz, the mean amplitude of the second population spike prior to stimulation was 29.7% ± 12.1 of the first, while after stimulation it was 149.8% ± 34.0 of the first (Fig. 2). At 3 Hz, the mean amplitude increased from 37.1% ± 16.5 to 106.3 % ± 4.7 following stimulation (n = 12). This loss persisted at 24 h and one week following stimulation, (mean amplitude of second population spike 92.7 % ± 12.8 over the first spike, n = 7) but was no longer significant one month after stimulation.

Granule cell dispersion

Folds in the granule cell layer were probably the result of shrinkage of the dentate gyrus of the hippocampus, but another frequent feature was the presence of granule cells in ectopic positions with dispersion outside the boundaries of the dentate gyrus (Fig. 3). This was seen much more frequently in pups than in adults, raising the possibility that this phenomenon is associated with the vigorous granule cell neuronogenesis (Bengzon et al., 1997) and neurotrophin induction (Kornblum et al., 1997) which follow seizures in the young.

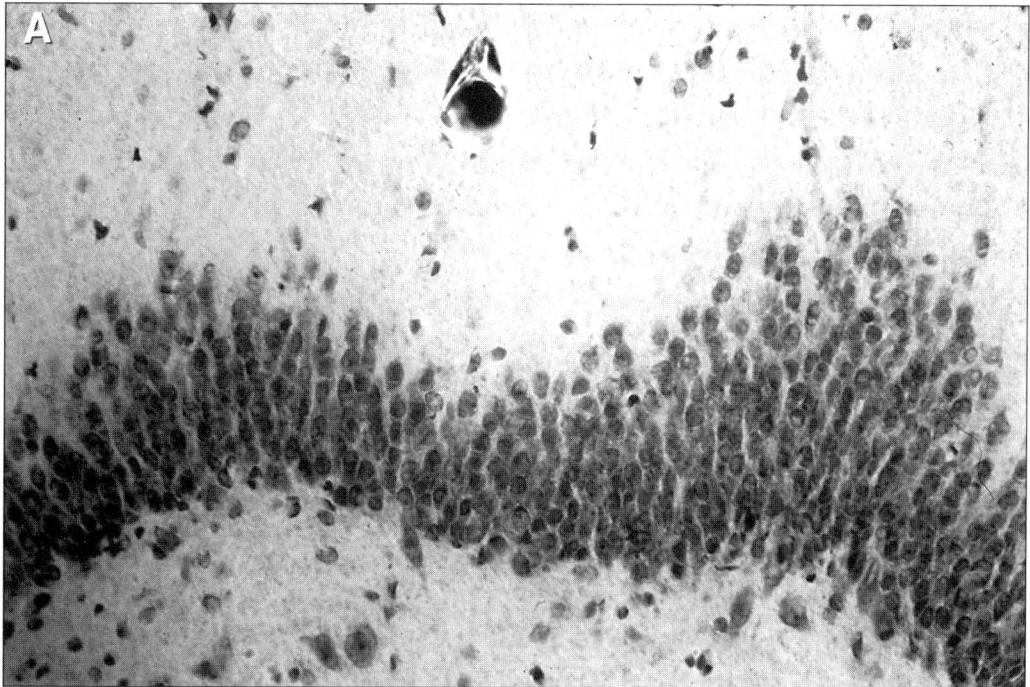

Fig. 3. One month after perforant path stimulation at P14, dispersion of dentate gyrus granule cells is evident. H&E, original magnification × 20.

Selective vulnerability of subpopulations of hilar interneurons

In animals killed one month after stimulation, cell counts in the stimulated hilus showed a significant reduction for cells stained with cresyl violet, with antisomatostatin antibodies, and with antineuropeptide Y antibodies, and a significant increase in staining density with anti-glial fibrillary acidic protein (GFAP) antibodies, but no significant difference was observed for cells stained with antiparvalubumin antibodies or with NADPH diaphorase stains, which localize nitric oxide synthase (NOS). The number of large (>5 µM) darkly staining neurons in the hilus was 54.2 ± 12.2 per section on the stimulated side versus 100.5 ± 10.2 per section on the unstimulated side ($P < 0.01$). When cell counts were limited to the tip of the hilus (Fig. 4), the number of large mossy cell-like neurons per section was reduced from 35.3 ± 4.7 (unstimulated side) to 9.7 ± 3.0 on the stimulated side ($P < 0.001$). There was a significant reduction in width of the hilus on the stimulated side (288 ± 20 µm), compared to the unstimulated side (415 ± 33 µm) while the granule cell layer was spared or had recovered. Somatostatin-immunoreactive cells on the stimulated side were reduced to 39 ± 12 per cent of the counts on the unstimulated side (Fig. 4A–B). These losses again were most marked in the polymorph area of the hilus. Neuropeptide Y (NPY)-immunoreactive neurons were also significantly reduced to 76 ± 6 per cent of the unstimulated side (Fig. 4C–D). NPY-immunoreactive cells in the subgranular layer appeared strikingly preserved. Parvalbumin-immunoreactive neurons were spared (Fig. 4E–F), while they are afflicted in adult SE, and so were cells staining for NADPH diaphorase or NOS. GFAP staining was more intense in the stimulated hilus, suggesting that gliosis had taken place (Fig. 4G–H). These results show that the selective vulnerability of subpopulations of interneurons, which is well documented after SE in the adult (Sloviter, 1987), is also present in the young, but that the cell populations involved are not identical. Damage at P14–16 appeared to disproportionately affect the somastostatin-immunoreactive cells, with lesser involvement of NPY-immunoreactive cells and

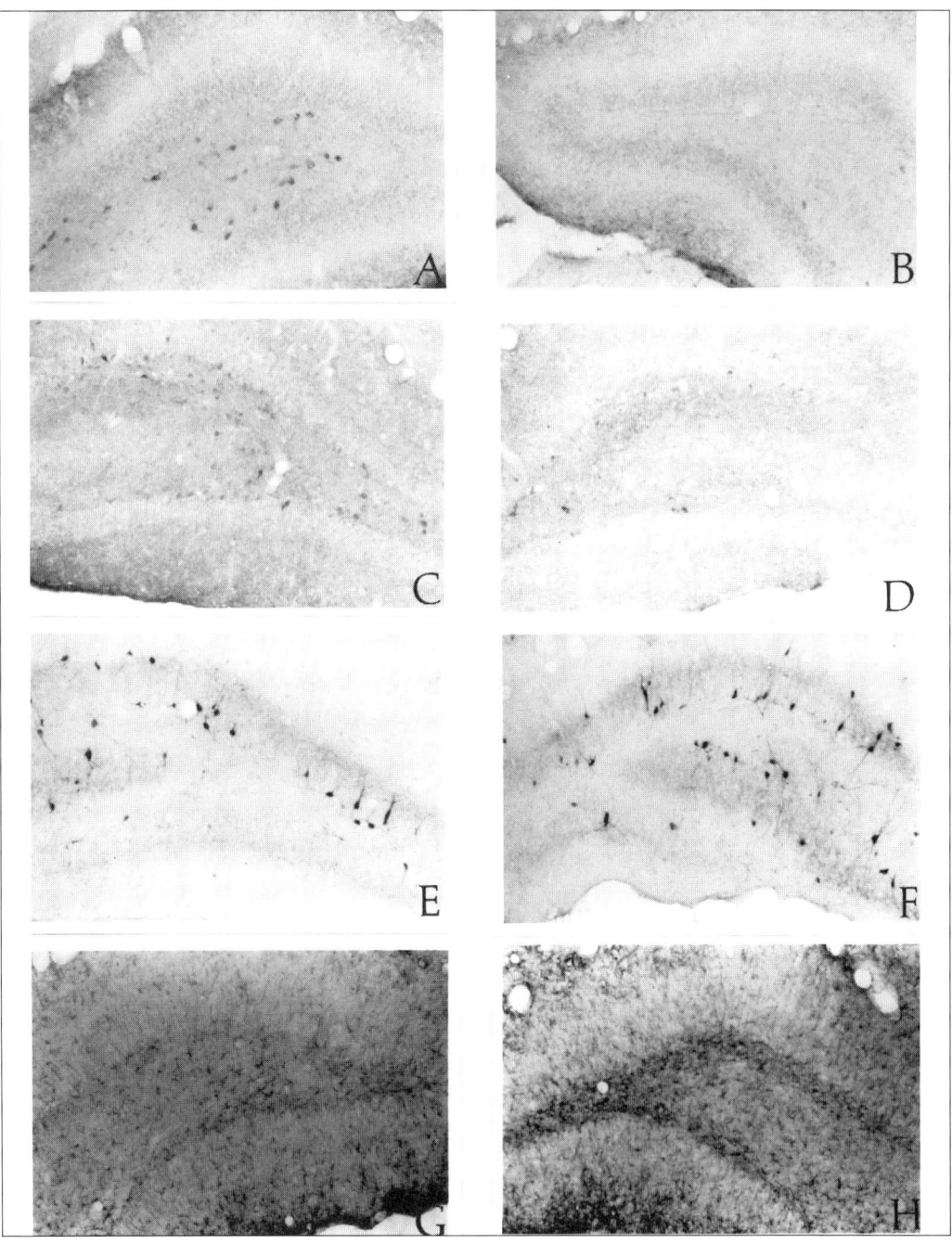

Fig. 4. Immunohistochemical staining one month after perforant path stimulation in young rats. Indirect immunohistochemical analysis showed significant losses in somatostatin-, and neuropeptide-Y-immunoreactive cells in the stimulated hilus (B & D) compared to the unstimulated hilus (A & C). No differences were seen in paravalbumin staining patterns between stimulated (F) and unstimulated (E) sides. GFAP staining showed increased staining in the stimulated hilus (H) compared to the unstimulated hilus (G). Reproduced from Thompson et al. (1998) with permission.

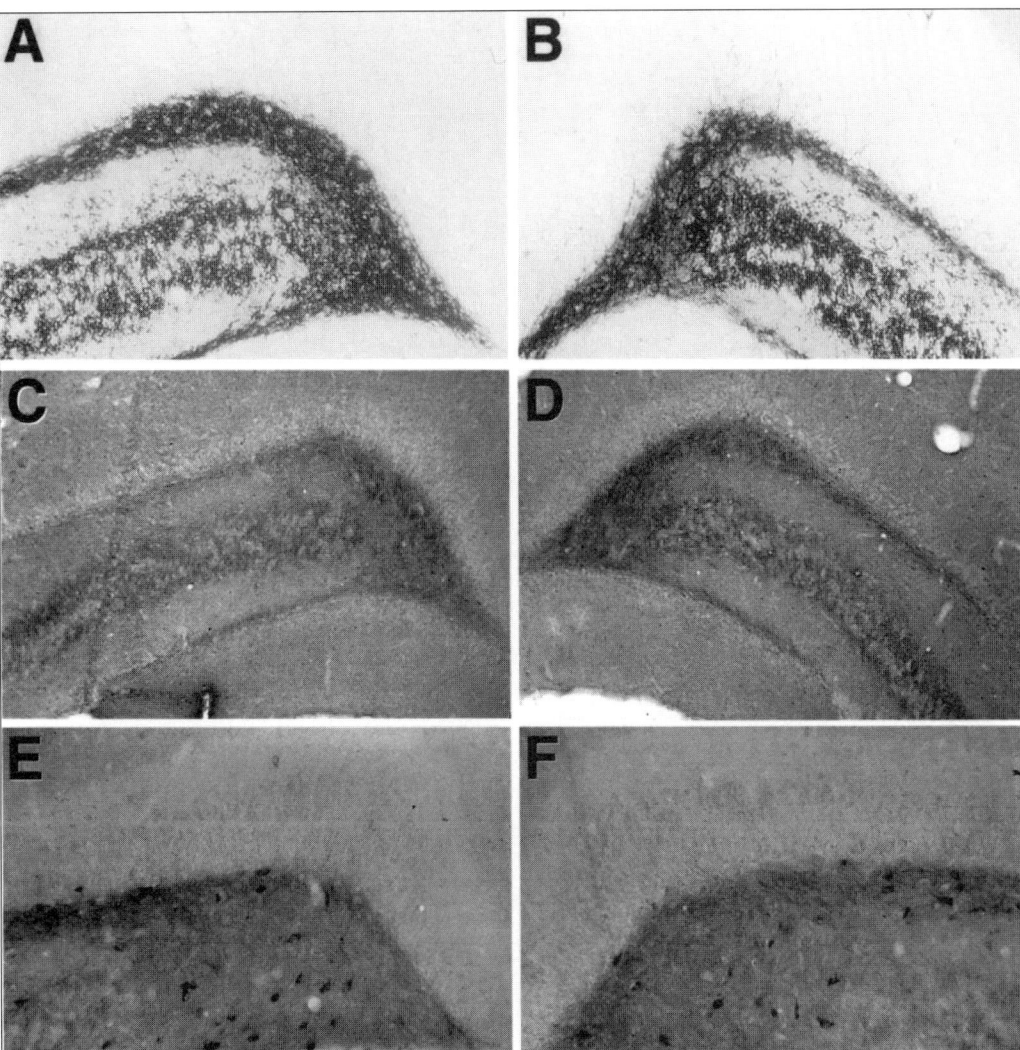

Fig. 5. One month after perforant path stimulation at P15, there is no difference in distribution of mossy fibres between the stimulated hippocampus and the contralateral, unstimulated hippocampus of the same rat with the Timm stain (B stimulated, A contralateral) or with dynorphin-like immunoreactivity (C contralateral, D stimulated). NPY-LI shows a reduced number of hilar cells on the stimulated side (F) compared to the contralateral hilus (E).

sparing of parvalbumin-immunoreactive cells. We cannot completely rule out a change in gene expression which made the peptidergic cells stop expressing their marker, but in view of the extensive acute neuronal injury affecting the same locations and of the overall reduction in neuronal numbers, cell death appears a more likely explanation for the differences observed at one month. The same subpopulations are also lost in the hippocampi of patients who come to surgery for intractable epilepsy (de Lanerolle et al., 1989). Many somatostatin-immunoreactive cells in the rat hilus have been shown to colocalize glutamate decarboxylase (GAD), while only 30 per cent of GAD-immunoreactive neurons colocalize somatostatin in this region. Many of the vulnerable NPY-immunoreactive neurons in the polymorph layer also colocalize GAD, and may have an inhibitory function. The loss of specific

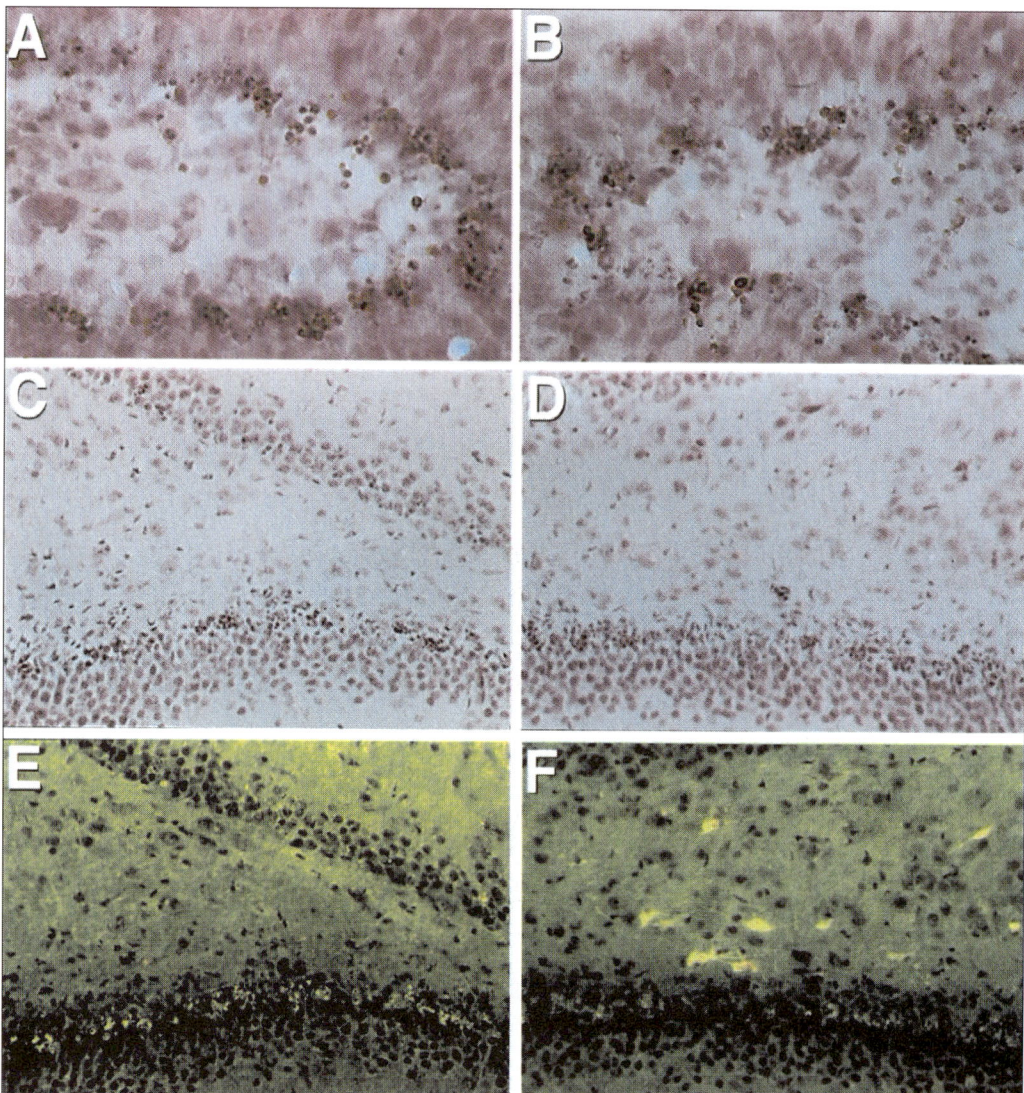

Fig. 6. In situ end-labelling 2 h after perforant path stimulation in the P15 rat. Labelled nuclei were seen in cells located within the inner layer of dentate granule cells bilaterally: (A, C & E) unstimulated hippocampus; (B, D & F) stimulated hippocampus. The cells within the hippocampus which contained labelled nuclei were eosinophilic (A–D) and fluorescent (E & F). Injured ISEL-positive cells in the granule cell layer were seen concomitantly with ISEL-negative injured cells within the hilus (D & F). From Thompson et al. (1998) with permission.

subpopulations of inhibitory hilar interneurons could account for the massive loss of GABAergic inhibition measured by the paired pulse method in our animals. Frequency-dependent paired pulse inhibition involves a mixture of feedback and feedforward circuits which are both $GABA_A$-mediated (Pollard *et al.*, 1994). The dentate gyrus is the gateway to excitatory hippocampal circuitry, and the hilar interneurons represent the single greatest brake to runaway excitation in the hippocampus, thus loss of those cells and the resulting loss of GABAergic inhibition could conceivably be epileptogenic. However, we observed only one animal which developed spontaneous SE during the first day after

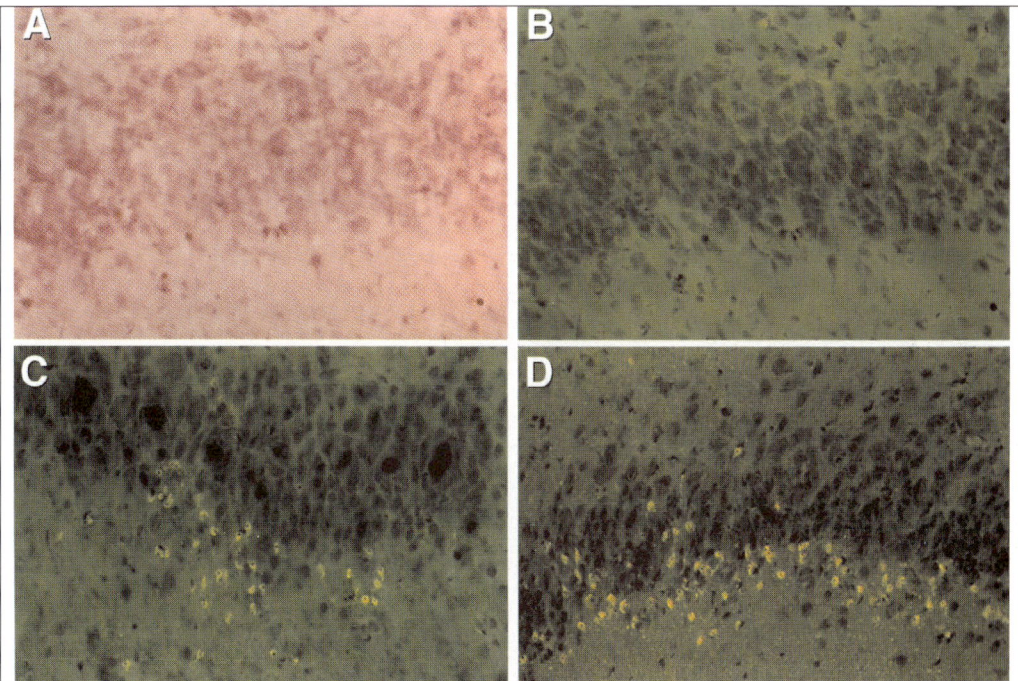

Fig. 7. (A) In situ end-labelling indicating the presence of DNA breaks is positive (red dots) within the prepyriform cortex 2 h after perforant path stimulation in a P15 rat. Sparse labelling was present in two of the three animals examined. (B) At the same time, histology (viewed under fluorescence as shown here or under regular light) is indistinguishable from controls. (C) and (D) 24 h (C) and 72 h (D) after perforant path stimulation, cytoplasmic fluorescence indicative of irreversible neuronal injury has developed in the same cell population that was ISEL positive earlier. From Thompson et al. (1998) with permission.

stimulation. This animal died in SE before its assigned perfusion time of 24 h and therefore was not included in the study. We did not see spontaneous seizures in the few chronic animals that we kept, but these animals were observed for only one month. Neither did we see mossy fibre sprouting by Timm staining or by dynorphin-like immunoreactivity, performed one month after stimulation (Fig. 5). At the time of that study, we were unaware of the fact that animals which develop chronic spontaneous seizures after lithium-pilocarpine SE at P15 do so with a delay of 4 to 6 months, much longer than that seen in adults after perforant path stimulation (usually less than one month, Shirasaka & Wasterlain, 1994). More animals and longer observation times after stimulation are needed to resolve that question of epileptogenicity.

Modes of neuronal death

Early nuclear DNA fragmentation was visualized using an in situ end labelling (ISEL) method derived from Gavrieli *et al.* (1992). This method labels both single- and double-stranded DNA breaks. While it is positive in apoptotic cells, it is not specific for apoptosis and can label reversibly injured cells. In the P15 rats after SE, hilar neurons were consistently and strikingly negative for ISEL. The combination of early development of cytoplasmic fluorescence and ISEL negativity raises the possibility that the death of hilar neurons was necrotic in nature. By contrast, inner layer granule cells and pyriform neurons showed early ISEL positivity which was scattered in pyriform cortex and laminar in distribution in granule cells (Fig. 6). Pyriform cortex neurons were ISEL-positive 2 h after stimulation, at a time when no cytoplasmic fluorescence was seen and the cells appeared relatively normal by light microscopy (Fig. 7). Twenty-four to 72 h later, increasing numbers of those cells showed 'ischaemic cell change' and cytoplasmic fluorescence. These results suggest that two different modes of cell death occur in the stimulated dentate gyrus and pyriform cortex. Hilar neurons show early cytoplasmic changes and no DNA breakdown, suggesting necrosis, while cell death in granule cells and pyriform neurons is characterized by early DNA breaks at a time when cell morphology is intact by light microscopy, followed by delayed neuronal degeneration. Definite studies have not been done in this model, but after lithium-pilocarpine SE at P15, early chromatin condensation by electron microscopy, evidence of caspase activation, ISEL and TUNEL positivity, and the presence of apoptotic bodies suggest that delayed neuronal death induced by seizures is apoptotic (see Chapter 18 of this book). There are interesting therapeutic implications of this duality of cell death, since late treatment is unlikely to rescue the cells which show early cytoplasmic changes, but could potentially salvage those which are undergoing apoptosis.

The presence of delayed neuronal death may also account for some of the discrepancies in the literature on neuronal vulnerability to seizures in immature animals. These young animals are very difficult to keep alive after SE, and to our knowledge our studies are the first to follow the temporal evolution of neuronal death after SE in the immature brain. Apoptotic neurons die quickly and quietly, and delayed neuronal death could easily be missed by the traditional method of early perfusion, since at early time points the neurons appear essentially normal by light microscopy. TUNEL positivity indicating double-stranded DNA breaks was quite widespread, not only in this model (in which the ISEL positive cells were also TUNEL positive) but also in the rabbit and marmoset models of SE described below. It is not possible to tell from this study whether the possibly necrotic nature of injury in hilar cells is cell-specific or reflects intense stimulation, since many hilar neurons receive direct excitatory input from the stimulated perforant path.

In summary, the presence of neuronal loss both one day and one month after stimulation shows that it is a severe and permanent result of seizure activity in this model. The unilaterality of hilar lesions proves that they result from neuronal firing and not from associated systemic complications. The loss of GABAergic inhibition and of GABAergic subpopulations of interneurons in the hilus demonstrate that SE at P15 can produce a state of hyperexcitability which might potentially be epileptogenic.

SE induced by pilocarpine or by lithium and pilocarpine

Pilocarpine SE in immature rats

While recent reviews have concluded that this model produces no damage in rat pups, in the original study of Cavalheiro *et al.* (1987) five of 14 rats between P10 and P21 showed lesions. Lithium-pilocarpine SE in immature rats, which produces very similar SE with a lower mortality, causes widespread neuronal loss in the vast majority of P15 rats (see Chapter 18 in this book). It is not clear why the models show different proportions of animals with neuronal loss after SE at P15, but it is clear that some animals show damage after SE at young ages in both models.

Lithium-pilocarpine SE in immature rabbits

We injected lithium (3 meq/kg i.p., 18 h before pilocarpine) and pilocarpine (200 mg/kg i.p.) in P10 rabbits, which are quite immature since the rabbit is a postnatal brain developer, and might be considered the rough equivalent of human neonates. This treatment induced severe limbic SE in those animals, with an average seizure duration of 1–3 h. Arterial blood pressure and blood gases were measured and did not decline during SE (Thompson *et al.*, 1998). Forty-eight h later, histological studies disclosed severe neuronal loss in the CA1 sector of hippocampus, with milder damage in hilus, in CA3, in amygdala, in pyriform and prepyriform cortex, and entorhinal cortex (Fig. 8). These results show that neuronal injury following SE is not restricted to the P15 rat, or to electrical stimulation models. In this rabbit model, neuronal injury was not the result of problems in oxygen delivery, since oxygen availability and blood pressure remained intact, but was probably the result of seizure activity.

CA1 neurons were strikingly TUNEL positive, suggesting the presence of extensive DNA breaks in those cells. Additional studies were not carried out to determine whether or not the mode of death was apoptotic.

Pilocarpine SE in immature marmosets

Marmosets aged 2–4 weeks were injected with lithium (3 meq/kg i.p., 18 h before pilocarpine) and pilocarpine (100 mg/kg i.p.). They were sacrificed 72 h after pilocarpine injection. Neuronal injury was severe in the reticular nucleus of the thalamus and in nucleus accumbens. Moderate neuronal loss was observed in amygdala, medial septum and caudate. Damage was mild in thalamus, in layers 4 and 5 of neocortex, in Ammon's horn, in the dentate hilus, and in pyriform and prepyriform cortex. TUNEL positivity was observed, suggesting the presence of extensive double stranded DNA breaks as well. These results suggest that SE can lead to neuronal loss in young primates as well as young rodents.

Expression of brain neurotrophins after SE in the immature brain

Most seizures induce the immediately early gene *c-fos* in adult rats, but not in the brain of P15 rats (Sperber *et al.*, 1991). Kainic acid seizures were reported not to induce neurotrophin mRNA in rats below P13 and to produce only very limited induction between P13 and P21 (Dugich *et al.*, 1992). Seizures were induced in Wistar rats of age P7 through adulthood (Kornblum *et al.*, 1997) with lithium (3 meq/kg i.p., 16 h before pilocarpine) and pilocarpine (100 mg/kg s.c.), and in a more limited group with kainic acid (3 mg/kg i.p. in P7 and P9 rats, $n = 7$ and 6 respectively). *In situ* hybridization for brain-derived neurotrophin factor (BDNF) mRNA was carried out in frozen sections, using a 540 base pair long antisequence which contained a 384 base pair sequence coding for rat BDNF exon 5. This sequence is present in all splice-variants of BDNF mRNA identified to date (Timmusk *et al.*, 1993). The sense sequence did not give any significant hybridization signal. ^{35}S-labelled cRNA was detected by autoradiography, and levels were quantified by densitometric analysis. Lithium-pilocarpine injection induced behavioural seizures at all ages studied, with animals P7–P14 exhibiting behavioural arrest, chewing, falling, clonus and tonic extension, and rats P14 and older also exhibiting clonic seizure activity with rearing. Behavioural and electrographic seizures started approximately 10 min after injections of pilocarpine, and SE-like continuous polyspike activity was the rule 20 min after injection. In response to this treatment, an increased BDNF mRNA expression was seen in the brain of all animals, but its distribution and magnitude varied greatly with age. At P7, elevations were restricted to hippocampal CA1 and to cingulate, pyriform and entorhinal cortices (Fig. 9). At P14, increases in BDNF mRNA were larger throughout the hippocampus, pyriform cortex, entorhinal cortex, amygdala, layers 2, 3, 5 and 6 of neocortex (with an additional narrow band in layer 4), in the superficial granule layer of cingulate cortex, midline thalamic nuclei, claustrum, and pyriform and anterior olfactory nuclei. Twenty one-day-old rats were similar to P14, and the same regions continued to show increases in older ages including adults. At P12, elevations in BDNF mRNA peaked 2 to 4 h after injection and lasted at least 8 h. Pretreatment with diazepam (25 mg/kg i.p.) blocked behavioural and electrographic seizures and completely blocked the changes in BDNF mRNA in P11 rats, suggesting that elevations were the result of seizure activity and not the direct effect of lithium and/or pilocarpine.

A limited number of P7 ($n = 7$) and P9 ($n = 6$) rats were subjected to kainic acid SE. They developed behavioural and electrographic seizures within 10 min of injection, and within 2 h of injection BDNF mRNA densities were markedly elevated within the CA3 pyramidal cell layer of the hippocampus (340 per cent elevation at P7). Two of six P9 animals also showed widespread extrahippocampal elevations of BDNF mRNA.

These results demonstrate that seizure activity in the immature brain elevates expression of BDNF massively, and suggest that elevation may be present in most cells which increase their firing rate in response to seizure activity. For example, the restricted region of BDNF mRNA activation seen in

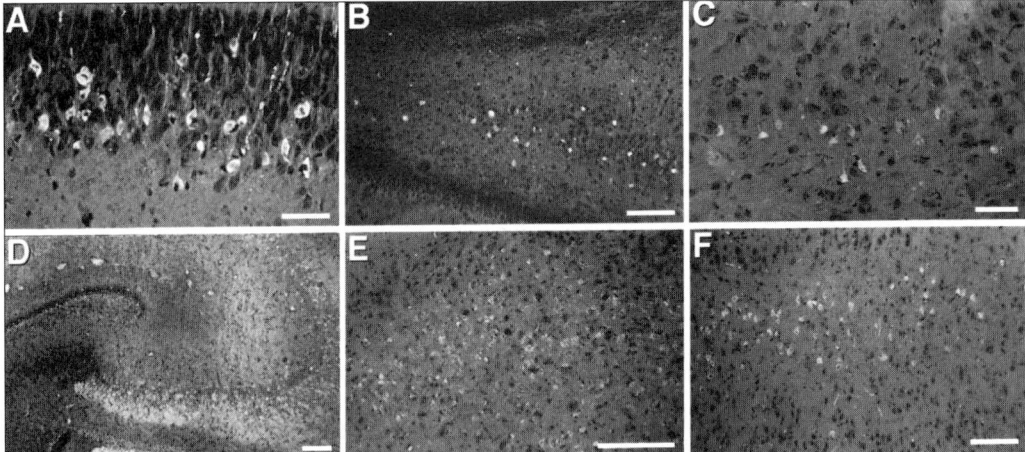

Fig. 8. Histological lesions in rabbits treated with Li-pilocarpine. Lesions in CA1 (A) were seen in all animals which had severe seizures. Other hippocampal areas involved were the hilus (B), area of CA3 and the subiculum (C). The most severe case of hippocampal damage is shown in (D) with total destruction of the CA1 and CA3 pyramidal cell layers. Extra-hippocampal structures were damaged in many of the experimental animals: examples are the amygdala (E) and the perihinal cortex (F). Scale bars represent μm (A), 200 μm (E) and 100 μm (F). (D) is a micrograph of a section stained with H and E viewed without fluorescent filters and u.v. exposure: all others are with filters. Reproduced from Thompson et al. (1997a) with permission.

our kainic acid animals precisely matches the areas reported to be activated with seizures at those ages by Tremblay *et al.* (1984) using the 2-deoxyglucose method to demonstrate increased metabolic activity. Neurotrophins enhance neuronal differentiation and neurite outgrowth *in vitro*, thus the possibility exists that they might modify brain growth following SE and lead to abnormal patterns of innervation which could contribute to epileptogenesis (Gall, 1993) and to abnormal brain development (Wasterlain, 1976). They may also contribute to cell protection, since BDNF has been shown to increase survival of injured neurons (Cheng & Mattson, 1994; Lindvall *et al.*, 1994; Larmet *et al.*, 1995). The possibility of deleterious effects also exists, since under some circumstances neurotrophins can enhance neuronal death (Koh *et al.*, 1995). BDNF expression may also be a factor in the neuronogenesis induced by SE (Bengzon *et al.*, 1997; Parent *et al.*, 1997) and in regenerative responses including mossy fibre sprouting, which is observed after many types of experimental SE.

Effect of recurrent single seizures on the developing brain

Even in the absence of histological lesions, repeated seizures in the immature brain can reduce brain growth (Wasterlain & Plum, 1973; Wasterlain, 1976; Wasterlain & Sankar, 1993), curtail the amount of myelin present in the brain (Dwyer & Wasterlain, 1982), and reduce markers of the establishment of synaptic connections (Jorgensen *et al.*, 1980). They also delay behavioural milestones significantly (Wasterlain, 1977), although permanent behavioural deficits have not been demonstrated but neither have they been tested for. Growth-dependent effects of seizures vary with the developmental stage of the animal in which they occur, and tend to be more severe at younger ages. The demonstration by Cavazos & Sutula (1990) that single seizures in the adult can cause neuronal loss is of unknown significance for the immature brain. The threshold for seizure intensity and severity that could cause neuronal loss in the immature brain has not been determined, and the mechanism of neuronal death with seizure repetition even in the adult is not understood. It may be important for future studies to determine whether electrographic seizure activity alone (such as that seen in electrical SE during slow-wave sleep), or focal seizure activity of a sustained nature, or repeated single seizures can induce

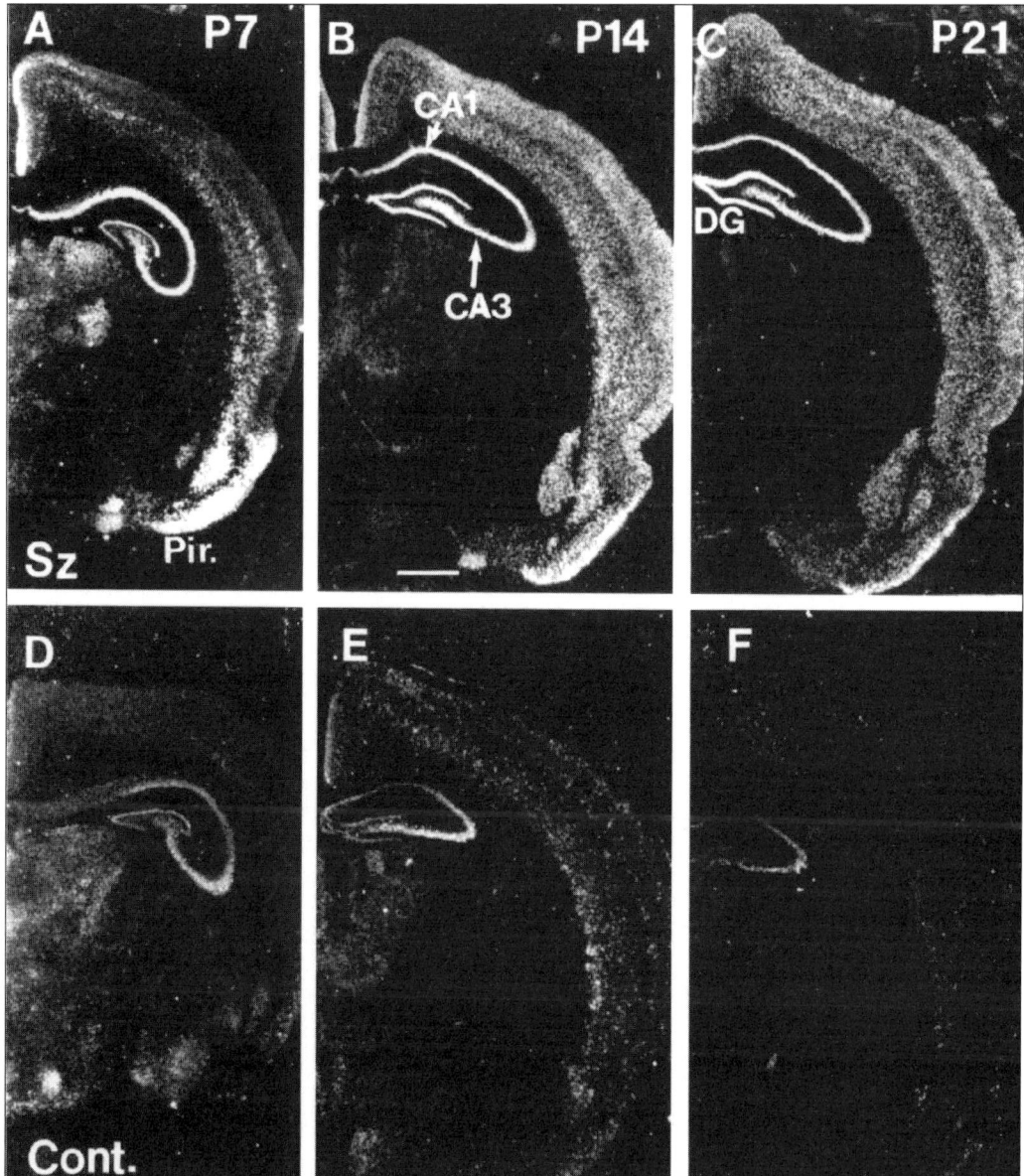

Fig. 9. Effects of lithium-pilocarpine treatment on BDNF mRNA expression in developing rat brain. Rats were treated on P7 (A & D), P14 (B & E), or P21 (C & F) with lithium-pilocarpine (A–C) or with vehicle (D–F) and killed 2 h later. Panels show dark-field photomicrographs of emulsion autoradiograms. Each experimental (sz) slide was processed and photographed under conditions indentical to the paired control (cont.) slide. However, sections A & D were exposed to the emulsion for a longer period of time than were B, C, E & F, which were all exposed for identical time periods. Note elevated hybridization densities in all experimental seizure tissue as compared with labelling in paired controls.

Abbreviations: CA1, area CA1 stratum pyramidale; CA3, area CA3 stratum pyramidale; DG, dentate gyrus stratum granulosum; Pir, piriform cortex.

Scale bar = 1 mm. Reproduced from Kornblum et al. (1997) with permission.

apoptosis or other modes of neuronal death in the immature brain, and whether such loss can be made up by neurogenesis, by reducing physiological programmed cell death, by enhanced growth factor production, or by other adaptive mechanisms.

Conclusions

These studies demonstrate that the immature brain is vulnerable to seizure-induced and stimulation-induced neuronal death, and suggest that specific populations of neurons are vulnerable to seizure-induced damage, and that these subpopulations may vary with age. Severe seizures in the young brain may cause both necrosis and apoptosis of neurons and trigger a massive elevation of neurotrophic factors which may play a role in the developmental effects of seizures.

Acknowledgements: We are indebted to B. Blackburn for preparation of the manuscript. Supported by the Research Service of the V.H.A., and by Research Grant NS13515 from NINDS.

References

Aicardi, J. (1986): Consequences and prognosis of convulsive status epilepticus in infants and children. *Jpn. J. Psych. Neurol.* **40**, 283–290.

Aicardi, J. & Baraton, J. (1971): A pneumoencephalographic demonstration of brain atrophy following status epilepticus. *Dev. Med. Child Neurol.* **13**, 660–667.

Aicardi, J. & Chevrie, J.J. (1970): Convulsive status epilepticus in infants and children: A study of 239 cases. *Epilepsia* **11**, 187–197.

Albala, B, Moshé, S. & Okada, R. (1984): Kainic-acid-induced seizures: A developmental study. *Dev. Brain Res.* **13**, 139–148.

Asarnow, R.F., LoPresti, C., Elliott, T., Cynn, V., Shields, W.D., Peacock, W.J., Shewmon, D.A., Sankar, R. & Guthrie, D. (1997): Developmental outcomes in children receiving resective surgery for medically intractable infantile spasms. *Dev. Med. Child Neurol.* (in press).

Bengzon, J., Kokaia, Z., Nanobashvili, A., Kokaia, M. & Lindvall, O. (1997): Apoptosis and proliferation of dentate gyrus neurons after single and intermittent limbic seizures. *Proc. Natl. Acad. Sci. USA* **94**, 10432–10437.

Brown, A.W. & Brierley, J.B. (1968): The nature, distribution and earliest changes of anoxic-ischaemic nerve cell damage in the rat brain as defined by the optical microscope. *Brit. J. Exp. Pathol.* **49**, 87–106.

Campochiaro, P. & Coyle, J.T. (1978): Ontogenic development of kainate neurotoxicity: correlates with glutamatergic innervation. *Proc. Natl. Acad. Sci. USA* **75**, 2025–2029.

Cavalheiro, E., Silva, D., Turski, W., Calderazzo-Filho, L., Bartolotto, Z. & Turski, L. (1987): The susceptibility of rats to pilocarpine is age dependent. *Dev. Brain Res.* **37**, 43–58.

Cavazos, J.E. & Sutula, T.P. (1990): Progressive neuronal loss induced by kindling: a possible mechanism for mossy fiber synaptic reorganization and hippocampal sclerosis. *Brain Res.* **527**, 1–6.

Cheng, B. & Mattson, M.P. (1994): NT–3 and BDNF protect CNS neurons against metabolic/excitotoxic insults. *Brain Res.* **640**, 56–67.

Chugani, H.I. & Phelps, M.E. (1986): Maturational changes in cerebral function in infants determined by 18FDG positron emission tomography. *Science* **231**, 840–843.

Corsellis, J.A.N. & Bruton, C.J. (1983): Neuropathology of status epilepticus in humans. In: *Status epilepticus: mechanisms of brain damage and treatment*, Delgado-Escueta, V.A., Wasterlain, C.G., Treiman, D.M. & Porter, R.J. (eds), pp. 129–139. New York: Raven Press.

de Lanerolle, N.C., Kim, J.H., Robbins, R.J. & Spencer, D.D. (1989): Hippocampal interneuron loss and plasticity in human temporal lobe epilepsy. *Brain Res.* **495**, 387–395.

De Lorenzo, R.J. (1998): Epidemiology of status epilepticus: incidence, causes and clinical presentation. In: *Status epilepticus*, Treiman, D.M. and Wasterlain, C.G. (eds). New York: Lipincott-Raven (in press).

Dugich, D.M., Tocco, G., Lapchak, P.A., Pasinettim G.M., Najam, I., Baudry, M. & Hefti, F. (1992): Regionally specific and rapid increases in brain-derived neurotrophic factor messenger RNA in the adult rat brain following seizures induced by systemic administration of kainic acid. *Neuroscience* **47**, 303–315.

Dwyer, B.E. & Wasterlain, C.G. (1982): Electroconvulsive seizures in the immature brain adversely affect myelin accumulation. *Exp. Neurol.* **78,** 616–628.

Franck, J.E. & Schwartzkroin, P.A. (1984): Immature rabbit hippocampus is damaged by systemic but not intraventicular kainic acid. *Dev. Brain Res.* **13,** 219–227.

Freeman, J.M. (1989): Status epilepticus: it's not what we've thought or taught. *Pediatrics* **83,** 444–445.

Gall, C.M. (1993): Seizure-induced changes in neurotrophin expression: implications for epilepsy. *Exp. Neurol.* **124,** 150–166.

Gavrieli, Y., Sherman, Y. & Ben-Sasson, S.A. (1992): Identification of programmed cell death in situ via specific labeling of nuclear DNA fragmentation. *J. Cell Biol.* **1193,** 493–501.

Hattori, H. & Wasterlain, C.G. (1990): Excitatory amino acids in the developing brain: ontogeny, plasticity and excitotoxicity. *Pediatric Neurol.* **6,** 219–228.

Jorgensen, O.S., Dwyer, B.E. & Wasterlain, C.G. (1980): Synaptic proteins after electroconvulsive seizures in immature rats. *J. Neurochem.* **35,** 1235–1237.

Koh, Y.T., Gwag, F.J., Lobnerm D. & Choi, D.W. (1995): Potentiated necrosis of cultured cortical neurons by neurotrophins. *Science* **268,** 573–575.

Kornblum, H.I., Sankar, R., Shin, D.H., Wasterlain, C.G. & Gall, C.M. (1997): Induction of brain derived neurotrophic factor mRNA by seizures in neonatal and juvenile rat brain. *Mol. Brain Res.* **44,** 219–228.

Larmet, Y., Reibel, S., Carnahan, J., Nawa, H., Marescaux, C. & Depaulis, A. (1995): Protective effects of brain-derived neurotrophic factor on the development of hippocampal kindling in the rat. *NeuroReport* **6,** 1937–1941.

Lindvall, O., Koksaia, Z., Bengzon, J., Elmer, E. & Koksaia, M. (1994): Neurotrophins and brain insults. *Trends Neurosci.* **17,** 490–496.

Maher, J. & McLachlan, R.S. (1995): Febrile convulsions. Is seizure duration the most important predictor of temporal lobe epilepsy? *Brain* **118,** 1521–1528.

Margerison, J.H. & Corsellis, J.A.N. (1996): Epilepsy and the temporal lobes: a clinical, electroencephalographic and neuropathological study of the brain with particular reference to the temporal lobes. *Brain* **89,** 680–708.

Maytal, J., Shinnar, S., Moshé, S.L. & Alvarez, L.A. (1989): Low morbidity and mortality of status epilepticus in children. *Pediatrics* **83,** 323–331.

McDonald, J., Silverstein, F. & Johnston, M. (1988): Neurotoxicity of N-methyl-D-aspartate is markedly enhanced in developing rat central nervous system. *Brain Res.* **459,** 100–103.

Moshé, S.L., Albala, B.J., Ackermann, R.F. & Engel, J. Jr. (1983): Increased seizure susceptibility of the immature brain. *Brain Res.* **283,** 81–85.

Nitecka, L., Tremblay, E., Charton, G., Bouillot, J.P., Berger, M. & Ben-Ari, Y. (1984). Maturation of kainic acid seizure-brain damage in the rat. II. Histopathological sequellae. *Neuroscience* **13,** 1073–1094.

Norman, R.M. (1969): The neuropathology of status epilepticus medicine, *Science and the Law* **4,** 46–51.

Ohtahara, S., Yamatogi, Y., Kobayashi, K., Nishibayashi, N. & Ohmori, I. (1998): Nonconvulsive status epilepticus in children with special reference to ESES syndromes. In: *Status epilepticus,* Treiman, D.M. & Wasterlain, C.G. (eds). New York: Lipincott-Raven (in press).

Okada, R., Moshé, S.L. & Albala, B.J. (1984): Infantile status epilepticus and future seizure susceptibility in the rat. *Dev. Brain Res.* **15,** 177–183.

Parent, J.M., Yu, T.W., Leibowitz, R.T., Geschwind, D.H., Sloviter, R.S. & Lowenstein, D.H. (1997): *J. Neurosci.* **17,** 3727–3738. Dentate granule cell neurogenesis is increased by seizures and contributes to aberrant network reorganisation in the adult rat hippocampus.

Pollard, H., Charriaut-Marlangue, C., Cantagrel, S., Repressa, A., Robain, O., Moreau, J. & Ben-Ari, Y. (1994): Kainate-induced apoptotic cell death in hippocampal neurons. *Neuroscience* **631,** 7–18.

Sagar, H.J. & Oxbury, J.M. (1987): Hippocampal neuron loss in temporal lobe epilepsy: correlation with early childhood convulsions. *Ann. Neurol.* **22,** 334–340.

Schiottz-Christiansen, E. & Bruhn, P. (1973): Intelligence, behaviour and scholastic achievement subsequent to febrile convulsions: An analysis of discordant twin pairs. *Devel. Med. Child Neurol.* **15,** 565–575.

Shirasaka, Y. & Wasterlain, C.G. (1994): Chronic epileptogenicity following focal status epilepticus. *Brain Res.* **655,** 35–44.

Sloviter, R.S. (1987): Decreased hippocampal inhibition and a selective loss of interneurons in experimental epilepsy. *Science* **235**, 73–76.

Sperber, E.F., Haas, K.Z., Stanton, P.K. & Moshé, S.L. (1991): Resistance of the immature hippocampus to seizure-induced synaptic reorganization. *Dev. Brain Res.* **60**, 88–93.

Swann, J.W., Smith, K.L. & Brady, R.J. (1991): Age-dependent alterations in the operations of hippocampal neural networks. *Ann. N.Y. Acad. Sci.* **627**, 264–276.

Thompson, K.W. & Wasterlain, C.G. (1997a): Lithium-pilocarpine status epilepticus in the immature rabbit. *Brain Res.* **100**, 1–4.

Thompson, K.W. & Wasterlain, C.G. (1997b): Partial protection of hippocampal neurons by MK–801 during perforant path stimulation in the immature brain. *Brain Res.* **751**, 96–101.

Thompson, K.W., Holm, A.M. & Wasterlain, C.G. (1998): Focal status epilepticus produces neuronal necrosis in the immature brain. *Neuroscience* **82**, 337–334.

Timmusk, T., Palm, K., Metsis, M., Reintam, T., Paalme, V., Saarma, M. & Persson, H. (1993): Multiple promoters direct tissue-specific expression of the rat BDNF gene. *Neuron* **10**, 475–489.

Tremblay, E., Nitecka, L., Berger, M. & Ben-Ari, Y. (1984): Maturation of kainic acid seizure-brain damage syndrome in the rat. I. Clinical, electrographic and metabolic observations. *Neuroscience* **4**, 1051–1072.

Van Esch, A., Ramlal, I.R., van Steensel-Moll, H.A., Steyerberg, E.W. & Derksen-Lubsen, G. (1996): Outcome after febrile status epilepticus. *Dev. Med. Child Neurol.* **38**, 19–24.

Verity, C.M., Ross, E.M. & Golding, J. (1993): Outcome of childhood status epilepticus and lengthy febrile convulsions: findings of national cohort study. *BMJ* **307**, 225–228.

Wasterlain, C.G. (1976): Effect of neonatal status epilepticus on rat brain development. *Neurology* **26**, 975–986.

Wasterlain, C.G. (1977): Effect of neonatal seizures on ontogeny of reflexes and behavior. An experimental study. *Eur. Neurol.* **15**, 9–19.

Wasterlain, C.G. & Plum, F. (1973): Vulnerability of the developing brain to electroconvulsive seizures. *Arch. Neurol.* **29**, 38–45.

Wasterlain, C.G. & Sankar, R. (1993): Excitotoxicity and the developing brain. In: *Epileptogenic and excitotoxic mechanisms*, Avanzini, G., Fariello, R., Heinemann, U. & Mutani, R. (eds), pp. 135–151. John Libbey: London.

Chapter 22

The resiliency of the immature brain to seizure induced damage

E.F. Sperber[1,2], I.M. Germano[3], L.K. Friedman[2], J. Velíšková[1] and M.T. Romero[4]

[1]*Departments of Neurology &* [2]*Neuroscience, Albert Einstein College of Medicine, Bronx, NY 10461, USA;*
[3]*Department of Neurosurgery, Mount Sinai School of Medicine, New York, NY 10029, USA;*
[4]*Department of Psychology, State University of New York at Binghamton, Binghamton, NY 13902, USA*

Summary

Temporal lobe epilepsy in adulthood is often attributed to childhood seizures resulting in mesial temporal sclerosis. However, the relationship between temporal lobe epilepsy, childhood seizures and hippocampal sclerosis may not be apparent as previously believed. 'Is the hippocampal sclerosis a consequence of seizures early in life?' or 'Is the sclerosis a result of an injury that becomes epileptogenic?' A series of experiments were carried out to address these questions. To determine if seizures early in life produce hippocampal sclerosis, several neuropathological techniques were used. Damage was assessed at various times (acutely and chronically), at two levels of structural analysis (light electron microscopy) and in different cell types (neurons and glia). To establish whether a prior injury may increase the likelihood of seizures later in life, brain damage was produced by either radio frequency lesions or administration of methylazoxymethanol acetate. Results indicate that the immature brain is less vulnerable to seizure-induced damage than the mature brain. However, if the immature brain is compromised then there is an increased probability of seizures and seizure-induced damage.

Introduction

Over 100 years ago it was recognized that there is a link between epilepsy and mesial temporal sclerosis in adult patients (Sommer, 1880). In the mid 1960s, Falconer *et al.* (1964) reported that the sole abnormality in approximately half his patients with intractable seizures undergoing temporal lobectomy was mesial temporal sclerosis. In addition, it was suggested that there was an increased history of febrile convulsions in adults with temporal lobe epilepsy and mesial sclerosis (Falconer, 1974; Mathison, 1975). Based on retrospective studies, Falconer proposed that mesial temporal sclerosis was a result of seizures early in life and over time the cause of adult epilepsy. However, in recent years, an ongoing debate has emerged regarding the relationship between seizures early in life and epilepsy in adulthood.

Prospective studies suggest that seizures in childhood may not necessarily be associated with seizures in adulthood. For instance, the likelihood of recurrent status epilepticus in children is small and appears to be dependent on age (Shinnar *et al.*, 1997) and aetiology (Berg & Shinnar, 1991; Dunn, 1988; Maytal & Shinnar, 1990; Shinnar *et al.*, 1992). Although seizure recurrence is low for most aetiologies (excluding remote symptomatic) it is particularly low in children with febrile seizures. It has been reported that of 28 children who had febrile seizures, none of these children had prior unprovoked seizures and only one had a recurrent seizure (Shinnar *et al.*, 1992). These findings are consistent with earlier epidemiological studies which indicate that only a small percentage of children with febrile seizures have recurrent episodes (Hauser & Kurland, 1975; Nelson & Ellenberg, 1976). These children frequently have atypical seizures associated with other neurological dysfunctions. Similarly, in children with neurological impairment, the incidence of recurrent status epilepticus is significantly greater as compared to children who are otherwise neurologically normal (Shinnar *et al.*, 1992). Therefore, it appears that the probability of recurrent seizures in childhood, particularly febrile seizures, may be less likely than previously suggested.

This raises the question, 'Is hippocampal sclerosis a result of seizures early in life?', as proposed by Falconer or 'Is the sclerosis a result of some prior damage which becomes epileptogenic over time?'. We addressed this question by first determining the extent to which the immature brain was vulnerable to seizure-induced damage. Damage was assessed over time (acutely and chronically), at various levels of structural analysis (light electron microscopy) and in different cell types (neurons as well as glia). The potential role of calcium binding proteins and heat shock proteins in neuroprotection was assessed. Secondly, to determine whether a prior injury may increase the likelihood of seizures later in life, brain damage was produced by either lesions or administration of a teratogen. Changes in seizure vulnerability were examined during development and in adulthood.

Seizure-induced damage is age related

Initial studies determined the extent to which the immature brain was vulnerable to seizure-induced damage. Five, 14-day-old and adult rats were in status epilepticus for 30 min following kainic acid treatment and the hippocampus was examined for cell loss 2 weeks later using a nissl stain (Sperber *et al.*, 1991). Extensive CA3 lesions were observed in adult brains, in marked contrast to the 5- and 14-day-old intact rat brain (Figs. 1A and D). These findings confirmed earlier studies with kainic acid (Holmes & Thompson, 1988; Nitecka *et al.*, 1984) and pilocarpine (Cavalheiro *et al.*, 1987) in young rat pups. In addition, two weeks after the seizure, hippocampal tissue from both age groups was stained for mossy fibre synaptic reorganization using the Timm silver sulphide stain (Timm, 1958). In response to cell loss or lesioning of its afferents, the dentate granule cell mossy fibres, which normally terminate on pyramidal cells, reorganize and send new synaptic terminals into the supragranular layer. In adult rats, following kainic acid status epilepticus, a dense band of newly sprouted mossy fibre terminals has been reported in the supragranular layer (Cronin & Dudek, 1988; Tauck & Nadler, 1985). In contrast, in the immature brain, no positive Timm staining was apparent in this area (Sperber *et al.*, 1991). This indicates that seizure-induced synaptic rearrangement in the hippocampus is age-related (Figs. 1B and E).

It is possible that there may have been cell loss shortly after the seizure, however, due to the greater plasticity of the immature brain, damage was no longer apparent when the brains were examined two weeks after the seizure. Therefore, the silver impregnation stain for lysosomal processes was used as a marker of acute neuronal degeneration (Nadler & Evenson, 1983). Extensive pyramidal cell degeneration was present in the adult CA3 area and hilus 24 h after kainic acid status epilepticus. Similar results have been reported by others (Gruenthal *et al.*, 1986; Sater & Nadler, 1987). In contrast, in 5- and 14-day-old rats, 24 h after kainic acid status epilepticus, there was an absence of acute neuronal degeneration and pyramidal cells appeared morphologically normal and intact throughout the hippocampus (Friedman *et al.*, 1997). This suggests that the developing brain is also resistant to acute neuronal degeneration (Figs. 1E and F).

It is conceivable that damage occurs in the immature brain, but it is so subtle that it can only be observed at the ultrastructural level. Therefore, the hippocampus was examined in both adult and 14-day-old rats two weeks after kainic acid status epilepticus using electron microscopy. Adult sections from kainic acid treated rats had several abnormalities. These included irregular cytoplasmic organelles, in addition to the presence of lucent vacuoles and an abundance of degenerating profiles. In contrast, the

Chapter 22 The resiliency of the immature brain to seizure induced damage

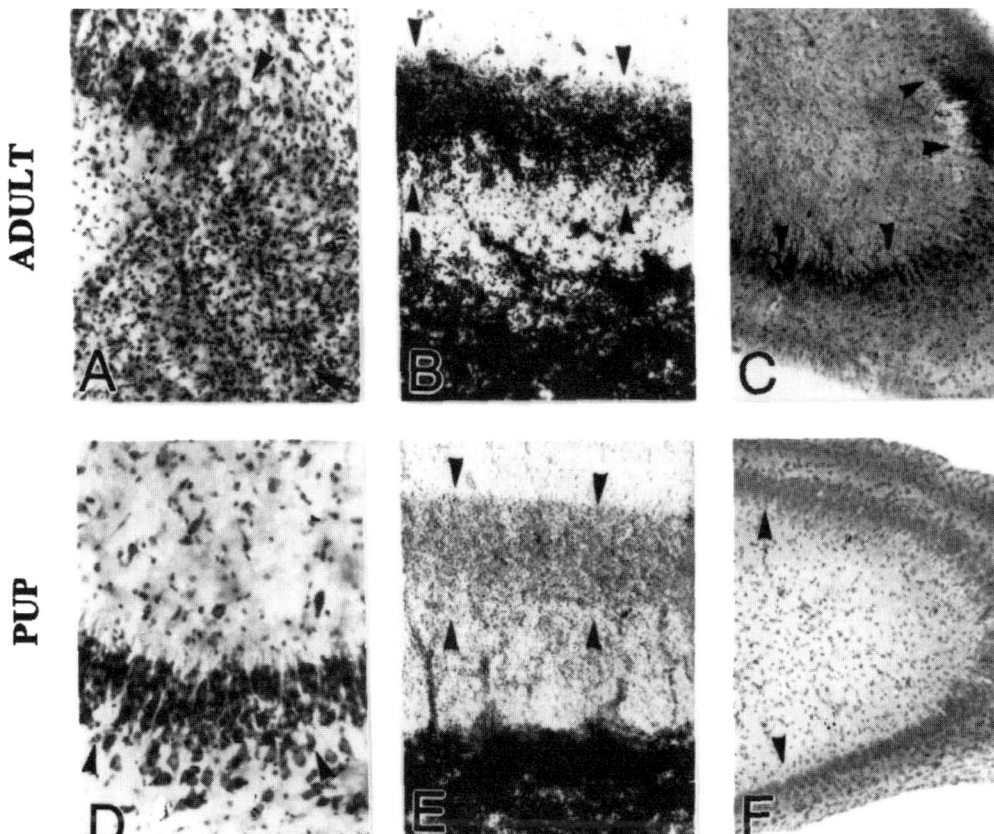

Fig. 1. Kainic acid seizure status epilepticus results in age-related hippocampal damage. In the adult rat hippocampus, extensive neuronal loss in the CA3 layer (A), mossy fibre synaptic reorganization in the dentate gyrus supragranular layer (B) and acute neuronal degeneration in the pyramidal cell layers (C) are visible. In contrast, in the 14-day-old rat hippocampus, there is no apparent neuronal loss (D), an absence of mossy fibre sprouting (E) and acute neuronal degeneration (F). (A & D: thionin stain; B & E: Timm silver sulphide stain; C & F: silver impregnation stain).

distribution and morphology of cells in the immature hippocampal tissue were similar to age-matched control rats. Both the cellular morphology and inclusions appeared normal with a complete absence of degenerating profiles. Therefore, it appears that even at the ultrastructural level, the immature rat brain is highly resistant to damage following kainic acid status epilepticus.

These results indicate that hippocampal neurons in the rat pup appears to be protected from seizure-induced injury. To determine whether neurons were uniquely resistant to neurodegeneration, a non-neuronal marker for damage was used to assess the susceptibility of immature hippocampal glial cells. In adult rats, seizures affect glial cells, as well as neurons. In particular, astrocytes are known to proliferate in response to an injury. By using immunocytochemistry it was possible to stain the glial fibrillary acidic protein (GFAP), a cytoskeleton protein which is specific to astrocytes. Hippocampal tissue from 14-day-old rats and adults 4 days after kainic acid induced status epilepticus were compared. Extensive reactive astrocytes were present throughout the adult hippocampus, particularly in the area of cell loss. The astrocytes appeared broken and truncated. In contrast, astrocytes in the young brain were normal in distribution and appearance including the presence of extensive fine dendritic arborizations. It therefore appears that there is a resiliency of astrocytes, as well as neurons to the consequences of seizures.

Potential neuroprotective mechanisms in the immature brain

Several studies have demonstrated a link between seizure-induced damage and intracellular calcium levels (Griffiths *et al.*, 1982). Due to their ability to sequester calcium, calcium binding proteins may play a role in neuroprotection. A neuroprotective role has been suggested in immature rats exposed to ischaemia (Goodman *et al.*, 1993). Therefore, the expression of calcium binding proteins, parvalbumin and calbindin was compared in adult and 2-week-old rats 4 days after kainic acid induced status epilepticus. The morphology and distribution of immunoreactive positive cells were examined in the stratum pyramidale, which is most susceptible to kainic acid status epilepticus induced degeneration and the adjacent stratum lucidum. In adult rats there was a decrease in the number of positively stained parvalbumin and calbindin expressing cells. In addition, a debris like pattern of staining was apparent in the lesioned pyramidal cell region by parvalbumin and in the adjacent stratum lucidum by calbindin. In contrast, staining in the immature rat had a distribution and morphology similar to control tissue. Results of these studies suggest that calcium binding proteins may be involved in neuroprotection in the young animal. It is possible that calcium binding proteins are functionally different in the immature and mature brain. However, studies must elaborate as to why calcium binding proteins did not have a similar protective function in adults. It is also possible that calcium binding proteins were not involved in neuroprotection since they were not altered by the seizure. Therefore, further studies are needed to determine the possible role of these proteins in neuroprotection.

Several studies also suggest a link between expression of the inducible form of heat shock protein (HSP72) and protection from damage following a variety of stressors (Barbe *et al.*, 1988; Kirino *et al.*, 1991; Kitagawa *et al.*, 1990). In adult rats, HSP72 is synthesized in response to seizure-induced neuronal damage (Lowenstein *et al.*, 1990; Vass *et al.*, 1989). Following kainic acid, HSP72 expression is correlated with the severity of the seizure and the distribution of areas susceptible to damage (Armstrong *et al.*, 1996; Gass *et al.*, 1995; Zhang *et al.*, 1996). Age-related changes in the expression of HSP72 were examined following kainic acid induced status epilepticus at 12, 24 and 36 h after kainic acid was injected. In adult rats, there was extensive positive staining in the hippocampus and throughout limbic structures. In contrast, there was little or no expression of HSP72 immunoreactivity in the 2-week-old rat. In the young rats, alterations in HSP72 were also examined, at 0, 1, 2 and 8 h after kainic acid status epilepticus. No change in HSP72 expression was observed at all the times examined suggesting that the absence of HSP72 expression in the developing rat was not due to a shift in the time course for the induction of HSP72 during development. Furthermore, arguement that HSP72 expression may not be induced in response to seizures until a later age seems unlikely, since positive expression of HSP72 has been observed in the fetal and neonatal rat following ischaemia (Dwyer *et al.*, 1989; Gilbert *et al.*, 1997). In any event, differential expression of the inducible form of heat shock proteins with age suggests that HSP72 induction may not necessarily be involved in neuroprotection in the young. In fact, the expression of HSP72 may even signal the onset of damage rather than protection from damage (Gass *et al.*, 1995).

Increased seizure vulnerability in the compromised brain

With regard to the previous question, 'Is hippocampal sclerosis in adulthood a result of seizures early in life?', studies with kainic acid induced status epilepticus indicate that this is unlikely since the normal immature brain appears to be quite resistant to seizure-induced damage. Our findings with kainic acid are similar to reports by others (Cavalheiro *et al.*, 1987; Holmes & Thompson, 1988; Nitecka *et al.*, 1984). In addition, we have also observed a similar resiliency of the immature brain using two additional seizure models: kindling (Haas *et al.*, personal data) and flurothyl status epilepticus (Sperber *et al.*, personal data). In both cases, 2-week-old rats again did not exhibit hippocampal cell loss or synaptic reorganization. Therefore, it appears that the normal immature brain is very resistant to seizure-induced damage.

This led to the question of whether the presence of a previous injury may alter the immature's resistance to seizures and seizure-induced damage? We first addressed the question of increased

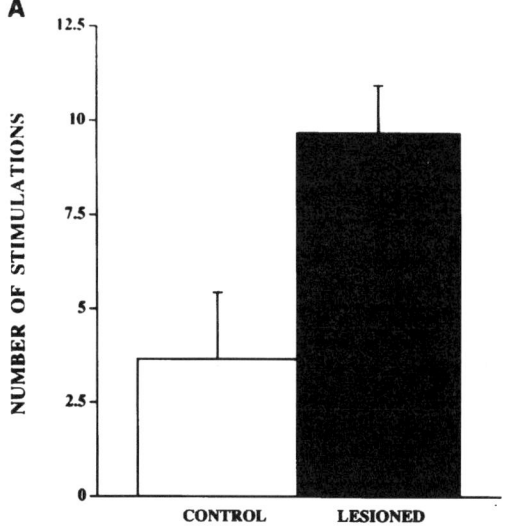

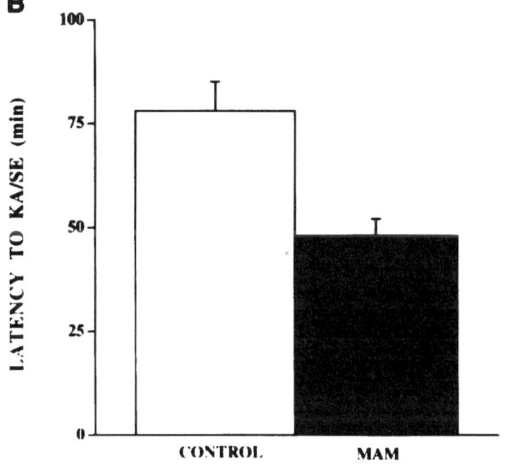

Fig. 2. The presence of brain damage increases susceptibility to seizures. During kindling (A), 14-day-old rats which were bilaterally lesioned in the hippocampus had significantly longer afterdischarge durations on more stimulation trials than non-lesioned control rats in adulthood. Fourteen-day-old rats pretreated with MAM (B) had significantly shorter latency to the onset of clonic–tonic seizures following kainic acid treatment.

seizure susceptibility in the compromised brain or as previously stated, 'Is the sclerosis a result of some prior damage which becomes epileptogenic overtime?'. Brain damage was produced either by *in utero* administration of methylazoxymethanol acetate (MAM) or lesioning the immature hippocampus. Seizure susceptibility to kindling and kainic acid status epilepticus was assessed later in life. The brains were also examined to determine if seizure-induced damage was present in animals with a compromised brain.

Adult rats demonstrated an increased seizure susceptibility in the presence of previous brain damage. Rats which received bilateral hippocampal lesions at 14 days of age were tested for changes in the development of kindled seizures. In adulthood, using a rapid kindling procedure (stimulated at 20-min intervals), lesioned rats reached a higher kindling stage than non-lesioned rats. Similarly, when kindled as adults, using a typical stimulation paradigm (2–3 h interstimulus intervals), lesioned rats had longer afterdischarge durations on more stimulation trials (Fig. 2A). This suggests that irrespective of the kindling paradigm, adult rats with discrete brain damage from early in life are more susceptible to kindling than rats with an intact brain. To determine whether the location or type of brain damage affects seizure outcome, rats with a more diffuse type of damage were studied.

Methylazoxymethanol acetate (MAM) is an antimitotic agent that produces diffuse brain damage when administered *in utero* (Johnston & Coyle, 1979; Spatz & Laquer, 1968). The pattern of damage is similar to neuronal migrational disorders in humans (Germano & Sperber, 1998; Mischel et al., 1995). Pathological characteristics include cortical disorganization, presence of heterotopia, abnormally oriented cells and decreased cortical thickness. In rats, both the incidence and severity of neuronal migrational disorders are time-dependent. The highest incidence, greatest behavioural consequences and most dramatic effects on brain development occur when MAM is administered on gestational day 15 (Balduini et al., 1991; Germano & Sperber, 1998).

Recent advances in neuroimaging techniques demonstrate a link between neuronal migrational disorders and epilepsy in humans. There appears to be a similar association between MAM exposure and seizure susceptibility in rats. Two-week-old rats that were exposed to MAM prenatally were assessed for changes in susceptibility to kainic acid induced status epilepticus. Rat pups with neuronal migrational disorders demonstrated a shorter latency to onset of clonic seizures, tonic seizures and clonic–tonic seizures (Fig. 2B). In addition, behavioural manifestations and development of the seizure are also affected by MAM (de Feo *et al.*, 1995; Germano & Sperber, 1998). Two-week-old MAM rats also have a higher incidence of seizures and mortality when exposed to hyperthermia (Germano *et al.*, 1996). In addition, MAM-treated rat pups also demonstrate a different pattern of kindling development. These rats reached stage 3.5 (alternating forelimb clonus) and stage 4 (bilateral forelimb clonus) faster than normal control rats. This suggests that seizure generalization occurs earlier in rats with neuronal migrational disorders.

Electrophysiological studies also demonstrate an increased epileptogenicity in hippocampal tissue from rats prenatally treated with MAM. *In vitro* slice recordings of cells in the ectopic area were compared to cells in normal hippocampal tissue. MAM-treated rats were found to have significantly more cells with a lower stimulation threshold (Baraban & Schwartzkroin, 1995). Thus, electrophysiological and behavioural studies suggest a heightened sensitivity to seizures in rats with brain damage.

The increased susceptibility to seizure which is present in immature rats exposed to MAM appears to be permanent. Studies using kainic acid demonstrate adult MAM rats have a shorter latency to seizure onset and more prolonged seizures in comparison to age-matched control animals (Germano & Sperber, 1998). Similarly, in adulthood, MAM rats with neuronal migrational disorders demonstrate a shorter latency to flurothyl-induced myoclonic jerks, forelimb clonus and lower seizure thresholds (Baraban & Schwartzkroin, 1996). While these studies report prenatal MAM increase susceptibility to kainic acid and bicuculline seizures during development and in adulthood, others have not (de Feo, *et al.*, 1995).

Studies indicate that MAM-treated rats are not only more susceptible to seizures but also to seizure-induced damage. Following kainic acid and hyperthermia-induced seizures, histological examination revealed that MAM rats had significantly more degenerated neurons than control animals. This is an interesting finding in the light of previously discussed studies indicating an increased resistance to seizure-induced damage in the normal developing rat. Taken together, these studies indicate that the normal intact immature brain is less vulnerable to seizure-induced damage. However, if the brain is already compromised then there is an increased probability of seizures and seizure-induced injury.

Is the immature brain completely resistant to damage?

Numerous studies from this laboratory and others demonstrate that although the immature brain is sensitive to seizures and status epilepticus, it is highly resistant to seizure-induced damage, as compared to mature rats (Cavalheiro *et al.*, 1987; Holmes & Thompson, 1988; Nitecka *et al.*, 1984). However, these studies do not necessarily indicate that the immature brain is completely resistant or impervious to seizure-induced damage. Transitory changes and acute neuronal injury have been reported in 11-day-old rats following kainic acid status epilepticus (Chang & Baram, 1994). In addition, it has also been demonstrated that some extreme conditions, such as electrical stimulation of perforant path for 16 h (Wasterlain *et al.*, 1996), and prolonged status epilepticus induced by corticotropin releasing hormone (Baram & Ribak, 1995) or lithium-pilocarpine (Sankar *et al.*, 1997), can result in hippocamapal damage in the immature brain. Despite these severe conditions, damage still emerges according to a developmental profile. Therefore, it appears that even with severe seizures, the immature brain is still resistant to seizure-induced damage, however there is a shift in the window of vulnerability to an earlier age.

Acknowledgements: The authors wish to thank Shalini Ahuja, Tahira Evelyne, Kristen Ullmeyer, Hansoo Keyoung, Ulrik Branner and Obida Lavin for their technical expertise. This research was partially supported by research grants from NINDS NS–30387 (EFS), Epilepsy Foundation of America (IMG and JV), March of Dimes 0097–2469 (LKF) and SUNY Sponsored Funds (MTR).

References

Armstrong, J.N., Plumier, J.L., Robertson, H.A. & Currie, R.W. (1996): The inducible 70,000 molecular/weight heat shock protein is expressed in degenerating denate hilus and piriform cortex after systematic administration of kainic acid in the rat. *Neuroscience* **74**, 685–693.

Balduini, W., Lombardelli, G., Perruzzi, G. & Cattabeni, F.. (1991): Treatment with methylazoxymethanol at different gestational days: Physical reflex, development, and spontaneous activity in the offspring. *Neurotoxicology* **12**, 179–188.

Baraban, S.C. & Schwartzkroin, P.A. (1995): Electrophysiology of CA1 pyramidal neurons in an animal model of neuronal migration disorders: prenatal methylazoxymethanol treatment. *Epilepsy Res.* **22**, 145–156.

Baraban, S.C. & Schwartzkroin, P.A. (1996): Flurothyl seizure susceptibility in rats following prenatal methylazoxymethanol treatment. *Epilepsy Res.* **23**, 189–194.

Baram, T.Z. & Ribak, C.E. (1995): Peptide-induced infant status epilepticus causes neuronal death and synaptic organization. *NeuroReport* **6**, 277–280.

Barbe, M.F., Tytell, M., Gower, D.G. & Welch, W.J. (1988): Hyperthermia protects against light damage in the rat retina. *Science* **241**, 1817–1820.

Berg, A.T. & Shinnar, S. (1991): The risk of seizure recurrence following a first unprovoked seizure: A quantitative review. *Neurology* **41**, 965–972.

Cavalheiro, E.A., Silva, D.F., Turski, W.A., Calderazzo-Filho, L.S., Bartolotto, Z. & Turski, L. (1987): The susceptibility of rats to pilocarpine-induced seizures is age dependent. *Dev. Brain Res.* **37**, 43–58.

Chang, D. & Baram, T.Z. (1994): Status epilepticus results in reversible neuronal injury in infant rat hippocampus: novel use of a marker. *Dev. Brain Res.* **77**, 133–136.

Cronin, J. & Dudek, F.E. (1988): Chronic seizures and collateral sprouting of dentate mossy fibers after kainic acid treatment in rats. *Brain Res.* **474**, 181–184.

de Feo, M.R., Mecarelli, O. & Ricci, G.F. (1995): Seizure susceptibility in immature rats with micrenecphaly induced by prenatal exposure to methylazoxymethanol acetate. *Pharm. Res.* **31**, 109–114.

Dunn, W.D. (1988): Status epilepticus in children: etiology, clinical features and outcome. *J. Child Neurol.* **3**, 167–173.

Dwyer, B.E., Nishimura, R.N. & Brown, I.R. (1989): Synthesis of the major inducible heat shock protein in rat hippocampus after neonatal hypoxia-ischemia. *Experimental Neurology* **104**, 28-31.

Falconer, M.A. (1974): Mesial temporal (Ammon's Horn) sclerosis as a common cause of epilepsy. Etiology, treatment, and prevention. *Lancet* **2**, 767–770.

Falconer, M.A., Serafetinides, E.A. & Corsellis, J.A.N. (1964): Etiology and pathogenesis of temporal lobe epilepsy. *Arch. Neurol.* **10**, 233–248.

Friedman, L.K., Sperber, E.F., Moshé, S.L., Bennett, M.V.L. & Zukin, R.S. (1997): Developmental regulation of glutamate and GABAA receptor gene expression in rat hippocampus following kainate-induced status epilepticus. *Dev. Neurosci.* **19**, 529–542.

Gass, P., Prior, P. & Kiessling, M. (1995): Correlation between seizure intensity and stress protein expression after limbic epilepsy in the rat. *Neuroscience* **65**, 27–36.

Germano, I.M. & Sperber, E.F. (1998): Transplacentally induced neuronal migration disorders: an animal model for the study of the epilepsies. *J. Neurosci. Res.* **51**, 473–488.

Germano, I.M., Zhang, Y.F., Sperber, E.F. & Moshé, S.L. (1996): Neuronal migration disorders increase seizure susceptibility to febrile seizures. *Epilepsia* **37**, 902–910.

Gilbert, K.L., Armstrong, J.N., Currie, R.W. & Robertson, H.A. (1997): The effects of hypoxia-ischemia on expression of c-Fos, c-Jun and Hsp70 in the young rat hippocampus. *Molec. Brain Res.* **48**, 87–96.

Goodman, J.H., Wasterlain, C.G., Massarweh, W.F., Dean, E., Sollas, A.L. & Sloviter, R.S. (1993): Calbindin-D28k immunoreactivity and selective vulnerability to ischemia in the dentate gyrus of the developing brain. *Brain Res.* **606**, 309–314.

Griffiths, T., Evans, M.C. & Meldrum, B.S. (1982): Intracellular sites of early calcium accumulation in rat hippocampus during status epilepticus. *Neurosci. Lett.* **30**, 329–334.

Gruenthal, M., Armstrong, D.R., Ault, B. & Nadler, V. (1986): Comparison of seizures and brain lesions produced by intracerebroventricular kainic acid and bicuculline methiodide. *Exp. Neurol.* **93**, 621–630.

Hauser, W.A. & Kurland, L.T. (1975): The epidemiology of epilepsy in Rochester, Minnesota, 1935–1967. *Epilepsia* **16**, 1–66.

Holmes, G.L. & Thompson, J.L. (1988): Effects of kainic acid on seizure susceptibility in the developing brain. *Dev. Brain Res.* **39,** 51–59.

Johnston, M.V. & Coyle, J.T. (1979): Histological and neurochemical effects of fetal treatment with methlazoxy methanol on rat neocortex in adulthood. *Brain Res.* **170,** 135–155.

Kirino, T., Tsujita, Y. & Tamura, A. (1991): Induced tolerance to ischemia in gerbil hippocampal neurons. *J. Cereb. Blood Flow Metab.* **11,** 299–307.

Kitagawa, K., Matsumoto, M., Tagaya, M., Hata, R., Ueda, H., Niinobe, M., Handa, N., Fukunaga, R., Kimura, K., Mikoshiba, K. & Kamada, T. (1990): Ischemic tolerance phenomenon found in the brain. *Brain Res.* **528,** 21–24.

Lowenstein, D.H., Simon, R.P. & Sharp, F.R. (1990): The pattern of 72-kDa heat shock protein-like immunoreactivity in the rat brain following flurothyl-induced status epilepticus. *Brain Res.* **531,** 173–182.

Mathison, G. (1975): Pathology of temporal lobe foci. In: *Advances in Neurology*, Penry, J.K. & Daly, D.D. (eds), vol. 11, pp. 163–185. New York: Raven Press.

Maytal, J. & Shinnar, S. (1990): Febrile status epilepticus. *Pediatrics* **86,** 611–616.

Mischel, P.S., Nguyen, L.P. & Vinters, H.V. (1995): Cerebral cortical dysplasia associated with pediatric epilepsy. Review of neuropathologic features and proposal for a grading system. *J. Neuropath. Exp. Neurol.* **54,** 137–53.

Nadler, J.V. & Evenson, D.A. (1983): Use of excitatory amino acids to make axon-sparing lesions of hypothalamus. *Methods Enzymol.* **103,** 393–400.

Nelson, K.B. & Ellenberg, J.H. (1976): Predictors of epilepsy in children who have experienced febrile seizures. *N. Engl. J. Med.* **295,** 1029–1033.

Nitecka, L., Tremblay, E., Charton, G., Bouillot, J.P., Berger, M.L. & Ben-Ari, Y. (1984): Maturation of kainic acid seizure-brain damage syndrome in the rat. II. Histopathological sequelae. *Neuroscience* **13,** 1073–1094.

Sankar, R., Shin, D.H. & Wasterlain, C.G. (1997): Serum neuron-specific enolase is a marker for neuronal damage following status epilepticus in the rat. *Epilepsy Res.* **28**(2), 129–136.

Sater, R.A. & Nadler, V. (1987): On the relationship between seizures and brain lesions after intracerebroventricular kainic acid. *Neurosci. Lett.* **84,** 73–78.

Shinnar, S., Maytal, J., Krasnoff, L. & Moshé, S.L. (1992): Recurrent status epilepticus in children. *Ann. Neurol.* **31,** 598–604.

Shinnar, S., Pellock, J.M., Moshé, S.L., Maytal, J., O'Dell, C., Driscoll, S.M., Alemany, M., Newstein, D. & DeLorenzo, R.J. (1997): In whom does status epilepticus occur? Age-related differences in children. *Epilepsia* **38,** 907–914.

Sommer, W. (1880): Erkrankung des Ammonshorns als aetiologisches Moment der Epilepsie. *Arch. Psychiatr. Nervenkr.* **10,** 631–675.

Spatz, M. & Laquer, G.L. (1968): Transplacental chemical induction of microencephaly in two strains of rats. *Proc. Soc. Exp. Biol.* **129,** 705–710.

Sperber, E.F., Haas, K.Z., Stanton, P.K. & Moshé, S.L. (1991a): Resistance to damage of the immature hippocampus in flurothyl induced status epilepticus. *Ann. Neurol.* **30,** 495.

Sperber, E.F., Haas, K.Z., Stanton, P.K. & Moshé, S.L. (1991b): Resistance of the immature to seizure-induced synaptic reorganization. *Dev. Brain Res.* **60,** 88–93.

Tauck, D.L. & Nadler, J.V. (1985): Evidence of functional mossy fiber sprouting in hippocampal formation of kainic acid-treated rats. *J. Neurosci.* **5,** 1016–1022.

Timm, F. (1958): Zur Histochemie der Schwermetalle, das Sulfid-Silber Verfahren. *Dtsch. Z. Gesamte. Gerichtl. Med.* **46,** 706–711.

Vass, K., Berger, M.L., Nowak, T.S.J., Welch, W.J. & Lassmann, H. (1989): Induction of stress protein HSP70 in nerve cells after status epilepticus in the rat. *Neurosci. Lett.* **100,** 259–264.

Wasterlain, C.G., Shirasaka, Y., Mazarati, A.M. & Spigelman, I. (1996): Chronic epilepsy with damage restricted to the hippocampus: possible mechanism. *Epilepsy Res.* **26**(1), 255–265.

Zhang, X., Boulton, A.A. & Yu, P.H. (1996): Expression of heat shock protein–70 and limbic seizure-induced neuronal death in the rat brain. *Eur. J. Neurosci.* **8,** 1432–1440.

Chapter 23

Effects of recurrent seizures in the developing brain

Gregory L. Holmes[1,2], Matthew Sarkisian[1], Yehezkel Ben-Ari[2] and Nicolas Chevassus-Au-Louis[2]

[1]*Department of Neurology, Harvard Medical School, Children's Hospital, Boston, Massachusetts, USA; and*
[2]*Institut National de la Sante de la Recherche Medicale, Unit 29, Paris, France*

Summary

A small, but significant portion of children with epilepsy have a progressive decline in cognitive abilities over time. From a clinical standpoint it is difficult to determine if these cognitive changes are due to the recurrent seizures, antiepileptic drug therapy, or underlying cause of the seizures. In animals, a number of studies have indicated that prolonged seizures are associated with less cognitive impairment than seizures of similar duration and intensity in mature animals. However, the immature brain is not invulnerable to seizure-induced brain damage and there is increasing evidence suggesting that recurrent seizures may result in long-term detrimental changes to the developing brain. Recent work from our laboratory has demonstrated that daily seizures, beginning as early as the first day can result in changes in the hippocampal network. These morphological changes in the developing brain are associated with changes in seizure threshold and cognitive impairment. These studies suggest that recurrent seizures during early development may result in long-term deleterious effects. The mechanisms responsible for these changes are not yet known.

Introduction

The high incidence of epilepsy in the first decade of life and the propensity of children toward febrile seizures are reflective of the increased susceptibility of the immature brain to seizures (Hauser & Hersdorffer, 1990; Holmes, 1997). While the majority of children with epilepsy do well, a small percentage of children with epilepsy have cognitive and behavioural problems. The mean IQ score in children with epilepsy is lower than the normal population and learning and behavioural problems are over-represented in children with epilepsy (Holmes & Moshé, 1990; Holmes, 1991a, b). While the cognitive and behavioural abnormalities are often explained by the aetiological factors responsible for the epilepsy, there are a number of clinical studies indicating that some children with poorly controlled epilepsy have progressive declines of IQ on serial intelligence tests and behavioural and psychiatric deterioration over time (Gomez *et al.*, 1982; Bourgeois *et al.*, 1983; Rodin *et al.*, 1986; Funakoshi *et al.*, 1988).

Clinical studies

Rodin *et al.* (1986) performed psychological studies on 64 patients with epilepsy who had an initial evaluation between five and 16 years of age and a re-evaluation after a period of at least five years. Patients who had seizures that remained uncontrolled had a significant decrease in performance IQ, whereas the IQ was stable or increased for patients in remission. The study indicated that the decreased IQ indicated slower mental growth rather than loss of previously acquired abilities. Phenobarbital, but not phenytoin, levels were inversely correlated with IQ.

In a prospective study of serial changes in the IQs of 72 children with seizures, Bourgeois *et al.* (1983) reported a mean IQ of 99.7 within two weeks of the initial diagnosis. In 45 patients, siblings without a history of epilepsy were also evaluated, and no substantial differences in IQs from their siblings were noted. However, in eight patients (11.1 per cent), there was a decrease in IQ of 10 points or more. The number of antiepileptic drugs (AEDs) to which the patient exhibited a toxic reaction and the age at seizure onset were the two best indicators of ultimate IQ. However, total number of seizures and degree of seizure control were not reliable predictors.

The importance of AEDs as a factor in the decline in intelligence was reinforced by Funakoshi *et al.* (1988) who performed prospective serial Wechsler Intelligence Scales for Children – Revised (WISC-R) testing in 45 children with epilepsy. The authors found that AEDs, phenobarbital in particular, resulted in a detrimental effect of the WISC-R scores. In children in whom seizures continued and AED dosage remained unchanged, both the verbal IQ and performance IQ scores decreased. It was concluded that either continuing seizures or AEDs may exert a detrimental effect on intelligence, although the authors could not exclude the underlying cerebral pathology associated with the epilepsy as a cause of the progressive intellectual deterioration.

A number of older twin studies have also suggested that recurrent seizures may be detrimental. Dodrill & Troupin (1976), in a study of identical twins with seizures, found that the twin with the larger number of seizures had a full-scale IQ 22 points below the twin with the better seizure control. Forty-seven twin pairs in which one of each twin pair had a history of febrile seizures were studied by Schiottz-Christensen & Bruhn (1973); the twin with febrile seizures had a lower IQ on the performance section of the WISC. Gomez *et al.* (1982) studied two sets of homozygous twins in which one twin in each set suffered frequent generalized seizures from early life and the second either had no seizures or had only short-lived ones. The twins with frequent seizures were mentally subnormal in follow-up, while their co-twins were normal. While the twins were identical, it is possible, and likely, that the twin with more severe seizures had a more severe form of tuberous sclerosis and therefore was more likely to have lower intelligence.

Animal studies

Even with well-designed longitudinal or twin studies the difficulties in reaching conclusions regarding the relationship of epilepsy during development with cognitive impairment are enormous. Differentiating effects of recurrent seizures from the effects of antiepileptic drugs may not be possible. Compounding the difficulties are the variables of seizure type, duration and frequency. Since in animal studies many of these variables can be controlled, there are some distinct advantages of addressing these questions in the laboratory.

Effect of prolonged seizures during development

The immature brain, like the mature brain, is vulnerable to seizure-induced brain injury (see Chapters 18 & 21 in this book). However, a number of studies have demonstrated that the degree of seizure-related injury is related to age at the time of the seizure, with younger animals faring better than more mature animals (Albala *et al.*, 1984; Nitecka *et al.*, 1984; Cavalheiro *et al.*, 1987; Holmes *et al.*, 1988; Sperber *et al.*, 1991; Hirsch *et al.*, 1992; Stafstrom *et al.*, 1992; Thurber *et al.*, 1992; Stafstrom *et al.*, 1993; Thurber *et al.*, 1994). In the adult animal status epilepticus causes neuronal loss in the hippocampal subfields CA1, CA3 and the dentate hilus (Meldrum & Brierley, 1973; Meldrum *et al.*, 1973; Nadler *et al.*, 1978; Olney *et al.*, 1979; Nadler, 1981; Sloviter & Damiano, 1981; Sloviter, 1983), leads to aberrant growth of granule cell axons (sprouting) in the supragranular zone of the fascia dentata (Tauck & Nadler, 1985; Represa *et al.*, 1987a; Okazaki *et al.*, 1995) and stratum infrapyramidale of CA3 (Represa *et al.*, 1987a), and results in long-term deficits in learning, memory and behaviour (Stafstrom *et al.*, 1993). The immature brain appears to be less vulnerable to damage associated with prolonged seizures than the mature brain. For example, a number of studies have demonstrated that prolonged seizures in immature animals result in less cell loss (Albala *et al.*, 1984; Cavalheiro *et al.*, 1987; Sperber *et al.*, 1991; Hirsch *et al.*, 1992; Stafstrom *et al.*, 1992) and sprouting (Sperber *et al.*, 1991; Baram & Ribak, 1995), and fewer deficits in learning, memory and behaviour than similar seizures in adults (Stafstrom *et al.*, 1993; Liu *et al.*, 1995).

While it is known that status epilepticus may be accompanied by severe metabolic aberrations including hypoxia, hypotension and acidosis, there is convincing evidence from both humans and animal studies that the prolonged seizures, *per se*, are responsible for the majority of the cell loss. The major cause of seizure-induced cell damage is excessive excitability secondary to release of excitatory amino acids, predominately glutamate (Olney *et al.*, 1986; Choi, 1988a).

If sufficient amounts of excitatory amino acids are given to animals, either systemically or intraventricular or intrahippocampal, lesions similar to the human condition of mesial temporal sclerosis can be produced. For example, when kainic acid (KA) is administered in a sufficient dosage to experimental animals prolonged seizures ensue (Ben-Ari *et al.*, 1979a,b; 1980a,b; Berger *et al.*, 1984). While animals that survive have widespread cerebral lesions, the hippocampus (hilus, CA1 and particularly CA3) are the structures most damaged. These hippocampal lesions are remarkably similar to those seen in human temporal lobe epilepsy. The neurotoxicity of KA appears to be primarily due to endogenous release of glutamate resulting from activation of the pre-synaptic KA receptors, as opposed to a direct neurotoxic effect. For example, diazepam will prevent distant damage induced by KA without altering the local neurotoxic damage secondary to KA itself (Ben-Ari *et al.*, 1979b). Antagonists of both the N-methyl-D-aspartate (NMDA) (Fariello *et al.*, 1989) and non-NMDA (Lees & Leong, 1992) receptors can reduce the histological damage associated with KA.

Sloviter & Dempster (1985) have demonstrated that neuronal injury induced in the hippocampus by stimulation of the perforant path shares many of the characteristics of excitotoxic injury. Immediately after 24 h of intermittent, unilateral perforant path stimulation, acute cell injury could be detected in the ipsilateral dentate hilus and areas CA3 of the hippocampal pyramidal cell layer. High concentrations of glutamate or aspartate injected directly into the brain replicated all of the qualitative features of acute seizure-induced damage, supporting the hypothesis that the sustained release of an excitatory amino acid is the initiating factor in seizure-associated cell injury.

Glutamate receptors, when activated by the appropriate ligands during seizures, allow a considerable influx of Ca^{2+} ions into the postsynaptic neurons (Hori *et al.*, 1985; Kudo & Ogura, 1986; Collingridge & Bliss, 1987). The flow of Ca^{2+} into the cell triggers a cascade of reactions resulting in activation of proteases, phospholipases and endonucleases, ultimately leading to the generation of active and potentially toxic metabolites (Choi, 1987, 1988b; Siesjö, 1988; Orrenius *et al.*, 1989). There is also evidence that cell death may be secondary to both necrosis and apoptosis (Pollard *et al.*, 1994; Sloviter *et al.*, 1996).

There is no reason to believe that similar events should not result in damage in the immature brain. However, there is evidence that the immature brain is less prone to glutamate toxicity than the mature brain. Liu *et al.* (1996) administered equal amounts of glutamate (0.5 mmol in 1.0 ml) unilaterally into the CA1 subfield of the hippocampus of rats at postnatal (P) days 10, 20, 30 and 60. Rats were sacrificed seven days later and their brains were examined for hippocampal cell loss. The size of the resultant hippocampal lesion was highly age-dependent. Minimal cell loss was noted in the P10 rats; lesions in the P20 rats were smaller than those at P30 and P60, which were similar in extent. This study demonstrated that the extent of glutamate neurotoxicity in the hippocampus was highly age-dependent, with immature brain more 'resistant' to glutamate toxicity than the mature brain.

The decreased vulnerability of the immature brain to glutamate may relate to differences in the postsynaptic action of glutamate. Ca^{2+} entry through NMDA receptor ionophores may exhibit age-dependent changes, as may each step in the intracellular cascade following Ca^{2+} entry (Bickler et al., 1993; Carmant et al., 1995). Bickler et al. (1993) noted an increase in intracellular Ca^{2+} of 240 per cent from P1–P2 days to P28 days following application of 500 mM glutamate in rat cerebral cortex slices. In a study of the effects of hypoxia, aglycemia and hypoxia–aglycemia on intrasynaptosomal free Ca^{2+} it was found that neither aglycemia nor hypoxia–aglycemia caused a rise in Ca^{2+} in rats that were P20 or younger while in older rats significant increases in Ca^{2+} were noted. These differences in intracellular Ca^{2+} could not be attributed to differences in ATP levels since the declines in ATP levels was similar in all age groups studied.

Carmant et al. (1995) measured inositol 1,4,5 trisphosphate (IP3), one of the intermediates in the complex cascade of phosphoinositide hydrolysis, following KA in immature and mature rats. IP3 is of particular interest in seizures and seizure-induced brain damage, because it controls intracellular Ca^{2+} stores and may also promote influx of external Ca^{2+} in conjunction with IP4 (Irvine, 1991; Mitani et al., 1993). Despite KA causing more severe seizures in the immature animals, there was no hippocampal damage or induction of phosphoinositide hydrolysis. In mature animals, seizures were mild but severe hippocampal damage was seen and was associated with a marked and sustained release of IP3. Intracellular Ca^{2+} buffering capabilities may also differ as a function of age. Sperber et al. (1995) noted that following KA there is a greater increase in the Ca^{2+} binding protein parvalbumin in hippocampal neurons of the immature brain than in the adult brain.

While it is clear that prolonged seizures can injure the brain at any age, age is an important variable in determining outcome. Whether the cognitive impairment seen in some children with recurrent seizures results from a similar mechanism is less clear.

Effect of recurrent seizures during development

In experimental studies recurrent seizures have been associated with adverse effects on learning and memory. There are a number of reports which have demonstrated impairment of working or reference memory in spatial tests after hippocampal, amygdala, septal or perforant path kindling (Lopes da Silva et al., 1986; Knowlton et al., 1989; Leung et al., 1990; Leung & Shen, 1991). Following pre-training in the 8-arm maze, Leung et al. (1990, 1991) kindled rats in the hippocampus and then measured relearning. Compared to non-stimulated controls and rats subjected to low-frequency stimulations kindled rats had significant deficits in memory. Lopes da Silva et al. (1986) also performed hippocampal kindling following training in the eight-arm maze. The authors found that both working (short-term) and reference (long-term) memory were impaired by the kindling.

However, a number of studies have demonstrated that kindling does not appear to impair memory when kindling either precedes or follows the learning task (McNamara et al., 1992; Nieminen et al., 1992; Feasy-Truger et al., 1993; Holmes et al., 1993; Letty et al., 1995). For example, Holmes et al. (1993) evaluated the long-term effects of kindling in P20, P40 and P60 day-old rats using hippocampal electrical stimulations. Rats were kindled to stage 5 seizures and then received an additional 15 seizures using the same kindling stimulation. At age 80 days, animals were tested in the Morris water maze and open field test, a measure of activity level. No differences were noted in time to platform in the water maze or activity level in the open field test between the kindled rats and controls in any of the three age groups. Likewise, Letty et al. (1995) also found that mature rats undergoing amygdala kindling had no deficits in the radial-arm maze, a test of spatial memory.

In addition to the kindling studies, investigators using other seizure models have evaluated the effects of recurrent seizures on cognition. Neill et al. (1996) administered the convulsant inhalant flurothyl to P15 rats three times a day for five consecutive days. When the rats were fully mature, they underwent behavioural testing using the water maze and auditory quality and location discrimination. The Morris water maze is a test where a rat has to remember where a submerged platform is located in a large tank of opaque water. The rat uses visuospatial clues to learn and remember where the platform is located. Normally the rat will quickly learn the location of the platform and swim quickly to it and climb out of the water. Rats with hippocampal lesions typically have impaired performance in this task. In the auditory quality discrimination test rats have to learn to correctly distinguish between two

Chapter 23 Effects of recurrent seizures in the developing brain

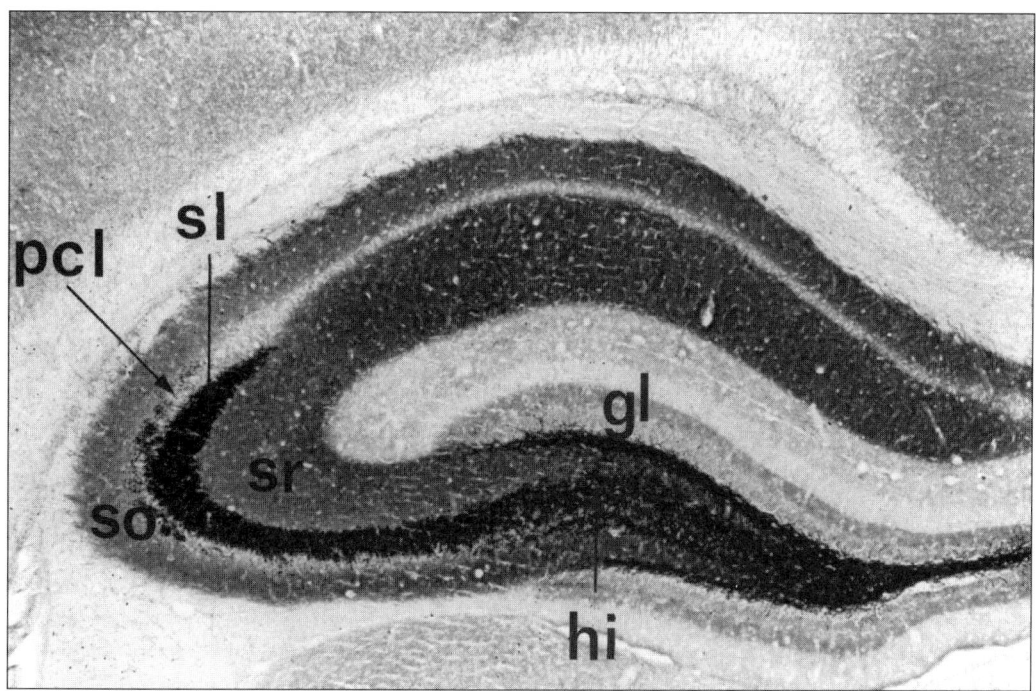

Fig. 1. Timm staining of hippocampus in a rat, sr = stratum radiatum, sl = stratum lucidum, pcl = pyramidal cell layer, so = stratum oriens).

sounds of different quality in order to obtain a food reward, whereas with auditory location the rat must learn to distinguish between sounds coming from two different locations to earn a reward.

With serial flurothyl administration seizure duration increased progressively and latency to seizure onset decreased. Compared to controls, flurothyl-treated rats had impaired performance in the water maze and on auditory location, but not on quality discrimination. Histological examination showed no gross cell loss in the hippocampus. This study demonstrated that serial seizures in the developing brain results in long-term detrimental effects on memory and learning. In addition, these results demonstrated that even in the absence of significant cell loss, recurrent seizures can adversely affect the developing brain.

In another study of the effects of recurrent seizures Holmes *et al.* (1990) subjected genetically epilepsy prone rats (GEPRs) to 66 audiogenic seizures between 45 and 75 days of age, administered at a rate of two to three stimulations a day. Compared to controls, GEPRs reached criteria less frequently in the T-maze (a test in which water-deprived rats must learn to go to alternate arms of a T-shaped maze in order to receive a water reward) and required longer times to find the platform in the Morris water maze. These results demonstrated that frequent, brief seizures can lead to long-term deficits in learning and memory. However, since GEPRs do not demonstrate the audiogenic seizure trait consistently until after 20 days of age, prepubescent animals could not be studied.

Together, these studies demonstrate that recurrent seizures may result in long-term behavioural changes during development. We have also observed that recurrent seizures during early development can result in a decreased seizure threshold and lead to the development of new synapses in the hippocampus.

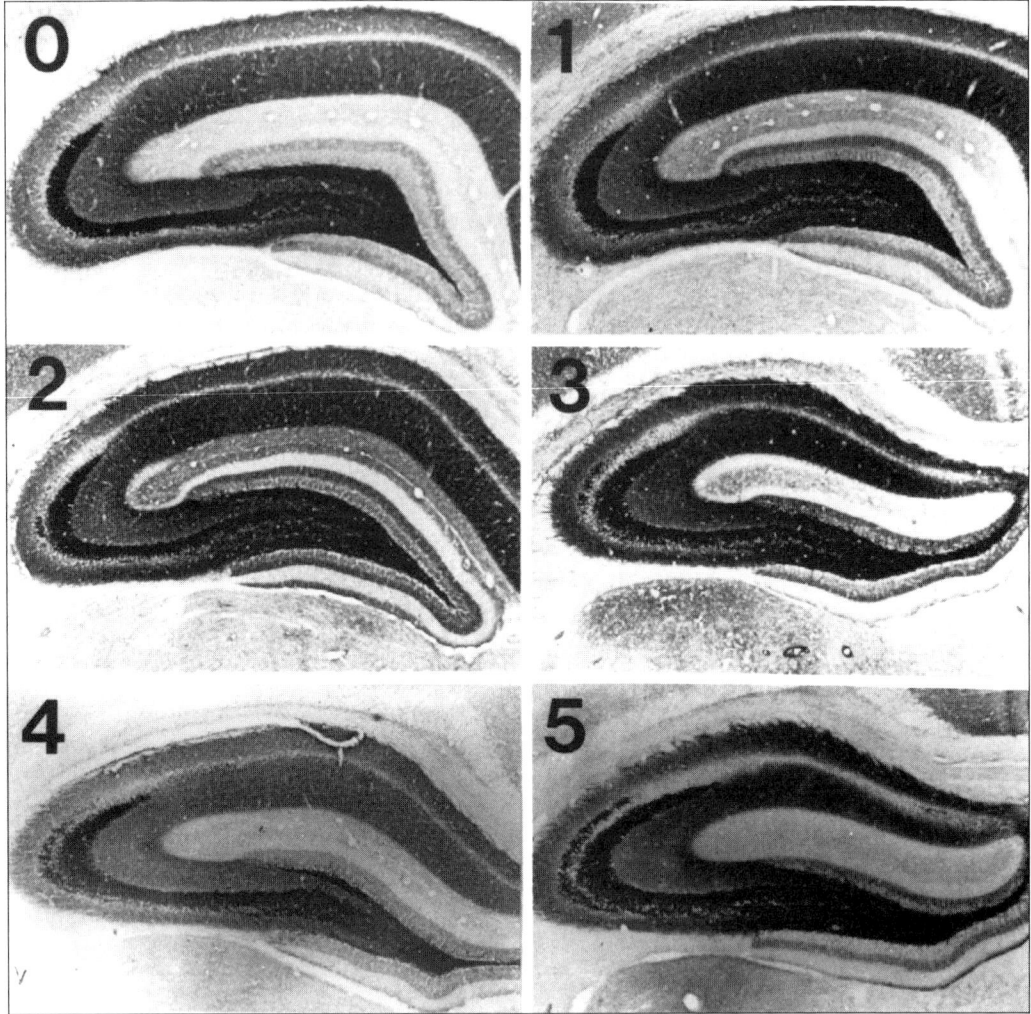

Fig. 2. Scoring scale for evaluation of mossy fibre synaptic reorganization in the CA3 region. The distribution of Timm granules in the stratum pyramidale and stratum oriens was rated on a scale of 0–5, with higher scores representing more staining.

Morphological changes following recurrent seizures

Reactive synaptogenesis, with aberrant growth or so-called sprouting of axon terminals, following prolonged or recurrent seizures, has been an area of interest to many investigators (Sutula, 1990, 1993; McNamara, 1994). Most of the attention in epilepsy has been directed towards supragranular mossy fibre sprouting. The mossy fibres are the zinc-staining axons of the dentate granule cells which innervate the CA3 pyramidal cell layer and hilar interneurons. Sprouting of mossy fibres has been described following prolonged seizures in a number of models including KA (Tauck & Nadler, 1985; Represa *et al.*, 1987a; Cronin & Dudek, 1988; Okazaki *et al.*, 1995) and pilocarpine (Okazaki *et al.*, 1995). In addition, sprouting has been observed in adult animals following electrical (Sutula *et al.*, 1988; 1996; Cavazos *et al.*, 1991) or pentylenetetrazol (PTZ) (Golarai *et al.*, 1992) kindling. Examination of pathological specimens removed from patients with temporal lobe epilepsy has also

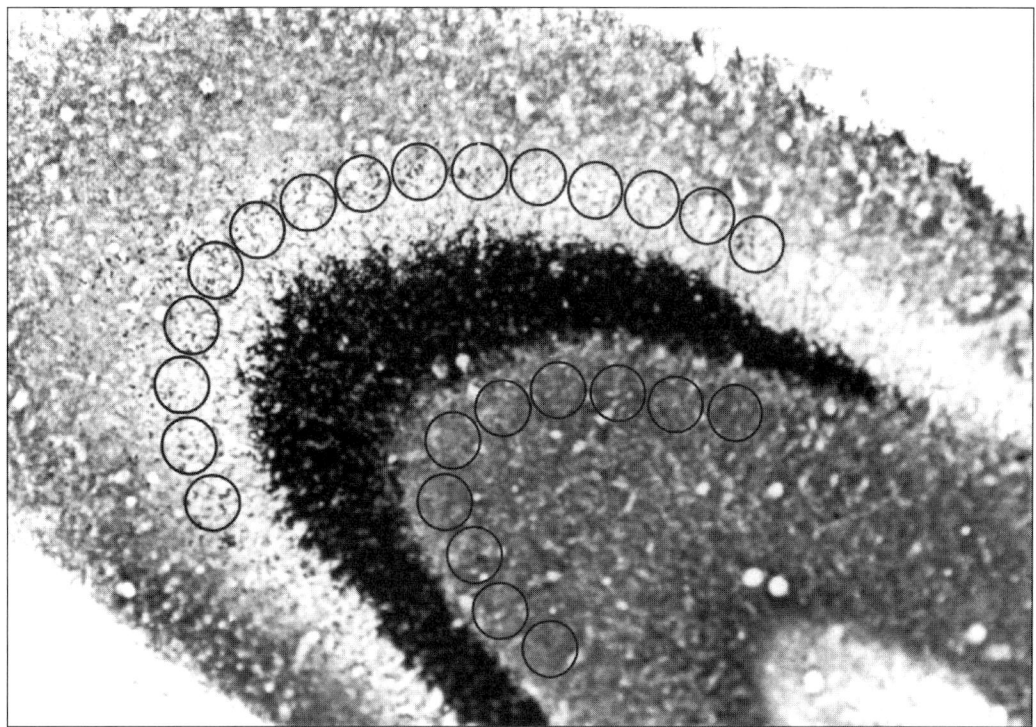

Fig. 3. Location of 15 circles placed sequentially along the junction between the stratum pyramidale and stratum oriens and 10 circles in the stratum radiatum. Circles did not overlap. In rare situations where artefact or disrupted tissue was noted, the circles were placed on immediately adjacent tissue.

demonstrated mossy fibre sprouting (Sutula et al., 1989; Houser et al., 1990; Babb et al., 1991; Isokawa et al., 1993; Masukawa et al., 1995). There is also now a considerable amount of indirect evidence that these new mossy fibre terminals represent functional synaptic connections (Tauck & Nadler, 1985; Represa & Ben-Ari, 1992; Represa et al., 1993; Okazaki et al., 1995; Wuarin & Dudek, 1996). Since the dentate granule cells use glutamate as a neurotransmitter, these aberrant synaptic conditions may contribute to the state of hyperexcitability that either provokes or facilitates abnormal discharges (Tauck & Nadler, 1985)

Although not as extensively studied as supragranular staining, sprouting of mossy fibre terminals has also been demonstrated in the CA3 region following treatment with KA (Represa et al., 1987a, b; 1993) and amygdala kindling (Represa & Ben-Ari, 1992, 1993; Van der Zee et al., 1995).

Figure 1 provides an example of mossy fibre staining using the Timm technique. In control Wistar rats mossy fibres originated from the soma of granule cells, and entered the hilus where branches formed a dense network. In the hilus a band of fibres is formed transversing the long axis of the hippocampus and pursuing a close course to CA3, ending in a dense band in the stratum lucidum. The stratum lucidum corresponds to the suprapyramidal region where mossy fibres innervate the apical dendrites of the pyramidal cells.

We wished to determine whether recurrent seizures were associated with changes in the synaptic pattern in both CA3 and in the dentate. To do this we administered convulsive doses of pentylenetetrazol (PTZ) to immature rats beginning at P1, P10 or P60. We also subjected another group of P10 rats to twice daily seizures for 15 days. Supragranular and terminal sprouting in the CA3 hippocampal subfield was assessed using both a rating scale and computer-assisted density measurements. Figure

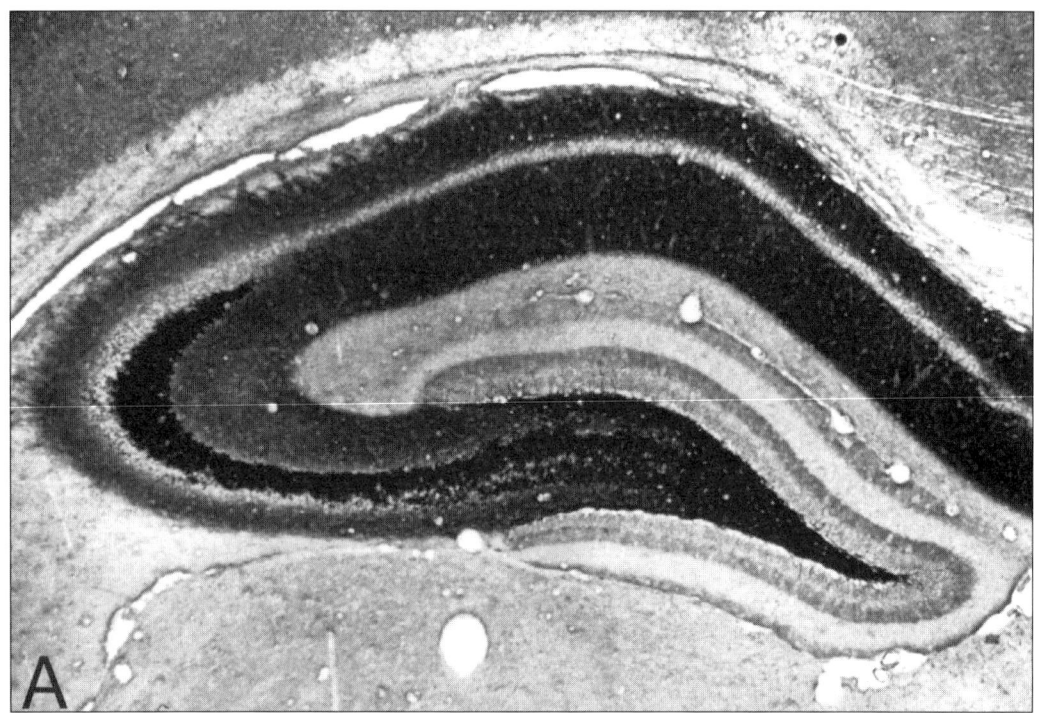
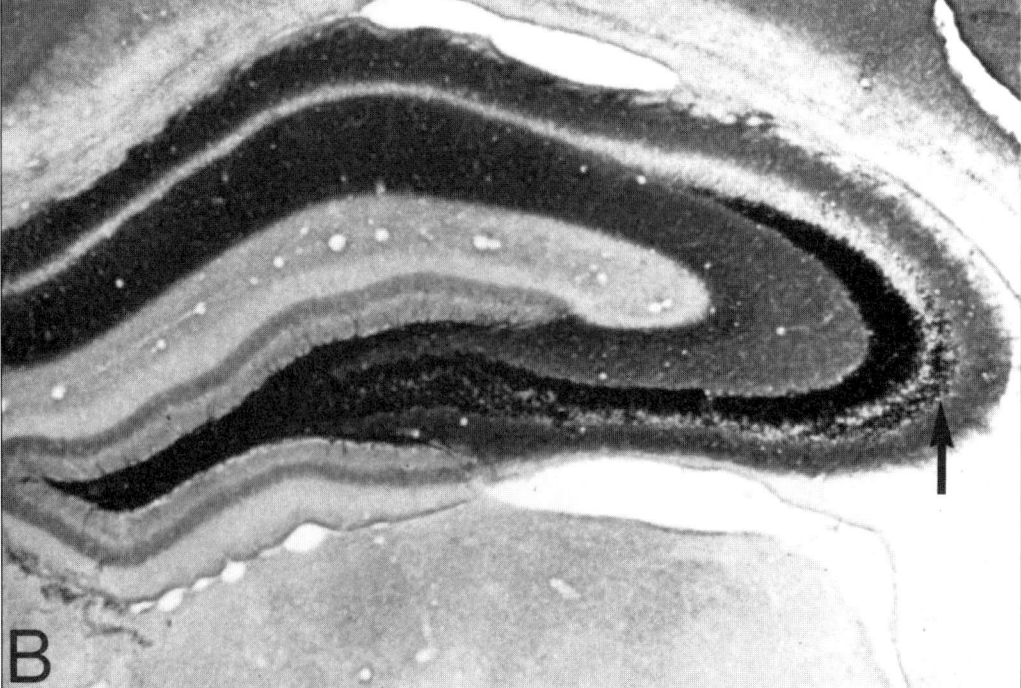

Fig. 4. Comparison of CA3 Timm staining in control (A, upper) and rat with recurrent seizures beginning on P10 (B, lower). Note prominent stratum pyramidale Timm staining in the rat with recurrent seizures.

Chapter 23 Effects of recurrent seizures in the developing brain

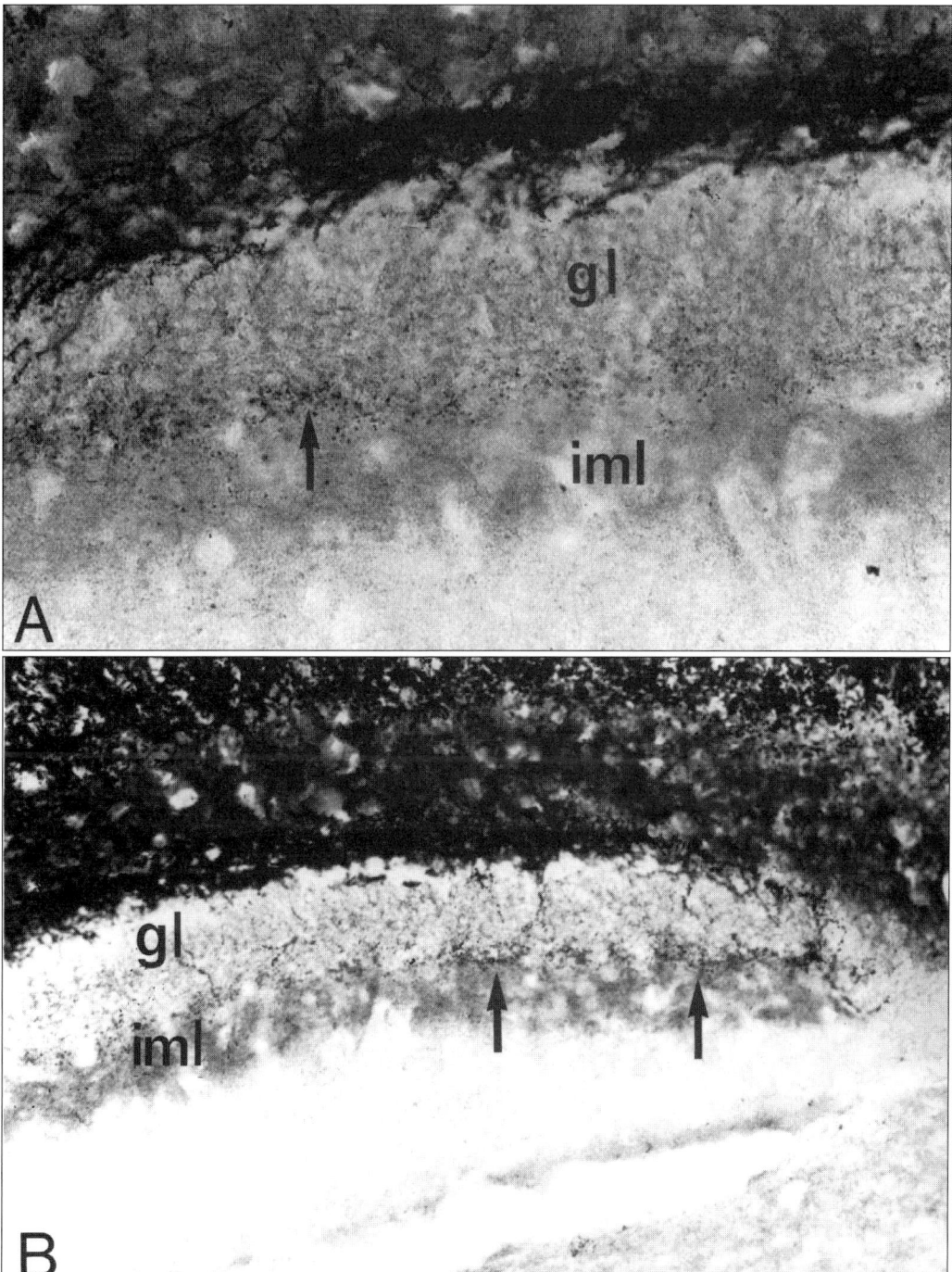

Fig. 5. Examples of supragranular Timm staining. All specimens came from rats having two seizures a day between P10 and P25 and are from the inferior blade of the dentate. (A, upper) Occasional Timm granules (arrow) are seen in the supragranular region (gl = granule cell layer, iml = inner molecular layer). (B, lower) Patchy groups of Timm staining (arrows).

2 demonstrates the scale used for the CA3 changes while a scale similar to that described by Sutula et al. (Sutula et al., 1988; Cavazos et al., 1991) was used for the supragranular staining.

For computer-assisted density measurements images were captured digitally to a monitor utilizing an image analysis system (Media Cybergenics, Silver Spring, MD). Once an image was captured to screen, it was then converted to a grey scale. We placed 15 circles of uniform area sequentially along the junction between the stratum pyramidale and stratum oriens and 10 circles in the stratum radiatum (Fig. 3). In addition, five circles were placed over the dentate granule cell layer and the three bands of the molecular layer and the corpus callosum. Once all circles were in place, a mean optical density for each region was obtained.

Prominent sprouting was seen in the stratum infrapyramidale layer of CA3 in all rats having 15 daily seizures regardless of the age when seizures began (Fig. 4). In rats receiving single daily seizures no differences from controls were noted in supragranular staining in any age group. However, in rats subjected to twice daily PTZ modest supragranular staining was found, particularly in the inferior blade of the dentate (Fig. 5). Although there was some modest cell loss found in the CA1 subfield in the P60 rats, no cell loss was noted in any of the immature rats with recurrent seizures.

This study demonstrates that like the mature brain, immature animals have neuronal reorganization following recurrent seizures with sprouting in both the CA3 subfield and supragranular region. It is important to mention that sprouting occurred in rats with no cell loss.

While supragranular sprouting following repetitive seizures in the immature brain has not been previously reported, sprouting in the immature brain has been previously described. While Sperber et al. (1991) did not find supragranular Timm's staining in P15 rats following KA-induced status epilepticus, Baram & Ribak (1995, 1996) reported supragranular sprouting following corticotrophin-releasing hormone-induced status epilepticus in P12 rats. Leite et al. (1996) in a study using intrahippocampal KA found that even rats as young as P7 had supragranular sprouting when sacrificed as adults. The authors did note that sprouting was more prominent when KA was given at older ages. In both the work by Baram & Ribak (1995, 1996) and Leite et al. (1996) cell loss was noted in association with the sprouting. Sprouting has also been observed in the hippocampus from children undergoing temporal lobe resection for medically intractable epilepsy (Mathern et al., 1994, 1996)(also see Chapter 16 in this book).

Both behavioural studies and morphological studies have now demonstrated that recurrent seizures can lead to adverse effects on brain development. However, the pathophysiological mechanisms responsible for both the sprouting and subsequent deficits in learning and memory reported in some studies are not clear. In addition to studying the type, duration and frequency of seizures required to cause damage, investigators will be challenged to identify the mechanisms of such seizure-related damage. Only then can rational treatment be developed.

Acknowledgements: This research was supported by INSERM, the Emily P. Rogers Research Fund, American Epilepsy Society, and grants to GLH from the NINDS (NS27984) and Fogarty Foundation.

References

Albala, B.J., Moshé, S.L. & Okada, R. (1984): Kainic-acid-induced seizures: A developmental study. *Dev. Brain Res.* **13**, 139–148.

Babb, T.L., Kupfer, W.R., Pretorius, J.K., Crandall, P.H. & Levesque, M.F. (1991): Synaptic reorganization by mossy fibers in human epileptic fascia dentata. *Neuroscience* **42**, 351–363.

Baram, T.Z. & Ribak, C.E. (1995): Peptide-induced infant status epilepticus causes neuronal death and synaptic reorganization. *NeuroReport* **6**, 277–280.

Ben-Ari, Y., Lagowska, J., Tremblay, E. & Le Gal La Salle, G. (1979a): A new model of focal status epilepticus: intra-amygdaloid application of kainic acid elicits repetitive secondarily generalized convulsive seizures. *Brain Res.* **163**, 176–179.

Ben-Ari, Y., Tremblay, E., Ottersen, O.P. & Naquet, R. (1979b): Evidence suggesting secondary epileptogenic lesions after kainic acid: pre-treatment with diazepam reduces distant but not local brain damage. *Brain Res.* **165**, 362–365.

Ben-Ari, Y., Tremblay, E. & Ottersen, O.P. (1980a): Injections of kainic acid into the amygdaloid complex of the rat: An electrographic, clinical and histological study in relation to the pathology of epilepsy. *Neuroscience* **5**, 515–528.

Ben-Ari, Y., Tremblay, E., Ottersen, O.P. & Meldrum, B.S. (1980b): The role of epileptic activity in hippocampal and 'remote' cerebral lesions induced by kainic acid. *Brain Res.* **191**, 79–97.

Berger, M.L., Tremblay, E., Nitecka, L. & Ben-Ari, Y. (1984): Maturation of kainic acid seizure-brain damage syndrome in the rat. III. Postnatal development of kainic acid binding sites in the limbic system. *Neuroscience* **13**, 1095–1104.

Bickler, P.E., Gallego, S.M. & Hansen, B.M. (1993): Developmental changes in intracellular calcium regulation in rat cerebral cortex during hypoxia. *J. Cereb. Blood Flow Metab.* **13**, 811–819.

Bourgeois, B.F.D., Prensky, A.L., Palkes, H.S., Talent, B.K. & Busch, S.G. (1983): Intelligence in epilepsy: A prospective study in children. *Ann. Neurol.* **14**, 438–444.

Carmant, L., Liu, Z., Werner, S.J., Mikati, M.A. & Holmes, G.L. (1995): Effect of kainic acid-induced status epilepticus on inositol-trisphosphate and seizure-induced brain damage in mature and immature animals. *Dev. Brain Res.* **89**, 67–72.

Cavalheiro, E.A., Silva, D.F., Turski, W.A., Calderazzo-Filho, L.S., Bortolotto, Z.A. & Turski, L. (1987): The susceptibility of rats to pilocarpine-induced seizures is age-dependent. *Dev. Brain Res.* **37**, 43–58.

Cavazos, J.E., Golarai, G. & Sutula, T.P. (1991): Mossy fiber synaptic reorganization induced by kindling: time course of development, progression, and permanence. *J. Neurosci.* **11**, 2795–2803.

Choi, D.W. (1987): Ionic dependence of glutamate neurotoxicity. *J. Neurosci.* **7**, 369–379.

Choi, D.W. (1988a): Calcium-mediated neurotoxicity: Relationship to specific channel types and role in ischemic damage. *TINS* **11**, 465–469.

Choi, D.W. (1988b): Glutamate toxicity and diseases of the nervous system. *Neuron* **1**, 623–624.

Collingridge, G.L. & Bliss, T.V.P. (1987): NMDA receptors – their role in long-term potentiation. *TINS* **10**, 288–293.

Cronin, J. & Dudek, F.E. (1988): Chronic seizures and collateral sprouting of dentate mossy fibers after kainic acid treatment in rats. *Brain Res.* **474**, 181–184.

Dodrill, C.B. & Troupin, A.S. (1976): Seizures and adaptive abilities: a case of identical twins. *Arch. Neurol.* **3**, 604–607.

Fariello, G.G., Golden, G.T., Smith, G.G. & Reyes, P.F. (1989): Potentiation of kainic acid epileptogenicity and sparing from neuronal damage by an NMDA receptor antagonist. *Epilepsy Res.* **3**, 206–213.

Feasy-Truger, K.J., Kargl, L. & ten Bruggencate, G. (1993): Differential effects of dentate kindling on working and reference spatial memory in the rat. *Neurosci. Lett.* **151**, 25–28.

Funakoshi, A., Morikawa, T., Muramatsu, R., Yagi, K. & Seino, M. (1988): A prospective WISC-R study in children with epilepsy. *Jpn. J. Psychiatry Neurol.* **42**, 562–564.

Golarai, G., Cavazos, J.E. & Sutula, T.P. (1992): Activation of the dentate gyrus by pentylenetetrazol evoked seizures induces mossy fiber synaptic reorganization. *Brain Res.* **593**, 257–264.

Gomez, M.R., Kuntz, N.L. & Westmoreland, B.F. (1982): Tuberous sclerosis, early onset of seizures, and mental subnormality: Study of discordant homozygous twins. *Neurology* **32**, 604–611.

Hauser, W.A. & Hersdorffer, D.C. (1990): *Epilepsy: frequency, causes and consequences.* New York: Demos.

Hirsch, E., Baram, T.Z. & Snead, O.C., III (1992): Ontogenic study of lithium-pilocarpine-induced status epilepticus in rats. *Brain Res.* **583**, 120–126.

Holmes, G.L., Thompson, J.L., Marchi, T. & Feldman, D.S. (1988): Behavioral effects of kainic acid administration on the immature brain. *Epilepsia* **29**, 721–730.

Holmes, G.L., Thompson, J.L., Marchi, T.A., Gabriel, P.S., Hogan, M.A., Carl, F.G. & Feldman, D.S. (1990): Effects of seizures on learning, memory, and behavior in the genetically epilepsy-prone rat. *Ann. Neurol.* **27**, 24–32.

Holmes, G.L. (1991a): Do seizures cause brain damage? *Epilepsia* **32**(Suppl. 5), S14-S28.

Holmes, G.L. (1991b): The long-term effects of seizures on the developing brain: clinical and laboratory issues. *Brain Dev.* **13**, 393–409.

Holmes, G.L., Chronopoulos, A., Stafstrom, C.E., Mikati, M.A., Thurber, S.J., Hyde, P.A. & Thompson, J.L. (1993): Effects of kindling on subsequent learning, memory, behavior, and seizure susceptibility. *Dev. Brain Res.* **73**, 71–77.

Holmes, G.L. (1997): Epilepsy in the developing brain: lessons from the laboratory and clinic. *Epilepsia* **38**, 12–30.

Holmes, G.L. & Moshé, S.L. (1990): Consequences of seizures in the developing brain. *J. Epilepsy* **3**(Suppl), 7–13.

Hori, N., ffrench-Mullen, J.M.H. & Carpenter, D.O. (1985): Kainic acid response and toxicity show pronounced Ca^{2+} dependence. *Brain Res.* **358**, 380–384.

Houser, C.R., Miyashiro, J.E., Swartz, B.E., Walsh, G.O., Rich, J.R. & Delgado-Escueta, A.V. (1990): Altered patterns of dynorphin immunoreactivity suggest mossy fiber reorganization in human hippocampal epilepsy. *J. Neurosci.* **10**, 267–282.

Irvine, R.F. (1991): Inositol tetrakisphosphate as a second messenger: confusions, contradictions and a potential resolution. *BioEssays* **13**, 419–427.

Isokawa, M., Levesque, M.F., Babb, T.L. & Engel, J., Jr. (1993): Single mossy fiber axonal systems of human dentate granule cells studied in hippocampal slices from patients with temporal lobe epilepsy. *J. Neurosci.* **13**, 1511–1522.

Knowlton, B.J., Shapiro, M.L. & Olton, D.S. (1989): Hippocampal seizures disrupt working memory performance but not reference memory acquisition. *Behav. Neurosci.* **103**, 1144–1147.

Kudo, Y. & Ogura, A. (1986): Glutamate-induced increase in intracellular Ca^{2+} concentration in isolated hippocampal neurons. *Brit. J. Pharmacol.* **89**, 191–198.

Lees, G.J. & Leong, W. (1992): The non-NMDA glutamate anatagonist NBQX blocks the local hippocampal toxicity of kainic acid, but not the diffuse extrahippocampal damage. *Neurosci. Lett.* **143**, 39–42.

Leite, J.P., Babb, T.L., Pretorius, J.K., Kuhlman, P.A., Yeoman, K.M. & Mathern, G.W. (1996): Neuron loss, mossy fiber sprouting, and interictal spikes after intrahippocampal kainate in developing rats. *Epilepsy Res.* **26**, 219–231.

Letty, S., Lerner-Natoli, M. & Rondouin, G. (1995): Differential impairments of spatial memory and social behavior in two models of limbic epilepsy. *Epilepsia* **36**, 973–982.

Leung, L.S., Boon, K.A., Kaibara, T. & Innis, N.K. (1990): Radial maze performance following hippocampal kindling. *Behav. Brain Res.* **40**, 119–129.

Leung, L.S. & Shen, B. (1991): Hippocampal CA1 evoked response and radial 8-arm maze performance after hippocampal kindling. *Brain Res.* **555**, 353–357.

Liu, Z., Gatt, A., Mikati, M. & Holmes, G.L. (1995): Long-term behavioral deficits following pilocarpine seizures in immature rats. *Epilepsy Res.* **19**, 191–204.

Liu, Z., Stafstrom, C.E., Sarkisian, M., Tandon, P., Yang, Y., Hori, A. & Holmes, G.L. (1996): Age-dependent effects of glutamate toxicity in the hippocampus. *Dev. Brain Res.* **97**, 178–184.

Lopes da Silva, F.H., Gorter, J.A. & Wadman, W.J. (1986): Kindling of the hippocampus induces spatial memory deficits in the rat. *Neurosci. Lett.* **63**, 115–120.

Masukawa, L.M., O'Connor, W.M., Lynott, J., Burdette, L.J., Uruno, K., McGonigle, P. & O'Connor, M.J. (1995): Longitudinal variation in cell density and mossy fiber reorganization in the dentate gyrus from temporal lobe epileptic patients. *Brain Res.* **678**, 65–75.

Mathern, G.W., Leite, J.P., Pretorius, J.K., Quinn, B., Peacock, W.J. & Babb, T.L. (1994): Children with severe epilepsy: evidence of hippocampal neuron losses and aberrant mossy fiber sprouting during postnatal granule cell migration and differentiation. *Dev. Brain Res.* **78**, 70–80.

Mathern, G.W., Babb, T.L., Mischel, P.S., Vinters, H.V., Pretorius, J.K., Leite, J.P. & Peacock, W.J. (1996): Childhood generalized and mesial temporal epilepsies demonstrate different amounts and patterns of hippocampal neuron loss and mossy fibre synaptic reorganization. *Brain* **119**, 965–987.

McNamara, J.O. (1994): Cellular and molecular basis of epilepsy. *J. Neurosci.* **14**, 3413–3425.

McNamara, R.K., Kirkby, R.D., dePace, G.E. & Corcoran, M.E. (1992): Limbic seizures, but not kindling, reversibly impair place learning in the Morris water maze. *Behav. Brain Res.* **50**, 167–175.

Meldrum, B.S. & Brierley, J.B. (1973): Prolonged epileptic seizures in primates: Ischaemic cell change and its relation to ictal physiological events. *Arch. Neurol.* **28**, 10–17.

Meldrum, B.S., Vigouroux, R.A. & Brierley, J.B. (1973): Systemic factors and epileptic brain damage. Prolonged seizures in paralysed artificially ventilated baboons. *Arch. Neurol.* **29**, 82–87.

Mitani, A., Yanase, H., Sakai, K., Wake, Y. & Kataoka, K. (1993): Origin of intracellular calcium elevation induced by *in vitro* ischemia-like condition in hippocampal slices. *Brain Res.* **601**, 103–110.

Nadler, J.V. (1981): Kainic acid as a tool for the study of temporal lobe epilepsy. *Life Sci.* **29**, 2031–2042.

Nadler, J.V., Perry, B.W. & Cotman, C.W. (1978): Intraventricular kainic acid preferentially destroys hippocampal pyramidal cells. *Nature* **271**, 676–677.

Neill, J., Liu, Z., Sarkisian, M., Tandon, P., Yang, Y., Stafstrom, C.E. & Holmes, G.L. (1996): Recurrent seizures in immature rats: effect on auditory and visual discrimination. *Dev. Brain Res.* **95**, 283–292.

Nieminen, A.S., Sirviö, J., Teittinen, K., Pitkänen, A., Airaksinen, M.M. & Riekkinen, P. (1992): Amygdala kindling increased fear-response, but did not impair spatial memory in rats. *Physiol. Behav.* **51**, 845–849.

Nitecka, L., Tremblay, E., Charton, G., Bouillot, J.P., Berger, M. & Ben-Ari, Y. (1984): Maturation of kainic acid seizure-brain damage syndrome in the rat. II. Histopathological sequelae. *Neuroscience* **13**, 1073–1094.

Okazaki, M.E., Evenson, D.A. & Nadler, J.V. (1995): Hippocampal mossy fiber sprouting and synapse formation after status epilepticus in rats: visualization after retrograde transport of biocytin. *J. Comp. Neurol.* **352**, 515–534.

Olney, J.W., Fuller, T. & De Gubareff, T. (1979): Acute dendrotoxic changes in the hippocampus of kainate treated rats. *Brain Res.* **176**, 91–100.

Olney, J.W., Collins, R.C. & Sloviter, R.S. (1986): Excitotoxic mechanisms of epileptic brain damage. *Adv. Neurol.* **44**, 857–877.

Orrenius, S., McConkey, D., Belloma, G. & Nicoterm, P. (1989): Role of Ca[$2+$] in toxic killing. *Trends Pharmacol. Sci.* **10**, 281–285.

Pollard, H., Charriaut-Marlangue, S., Cantagrel, S., Represa, A., Robain, O., Moreau, J. & Ben-Ari, Y. (1994): Kainate-induced apoptotic cell death in hippocampal neurons. *Neuroscience* **63**, 7–18.

Represa, A. & Ben-Ari, Y. (1992): Kindling is associated with the formation of novel mossy fiber synapses in the CA3 region. *Exp. Brain Res.* **92**, 69–78.

Represa, A., Tremblay, E. & Ben-Ari, Y. (1987a): Kainate binding sites in the hippocampal mossy fibers: localization and plasticity. *Neuroscience* **20**, 739–748.

Represa, A., Tremblay, E. & Ben-Ari, Y. (1987b): Aberrant growth of mossy fibers and enhanced kainic acid binding sites induced in rats by early hyperthyroidism. *Brain Res.* **423**, 325–328.

Represa, A., Jorquera, I., Le Gal La Salle, G. & Ben-Ari, Y. (1993): Epilepsy induced collateral sprouting of hippocampal mossy fibers: does it induce the development of ectopic synapses with granule cell dendrites? *Hippocampus* **3**, 257–268.

Ribak, C.E. & Baram, T.Z. (1996): Selective death of hippocampal CA3 pyramidal cells with mossy fiber afferents after CRH-induced status epilepticus in infant rats. *Dev. Brain Res.* **91**, 245–251.

Rodin, E.A., Schmaltz, S. & Twitty, G. (1986): Intellectual functions of patients with childhood-onset epilepsy. *Dev. Med. Child Neurol.* **28**, 25–33.

Schiottz-Christensen, E. & Bruhn, P. (1973): Intelligence, behavior, and scholastic achievement subsequent to febrile convulsions: An analysis of discordant twin-pairs. *Dev. Med. Child Neurol.* **15**, 565–575.

Siesjö, B.K. (1988): Historical review: calcium, ischemia, and death of brain cells. *Ann. N. Y. Acad. Sci.* **522**, 638–661.

Sloviter, R.S. (1983): 'Epileptic' brain damage in rats induced by sustained electrical stimulation of the perforant path. I. Acute electrophysiological and light microscopic studies. *Brain Res. Bull.* **10**, 675–697.

Sloviter, R.S. & Damiano, B.P. (1981): Sustained electrical stimulation of the perforant path duplicates kainate-induced electrophysiological effects and hippocampal damage in rats. *Neurosci. Lett.* **24**, 279–284.

Sloviter, R.S. & Dempster, D.W. (1985): 'Epileptic' brain damage is replicated qualitatively in the rat hippocampus by central injection of glutamate or aspartate but not by GABA or acetylcholine. *Brain Res. Bull.* **15**, 39–60.

Sloviter, R.S., Dean, E., Sollas, A.I. & Goodman, J.H. (1996): Apoptosis and necrosis induced in different hippocampal neuron populations by repetitive perforant path stimulation in the rat. *J. Comp. Neurol.* **366**, 516–533.

Sperber, E.F., Haas, K.Z., Stanton, P.K. & Moshé, S.L. (1991): Resistance of the immature hippocampus to seizure-induced synaptic reorganization. *Dev. Brain Res.* **60**, 88–93.

Sperber, E.F., Weireter, K.K., Kubova, H. & Romero, M.-T. (1995): Age-related changes in parvalbumin immunoreactivity following kainic acid seizure. *Soc. Neurosci. Abstr.* **21**, 1473

Stafstrom, C.E., Thompson, J.L. & Holmes, G.L. (1992): Kainic acid seizures in the developing brain: status epilepticus and spontaneous recurrent seizures. *Dev. Brain Res.* **65**, 227–236.

Stafstrom, C.E., Chronopoulos, A., Thurber, S., Thompson, J.L. & Holmes, G.L. (1993): Age-dependent cognitive and behavioral deficits following kainic acid-induced seizures. *Epilepsia* **34**, 420–432.

Sutula, T.P. (1990): Experimental models of temporal lobe epilepsy: new insights from the study of kindling and synaptic reorganization. *Epilepsia* **31**(Suppl. 3), S45-S54.

Sutula, T.P. (1993): The pathology of the epilepsies: Insights into the causes and consequences of epileptic syndromes. In: *Pediatric epilepsy: diagnosis and treatment*, Dodson, W.E. & Pellock, J.M. (eds), pp. 37–44. New York: Demos

Sutula, T., Xiao-Xian, H., Cavazos, J. & Scott, G. (1988): Synaptic reorganization in the hippocampus induced by abnormal functional activity. *Science* **239**, 1147–1150.

Sutula, T., Cascino, G., Cavazos, J., Parada, I. & Ramirez, L. (1989): Mossy fiber synaptic reorganization in the epileptic human temporal lobe. *Ann. Neurol.* **26**, 321–330.

Sutula, T., Koch, J., Golarai, G., Watanabe, Y. & McNamara, J.O. (1996): NMDA receptor dependence of kindling and mossy fiber sprouting: evidence that the NMDA receptor regulates patterning of hippocampal circuits in the adult brain. *J. Neurosci.* **16**, 7398–7406.

Tauck, D. & Nadler, J.V. (1985): Evidence of functional mossy fiber sprouting in the hippocampal formation of kainic acid-treated rats. *J. Neurosci.* **5**, 1016–1022.

Thurber, S., Chronopoulos, A., Stafstrom, C.E. & Holmes, G.L. (1992): Behavioral effects of continuous hippocampal stimulation in the developing rat. *Dev. Brain Res.* **68**, 35–40.

Thurber, S., Mikati, M.A., Stafstrom, C.E., Jensen, F.E. & Holmes, G.L. (1994): Quisqualic acid-induced seizures during development: A behavioral and EEG study. *Epilepsia* **35**, 868–875.

Van der Zee, C.E.E.M., Rashid, K., Le, K., Moore, K.-A., Stanisz, J., Diamond, J., Racine, R.J. & Fahnestock, M. (1995): Intraventricular administration of antibodies to nerve growth factor retards kindling and blocks mossy fiber sprouting in adult rats. *J. Neurosci.* **15**, 5316–5323.

Wuarin, J.-P. & Dudek, E.F. (1996): Electrographic seizures and new recurrent excitatory circuits in the dentate gyrus of hippocampal slices from kainate-treated epileptic rats. *J. Neurosci.* **16**, 4438–4448.

PART VI
Consequences of treatment on brain development

Chapter 24

Anti-epileptic drugs and cognitive function

Catherine Billard

Hôpital Clocheville, Department of Neuropaediatrics, 49 Bld Béranger, 37044 Tours Cedex 1, France

Introduction

All relevant studies published to date describe cognitive impairment in epileptic children with particular focus on areas such as attention, memory, speed of mental and motor processing, and verbal and visuo-spatial intellectual performance (Aldenkamp *et al.*, 1990; Jambaqué *et al.*, 1991; Dreifuss, 1992; Mitchell *et al.*, 1992). Presentation varies widely in frequency and severity, as do the types of epilepsy and epileptic children themselves.

However in the interpretation of studies on cognition and epilepsy, several confounding factors concerning epilepsy must be taken into account, including:

- Aetiology (especially brain lesions),
- Age of onset and duration,
- Severity (type, frequency, severity and duration of seizures and post-ictal state, but also frequency, and localization of diurnal and probably nocturnal EEG interictal paroxysms),
- Various environmental, social and psycho-affective factors,
- The eventual direct cognitive effect of the antiepileptic drugs.

Overall, the interaction between these different factors is very complex and well illustrated by the variation of the adverse effects of drugs according to the underlying lesions, as described by Durwen & Elger (1993). Only patients with left temporal epilepsy showed an improvement, in verbal memory only, after withdrawal of antiepileptics ('withdrawal effect'); patients with right temporal epilepsy showed no change in either type of memory. These findings constitute a further argument to suggest that the biological factors provided by drugs may contribute to the 'revealing' or 'aggravating' neuro-psychological consequences of an underlying anatomical lesion. So adverse effects, if existing, will always be those corresponding to the population studied and can never be extrapolated to another population.

Nevertheless the growing interest in 'quality of life' and the multiplication of new drugs constitute additional arguments for a very detailed evaluation of the precise role of drugs in cognitive impairment. Such work requires an 'ideal epileptic' situation which would make it possible to isolate this factor from all the others impinging on cognitive function in epileptic children.

Meta-analysis of more than 300 studies dating back over 25 years requires a precise and critical examination of the methodological difficulties, with reference to the choice of population, tests and statistical interpretation.

Choice of population

Three approaches have been adopted: studying healthy volunteers, non-epileptics or epileptics.

Healthy volunteers constitute a theoretically ideal population in the sense that other intercurrent factors related to epilepsy are eliminated. However such an approach involves using only adults and sub-therapeutic doses for short periods (usually two weeks maximum). It therefore overestimates the transitory effects and underestimates the chronic effects that interest us more.

Studies of chronic effects in non-epileptic patients relate, for adults, either to post-trauma epilepsy prevention or space medicine. The situation in children that is closest to this is prevention of the recurrence of febrile convulsions.

However, most studies have concerned epileptic patients using different methodologies. Retrospective, non-randomized, cross-sectional studies which associate, without being able to differentiate in any way, all the intercurrent factors, essentially showed that the studies describing the damaging cognitive effects of drugs are less numerous than those describing no effects. The two most interesting methodologies are prospective randomized studies and withdrawal studies. Randomized prospective studies compared, if possible blindly, two drugs or a drug and a placebo, either in parallel groups (where the two therapeutic situations concern different patients), or in a cross-over study (where the two therapeutic situations are alternated in the same patient). Although the methodolodgy of parallel groups is among the best, it is not beyond criticism and needs to carefully evaluate whether the two groups are identical in terms of epilepsy. On the other hand, it is never possible in a cross-over study to ensure that there is no 'carry over' effect, i.e. that the patient is not experiencing the consequences of the first therapy during the second therapeutic period. In withdrawal studies the side-effects of the drug are carefully assessed indirectly according to the improvement after withdrawal of antiepileptic drugs in patients who no longer experience seizures. Such studies effectively remove the seizure factor and probably the interictal paroxysmal factor, but whatever efforts are made to match populations at the outset, the absence of randomization of the drug cannot exclude the influence of the type of epilepsy on the results. A control group is obviously essential in order to judge the improvement related to repeated testing (test–retest effect). Above all, absence of improvement on withdrawal of the drug makes it very difficult to conclude whether there was no untoward effect or whether there is still an untoward effect which persists after withdrawal.

Choice of test

If the battery of neuro-psychological tests is too limited, there is a risk of not revealing mild effects. If the testing is too wide, there is a risk of bringing out 'subtle' effects which, while interesting, have little practical value. Everyone agrees that a method which is as rigorous as possible should be used, with comparison of a wide neuro-psychological battery with behaviour and psychosocial scales.

The battery needs, firstly the evaluation of the intellectual performance which is essential for the comparison of two populations; secondly, evaluation of motor (tapping) and mental performances ('computerized visual search', see Alpherts & Aldenkamp, 1990), attention, concentration and impulsivity (Stroop's test, reaction times; see Mitchell *et al.*, 1993), various aspects of memory and finally educational consequences, particularly in terms of written language and mathematics. Several types of battery have been described and they are fairly comparable. The use of computer programs has been developed and this has the huge advantage of providing material which can be used in many centres (e.g. FePsy; see Alpherts & Aldenkamp, 1990). Further research will probably use combined computerized tests, EEG and auditory related event potentials. Comparison with behaviour and psychosocial scales appropriate for children is indispensible for the interpretations of the consequences in everyday life.

Interpretation of the results

A statistically significant result does not imply a real consequence in everyday life but, contrariwise, absence of significant findings always warrants reflection in relation to the size of the population and to individual effects, which are sometimes considerable (Mitchell & Chavez, 1987).

All these considerations emphasize the necessity of careful and critical reading of each article included in the survey.

Results in the literature in terms of the analysis of each medication

Despite exercising caution in the evaluation of reports in the literature, the existence of adverse cognitive effects of antiepileptic drugs, which are psychotropic, is highly probable.

Experimental data

The experimental data must above all not be extrapolated to humans. However, various deleterious effects have been described on learning in rats (dose dependent) with phenytoin, ethosuxinimide, valproate and phenobarbital (Diaz, 1983; Yanai et al., 1979). In particular, chronic administration of phenytoin and phenobarbital has effects on cerebral growth. Conversely, the situation is complex with carbamazepine as it is more deleterious in non-epileptic rats (Mondadori & Classen, 1984). The adverse consequences of the exposition of foetuses whose mothers have been treated with phenobarbital and phenytoin but not with carbamazepine must be borne in mind (Scolnick et al., 1994). For more data on the effects of antiepileptic drug treatments in animals, see Chapter 25 in this book.

The problem of multiple therapy

Several studies in both children and adults (Thompson & Trimble, 1982) provide arguments for improvement in cognitive function and a decrease in adverse effects with reduction in the number of antiepileptic drugs. Cull (1988) compared four matched groups, one of non-epileptic subjects, a second of epileptic subjects with unchanged treatment, a third with reduced treatment and a fourth with increased therapy. Performance did not improve when therapy was increased, although reduction in antiepileptic drugs clearly improved performance, particularly with regard to attention (code subtest and reaction time).

Phenobarbital

Phenobarbital is the drug which has been most often studied in children. The negative reputation of the influence of phenobarbital on behaviour is widely known. Despite some contradictory conclusions, the majority of papers emphasize the adverse effects on behaviour, together with mental abilities, with phenobarbital compared to the other AEDs. Wolf & Forsythe (1978) studied the side-effects of phenobarbital, which is used for the prevention of recurrence of convulsions, and described such side-effects in 48 per cent of the treated group against 18 per cent in the non-treated group. Camfield et al. (1979) in a similar randomized study described more dose-related and unacceptable side-effects with phenobarbital compared to placebo. Domizio et al. (1993) performed an extensive study by interviewing 300 epileptic child out-patients and reached the same conclusions: the group treated with phenobarbital had a significantly higher level of severe complaints (76 per cent) (hyperactivity, instability, sleep disturbance) against 31 per cent in the group not treated with phenobarbital.

The rigorous methodology of Vining et al. (1987) provided a further argument. In a double-blind, cross-over study, they compared two periods of a six-month treatment in 21 epileptic children using valproate then phenobarbital or phenobarbital then valproate. Of the 48 items of the behaviour scale scored during and at the end of each period, 11 items scored significantly against phenobarbital. The nature of these items evoked truly disabling consequences of the behaviour changes: inability to finish tasks, inability to stop repeated activities, unhappiness, depression, disobedience, excitability, anxiety with many somatic complaints, sleep disorders and difficulties with making friends. Taken together, they represented the main features of the hyperkinetic syndrome. The behaviour problems did not appear to be obvious to the parents, emphasizing the possibility of side-effects not revealed but clearly deleterious.

Concerning phenobarbital and cognitive abilities, Vining *et al.* (1987) also studied the performance of the same patients with 35 items to test attention skills, memory, intelligence and school learning. Eight of 35 subtests also scored significantly against phenobarbital (PIQ, FIQ, block design, picture completion, vocabulary, arithmetic subtests, pair learning memory and mathematical abilities). On the other hand, attention measured by continuous reaction time was not significantly different with either therapy. These results are particularly interesting because the patients withdrawn from the study are few, i.e. seven, of whom four were related to the severe behaviour effects associated with phenobarbital.

In contrast to this study, Mitchell & Chavez (1987) did not reveal any significantly obvious differences between phenobarbital and carbamazepine. Thirty-one children with mild epilepsy were randomized into groups treated by either drug. Testing was performed blindly. The behaviour scale and neuro-psychological battery, applied at baseline and then after 6 months and one year of treatment, revealed no difference. The results warrant several comments. On the one hand, the population was small and the number lost to follow-up or withdrawn was high; only 21 of the 31 were assessed at 6 months and 17 at one year. On the other hand, the neuro-psychological battery was reduced to the measurement of intellectual quotient by various tests according to age. Thirdly, and this was one of the author's comments, the absence of group effect sometimes did not prevent huge individual differences: one child was withdrawn from the study because his IQ fell by 20 when receiving carbamazepine, without aggravating the seizure frequency, and the points were regained during treatment with phenobarbital.

Phenobarbital is the only antiepileptic drug whose effects on cognition have been studied in young children because of its frequent use in the prevention of recurrence of febrile convulsions. Camfield *et al.* (1970) found no difference in overall Development Quotient (DQ, Stanford Binet) at the end of follow-up in 8–12-month-old infants treated for febrile convulsions. On the other hand, memory was significantly less competent in the phenobarbital group. In particular, the infants treated for 12 months subsequently had a significant deficit on comprehension subtests, and it is not known how this might relate to eventual learning in school.

Farwell *et al.* (1990) carried out an extremely ambitious study. They randomized 217 infants with febrile convulsions aged 8–36 months, into two well-matched groups, one being treated with phenobarbital and the other with placebo. The follow-up comprised testing of DQ before randomization, further testing after two years of treatment and final DQ testing six months after withdrawal of treatment. The results were clearly against phenobarbital, both in evaluation of intention to treat and actual treatment. The phenobarbital group had a DQ which was significantly lower at two years than the placebo group (97 vs. 102), and this significant difference persisted at the examination performed six months after withdrawal of treatment. In agreement with these results, the patients of the phenobarbital group who maintained their treatment for two years had a mean DQ which was significantly lower than those who had not maintained it (95 vs. 102), whereas a similar difference was not found in the placebo group (105 vs. 103). Finally, in the phenobarbital group, the children whose parents confirmed regular administration of the drug had significantly lower DQs than those whose treatment had not been regular (94 vs. 101). Although the statistical analysis has been critized (Lee *et al.*, 1991), all these concordant results, associated with the absence of significant difference in frequency of recurrence in the two groups, tended to show that phenobarbital is a drug of dubious effectiveness in this situation and of limited tolerance. In fact, although methodological bias, such as frequency of loss to follow-up, prevents conclusions concerning the study by Farwell *et al.* (1990), it is nevertheless clear that there may be behavioural side-effects with phenobarbital and worrying effects on mental function. The issue is to distinguish to what extent the first explain the second, particularly in young children.

Phenytoin

Phenytoin has a controversial reputation in adults, with contradictory reports in the literature. Supporters of its adverse effects (Trimble & Thompson, 1983) go as far as to describe a true phenytoin encephalopathy (Dreifuss, 1992), while supporters of the absence of adverse effects consider it beneficial if used at the correct dosage (Meador et al., 1990). Dodrill (1992), who revised his first study by separating several groups according to plasma concentrations, clearly showed that the untoward cognitive effects of phenytoin were only related to above therapeutic, or even toxic, concentrations.

Phenytoin has the reputation of a 'disaster' drug for adolescents (Gallassi et al., 1992) and children, and this aspect is well summarized in Committee on drugs (1985).

If account is taken of the studies performed with strict methodology, the findings are as follows: Aldenkamp et al. (1993) performed a large multicentre, non-randomized study, assessing cognitive functions before and after complete withdrawal of phenytoin, carbamazepine or valproate on monotherapy. They found poorer performance in children treated with phenytoin both during treatment and after withdrawal of treatment. This deleterious effect was slight since it was only significant for the motor skill of hand tapping with the dominant hand. This certainly does not permit their conclusion that phenytoin is deleterious, and remains so after withdrawal. The lack of randomization at the outset of treatment may have contributed to these mild differences observed. It is possible that the choice of phenytoin or carbamazepine was linked rather to the severity of the epilepsy at the onset than to chance. In particular, they compared carbamazepine and phenytoin in patients in a subgroup of benign epilepsy with centrotemporal spikes, and found no difference in the performance between 9 patients treated with phenytoin and 18 treated with carbamazepine.

In contrast, the randomized study of Forsythe et al. (1991) tested blindly and without recurrence of crises, did not show a clear deleterious effect of phenytoin. Sixty-nine newly diagnozed epileptic children were prospectively randomly assigned to phenytoin, carbamazepine or valproate, and were assessed with an extensive battery of cognitive tests before and three subsequent times over a year. Only the speed of mental processing was transiently reduced in the subgroup treated with phenytoin but memory was not impaired for phenytoin and valproate, in contrast to carbamazepine.

Finally there seems to be no influence of blood levels of drug on cognitive function within therapeutic levels. Aman et al. (1994) found no difference in a wide battery of cognitive functions tested in outpatient epileptic children treated with phenytoin, whether the testing was according to residual levels or peak levels, and despite a 50 per cent difference in plasma concentrations.

In conclusion, the findings in children are as controversial as in adults, but the damaging effects suggested by Aldenkamp et al.'s withdrawal study (1993) in which the treatment was non-prospective and non-randomized do not seem clearly confirmed by prospective studies. Individual variations are certainly great and depend, in particular, on the severity of the epilepsy, and it is certainly true that the choice of phenytoin is often dependent on the severity. It is regretable that, in contrast to phenobarbital, there has as yet been no study comparing phenytoin with placebo and no study in young children, particularly because intra-utero exposition to phenobarbital seems to be damaging to the cognitive development of children (Scolnick et al., 1994).

Carbamazepine and valproate

Compared to the poor reputations of phenobarbital and phenytoin, those for carbamazepine and valproate are encouraging. Studies in healthy volunteers and open studies in adults of replacement of various treatments with carbamazepine (Smith et al., 1987) have indicated, without being proved, an almost complete absence of adverse effects for carbamazepine. No comparison of carbamazepine with placebo has been done. As we have seen, when Mitchell & Chavez (1987) compared carbamazepine as a randomized, prospective treatment in mild epilepsy with phenobarbital, they found no significant difference for the whole group but an individual severe and non-explained deleterious effect. Stores *et al.* (1992) found no clear difference, in an extensive behaviour scale and wide neuro-psychological battery, between carbamazepine and valproate prescribed prospectively but not randomly, for newly diagnosed epilepsy. The first results of Blennow *et al.* (1990), and more specifically those of Aldenkamp *et al.* multicentre study (1993) showed no clear modification of performance after withdrawal of carbamazepine, suggesting an absence of adverse effects. Two controlled, randomized studies of the replacement of ineffective or poorly tolerated phenobarbital by either phenytoin or carbamazepine in groups of children or adults (Bittencourt *et al.*, 1993) came to approximately the same conclusion, i.e. an improvement in memory and/or attention with replacement by carbamazepine, without distinguishing whether this is related to withdrawal of phenobarbital or improvement of epilepsy or direct effect of carbamazepine.

The only study suggesting slight but significant adverse effects was the prospective, randomized study of Forsythe *et al.* (1991) which used a wide battery of tests to compare three populations of recently diagnosed epileptic children treated with phenytoin, carbamazepine or valproate. Total memory performance scores were lower with carbamazepine in comparison with valproate and not different with phenytoin. This situation persisted throughout treatment, with a negative correlation with plasma concentrations despite levels which were never above therapeutic (8 mg/l). The relationship between plasma concentration and cognitive function has been studied in various ways. In an open monotherapy study O'Dougherty *et al.* (1987) suggested a slight benefit with carbamazepine on speed of eye–hand coordination but a negative correlation between performance and levels of concentration. At low levels the memory processes were quicker and at high levels performance scores in learning of new information and in a memory scanning test were decreased. On the other hand, a study by Aman *et al.* (1990) on outpatients receiving carbamazepine monotherapy in two conditions of different plasma concentrations by modifying the time of the test in relation to the time of administration, one at residual levels and the other at peak levels, found no difference in performance according to plasma concentrations. At the same time, several controlled, randomized studies have compared the classical form of carbamazepine to the sustained-released form (Pieters *et al.*, 1992) without showing any objective difference but a subjective preference for the release form.

In conclusion, although no study has compared carbamazepine to placebo and no study has been done on young children, the damaging effects of carbamazepine appear to be moderate or even nil, even though there are sometimes subjective side-effects (Bittencourt *et al.*, 1993).

Since it came onto the market, valproate has enjoyed a favourable reputation, attractively summarized as 'bright and lively'. Studies on healthy volunteers (Thompson & Trimble, 1982) and open studies (Harding *et al.*, 1980) would seem to indicate few harmful side-effects, and even an improvement in reaction time with valproate. Controlled and randomized adult studies have shown that the cognitive effects with valproate are minimal and reversible, but essentially at high doses (Trimble & Thompson, 1984), there are slight untoward but reversible effects on attention, memory and motility (Gallassi *et al.*, 1990); or minimal effects on learning, contrasting clearly with the harmful effects observed in the same conditions with clonazepam (Sommerbeck *et al.*, 1977).

No study in children has been randomized against placebo, as is the case for carbamazepine or phenytoin, and no conclusion can be made apart from comparison with a reference product, which has already been described. To summarize, performance such as behaviour under valproate in Vining *et al.*'s cross-over study (1987) was always better than that observed under phenobarbital. No harmful effects were evidenced in Forsythe *et al.* study (1991) comparing phenytoin and carbamazepine, nor in Stores *et al.* (1992) non-randomized study comparing carbamazepine. No clear improvement on withdrawal of drugs was evidenced in the two 'withdrawal' studies of Blennow *et al.* (1990) and Aldenkamp *et al.* (1993).

Aman *et al.* (1987) researched the effects on cognitive functions according to plasma concentrations and showed that valproate is deleterious on concentration, memory and motility at high concentrations in comparison with low concentrations. Perhaps this reinforces the thesis given in Hara & Fukuyama's non-randomized and non-controlled study (1989) that valproate may have a more harmful effect than carbamazepine on sustained attention in children of normal intelligence.

As shown in a cross-over study, even when the sustained release form is clearly chosen, it does not provide improvement in cognitive functions compared with the conventional form (Brouwer et al., 1992).

In conclusion, although it can be said that some studies concerning the cognitive consequences of carbamazepine and valproate are contradictory, all the conclusions emphasize the absence of untoward behavioural effects and the milder nature of the effects in terms of cognitive functions in comparison with the two previous drugs.

New drugs

In terms of new drugs, no conclusive tests have been carried out on children. As new AEDs should protect neurons from excitotoxic cell damage and harmful neuronal reorganization which occur after brain injury, it is essential to evaluate their cognitive effects.

In adults, vigabatrin appears to have no harmful effects on cognitive functions according to Gilham et al., randomized, double-blind, cross-over study compared to placebo (1993), or according to Dodrill et al.'s randomized, double-blind, parallel study also compared to placebo (1993). In children, a controlled, randomized pilot study compared monotherapy with vigabatrin versus carbamazepine in recently diagnosed epilepsy (Kalviainen et al., 1991). The results suggested an improvement of sustained concentration and mental processes with vigabatrin. The large open series of St Vincent de Paul in Paris (Jambaqué et al., personal communication) raises the possibility of hyperkinetic syndrome essentially in mentally retarded children. Nevertheless the improvement of vigilance observed in adults makes further studies necessary in order to know whether vigabatrin has a positive effect stimulating vigilance, compared to the drowsiness seen with carbamazepine, or if it has a negative effect inducing hyperkinetic syndrome. Oxcarbazepine was compared with phenytoin in a randomized, double-blind monotherapy study in adults (Aikia et al., 1992) and no deleterious effects were revealed by a wide battery of neuro-psychological tests. In a double-blind, cross-over study versus placebo, it was shown that lamotrigine did not significantly alter cognitive function (Banks & Beran, 1991) and seems to produce less drowsiness than carbamazepine or phenytoin. The open studies in children and the placebo controlled study in symptomatic generalized epilepsies emphasizes a frequent and clear well-being and improvement of vigilance in children treated with lamotrigine (Hosking et al., 1993).

Stiripentol may have a positive psychotropic effect in association with carbamazepine, in reducing the epoxy ratio (Loiseau et al., 1988). Nothing is known concerning gabapentin, tiagabine and topiramate in children.

Conclusion

The findings reported in the literature are numerous but contradictory and stem from methods which are difficult to compare and never beyond criticism. Nevertheless, some points warrant emphasis. Multiple therapy, phenobarbital and probably phenytoin appear to be the most harmful in terms of cognitive function and particularly at high doses. Carbamazepine and valproate are likely to provide slight statistical effects but seem to be less deleterious. The numerous reports of studies with phenobarbital and phenytoin have their principal interest in suggesting further studies with the new drugs using a more clearly defined methodological basis.

In certain studies, the findings should not be taken as interesting or even essential theoretical indications with regard to a new drug, but this in no way eliminates the possibility of extremely unpleasant individual effects of a drug with a good reputation or, on the other hand, the possibility of good individual tolerance of a drug with a poor reputation.

Clinical follow-up and clinical assessment of the risk/benefit ratio is always more important than theoretical results. Although Dodrill (1992) studied the long-term effects of prolonged treatment (up to 5 years) in adults, there is nothing similar available involving children, whereas studies concerning phenobarbital suggest, in particular during use in infants, the possibility of untoward effects which persist beyond the treatment time. The issue of knowing whether the harmful effects of certain drugs are seen essentially in certain particular types of epilepsies or at a certain age is a completely unanswered question. Recent studies comparing cognitive tests and auditory related potentials (Chen, 1995), showed modification in latencies or amplitudes of potentials where there is no deterioration of tests, suggesting perhaps a subtle but interesting way to monitor drugs.

We conclude with two apparently contradictory remarks. Despite the difficulties and despite the modesty of the conclusions, studying the effect on cognitive function in children is essential in the development programme of an antiepileptic drug. The goal of modern drug treatment should not only be the cessation of seizures, but also the prevention of cognitive dysfunction.

References

Aikia, M., Kalvianen, R., Sivenius, J., Halonen, T. & Riekkinen, P.J. (1992): Cognitive effects of Oxcarbazepine and phenytoin monotherapy in newly diagnosed epilepsy: one year follow-up. *Epilepsy Res.* **11**, 199–203.

Aldenkamp, A.P., Alpherts, W.C.J., Dekker, M.J.A. & Overweg, J. (1990): Neuropsychological aspects of learning disabilities in epilepsy. *Epilepsia* **31** (suppl. 4), S9–S20.

Aldenkamp, A.P., Alpherts, W.C.J., Blennow, G. *et al.* (1993): Withdrawal of antiepileptic medication in children; effects on cognitive function: the multicenter Holmfrid study. *Neurology* **43**, 41–50.

Alpherts, W.C.J. & Aldenkamp, A.P. (1990): Computerized neuropsychological assessment of cognitive functioning in children with epilepsy. *Epilepsia* **31** (suppl. 4), S35–S40.

Aman, M.G., Werry, J.S., Paxton, J.W. & Turbott, S.H. (1987): Effect of sodium valproate on psychomotor performance in children as a function of dose, fluctuations in concentration, and diagnosis. *Epilepsia* **28**, 115–124.

Aman, M.G., Werry, J.S., Paxton, J.W., Turbott, S.H. & Stewart, A.W. (1990): Effects of Carbamazepine on psychomotor performance in children as a function of drug concentration, seizure type, and time of medication. *Epilepsia* **31**, 51–60.

Aman, M.G., Werry, J.S., Paxton, J.W. & Turbott, S.H. (1994): Effects of phenytoin on cognitive-motor performance in children as a function of drug concentration, seizure type, and time of medication. *Epilepsia* **35**, 172–180.

Banks, G.K. & Beran, R.G. (1991): Neuropsychological assessment in lamotrigine treated epileptic patients. *Clin. Exp. Neurol.* **28**, 230–237.

Bittencourt, P.R., Antoniuk, S.A., Bigarella, M.M. *et al.* (1993): Carbamazepine and phenytoin in epilepsies refractory to barbiturates: efficacy, toxicity and mental function. *Epilepsy Res.* **16**, 147–155.

Blennow, G., Heijbel, J., Sandstedt, P. & Tonnby, B. (1990): Discontinuation of antiepileptic drugs in children who have outgrown epilepsy: effects on cognitive function. *Epilepsia* **31** (suppl. 4), S50–S53.

Bourgeois, B.L. (1991): Relationship between anticonvulsant drugs and learning disabilities. *Seminars in Neurology* **11**, 14–19.

Brouwer, O.F., Pieters, M.S.M., Edelbroak, P.M. *et al.* (1992): Conventional and controlled release valproate in children with epilepsy: a cross-over study comparing plasma levels and cognitive performances. *Epilepsy Res.* **13**, 245–253.

Camfield, C.S., Chaplin, S. & Doyle, A.B. (1979): Side effect of phenobarbital in toddlers: behavior and cognitive aspects. *J. Pediatr.* **95**, 361–365.

Camfield, P.R., Camfield, C.S. & Tibbles, J.A. (1982): Carbamazepine does not prevent febrile seizures in phenobarbital failures. *Neurology* **32**, 288–289.

Chen, Y.J., Kang, W.M. & So, W.C.M. (1996): Comparison of antiepileptic drugs on cognitive function in newly diagnosed epileptic children: a psychometric and neurophysiological study. *Epilepsia* **37**, 81–86.

Committee on Drugs, American Academy of Pediatrics (1985): Behavioral and cognitive effects of anticonvulsivant therapy. Committee on drugs. *Pediatrics* **76**, 644–647.

Cull, C.A. (1988): Cognitive function and behaviour in children. In: Trimble, M.R. & Reynolds, E.H., eds., *Epilepsy, behaviour and cognitive function*. Chichester: John Wiley, pp. 97–111.

Diaz, J. (1983): Research note: disruption of the brain growth spurt in adolescent rats by chronic phenobarbital administration. *Exp. Neurol.* **79**, 559–563.

Dodrill, C.B. (1992): Problems in the assessment of cognitive effects of antiepileptic drugs. *Epilepsia* **33** (suppl. 6), S29–S32.

Dodrill, C.B., Arnett, J.L., Sommerville, K.W. & Sussman, N.M. (1993): Evaluation of the effects of vigabatrin on cognitive abilities and quality of life in epilepsy. *Neurology* **43**, 2501–2507.

Domizio, S., Verrotti, A., Ramenghi, L.A., Sabatino, G. & Morgese, G. (1993): Anti-epileptic therapy and behaviour disturbances in children. *Child Nerv. Syst.* **9**, 272–274.

Dreifuss, F.E. (1992): Cognitive function – victim of disease or hostage to treatment? *Epilepsia* **33** (suppl. 1), S7–S12.

Durwen, H.F. & Elger, C.E. (1992): Verbal learning differences in epileptic patients with left and right temporal lobe foci – a pharmacologically induced phenomenon? *Acta Neurol. Scand.* **87**, 1–8.

Farwell, J.R., Lee, Y.J., Hirtz, D.G., Sulzbacher, S.I., Ellenberg, J.H. & Nelson, K.B. (1990): Phenobarbital for febrile seizures – effects on intelligence and on seizure recurrence. *N. Engl. J. Med.* **322**, 364–369.

Forsythe, I., Butler, R., Berg, I. & McGuire, R. (1991): Cognitive impairment in new cases of epilepsy randomly assigned to carbamazepine, phenytoin and sodium valproate. *Dev. Med. Child Neurol.* **33**, 524–534.

Gallassi, R., Morreale, A., Lorusso, S., Procaccianti, G., Lugaresi, E. & Barruzzi, A. (1990): Cognitive effects of Valproate. *Epilepsy Res.* **5**, 160–164.

Gallassi, R., Morreale, A., Di Sarro, R., Mara, M., Lugaresi, I.E. & Baruzzi, A. (1992): Cognitive effects of antiepileptic drug discontinuation. *Epilepsia* **33** (suppl. 6), S41–S44.

Gilham, R.A., Blacklaw, J., McK P.J. & Brodie, M.J. (1993): Effect of Vigabatrin on sedation and cognitive function in patients with refractory epilepsy. *J. Neurol. Neurosurg. Psychiatry* **56**, 1271–1275.

Harding, G.F., Alford, C.A. & Powell, T.E. (1985): The effect of Sodium Valproate on sleep, reaction time and visual evoked potential in normal subjects. *Epilepsia* **26**, 597–601.

Hara, H. & Fukuyama, Y. (1989): Sustained attention during the interictal period of mentally normal children with epilepsy or febrile convulsions, and the influence of anticonvulsants and seizures on attention. *Jpn. J. Psychiatry Neurol.* **43**, 411–416.

Jambaqué, I., Dellatolas, G., Dulac, O. & Signoret, J.L. (1991): Verbal and visual memory impairment in children with epilepsy. *Neuropsychologia* **31**, 1321–1337.

Kalviainen, R., Aikia, M., Partanen, J., Sivenius, J., Mumford, J., Saksa, M. & Riekkinen, P.J. (1991): Randomized controlled pilot study of vigabatrin versus carbamazepine monotherapy in newly diagnosed patients with epilepsy: an interim report. *J. Child Neurol.* **6**, S60–S69.

Lee, Y.J., Ellenberg, J.H., Hirtz, D.G. & Nelson, K.B. (1991): Analysis of clinical trials by treatment actually received: is it really an option? *Statistics in Medicine* **10**, 1595–1605.

Loiseau, P., Strube, E., Torr, J., Levy, R.H. & Dodrill, C. (1988): Evaluation neuropsychologique et thérapeutique du stiripentol dans l'épilepsie. *Rev. Neurol.* **144**, 165–172.

Meador, K.J., Loring, D.W., Huh, K., Gallagher, B.B. & King, D.W. (1990): Comparative cognitive effects of anticonvulsants. *Neurology* **40**, 391–394.

Mitchell, W.G. & Chavez, J.M. (1987): Carbamazepine versus phenobarbital for partial onset seizures in children. *Epilepsia* **28**, 56–60.

Mitchell, W.G., Zhou, Y., Chavez, J.M. & Guzman, B.L. (1992): Reaction time, attention, and impulsivity in epilepsy. *Pediatric Neurol.* **8**, 19–24.

Mitchell, W.G., Zhou, Y., Chavez, J.M. & Guzman, B.L. (1993): Effects of antiepileptic drugs on reaction time, attention, and impulsivity in children. *Pediatrics* **9**, 101–105.

Mondari, C. & Classen, W. (1984): The effects of various antiepileptic drugs on E-shock induced amnesia in mice: dissociability of effects on convulsions and effects on memory. *Acta Neurol. Scand.* **66** (suppl. 99), 119–124.

O'Dougherty, X., Wright, F.S., Cox, S. & Walson, P. (1987): Carbamazepine plasma concentration. Relationship to cognitive impairment. *Arch. Neurol.* **44**, 863–867.

Pieters, M.S.M., Jennekens, S., Schinkel, A., Stijnen, T. *et al.* (1992): Carbamazepine (CBZ) controlled release compared with conventional CBZ: a controlled study of attention and vigilance in children with epilepsy. *Epilepsia* **33**, 1137–1144.

Scolnik, D., Nulman, I., Rovet, J., Gladstone, D., Czuchta, D., Gardner, A., Gladstone, R., Ashby, P., Weksberg, R., Einarson, T. & Koren, G. (1994): In utero exposure to Phenytoin and Carbamazepine. *JAMA* **271**, 767–770.

Smith, D.B. (1988): Cognitive effects of antiepileptic drugs. *Advan. Neurol.* **55**, 197–212.

Smith, D.B., Mattson, R.H., Cramer, J.A., Collins, J.F., Novelly, R.A., Craft, B. & The Veterans Administration Epilepsy Cooperative Study Group (1987): Results of a nationwide veterans administration cooperative study comparing the efficacy and toxicity of Carbamazepine, Phenobarbital, Phenytoin, and Primidone. *Epilepsia* **28** (suppl. 3), S50–S58.

Sommerbeck, K.W., Theilgaard, A., Rasmussen, K.E., Lohren, G., Gram, L. & Wulff, K. (1977): Valproate sodium: evaluation of so-called psychotropic effect. A controlled study. *Epilepsia* **18**, 159–167.

Stores, G., Williams, P.L., Styles, E. & Zaiwalla Z (1992): Psychological effects of sodium valproate and carbamazepine in epilepsy. *Arch. Dischild.* **67**, 1330–1337.

Thompson, P.J. & Trimble, M.R. (1982): Anticonvulsivants drugs and cognitive functions. *Epilepsia* **23**, 531–541.

Tomson, T., Allkist, T.O., Nilsson, B.Y., Svnsson, J.O. & Brtilsson, L. (1990): Carbamazepine 10,11 epoxide in epilepsy. A pilot study. *Arch. Neurol.* **47**, 888–892.

Trimble, M.R. (1990): Antiepileptic drugs, cognitive function, and behavior in children: evidence from recent studies. *Epilepsia* **31** (suppl. 4), S30–S34.

Trimble, M.R. & Thompson, P.J. (1983): Anticonvulsant drugs, cognitive function, and behavior. *Epilepsia* **24** (suppl. 1), S55–S63.

Trimble, M.R. & Thompson, P.J. (1984): Sodium valproate and cognitive function. Epilepsia **25**(suppl. 1), S60–S64.

Vining, E.P.G., Mellits, E.D., Dorsen, M.M., Cataldo, M.F., Quaskey, S.A., Spielberg, S.P. & Freeman, J.M. (1987): Psychologic and behavioral effects of antiepileptic drugs in children: a double-blind comparison between phenobarbital and valproic acid. *Pediatrics* **80**, 165–174.

Wolf, F.M. & Forsythe, A. (1978): Behavior disturbance, phenobarbital and febrile seizures. *Pediatrics* **61**, 728–731.

Yanai, J., Rosslli-Austin, L. & Tabakoff, R. (1979): Neuronal deficits in mice following prenatal exposure to phenobarbital. *Exp. Neurol.* **64**, 237–244.

Chapter 25

Consequences of early chronic antiepileptic treatments in animals

A. Pereira de Vasconcelos[1], H. Schroeder[2] and A. Nehlig[1]

[1]*INSERM U 398, Strasbourg;* [2]*Laboratory of Biochemistry, University Hospital, Nancy, France*

Introduction

Antiepileptic drugs (AEDs), such as benzodiazepines (BDZ), are largely administered to neonates, children and epileptic women, even during pregnancy, for prophylaxis and treatment of convulsive seizures (Burdette, 1990). In addition, phenobarbital (PhB) is widely used for treatment of hyperbilirubinemia and hypoxia–ischaemia in neonates (Yaffe & Catz, 1971). As a consequence of their clinical administration, AEDs have been associated with a number of complications in the newborn infant, for example, the 'floppy infant syndrome' with DZP (Grimm, 1984). Indeed, all AEDs cross the placenta and accumulate in breast milk, causing indesirable effects such as poor weight gain, drowsiness and adverse effects on psychomotor development (Kaneko, 1991). Moreover, because of the high incidence of epilepsy in the first decade of life and the propensity of children to develop febrile seizures, the use of AEDs for prolonged periods has raised questions about their potential toxicity and interference with normal development. Indeed, deleterious effects of early AED exposure such as intellectual deterioration have been shown, particularly with PhB, although these effects are not easily dissociable from those of recurrent seizures and/or from the cerebral pathology underlying epilepsy (Funakoshi *et al.*, 1988). Animal studies have shown that early PhB exposure induces long-lasting cerebral morphological changes characterized by specific neuronal damage located in the hippocampus and cerebellum. This cellular loss appears whether barbiturate treatment has been pre- or postnatal, indicating that PhB is able to disturb neuronal differentiation as well as to destroy already formed neurons (Yanai *et al.*, 1979; Yanai & Bergman, 1981; Hannah *et al.*, 1982; Yanai, 1984). After early BDZ exposure, no extensive brain damage has been shown and morphological changes are restricted mainly to gliosis and perivascular cuffing which occur only after a prenatal exposure (Frieder *et al.*, 1984). Early BDZ or barbiturate treatment has also been associated with long-term behavioural alterations in adult rats characterized by disturbances in locomotor activity, learning and social behaviour (Fonseca *et al.*, 1976; Middaugh *et al.*, 1981; Pick & Yanai, 1984, 1985; Tucker, 1985; Alleva & Bignami, 1986; Barbier *et al.*, 1991; Chesley *et al.*, 1991; Dell'Omo *et al.*, 1993). The consequences of perinatal AED exposure on the biochemistry of the immature brain have not been extensively studied. Short- and long-term changes mainly in GABA, choline and serotonin systems were recorded after early exposure to BDZ (Frieder & Grimm, 1985; Livezey *et al.*, 1986).

So, in order to better understand the effects of early exposure to AEDs on brain development, we studied the maturation of cerebral functional activity, particularly the biosynthesis of the cerebral neurotransmitter amino acids involved in the pathophysiology of epilepsy, i.e. glutamate, aspartate, glutamine and GABA. At the regional level, we studied the short- and long-term effects of such treatments on local cerebral glucose utilization (LCGU) and the correlation between metabolic changes and long-term consequences on maze behaviour in adult rats exposed postnatally to either PhB or DZP. Since the early exposure to AED leads to growth retardation, an additional group exposed to undernutrition by raising the number of pups in the litters was included.

General effects of an early chronic AED treatment in the rat – circulating levels of the drugs

Pharmacological treatments

Adult Sprague–Dawley rats, one male and two females, were housed together in mating groups for 5 days. After delivery litter sizes were reduced to 12 pups. PhB (5-ethyl–5-phenylbarbituric acid, sodium salt, Fluka), 50 mg/kg from day 2 (P2) to P35 and DZP (valium, 10 mg/2 ml injectable ampoules, Roche), 10 mg/kg from P2 to P21 were administered subcutaneously once daily (day of birth = day 0). Control animals received an equivalent volume of the dissolution vehicle (saline for PhB-paired controls and propylene glycol 40 per cent, ethanol 10 per cent, benzyl alcohol 1.5 per cent, sodium benzoate 5 per cent, for DZP-paired controls). Rats were studied at P5–7, P10, P14, P21, P35 and the adult stage. In an additional group, the litter size was increased to 16 pups in order to achieve the same body weight reduction as in PhB- or DZP-exposed groups.

There was no difference in the rate of neonatal mortality in controls and PhB- or DZP-exposed rats, demonstrating that the doses used were far below the LD 50. In addition, an early exposure to either PhB or DZP did not induce prominent differences in physical maturation signs or general behaviour, except for a transient sedation which lasted 2–3 hours on the first few days of treatment and progressively disappeared with maturation.

Plasma drug measurements

Plasma PhB levels ranged from 41 to 80 µg/ml at all developmental ages studied, i.e. between P7 and P35 (Pereira de Vasconcelos & Nehlig, 1987). Plasma DZP concentrations ranged from 0.2 to 1.2 µg/ml, peaked at 1–2 hours after injection and were not detectable after 4–6 hours post-injection (Schroeder et al., 1994a). These values are close to therapeutic levels in the anticonvulsant range found in neonates and children (Booker, 1982; Farrel, 1986).

Effects of an early chronic AED treatment on body and brain growth

At all developmental ages studied, the body and brain weights were reduced by 6–26 per cent, in both PhB- and DZP-treated rats. This body and brain growth retardation persisted until adulthood (Pereira de Vasconcelos & Nehlig, 1987; Schroeder et al., 1994a). These results are in agrement with previous studies using either PhB (Schain & Watanabe, 1975; Diaz et al., 1977), DZP, lorazepam or clonazepam (Frieder et al., 1984; File, 1986; Wang & Huang, 1990). Likewise, clinical studies also show a decrease in birth weight and postnatal growth in babies born from a mother exposed to barbiturates, DZP or oxazepam (Gaily & Granström, 1989; Laegreid et al., 1992).

Undernutrition induced a significant 20–24 per cent decrease in body weight at all ages, whereas brain weight was only slightly decreased at P5 (Schroeder et al., 1994a). These results confirm the relative protection of the brain during early undernutrition (Dobbing, 1970) and the relatively selective effects of early AED exposure on brain growth.

Effects of an early AED exposure on the maturation of brain energy metabolism: incorporation of glucose and β-hydroxybutyrate carbon into amino acids

The fundamental characteristic of the mature brain energy metabolism *in vivo* is the rapid and important incorporation of glucose carbon into cerebral amino acids. This metabolic pathway develops sharply from P10 to P15 in the rat and reaches by P22 rates similar to those recorded in adult brain (Gaitonde & Richter, 1965; De Vivo et al., 1975; for review, see Nehlig & Pereira de Vasconcelos, 1993). On the other hand, as a result of the high lipid content of maternal milk, the infant rat develops a marked ketosis within a few hours following birth, and ketone bodies, i.e. acetoactetate (ACA) and β-hydroxybutyrate (βHB) are actively taken up and utilized by the immature brain (Hawkins et al., 1971; for review, see Nehlig & Pereira de Vasconcelos, 1993). Thus, in the developing rat brain, ketone bodies appear to be substrates more efficient than glucose for energy metabolism (Cremer, 1982) and for both amino acid (De Vivo et al., 1975) and lipid biosynthesis (Patel & Owen, 1977).

Circulating levels of glucose and ketone bodies

The neonatal treatment with both AEDs induced significant decreases in plasma glucose levels ranging from 6–14 per cent at all ages except at P7 and P35 in PhB- and at P10 in DZP-treated animals, where no difference was noticed among groups. Plasma βHB and ACA levels were affected only after PhB exposure with increases ranging from 27 to 99 per cent (Pereira de Vasconcelos & Nehlig, 1987; Schroeder et al., 1994a). These results show that early PhB, and to a lesser extent DZP, affect circulating levels of cerebral energy metabolism substrates in the developing brain.

Undernutrition did not affect glycaemia, but induced massive increases in blood βHB, up to 360 per cent at all ages (Schroeder et al., 1994a), as previously reported (Hawkins et al., 1971). Thus, the metabolic effects related to the administration of DZP mostly reflects direct effects not mediated by undernutrition. Early PhB increased blood ketone body levels, however these effects were less marked than the ones recorded in undernourished rats showing that the effects of PhB are rather direct effects, only partly related to sedation-induced undernutrition. This specific retardation of brain growth was also shown in PhB-exposed rat pups which were artificially reared to avoid body weight deficits (Diaz et al., 1977).

Cerebral amino acid content

Early chronic PhB or DZP exposure only slightly affected brain amino acid concentration during postnatal development of the rat. Indeed, with PhB, the effects were restricted to the cerebral cortex, affecting glutamate at P14 and P21, glutamine at P10 and P35, and aspartate and GABA at P14 and P35 (Pereira de Vasconcelos & Nehlig, 1987). DZP treatment increased only the cerebellar concentration of GABA at P10 and P21 (Schroeder et al., 1994a).

Glucose utilization by the developing brain

During development, 30 min after the administration of radioactive glucose in controls, the percentage of labelling remaining in the glucose fraction decreased with postnatal age, while the percentage of radioactivity in the amino acid fraction increased to reach more than 80 per cent at P21 (Fig. 1) (Gaitonde & Richter, 1965). An early chronic AED exposure affected the distribution of radioactivity with a percentage of labelling in the glucose fraction and in the amino acid fraction significantly higher and lower, respectively, in P7–P14 PhB-treated rats and in P5 and P10 DZP-treated rats compared to controls (Fig. 1). The DZP and the PhB treatment had no effect on the distribution of the radioactivity between glucose and amino acids after P14 and P21, respectively (Fig. 1) (Pereira de Vasconcelos & Nehlig, 1987; Schroeder et al., 1994a).

After the injection of radioactive glucose, the incorporation of radioactivity in the individual cerebral amino acids, i.e. glutamate, glutamine, aspartate and GABA, was not widely affected after PhB. Decreases concerned mostly cortical and cerebellar GABA, aspartate and glutamine at P10 and P35 and cortical glutamine at P21 after PhB (Pereira de Vasconcelos & Nehlig, 1987). After DZP, the biosynthesis of the different amino acids was only slightly affected until P14. Decreases were recorded in cortical GABA at P10 and subcortical glutamate, glutamine and GABA at P14 after DZP exposure. Surprisingly, at P21, the biosynthesis of amino acids from glucose was increased after DZP treatment (Schroeder et al., 1994a).

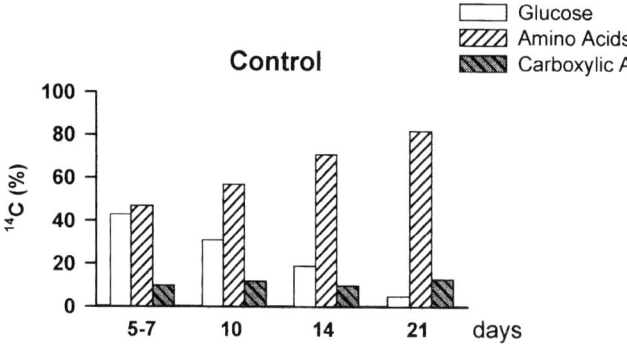
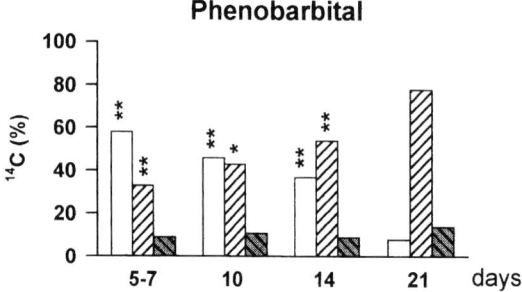
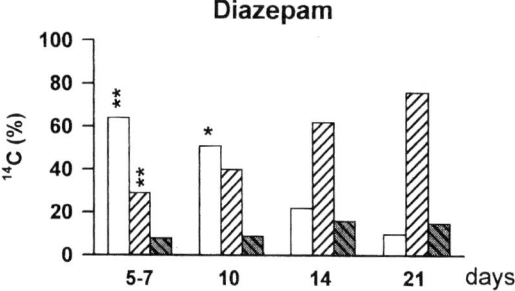

Fig. 1. Influence of PhB and DZP on postnatal evolution of the distribution of ^{14}C from [U-^{14}C]glucose between the three fractions of the acid-soluble extract in the cerebral cortex of the rat. Values are means ± S.D. of 3–6 experiments.
*$P < 0.05$, **$P < 0.01$, statistically significant differences from control (Student's t test).

Brain amino acid biosynthesis from β-hydroxybutyrate

After the injection of radioactive βHB, the incorporation of radioactivity in cerebral amino acids was increased in PhB-treated rats in all cortical amino acids at all ages. In the cerebellum, increases concerned aspartate and GABA at P10 and glutamate, glutamine and GABA at P21 (Pereira de Vasconcelos et al., 1987). Conversely, early DZP exposure had very limited effects on the biosynthesis of cerebral amino acids from βHB, only cortical glutamate at P5 and P10 and cerebellar GABA at P5 and aspartate at P21 were affected by the treatment (Schroeder et al., 1994a).

Conclusions of the biochemical studies

AED treatment in the developing brain delays the overall rate of glucose utilization, especially the maturation of the rapid incorporation of glucose carbon into amino acids which is an index of cerebral

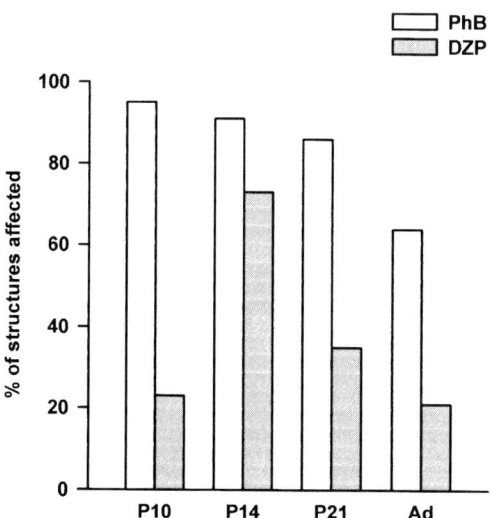

Fig. 2. Short- and long-term effects of PhB and DZP on local cerebral glucose utilization (LCGU). Rats received a daily subcutaneous injection of either PhB at the dose of 50 mg/kg from P2 to P35 or DZP at the dose of 10 mg/kg from P2 to P21. Values represent the percentage of structures showing significant decreases in LCGU compared to controls.

maturation (Gaitonde & Richter, 1965). The consequences of early chronic DZP exposure on cerebral amino acid metabolism are mostly manifest at P5 and P10, whereas PhB seems to interfere with the active phase of maturation of the glucose metabolic pathway, i.e. between P10 and P14 (Gaitonde & Richter, 1965). The absence of differences in the rate of incorporation of glucose carbon into amino acids at older ages, i.e. from P14, could reflect either a tolerance and/or the more active clearance and shorter half-life of the drug. Indeed, tolerance to the anticonvulsant, anxiolytic and sedative effects of AEDs has been well documented (Haigh & Feely, 1988; File,1990).

The critical questions arising from these results are whether the developing brain can have a choice in substrate supply, such that glucose and ketone bodies may be used interchangeably in meeting the metabolic needs of respiration, energy metabolism and myelinogenesis. Could this apparent prolonged period of immaturity induced by early AED exposure, especially PhB, have long-term consequences on brain function and behaviour?

Short- and long-term effects of early AED exposure on local cerebral glucose utilization

In order to assess the possible role of the relative imbalance between glucose and ketone body supply on brain development, we studied the effects of PhB and DZP on local cerebral glucose utilization (LCGU) in young animals both during drug exposure, i.e. at P10, P14 and P21, and in adults, at about 40 days after the end of the treatment. LCGU was measured by the quantitative autoradiographic [^{14}C]2-deoxyglucose method (Sokoloff *et al.*, 1977) adapted to the immature rat (Nehlig *et al.*, 1988).

PhB treatment induced a statistically significant decrease in LCGU in most structures studied and at all developmental ages which persisted in the adult rat. These changes translated into a 12 to 28 per cent decrease in the average rate of glucose utilization for whole brain (Pereira de Vasconcelos *et al.*, 1990a). The decreases in LCGU affected 86–100 per cent of the 58 structures studied during the period of treatment between P10 and P21 in PhB-treated rats. In the adult rats, i.e. at 35 days after the end

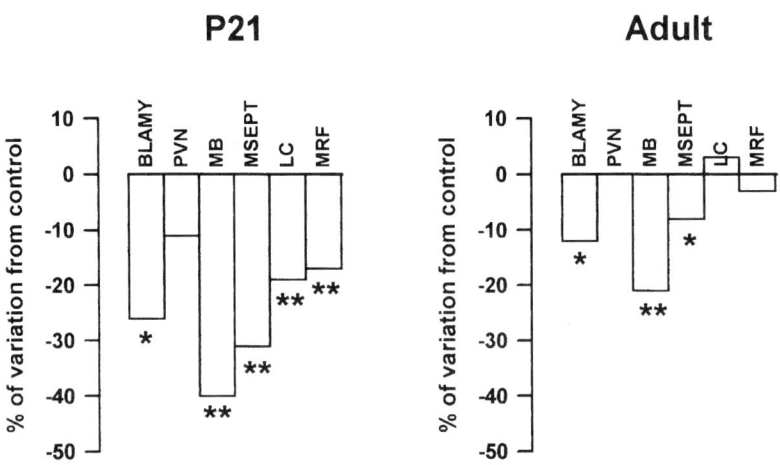

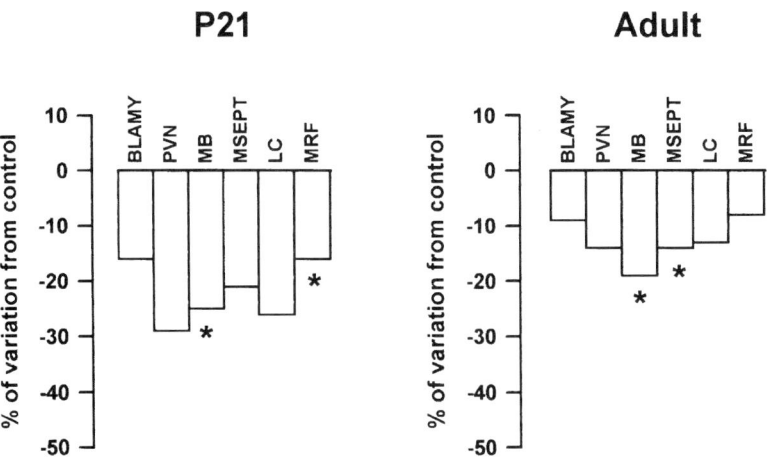

Fig. 3. Effects of early PhB or DZP exposure at P21 and at the adult stage in areas involved in the control of anxiety. Rats received a daily subcutaneous injection of either PhB at the dose of 50 mg/kg from P2 to P35 or DZP at the dose of 10 mg/kg from P2 to P21 and were tested between P60 and P80. Values represent the percentage of variation from control levels.

Abbreviations: BLAMY: basolateral amygdala; PVN: paraventricular nucleus; MB: mammillary body; MSEPT: medial septum; LC: locus coeruleus; MRF: mesencephalic reticular formation. *$P < 0.05$, **$P < 0.001$, statistically significant differences from control (Student's t test).

PHENOBARBITAL

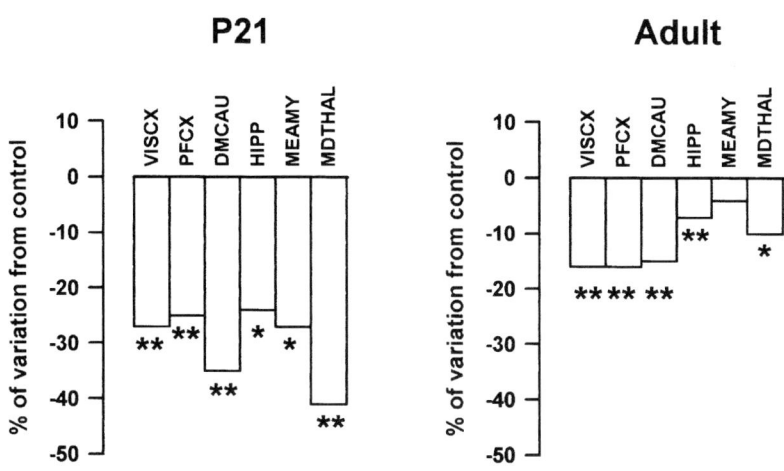

DIAZEPAM

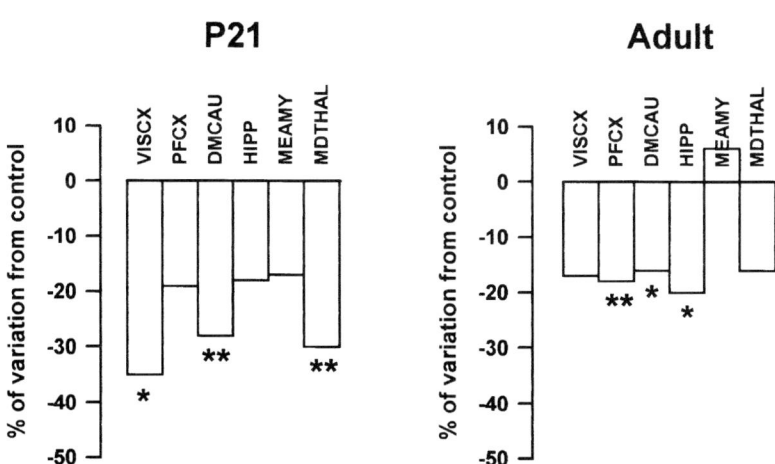

Fig. 4. Effects of early PhB or DZP exposure at P21 and at the adult stage in areas involved in the control of memory. Rats received a daily subcutaneous injection of either PhB at the dose of 50 mg/kg from P2 to P35 or DZP at the dose of 10 mg/kg from P2 to P21 and were tested between P60 and P80. Values represent the percentage of variation from control.
Abbreviations: VISCX: visual cortex; PFCX: prefrontal cortex; DMCAU: dorsomedian caudate nucleus; HIPP: dorsal hippocampus; MEAMY: medial amygdala; MDTHAL: mediodorsal thalamus.
*$P < 0.05$, **$P < 0.001$, statistically significant differences from control (Student's t test).

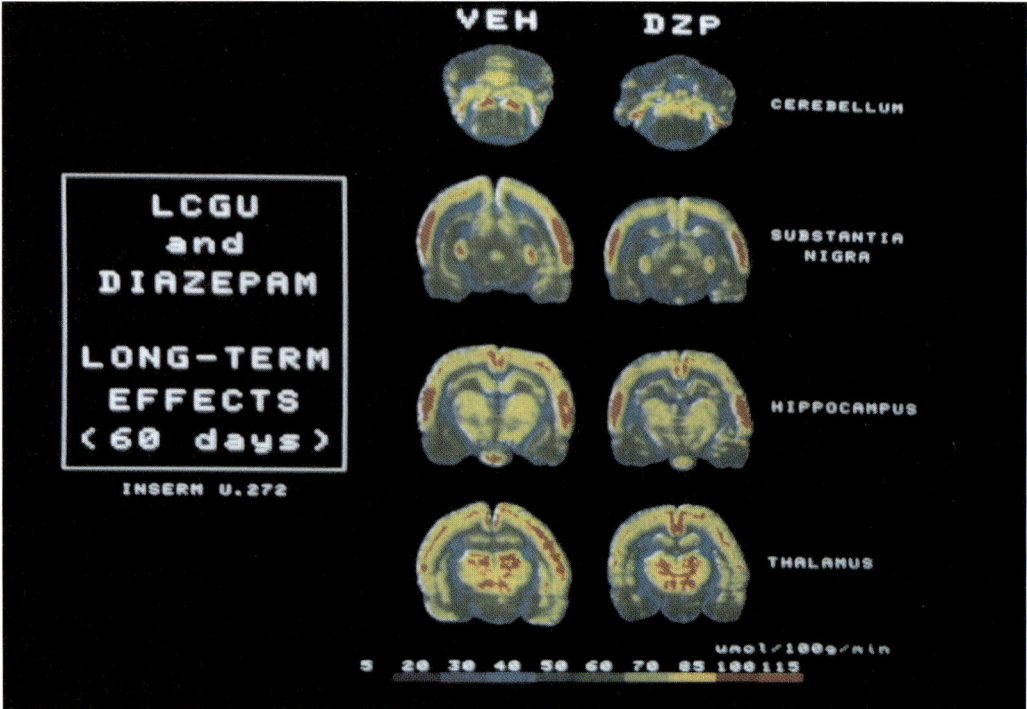

Fig. 5. Colour-coded autoradiograms of LCGU at different antero–posterior levels of the brain in controls and DZP-treated rats. Rats were exposed to 10 mg/kg/day DZP from P2 to P21 and injected with 2-deoxyglucose 40 days after the end of the treatment. Long-term effects of early DZP exposure translate mainly into decreases in LCGU restricted to the dorsal hippocampus and mammillary body.

of the treatment, LCGU remained depressed in 62 per cent of the structures belonging to all the functional systems (Figs. 2–4).

Conversely to PhB, DZP induced metabolic decreases only in a limited number of areas, one-third or less of the structures at P10, P21 and in adults (Fig. 2). Within the structures affected by DZP were mainly sensory and limbic regions and the mammillary body at P10, and sensory, limbic and motor areas at P21 and in adults (Figs. 3–5, Schroeder *et al.* 1994b). However, at P14, most structures (73 per cent) belonging to all functional systems studied were significantly decreased by DZP (Fig. 2). At that age, the rat brain is undergoing its period of 'rapid growth spurt' with an active maturation of neuronal cell bodies, multiplication of glial cells and synaptogenesis (Dobbing, 1970) which could render the brain more sensitive to the effect of the treatment.

Sensory functions

The AED exposure-induced depression of glucose utilization appears at the critical period of the maturation of glucose metabolism, i.e. between P10 and P15 in the rat (Gaitonde & Richter, 1965). The reductions in LCGU raise the question of the influence of AEDs on the acquisition of functions such as sensory functions which takes place around P12 for audition (Crowley & Hepp-Reymond, 1966; Myslivecek, 1970) and P15 for vision (Rose & Ellingson, 1970). Considering that a rise in metabolic rate in a particular structure generally marks the time at which it begins to contribute to an animal's function or behaviour (Nehlig *et al.*, 1988), the absence of a significant increase between P10 and P14 in the metabolic level of 4 out of the 5 auditory areas studied in PhB-treated rats may reflect alterations in the normal development of audition. Similar results were obtained in the visual system whose structures show no significant increases between P17 and P21 in PhB-treated rats whereas LCGU increased in these structures in control animals (Pereira de Vasconcelos et al., 1990a). Although more restricted, the effects of early DZP treatment on LCGU show that sensory structures appear also to be particularly sensitive. Within auditory areas, there were metabolic decreases at all ages including the adult rat after DZP treatment (Schroeder et al., 1994b), confirming previous results showing that early exposure to DZP interferes with the development of the auditory function (Kellogg et al., 1983). In addition, the acute injection of DZP to adult rats reduces the reaction to sound (Carlsson et al., 1976) and the metabolic activity in auditory areas (Nehlig et al., 1987). Likewise, in DZP-treated rats, all visual structures showed decreases in LCGU between P14 and P21, which corresponds to the period of the acquisition of this function (Rose & Ellingson, 1970; Schroeder et al., 1994b). Thus, because the rat is born very immature, especially blind and deaf, the metabolic decreases in sensory areas during the whole period of AED exposure which persist after the end of the treatment in adults, may be indicative of the great vulnerability of these fast growing brain structures to AEDs.

Structures related to anxiolytic and amnesic effects

BDZ have well-known anxiolytic properties which are related to their depressant action on structures such as the hippocampus, amygdala, mammillary body and associated regions, the amygdala being a key structure involved in the control of anxiety (Davies, 1992). In the present study, an early DZP exposure has little or no effects on the anxiety-related structures except at P14, the age at which most structures are affected by the treatment (Fig. 4). The only structure mediating anxiety whose metabolic activity is depressed at all ages by DZP is the mammillary body (Figs. 3 and 5) (Schroeder et al., 1994b). Likewise, the latter structure appears to be sensitive to the BDZ as shown in all metabolic studies using acute, subacute or chronic treatment of BDZ in adult animals (Kelly et al., 1986; Nehlig et al., 1987).

A well-known secondary effect of DZP is amnesia. The cerebral structures involved in the memory process are mainly the hippocampus, amygdala, mammillary body, dorsomedian thalamus, and prefrontal and cingulate cortices (Thompson, 1992). A depression in LCGU in these structures was evidenced for most of them in P14 DZP-exposed rats (Fig. 4). At P21, the mammillary body, the dorsomedian thalamus and cingulate cortex were still decreased by the early DZP treatment. Furthermore, LCGU remained reduced in the mammillary body, prefrontal and cingulate cortices in adult DZP-exposed rats (Figs. 3–5).

Conversely to DZP, PhB induced widespread short- and long-term decreases in LCGU rates and affected all of the structures involved in the control of anxiety and memory. These long-lasting metabolic changes after early PhB exposure could indeed have long-term consequences on brain function and behaviour, particularly those related to memory and spatial orientation involving the hippocampus and related areas.

These data show that an early AED exposure is able to induce short- and long-term depressions of cerebral glucose utilization that are widespread and homogeneous after PhB exposure and restricted mainly to sensory and limbic areas after DZP exposure. The consequences of the early DZP exposure are more or less related to the structures involved in the control of anxiety and memory.

Long-term behavioural consequences of early AED exposure: learning in T- and eight-arm mazes

The retardation in the maturation of cerebral energy metabolism, particularly marked after PhB, is accompanied by an acute depression in local cerebral glucose utilization which persists until adulthood. Moreover, early PhB exposure is able to induce long-lasting cellular destructions in the hippocampus and cerebellum (Hannah et al., 1982; Yanai, 1984). All these changes may have long-term consequences on brain function, especially behaviour and learning capacities. Thus, in adult rats exposed early in their life to either PhB or DZP, we studied the behaviour in a T-maze and an eight-arm maze. These two mazes are currently used to test spatial orientation, learning and memory

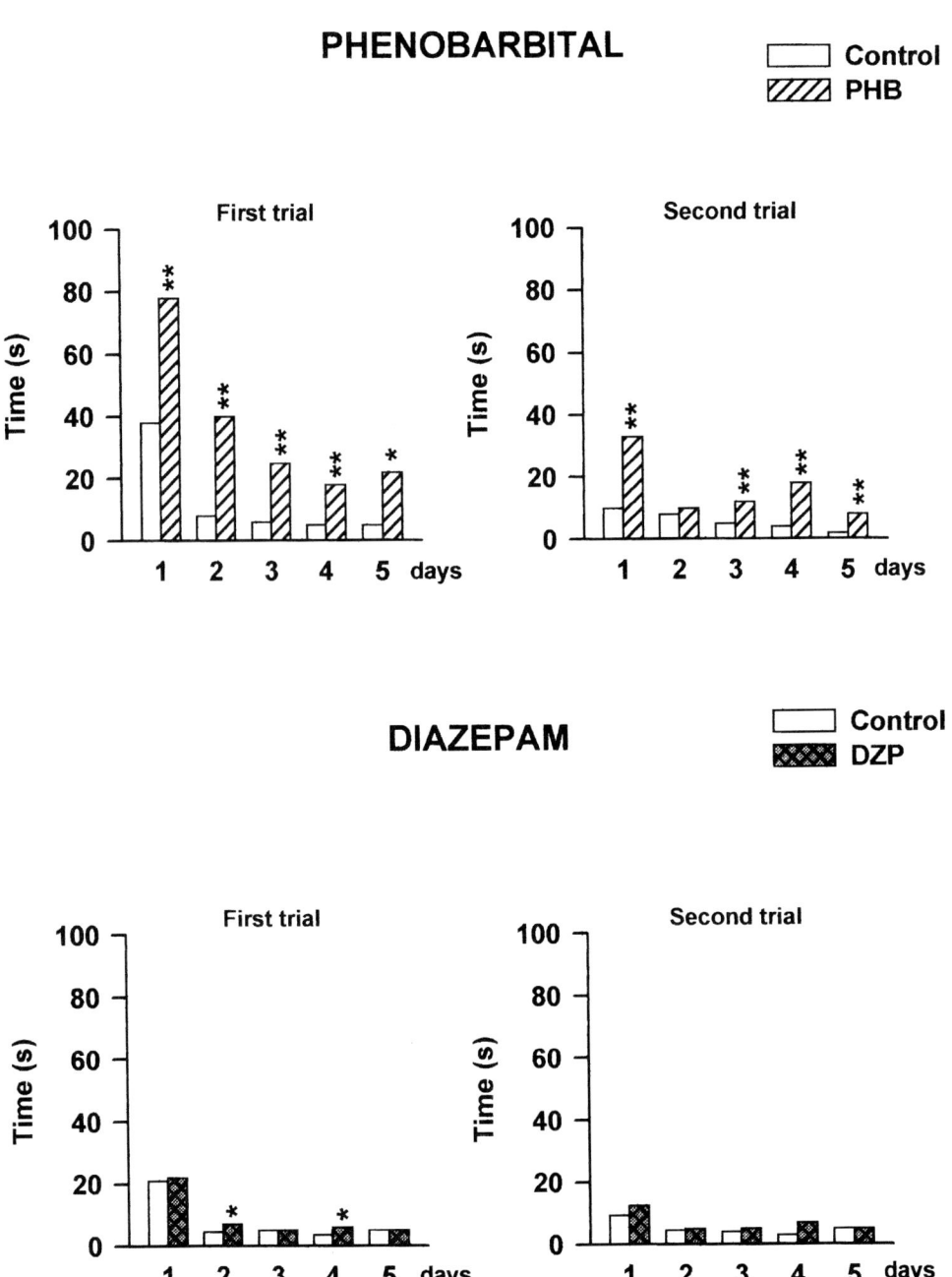

Fig. 6. Effects of early postnatal PhB or DZP treatment on the time necessary to reach one goal arm in the T-maze in the 30 s delay condition. The rats were treated from P2 to P35 with PhB at the dose of 50 mg/kg and from P2 to P21 with DZP at the dose of 10 mg/kg, and were tested at P60 and P70. The data represent medians of 14 to 27 animals.
*$P < 0.05$, **$P < 0.01$, statistically significant differences from control (Mann–Whitney U test).

PHENOBARBITAL

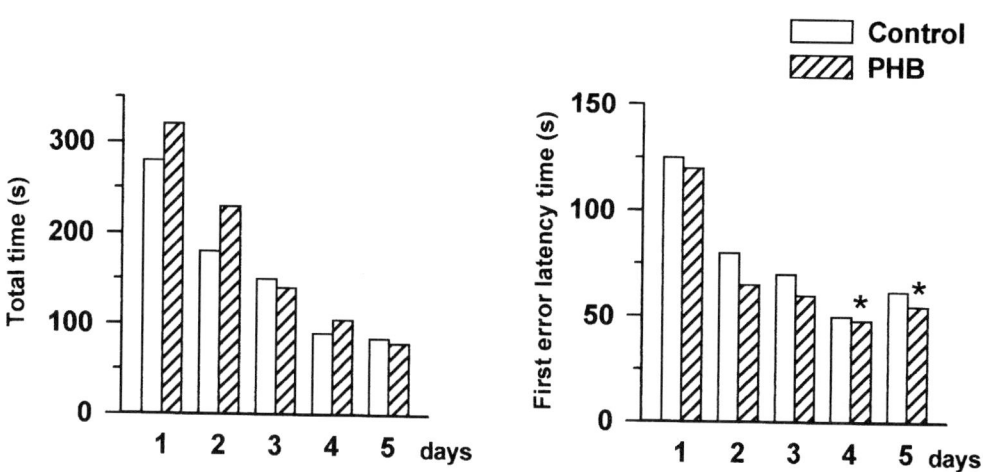

DIAZEPAM

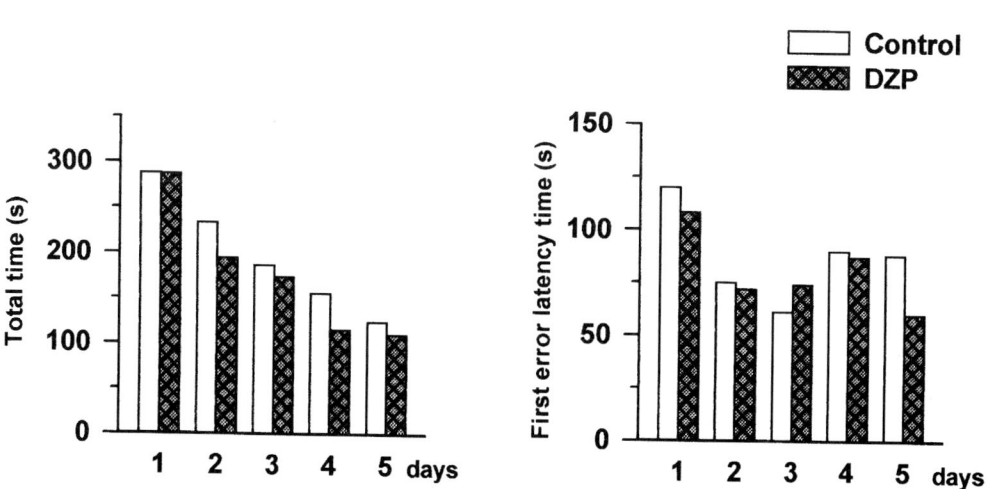

Fig. 7. Effects of early postnatal PhB or DZP treatment on eight-arm maze behaviour. The rats were treated from P2 to P21 with DZP at the dose of 10 mg/kg or from P2 to P35 with PhB at the dose of 50 mg/kg and were tested at P60 and P90 for DZP and PhB-treated rats, respectively. The data represent medians of 16 to 28 animals.
*$P < 0.05$, statistically significant difference from controls (Mann–Whitney U test).

(Montgomery, 1952; Olton & Samuelson, 1976) and have a spontaneous alternation component which is well-known to be related to the hippocampus (Douglas, 1975; Olton & Samuelson, 1976; Isaacson, 1982).

Spontaneous alternation in a T-maze

Spontaneous alternation is defined as the tendency of adult animals to alternate successive responses when facing equivalent choices. Two procedures were used, one with no interposed delay between the two trials (no delay condition) and one with a 30 s intertrial retention in the start box (delay condition). PhB did not affect the mean percentage of spontaneous alternation rate on the 5-day test in the no delay condition but, as soon as a delay was introduced between the two trials, this rate was significantly decreased by 25 per cent in PhB-treated rats. In addition, the time to perform trials, i.e. to reach any one of the two goal arms of the T-maze, was greatly increased in PhB-treated rats compared to controls, and the tendency to increase their time to perform trials was so high that 30–50 per cent of PhB-treated rats were excluded from the study which allows a 5 min time to reach the goal arm (Fig. 6) (Pereira de Vasconcelos et al., 1990b). Early DZP exposure affected the rate of spontaneous alternation only in the no delay condition and during the first two days of testing. The time necessary to perform the trials was similar or slightly increased by early DZP exposure (Fig. 6) (Schroeder et al., 1997).

The spontaneous alternation has been shown to relate to the integrity of the hippocampus and short-term memory function (Isseroff, 1979) and is reduced to chance value after large cerebral lesions of the hippocampus (Douglas, 1975; Isaacson, 1982). Previous studies have shown that the degree of impairment in this behaviour following chronic barbiturate treatment varies according to the period of exposure to the drug as well as the species considered, with no effect of a neonatal exposure in the rat (Middaugh et al., 1981; McBride et al., 1985) whereas deficits after a neonatal PhB treatment in mice appear to be correlated to the extensive damage in the hippocampus (Yanai & Bergman, 1981; Pick & Yanai, 1984). In the present study, the deficits in spontaneous alternation in PhB-exposed rats may reflect the short- and long-term depresssion in LCGU in hippocampus and related areas in PhB-treated rats (Fig. 4) (Pereira de Vasconcelos et al., 1990a,b) and could possibly reflect deficits of memory function (Isseroff, 1979). In addition, some PhB-treated rats exhibited a very hesitating behaviour, whereas others behaved as the controls. This wide heterogeneity of behaviour has also been noticed in children exposed to barbiturates and may originate in a difference in the sensitivity to PhB (Behrman & Vaughan, 1987). In contrast, the reduced performance recorded in DZP-exposed rats only on the first two days of testing and associated with a decreased time to perform the first trial (Schroeder et al., 1997) rather reflects to changes in emotionality patterns and a chronic state of hyperactivity/hyperarousal leading to poor focus of attention on the task to complete, as previously shown after pre- or postnatal BDZ exposure (Fox et al., 1977; Frieder et al., 1984; Livezey et al., 1986).

Eight-arm maze

To perform that test, animals were food-deprived to 85 per cent of their body weight. Food pellets were positioned at the far end of each arm and the animals were left in the maze until they had either entered all the eight arms or until 15 min had elapsed, whichever occurred first. An early AED exposure induced little change in the different parameters measured in the eight-arm maze. In both drug-exposed groups, the total time to perform was not affected during the 5 days of testing and the first error latency time was decreased only after PhB treatment on day 4 and 5 of the test (Fig. 7). There was also no difference in the number of errors performed between controls and PhB-treated rats (Pereira de Vasconcelos et al., 1990b). In addition, in the eight-arm maze, the animals are food-restricted prior to testing and get a food reward for each correct goal arm. This motivation, which does not exist in the T-maze, appears to be a good stimulation for PhB-treated rats.

DZP-treated rats had the tendency to be faster than control rats to perform their trials in the eight-arm maze, the difference reaching significance only on day 4 (Schroeder *et al.*, 1997). As previously shown in a T-maze, the disinhibition and hyperactivity of DZP-exposed rats are reflected by a higher exploratory activity (Fox *et al.*, 1977; Frieder *et al.*, 1984; File, 1986; Chesley *et al.*, 1991) which could reflect the decrease in the level of emotionality when the animal is placed in an unfamiliar environment as well as the absence of deficits in spatial orientation and memory after a postnatal exposure to BDZ (File, 1986; Livezey *et al.*, 1986; Wang & Huang, 1990).

Conclusion

Early postnatal exposure to PhB or DZP has acute effects on the maturation of cerebral energy metabolism and long-term consequences on both energy metabolism and behaviour. Indeed, PhB delays the appearance of the rapid incorporation of glucose carbon into cerebral amino acids and simultaneously favours the use of ketone body. These changes are accompanied by short- and long-term widespread depressions in local cerebral glucose utilization and long-term impairment of learning abilities of adult rats which reach variable levels of severity according to the individuals considered. In contrast, DZP affects the maturation of cerebral energy metabolism to a lesser extent with effects being more restricted, both in terms of duration and number of cerebral areas affected. Long-term behavioural effects of early DZP are quite subtle and translate mainly into hyperactivity and changes in the level of emotionality. These data are in good accordance with the generally believed lower toxicity of DZP compared to PhB. Indeed, while PhB is able to disturb not only neuronal differentiation but also to destroy already formed neurons (Yanai, 1984), DZP induces only neuronal damage when applied prenatally, affecting only differentiating neurons (Frieder *et al.*, 1984). However, both of these AEDs induce metabolic alterations that could interfere with the normal acquisition of specific functions or behaviours, and even moderate, these changes in the immature brain may have long-term consequences that still remain to be further clarified. Indeed, the vulnerability of the immature brain is obviously not only associated with brain damage in terms of neuronal loss, but also may rather include changes in synaptogenesis and final dendritic arborization, leading to possible aberrant connections, as previously suggested in a non-lesional model of pentylenetretrazol seizures in the immature rat (Nehlig & Pereira de Vasconcelos, 1996). In that way, both AEDs, but particularly DZP because of its wide use during pregnancy and in paediatric patients, have to be carefully considered for their potential long-lasting deleterious effects on the immature brain.

References

Alleva, F. & Bignami, G. (1986): Prenatal benzodiazepine effects in mice: postnatal behavioral development, response to drug challenges and adult discrimination learning. *Neurotoxicology* **7**, 303–318.

Barbier, P., Breteaudeau, J., Autret, E., Bertrand, P., Foussard-Blampin, O. & Breteau, M. (1991): Effects of prenatal exposure to diazepam on exploration behavior and learning retention in mice. *Dev. Pharmacol. Ther.* **17**, 35–43.

Behrman, R.E. & Vaughan, V.C. (1987): *Nelson textbook of pediatrics* (13th edn). Philadelphia: Saunders.

Booker, H.E. (1982): Phenobarbital relation of plasma concentration to seizure control. In: Woodbury, D.M., Penry, J.K. & Pippenger, C.E. (eds.), *Antiepileptic drugs*, pp. 341–350. New York: Raven Press.

Burdette, D.E. (1990): Benzodiazepines. In: Dam, M. & Gram, L. (eds), *Comprehensive epileptology*. New York: Raven Press, pp. 547–561.

Carlsson, C., Hägerdal, M., Kaasik, A.E. & Siesjö, B.K. (1976): The effects of diazepam on cerebral blood flow and oxygen consumption in rats and its synergistic interaction with nitrous oxide. *Anesthesiology* **45**, 319–325.

Chesley, S., Lumpkin, M., Schatzki, A., Galpern, W.R., Greenblatt, D.J., Shader, R.I. & Miller, L.G. (1991): Prenatal exposure to benzodiazepines: I. Prenatal exposure to lorazepam in mice alters open-field activity and $GABA_A$ receptor function. *Neuropharmacology* **30**, 53–58.

Cremer, J.E. (1982): Substrate utilization and brain development. *J. Cereb. Blood Flow Metabol.* **2**, 394–407.

Crowley, D.E. & Hepp-Reymond, M.C. (1966): Development of cochlear function in the ear of the infant rat. *J. Comp. Physiol. Psychol.* **62**, 427–432.

Davies, M. (1992): The role of amygdala in fear and anxiety. *Annu. Rev. Neurosci.* **15**, 353–375.

De Vivo, D.C., Leckie, M.P. & Agrawal, H.C. (1975): D-β-hydroxybutyrate: a major precursor of amino acids in developing brain. *J. Neurochem.* **25**, 161–170.

Dell'Omo,G., Wolfer, D., Alleva, E. & Lipp, H.P. (1993): Impaired aquisition of swimming navigation in adult mice exposed prenatally to oxazepam. *Psychopharmacology* **111**, 33–38.

Diaz, J., Schain, R.J. & Bailey, B.G. (1977): Phenobarbitone-induced brain growth retardation in artificially reared rat pups. *Biol. Neonate* **32**, 77–82.

Dobbing, J. (1970): Undernutrition and the developing brain. In: Himwich, W.A. (ed.), *Developmental neurobiology*. Springfield, IL: Charles C. Thomas, pp. 241–261.

Douglas, R.J. (1975): The development of hippocampal function. In: Isaacson, R.L. & Puibran, K.H. (eds), *The hippocampus*. New York: Plenum, pp. 327–361.

Farrel, K. (1986): Benzodiazepines in the treatment of children with epilepsy. *Epilepsia* **27**(suppl. 1), S45–S51.

File, S.E. (1986): The effects of neonatal administration of lorazepam on passive avoidance and on social, aggressive behavior, learning and convulsions. *Neurobehav. Toxicol. Teratol.* **8**, 301–306.

File, S.E. (1990): The history of the benzodiazepine dependence: a review of animal studies. *Neurosci. Biobehav. Rev.* **14**, 135–146.

Fonseca, N., Sell A.B. & Carlini, E.A. (1976): Differential behavioral responses of male and female adult rats treated with five psychotropic drugs in the neaonatal stage. *Psychopharmacologia* **46**, 263–268.

Fox, K.A., Abendsehein, D.R. & Laheen, R.B. (1977): Effects of benzodiazepines during gestation and infancy on Y-maze performance of mice. *Pharmacol. Res. Commun.* **9**, 325–338.

Frieder, B. & Grimm, V.E. (1985): Some lasting neurochemical effects of prenatal or early postnatal exposure to diazepam. *J. Neurochem.* **45**, 37–42.

Frieder, B., Meshorer, A. & Grimm, V.E. (1984): The effect of exposure to diazepam through the placenta or through the mother's milk. *Neuropharmacology* **23**, 1099–1104.

Funakoshi, A., Morikawa, T., Muramatsu, R., Yagi, R. & Seino, M. (1988): A prospective WISC-R study in children with epilepsy. *Jpn. J. Psychiatry Neurol.* **42**, 562–564.

Gaily, E. & Granström, M.L. (1989): A transient retardation of early postnatal growth in drug-exposed children of epileptic mothers. *Epilepsy Res.* **4**, 147–155.

Gaitonde, M.K. & Richter, D. (1965): Changes with age in the utilization of glucose carbon in liver and brain. *J. Neurochem.* **13**, 1309–1318.

Grimm, V. (1984): A review of diazepam and other benzodiazepines in pregnancy. In: Yanai, J. (ed.), *Neurobehavioral teratology*. Amsterdam: Elsevier, pp. 153–162.

Haigh, J.R.M. & Feely, M. (1988): Tolerance to the anticonvulsant effect of benzodiazepines.*Trends Neurosci.* **9**, 361–366.

Hannah, R.S., Roth, S.H. & Spira, A.W. (1982): The effect of chlorpromazine and phenobarbital on cerebellar Purkinje cells. *Teratology* **26**, 21–25.

Hawkins, R.A., Williamson, D.H. & Krebs, H.A. (1971): Ketone-body utilization by adult and suckling rat brain *in vivo*. *Biochem. J.* **122**, 13–18.

Isaacson, R.L. (1982): *The limbic system*. New York: Plenum Press.

Isseroff, A. (1979): Limited recovery of spontaneous alternation after extensive hippocampal damage: Evidence for a memory impairment. *Exp. Neurol.* **64**, 284–294.

Kaneko, S. (1991): Antiepileptic drug therapy and reproductive consequences: functional and morphological effects. *Reprod. Toxic.* **5**, 179–198.

Kellogg, C.K., Ison, J. & Miller, M.K. (1983): Prenatal diazepam exposure: effects on auditory temporal resolution in rats. *Psychopharmacology* **79**, 332–337.

Kelly, P.A.T., Ford, I. & McCulloch, J. (1986): The effect of diazepam upon local cerebral glucose use in the conscious rat. *Neuroscience* **19**, 257–265.

Laegreid, B.L., Hagberg, G. & Lunberg, A. (1992): The effects of benzodiazepines on the fetus and the newborn. *Neuropediatrics* **23**, 18–23.

Livezey, G.T., Marczynski, T.J. & Isaac, L. (1986): Prenatal diazepam: chronic anxiety and deficits in brain receptors in mature progeny. *Neurobehav. Toxicol. Teratol.* **8**, 425–432.

McBride, M.C., Rosman, N.P., Davidson, S.J. & Oppenheimer, E.Y. (1985): Long-term behavioural effects of phenobarbital in suckling rats. *Exp. Neurol.* **89**, 59–70.

Middaugh, L.D., Simpson, L.W., Thomas, T.N. & Zemp, J.W. (1981): Prenatal maternal phenobarbital increases reactivity and retards habituation of mature offspring to environmental stimuli. *Psychopharmacology* **74**, 349–352.

Montgomery, K.C. (1952): A test of two explanations of spontaneous alternation. *J. Comp. Physiol. Psychol.* **45**, 287–293.

Myslivecek, J. (1970): Electrophysiology of the developing brain. Central and eastern European contributions. In: Himwich, W. (ed.), *Developmental neurobiology*. Springfield, IL: Charles Thomas, pp. 475–527.

Nehlig, A. & Pereira de Vasconcelos, A. (1993): Glucose and ketone body metabolism in the neonatal rat brain. *Prog Neurobiol.* **40**, 163–221.

Nehlig, A. & Pereira de Vasconcelos, A. (1996): The model of pentylenetetrazol-induced status epilepticus in the immature rat: short- and long-term effects. *Epilepsy Res.* **26**, 93–103.

Nehlig, A., Daval, J.L., Pereira de Vasconcelos, A. & Boyet, S. (1987): Caffeine-diazepam interaction and local cerebral glucose utilization in the conscious rat. *Brain Res.* **419**, 272–278.

Nehlig, A., Pereira de Vasconcelos, A. & Boyet, S. (1988): Quantitative autoradiographic measurement of local cerebral glucose utilization in freely moving rats during postnatal development. *J. Neurosci.* **8**, 2321–2333.

Olton, D.S. & Samuelson, R.J. (1976): Remembrance of places passed: spatial memory in rats. *J. Exp. Psychol. Anim. Behav. Proc.* **2**, 97–116.

Patel, M.S. & Owen, O.E. (1977): Development and regulation of lipid synthesis from ketone bodies by rat brain. *J. Neurochem.* **28**, 109–114.

Pereira de Vasconcelos, A. & Nehlig, A. (1987): Effects of early phenobarbital treatment on the maturation of energy metabolism in the developing rat brain. I. Incorporation of glucose carbon into amino acids. *Dev. Brain Res.* **36**, 219–229.

Pereira de Vasconcelos, A., Schroeder, H. & Nehlig, A. (1987): Effects of early phenobarbital treatment on the maturation of energy metabolism in the developing rat brain. II. Incorporation of β-hydroxybutyrate into amino acids. *Dev. Brain Res.* **36**, 231–236.

Pereira de Vasconcelos, A., Boyet, S. & Nehlig, A. (1990a): Consequences of chronic phenobarbital treatment on local cerebral glucose utilization in the developing rat. *Dev. Brain Res.* **53**, 168–178.

Pereira de Vasconcelos, A., Colin, C., Desor, D., Divry, M. & Nehlig, A. (1990b): Influence of early neonatal phenobarbital exposure on cerebral energy metabolism and behavior. *Exp. Neurol.* **108**, 176–187.

Pick, C.G. & Yanai, J. (1984): Long term reduction in spontaneous alternations after early exposure to phenobarbital. *Int. J. Dev. Neurosci.* **2**, 223–228.

Pick, C.G. & Yanai, J. (1985): Long term reduction in eight arm maze performance after early exposure to phenobarbital. *Int. J. Dev. Neurosci.* **3**, 223–227.

Rose, G.H. & Ellingson, R.J. (1970): Ontogenesis of evoked potentials. In: Himwich, W.A. (ed.), *Developmental neurobiology* Springfield, IL: Charles Thomas, pp. 393–400.

Schain, R.J. & Watanabe, K. (1975): Effect of chronic phenobarbital administration upon brain growth of the infant rat. *Exp. Neurol.* **47**, 509–515.

Schroeder, H., Collignon, A., Uttscheid, L., Pereira de Vasconcelos, A. & Nehlig, A. (1994a): Effects of early chronic diazepam treatment on incorporation of glucose and β-hydroxybutyrate into cerebral amino acids: relation to undernutrition. *Int. J. Dev. Neurosci.* **12**, 471–484.

Schroeder, H., Nolte, A., Boyet, S., Koziel, V. & Nehlig, A. (1994b): Short- and long-term effects of neonatal diazepam exposure on local cerebral glucose utilization in the rat. *Brain Res.* **660**, 144–153.

Schroeder, H., Humbert, A.C., Desor, D. & Nehlig, A. (1997): Long-term consequences of neonatal exposure to diazepam on cerebral glucose utilization, learning, memory and anxiety. *Brain Res.* **766**, 142–152.

Sokoloff, L., Reivich, M., Kennedy, C., DesRosiers, M.H., Patlak, C.S., Pettigrew, K.D., Sakurada, O. & Shinohara, M. (1977): The [^{14}C] deoxyglucose method for the measurement of local cerebral glucose utilization: theory, procedure, and normal values in the conscious and anesthetized albino rat. *J. Neurochem.* **28**, 897–916.

Thompson, R.F. (1992) Memory. *Curr. Opin. Neurobiol.* **2**, 203–208.

Tucker, J.C. (1985): Benzodiazepines and the developing rat: a critical review. *Neurosci. Biobehav. Rev.* **9**, 101–111.

Wang, L.I. & Huang, Z. (1990): Effect of clonazepam on brain development of mice. *Dev. Pharmacol. Ther.* **15**, 21–25.

Yaffe, S.J. & Catz, C.S. (1971): Pharmacology of the perinatal period. *Clin. Obstet. Gynecol.* **14**, 722–744.

Yanai, J. (1984): An animal model for the effect of barbiturate on the development of the central nervous system. In: Yanai, J. (ed.), *Neurobehavioral teratology*. Amsterdam: Elsevier, pp. 111–132.

Yanai, J. & Bergman, A. (1981): Neuronal deficits in mice following neonatal exposure to barbiturates. *Exp. Neurol.* **73**, 199–208.

Yanai, J., Rosselli-Austin, L. & Tabakoff, B. (1979): Neuronal deficits in mice following prenatal exposure to phenobarbital. *Exp. Neurol.* **65**, 237–244.

PART VII
Concluding remarks and future plans

Chapter 26

Concluding remarks and future plans

Solomon L. Moshé

Departments of Neurology, Neuroscience and Paediatrics, Laboratory of Developmental Epilepsy and Montefiore/AECOM Epilepsy Management Center, Albert Einstein College of Medicine and Montefiore Medical Center, Bronx, NY 10461, USA

This international conference brought together basic scientists and clinicians in an attempt to address the issues of brain development and epileptic disorders. Seizures and epilepsy are common problems in infancy and childhood and, despite several years of active research, there are several questions that remain (Table 1).

Table 1. Pertinent questions concerning seizures and epilepsy in normal brain

1.	Why is the immature brain more susceptible to seizures in response to environmental stimuli that fail to induce seizures in the mature brain?
2.	What are the structures involved in the generation of seizures early in life? Are these structures different from the structures involved in the generation of seizures later on, i.e. after adolescence?
3.	Are the electrographic and behavioural manifestations age-specific?
4.	What are the structures involved in the propagation and control of seizures early in life? Are these structures different from the structures involved in the propagation and control of seizures later on, i.e. after adolescence?
5.	Are there developmental windows of altered seizure susceptibility?
6.	Are the consequences of seizures age-specific? Do the consequences depend on site of origin of seizures, seizure type or seizure duration?
7.	Do provoked seizures lead to the development of subsequent epilepsy? If yes, where is the site of origin of the persistent epileptic disorder?
8.	Are the antiseizure and antiepileptic effects of various drugs age-specific?
9.	What are the consequences of chronic treatment on the developing brain?

Both groups realize the need for cross fertilization in order to understand the pathophysiology and consequences of epileptic seizures, as well as the problems that arise while caring for infants and children with epilepsy. Many times clinicians and basic scientists work *ex vacuo*, failing to communicate with each other or even ignoring each other. Yet both have in mind a common pursuit, to improve the care of patients with epilepsy. The conference included several outstanding, eloquent presentations and fierce arguments but the main winner was the whole group. The group was able to discuss together the common problems and perhaps open new avenues for research and, of course, in the long run improve the care of children with epilepsy.

There is an urgency to develop pertinent animal models to study the questions that have risen from clinical practice. This conference provided the forum for these questions to be asked. There was a videotape session for basic scientists to show them what seizures look like in infants and children. These seizures are quite different from seizures observed in experimental dishes or in rats, but the tapes also revealed the difficulties in describing seizures characterized predominantly by motor manifestations in very young infants. Are these seizures focal, multifocal, bilateral or generalized? Are they cortical or subcortical in origin? The same session included the presentation of a videotape showing seizures in developing rats and again the same limitations that apply to the study of the phenomenology of human seizures are pertinent for the study of seizures in developing animals.

The main clinical syndromes that were discussed were infantile spasms and the Lennox–Gastaut syndrome. Both syndromes are of multiple aetiologies and have variable outcome and functional consequences. The clinicians among the participants would like to know why these particular types of seizures occur during discrete periods of development and what are the structures involved to account for the unique behavioural and electrographic features. We heard evidence and theories on how even brief seizures can alter the intellectual development of the babies, although the problem may be quite complicated by the influence of the underlying disease (Table 2).

Table 2. Issues of epileptogenesis in genetically altered or compromized brains

1.	What is the role of heredity in the development of seizures and epilepsy?
2.	What is the role of a brain injury early in life in the development of seizures and epilepsy?
3.	How are the issues raised in Table 1 affected by the presence of altered genetic predisposition to seizures?
4.	How are the issues raised in Table 1 affected by the presence of altered brain structure and function?
5.	What is the combined effect of genetic predisposition, abnormal brain development and subsequent injuries on the issues raised in Table 1?
6.	Can models of epilepsy be developed to study catastrophic epilepsies of infancy and childhood, i.e. infantile spasms and Lennox–Gastaut syndrome?

Basic science research is guided by clinical queries and from ongoing dialogue. During the past few years, our knowledge of how genes influence brain development has expanded. Genes have been discovered that are involved in the expression of spike-and-wave discharges, as well as ataxia, in mice. In the future we will be able to screen for abnormal genes that may be responsible for the development of seizures in humans. Furthermore, genes are involved in the formation of the brain; changes in their expression may lead to the development of severely malformed brains. This is important because we have now begun to investigate seizures that emerge from normal brains as well as from abnormal brains.

While studying normal brains, it is important to understand whether there are windows of increased excitability and what is the underlying role in the maturation of inhibitory or excitatory systems in the expression of seizures. Since basic science research is increasingly becoming more and more specialized, it is in symposia like this one that the participants will have the chance to correlate anatomical findings of the developmental changes in GAD-containing neurons in the hippocampus with the physiologic effects of GABA. It is an intriguing notion that the GABAergic system may not only be involved in neurotransmission, but its effects on neuronal excitation and inhibition may be age specific and GABA may have a trophic influence on other neurons as well.

Are these effects limited to the hippocampus and specifically to the CA3 region, or are they a widespread phenomenon? In infants and children many seizures may arise from neocortical structures rather than the hippocampus, as is often the case in adults. Studies from animal models and neocortical slices obtained from the brain undergoing epilepsy surgery indicate that there are many similarities between the models and the epileptic disorders that we see in human patients, at least concerning several properties of recorded neurons. In studies involving human tissue, it is also evident that there are still many limitations, including sampling or the availability of techniques, that limit our ability to study this precious tissue for clues for the reasons underlying the permanence of an epileptic state.

Sampling may also be a factor for the notion that seizures originating from limbic structures are rare in humans. Although clinicians are usually dismayed when the hippocampus is discussed in terms of epileptogenesis in the developing brain, it should be pointed out that on many occasions, such as neonatal seizures or even catastrophic epileptic syndromes such as infantile spasms or the Lennox–Gastaut syndrome, the site of origin of epileptic discharges is not known and most often we are restricted by EEG sampling only from neocortical structures in brains with limited propagation patterns. Therefore, it important to continue the study of systems such as the entorhinal–hippocampal circuit and investigate the role of newly identified receptors (such as metabotropic excitatory receptors) in mediating hippocampal hyperexcitability and seizures. Even within the hippocampus, there may be significant differences in the function of excitatory or inhibitory systems with age.

These studies emphasize the need to avoid generalizations. On the other hand, we may need to use extremely simple models to ask an initial set of questions, and later expand this to animals and eventually to studies of the human brain. However, this process cannot and must not be considered linear, but information should be obtained concurrently with open channels of communication. One such example is the increasing need to study how hormones alter the epileptic process, especially since hormone therapy may have a crucial role in the control of certain age-specific disorders, and hormonal changes that occur with puberty may influence the exacerbation or remission of specific epileptic syndromes. There is evidence that gonadal hormones may influence the functionality of subcortical structures involved in the control of seizures with age. Similar changes can be postulated for the unique role of the adrenocortical system in infantile spasms, and the urgent need to develop a model to better study this unique human syndrome. Under all these circumstances, the role of malnutrition cannot be underestimated.

Many seizure disorders are associated with dysplastic brains and migration defects. Homeobox genes may be important for the development of some of the brain abnormalities that we observe in patients. There are a variety of such clinical syndromes, therefore it is important to develop a variety of models such as those produced by the injection of toxins (ibotenic acid) or antimitotic agents (methylazoxymethanol) *in utero*. Structural brain abnormalities reminiscent of human dysplastic lesions can be produced by freezing lesions. All these are models of dysplasias and in none of these models have spontaneous seizures been observed; in some cases there may not even be changes in excitability. We now have an understanding of how dysplasias may occur and how normal tissue unexpectedly finds its way into these dysplastic areas. Many questions remain, such as what happens to the tissue that has been replaced. It is interesting that in some of these potentially epileptic lesions there are decreases in GABA, the inhibitory neurotransmitter, which are often associated with seizures. These models can also be used to study the interaction of environmental factors on an abnormal substrate. Perhaps a combination of stressful stimuli such as hyperthermic seizures or hypoxic injuries may lead to the development of better models to study the intractable seizures shown in this conference such as infantile spasms and the Lennox–Gastaut syndrome. In fact, after all only some of the children with dysplastic brains will develop epilepsy. Another group of patients that may develop epilepsy are neonates who suffer hypoxic/anoxic injury at birth. The mechanisms under which this injury may eventually produce permanent epilepsy are poorly understood; however, progress has been made that may lead to the development of new treatments to prevent this rare but often devastating condition.

What are the effects of seizures on the developing brain? There are clinical observations from mostly retrospective studies indicating that seizures may produce damage in the developing hippocampus leading to subsequent epilepsy. Is this the case for all seizures or are there certain seizures that may be more harmful than others? In the model of epilepsy produced by injections of intrahippocampal tetanus toxin early in life, spontaneous seizures appear later on and are associated with the appearance of abnormal neurons in the area of injection reminiscent of the neurons observed in the tissue of patients with chronic epilepsy. Yet many questions remain: are these the result of seizures early in life or the results of the spontaneous seizures as they develop later on? What are the anatomical changes of damage that we should be looking for? When does the type of hippocampal damage frequently observed in humans with temporal lobe epilepsy actually occur? Analysis of resected tissue from young children with intractable epilepsy has failed to show the classical pattern of mesial temporal sclerosis, substantiating observations obtained from several models of status epilepticus and recurrent seizures in developing animals. The human studies reveal unique patterns of alterations including synaptic reorganization without any evidence of hippocampal CA3 or hilar cell loss. These types of data suggest that we should be searching for age-specific changes and continuously ask about the functional consequences of any newly identified process. For example, is this synaptic reorganization always detrimental to the developing brain? Because the permanent epileptic state may take many years to emerge in humans, how can we better study kindling mechanisms that not just involve the notion that seizures become progressively more intense, which may not be the case in humans? A kindling mechanism may underlie the development of partial seizures late in life after an initial bout of severe status epilepticus in infancy.

Some acute seizures in human infants lead to acute devastating consequences including the destruction of many cortical areas. Fortunately, these seizures occur infrequently in humans but nevertheless understanding of the pathophysiology and the circumstances under which this hyperacute injury may occur is essential. The recent emergence of models mimicking this clinical situation may provide significant insights as to how the damage occurs. Studies of blood flow and metabolism may provide compelling evidence as to how a mismatch in flow and metabolism may produce extensive injury, although the process via which the actual injury occurs remains unclear.

The metabolic studies have revealed that subcortical structures including the basal ganglia undergo significant changes during seizures. These studies parallel human studies that have been performed in patients with infantile spasms and Lennox–Gastaut, indicating that subcortical structures may have a role in the propagation and suppression of seizures. If subcortical structures are crucial in the propagation and control of seizures then perhaps we can develop new treatments that can take into account the maturation of these brain circuits that are involved in seizure suppression which also appear to be gender dependent. Novel treatments should be designed keeping in mind not only that the goal is to stop an ongoing seizure or prevent seizure recurrences but also that these new treatments do not harm the developing brain. Several of the currently available treatments may have detrimental effects, although it should be pointed out that most of these studies have been performed in patients with difficult to control seizure disorders and, in these patients, the detrimental effects of the drugs may become more obvious. On occasion, epilepsy surgery should be considered as a form of early intervention to prevent the development of a vicious cycle.

This conference was an important step forward in bridging the gap between clinicians and basic scientists. The presentations and the ensuing discussions reflected the significant progress we have made in the field of developmental epilepsies but also pointed out the limitations of the currently available techniques. I remain extremely optimistic that conferences such as this one will greatly enhance our understanding on how the brain functions and how its dysfunction leads to the development of seizures that may or may not have devastating consequences on the brain depending on the morphology of the underlying brain. In fact, we have come a long way from just simple observations in humans to creating complicated models of normal and abnormal brain development and examining a variety of seizure models that may be similar to the human condition, although one should not forget that these are only models. By creating such models we can begin to ask more fundamental questions and then by adding the blocks, we can piece information together to understand the complicated human condition that is called the epilepsies.

Acknowledgement: Supported in part by grant NS–20253 from the NINDS. Dr Moshé is the recipient of Martin A. and Emily L. Fisher fellowship in Neurology and Paediatics..

Author Index

Adelson, P. David	171	Liu, Hantao	237
Albani, Francesca	3	Luhmann, Heiko J.	71
Baram, Tallie Z.	145	Maquet, Pierre	135
Barbaria, Elena	3	Mareš, Pavel	157
Ben-Ari, Yehezkel	81, 263	Marescaux, Christian	135
Billard, Catherine	279	Massa, Rita	123
Boncinelli, Edoardo	3	Mathern, Gary W.	171
Cavalheiro, Esper A.	211	Mazarati, Andrey M.	237
Caviness, Verne S., Jr	55	Metz-Lutz, Marie-Noëlle	113, 135
Chevassus-Au-Louis, Nicolas	81, 263	Misson, Jean-Paul	55
Chiron, Catherine	93	Moshé, Solomon L.	307
Congar, P.	81	Motte, Jacques	221
Coulter, Douglas A.	187	Nehlig, Astrid	221, 289
da Silva Fernandes, Maria José	221	Pierson, Martha	25
de Vasconcelos, A. Pereira	289	Pinard, Jean-Marc	93
Deonna, Thierry	113	Pirard, Sandrine	55
Dravet, Charlotte	103	Plouin, Perrine	93
Dubé, Céline	221	Pretorius, James K.	171
Dubru, Jean-Marie	55	Rafiki, A.	81
Dulac, Olivier	93	Reiprich, Robert-Alexander	71
Dupuy-Davies, Shannon T.	13	Represa, A.	81
Faiella, Antonio	3	Robain, Olivier	93
Franck, Georges	135	Romero, M.T.	255
Friedman, L.K.	255	Sankar, Raman	199, 237
Gaïarsa, J.L.	81	Sarkisian, Matthew	263
Germano, I.M.	255	Schroeder, H.	289
Hatalski, Carolyn G.	145	Schwarz, Petra	71
Hirsch, Edouard	135	Shirasaka, Yukiyoshi	237
Holmes, Gregory L.	263	Sperber, E.F.	255
Houser, Carolyn R.	13	Stichel, Christine C.	71
Jambaque, Isabelle	93	Swann, John	25
Jensen, Frances E.	161	Takahashi, T.	55
Jorquera, I.	81	Thompson, Kerry W.	237
Karpuk, Nik	71	Vasconcelos, Anne Pereira de	221
Katsumori, Hiroshi	237	Velíšková, Jana	39, 255
Kornblum, Harley	237	Wasterlain, Claude G.	237
Leite, Joao P.	171	Zhang, Nianhui	13
Leroy, Patricia	55	Zortea, Michela	3